I0478887

Bladder Cancer: Causes, Symptoms, Stages and Treatment

Bladder Cancer: Causes, Symptoms, Stages and Treatment

Edited by Derek Russoe

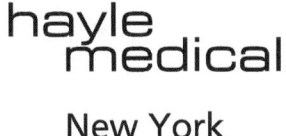

hayle
medical

New York

Hayle Medical,
750 Third Avenue, 9th Floor,
New York, NY 10017, USA

Visit us on the World Wide Web at:
www.haylemedical.com

© Hayle Medical, 2020

This book contains information obtained from authentic and highly regarded sources. Copyright for all individual chapters remain with the respective authors as indicated. All chapters are published with permission under the Creative Commons Attribution License or equivalent. A wide variety of references are listed. Permission and sources are indicated; for detailed attributions, please refer to the permissions page and list of contributors. Reasonable efforts have been made to publish reliable data and information, but the authors, editors and publisher cannot assume any responsibility for the validity of all materials or the consequences of their use.

ISBN: 978-1-63241-834-0

Trademark Notice: Registered trademark of products or corporate names are used only for explanation and identification without intent to infringe.

Cataloging-in-Publication Data

Bladder cancer : causes, symptoms, stages and treatment / edited by Derek Russoe.
p. cm.
Includes bibliographical references and index.
ISBN 978-1-63241-834-0
1. Bladder--Cancer. 2. Bladder--Cancer--Etiology. 3. Bladder--Cancer--Diagnosis.
4. Bladder--Cancer--Treatment. I. Russoe, Derek.
RC280.B5 B53 2020
616.994 62--dc23

Table of Contents

Preface

Any cancer that arises in the tissues of the urinary bladder can be termed as bladder cancer. Some of its common types are transitional cell carcinoma, squamous cell carcinoma and adenocarcinoma. These cancers typically cause hematuria, dysuria, frequent urination, etc. Individuals with advanced bladder cancer experience lower-extremity swelling, flank pain and pelvic or bony pain. Tobacco smoking is the chief contributor to urinary bladder cancer. The diagnosis of bladder cancer is done through an examination of the bladder, aided by a cystoscopy. It can also be diagnosed with a Hexvix/Cysview guided fluorescence cystoscopy. The treatment strategy employed for the management of bladder cancer is dependent on the degree of the invasion of the cancer. It can involve a combination of surgery, chemotherapy, immunotherapy and radiation therapy. This book covers in detail the causes, symptoms, stages and treatment of bladder cancer. From theories to research to practical applications, case studies related to all contemporary topics of relevance to this condition have been included in this book. The extensive content of this book provides the readers with a thorough understanding of bladder cancer.

This book unites the global concepts and researches in an organized manner for a comprehensive understanding of the subject. It is a ripe text for all researchers, students, scientists or anyone else who is interested in acquiring a better knowledge of this dynamic field.

I extend my sincere thanks to the contributors for such eloquent research chapters. Finally, I thank my family for being a source of support and help.

Editor

Laparoscopic versus Open Radical Cystectomy for Elderly Patients over 75-Year-Old: A Single Center Comparative Analysis

Shuxiong Zeng[1,♀], Zhensheng Zhang[1,♀], Xiaowen Yu[2], Ruixiang Song[1], Rongchao Wei[1], Junjie Zhao[1], Linhui Wang[1], Jianguo Hou[1], Yinghao Sun[1], Chuanliang Xu[1]*

1 From the Department of Urology, Changhai Hospital, Second Military Medical University, Shanghai, P. R. China, 2 From the Department of Geriatrics, Changhai Hospital, Second Military Medical University, Shanghai, P. R. China

Abstract

Purpose: To explore the morbidity, mortality and oncological results of laparoscopic radical cystectomy (LRC) in the elderly patients over 75-year-old in contrast with open radical cystectomy (ORC).

Materials and Methods: We analyzed 46 radical cystectomies from January 2009 to December 2013 in patients over 75-year-old in our institute, 21 patients in the LRC group and 25 in the ORC group. Demographic parameters, operative variables and perioperative outcome were retrospectively collected and analyzed between the two groups. Perioperative morbidity and mortality were categorized as early (within 90 days after surgery) or late (more than 90 days) according to the time of occurrence.

Results: Patients in both groups had comparable preoperative characteristics. A significant longer operative time (418 vs. 337 min, p = 0.018) and less estimated blood loss (400 vs. 500 ml p = 0.038) were observed in LRC group compared with ORC group. Infection and ileus were the most common early complications after surgery. Patients underwent ORC suffered from significantly more postoperative ileus (28.0% vs. 4.8%, P = 0.038) and infection (40% vs. 9.5%, P = 0.019) than LRC group within 90 days after surgery. The mortality rate was 4.7% (1/21) and 4% (1/25) for LRC group and ORC group respectively. At a median follow-up of 21 months (range 2–61 months), the Kaplan-Meier survival curves and log-rank analysis demonstrate that there were no significant differences between the LRC and ORC groups in the 3-year overall, cancer-specific, or recurrence-free survival rates.

Conclusions: It is suggested that LRC should be recommended as the primary intervention to treat muscle invasive or high risk non-muscle invasive bladder cancer in elderly patients with a relative long life expectancy.

Editor: Peter C. Black, University of British Columbia, Canada

Funding: The authors have no support or funding to report.

Competing Interests: The authors have declared that no competing interests exist.

* E-mail: xuchuanliang@medmail.com.cn

♀ These authors contributed equally to this work.

Introduction

With marked improvements in medical technology and health care, the average life span of the general population in most countries has progressively increased. It was reported that by 2030 in America, there will be about 72.1 million older persons, over twice their number in 2000. [1] Because of a strong link between age and bladder cancer, the incidence of bladder cancer ranked the fourth (3.69%, 1/27) and sixth (0.98%, 1/106) among all cancers in male and female over 70 years old in America, respectively. [2] Meanwhile, the incidence of bladder cancer was rising with the increasing number of older people in China, ranking 1st in the Chinese urinary malignant tumor and reaching a peak over age 85 with an incidence of 69.7/100,000 [3]. So it is important but still a conundrum for most urologists to treat elderly patients with muscle invasive or high risk non-muscle invasive bladder cancer. [4,5].

Although open radical cystectomy (ORC) with different types of urine diversion have been proved safe for elderly patients and remains the standard of care for the treatment of muscle invasive bladder cancer, it is associated with significant short and long-term morbidity. [5,6,7] Elderly patients, especially those older than 75 years old, are always associated with several comorbidities, thus putting these patients at an even greater risk of complications or mortality. [8,9] As a result, older patients may potentially be guided toward conservative therapies such as radiation therapy with or without chemotherapy, or palliative transurethral resection. [7] It is imperative for us to find ways minimizing the perioperative morbidity and mortality in elderly patients. Recently, laparoscopic surgery has been widely accepted as a minimally invasive treatment to reduce the morbidity after conventional surgery, and a number of studies have demonstrated the feasibility of laparoscopic radical cystectomy (LRC) was technically feasible and oncological safe since the first report by Parra et al. [10] in 1992 [11–15].

The elderly patient poses several challenges to LRC surgery such as whether elderly patients can tolerate longer operation time, pneumoperitoneum, and peculiar surgical position as well as younger patients. Few studies, however, have focused the feasibility of LRC on the elderly patients older than 75-year-old compared with ORC. To explore the morbidity, mortality and oncological results of LRC in the elderly patients more than 75-year-old, we thus conducted such a retrospective single center study with a control group of ORC elderly patients.

Materials and Methods

Between January 2009 and December 2013, 310 consecutive patients underwent LRC or ORC and urinary diversion in our institution, the median age was 64 years old (range 31 to 89). Of these patients, 54 patients were older than 75-year-old, 24 and 30 were included in the LRC group and ORC group respectively. All the participants were informed that their clinical information may be used in later clinical study when they enter hospital and their written informed consents were obtained. This study was approved by the ethical board of Changhai Hospital, all procedures performed in accordance with the ethical principles expressed in the 1995 Declaration of Helsinki. Patients' information was anonymized prior to analysis. The indication for radical cystectomy was histologically diagnosed muscle-invasive bladder cancer by transurethral resection, or biopsy confirmed recurrent multi-focal high-grade superficial bladder cancer or bladder cancer in situ that were refractory to repeated transurethral resection. The clinical and follow-up data were retrospectively collected and analyzed from our bladder cancer database. We failed to contact 3/24 and 5/30 patients in LRC group and ORC group respectively to confirm the survival status and late complications, thus they are excluded from the study.

All patients underwent a thorough preoperative examination including routine laboratory test, chest radiography, and intravenous pyelogram, echocardiography, lung function test, computerized tomography or magnetic resonance imaging and abdominal ultrasonography. Patients were graded according to the American Society of Anesthesiologists (ASA) class. Common comorbidities such as hypertension, coronary artery disease, chronic obstructive pulmonary disease, diabetes mellitus and other chronic diseases were recorded.

Two days before surgery all patients began Semi-liquid diet and metronidazole intake. The day before surgery, patients began liquid diet and underwent bowel preparation with 50% magnesium sulfate 12 hours before surgery. All patients wore compression stockings before entering operation room and broad-spectrum systemic antibiotic was given intravenously during induction of anesthesia. The procedure of LRC and ORC with bilateral pelvic and iliac lymphadenectomy for man and woman was performed according to the procedures described by Campbell-Walsh Urology. [16] The urinary diversion of LRC was reconstructed extracorporeally through a 5 to 6 cm supraumbilical extended incision of the camera port. All the surgeons (XCL, WLH, HJG) are urological professor performing cystectomy more than 25 cases annually, two of the surgeons (XCL, WLH) in this series performed both ORC and LRC surgery, while the other one performed only open surgery (HJG).

The demographic parameters included age, gender, body mass index (BMI), comorbid conditions, surgery history, laboratory test results, multidisciplinary consultations needed. Operative variables namely operative time (defined as anesthesia from begin to end) and estimated blood loss (EBL), and transfusion. Perioperative outcome such as time to liquid intake, time to exsufflation, time to canalization and hospital stay after surgery. Early complication was defined within 90 days and late complications occurred more than 90 days after operation. [5] Oncological outcomes, including survival and recurrence were evaluated. The pathological tumor stage and grade were examined according to the TNM classification and the World Health Organization system in 2004, respectively. [17,18].

Chi-square test, Mann-Whitney U test and Student t test were used to compare categorical, nonparametric, and parametric data respectively between the two groups. Overall, disease-specific and recurrence-free survival were analyzed using Kaplan-Meier survival method and log-rank tests. Differences were considered significant at p<0.05. Statistical analysis was performed with the use of the Statistical Package for Social Scientists, version 19.0 (IBM Inc).

Results

As was shown in Table 1, patients in the LRC group and ORC group had comparable preoperative characteristics with regards to patients' age, gender, BMI, ASA class, comorbid conditions, surgical history and the results of blood test. Pathological results were also comparable between the two groups as was showed in Table 2.

There was no conversion to open surgery in LRC group. The operative and postoperative characteristics were shown in Table 3. A significant difference was observed at the two groups regarding to operative time and EBL. The LRC group required a significant longer operative time, with a mean operative time of 418 min compared with 337 min for ORC group (P = 0.018). The median EBL was 400 ml for LRC and 500 ml for the ORC (P = 0.038). Compared with preoperative data, serum albumin significantly decreased 7.2±5.8 g/L and 8.7±4.4 g/L (both P<0.001) for LRC group and ORC group respectively and so was hemoglobin which significantly decreased 15.5±19.31 g/L and 27.8±19.3 g/L (both P<0.001) respectively. However, there was no significantly change for serum creatinine in both groups. Seven patients in LRC group and 16 in the ORC group required multidisciplinary consultation after operation (P = 0.038), which was resulted from more complications occurred in the ORC group.

Postoperative complications were noted in Table 4. Infection and ileus were the most common early complications after surgery. Patients underwent ORC suffered from significantly more postoperative ileus (28.0% vs. 4.8%, P = 0.038) and infection (40% vs. 9.5%, P = 0.019) than LRC group within 90 days after surgery. In 2 LRC group and 5 ORC group patients (Table 3), a postoperative complications required re-operation. There was one patient (4.7%) in LRC group died from operation related complications. An 84 years old man died of multiple organ dysfunction caused by ileus 5 months after discharging from hospital. One (4%) 77-year-old male patient in the ORC group died of sepsis resulted from ileus within 3 months after operation.

The median follow-up was 20 months (range 2–55 months) and 21 months (range 3–61 months) for LRC group and ORC group respectively. There were 17 (81.0%) and 19 (76.0%) patients alive for LRC group and ORC group at the last follow-up, respectively. All patients in LRC group and the majority of patients (94.7%, 18/19) are disease-free. Cancer specific death occurred in 3/4 (75.0%) and 5/6 (83.3%) in LRC group and ORC group, respectively. Kaplan-Meier survival curves, as was shown in

Table 1. Baseline patient characteristics.

	LRC	ORC	P value
Age, median (IQR)	77 (75,79)	78 (75,80)	0.750*
Gender, men/women	19/2	21/4	0.673**
BMI, mean±SD (kg/m²)	23.5±2.3	23.4±2.5	0.959*
Hb, mean±SD (g/L)	120.1±25.6	125.0±23.0	0.501*
SCR, mean±SD(umol/L)	96.8±62.0	90.1±31.3	0.641*
ALB, mean±SD (g/L)	37.1±4.2	36.8±3.2	0.756*
MC needed before surgery (n%)	6 (28.6%)	9 (36%)	0.592**
ASA class (n%)			
2	10 (47.6%)	15 (60.0%)	0.401**
3	11 (52.4%)	10 (40.0%)	
Surgery history (n%)			
Abdominal surgery	3 (14.3%)	5 (20.0%)	0.710**
Nephrectomy	1 (4.8%)	3 (12%)	0.614**
Comorbid conditions			
Coronary heart disease	2 (9.5%)	1 (4.0%)	0.585**
Hypertension	5 (23.8%)	11 (44%)	0.152**
Diabetes mellitus	7 (33.3%)	4 (16%)	0.170**
COPD	2 (9.5%)	1 (4.0%)	0.585**
Other chronic diseases	1 (4.8%)	2 (8.0%)	1.000**

LRC = laparoscopic radical cystectomy; ORC = open radical cystectomy; IQR = Interquartile range; BMI = body mass index; Hb = hemoglobin; SCR = Serum creatinine; ALB = serum albumin; MC = multidisciplinary consultation; ASA = American society of anesthesiologists; COPD = chronic obstructive pulmonary disease.
*Student t test was used for statistical analysis.
**Chi-square tests was used for statistical analysis.

Figure 1, demonstrate that there were no significant differences between the LRC and ORC groups in the 3-year overall, cancer-specific, or recurrence-free survival rates.

Discussion

In most countries life expectancy of the general population is increasing, however, it was estimated that nearly 1 in 3 people older than 70-year-old may suffer from a wide variety of malignant tumors, including bladder cancer, which were the main factor affecting the health of elderly people. [2] The incidence of bladder

Table 2. Pathological results.

	LRC	ORC	P value**
Pathological stage (n%)			0.883**
T0, Ta, Tis, T1	8 (38.1%)	12 (48.0%)	
T2	5 (23.8%)	6 (24.0%)	
T3	3 (14.3%)	3 (12.0%)	
T4	5 (23.8%)	4 (16.0%)	
Grade (n%)			1.000**
Low grade	0	1 (4%)	
High grade	21 (100%)	24 (96.0%)	
Lymph node status(n%)			0.585**
negative	19 (90.5%)	24 (96.0%)	
positive	2 (9.5%)	1 (4.0%)	
Lymph node number	12	13	0.684*
Positive surgical margins	0	0	1.000

*Student t test was used for statistical analysis.
**Chi-square tests was used for statistical analysis.

Table 3. Operative and postoperative characteristics.

	LRC	ORC	P value
Operative time, mean±SD (min)	413±103.6	337±105.0	0.018*
EBL (ml), median (IQR)	400 (250,500)	500 (350,800)	0.038#
Transfusion needed (n%)	6 (28.6%)	10 (40%)	0.418**
Division (n%)			0.469**
Ileal conduit	14 (70.0%)	22 (84.6%)	
Ureterocutaneostomy	5 (25.0%)	3 (11.5%)	
Orthotopic neobladder	1 (5.0%)	1 (3.8%)	
Hb, mean±SD (g/L)	104.6±16.0	97.2±15.3	0.115*
SCR, mean±SD (umol/L)	101.7±56.8	99.8±45.7	0.900*
ALB, mean±SD (g/L)	29.9±4.2	28.0±4.0	0.133*
MC needed after operation (n%)	7 (33.3%)	16 (64.0%)	0.038*
Time to liquid intake, mean±SD (d)	4.5±2.5	5.1±2.1	0.361*
Time to nasogastric tube removal, mean±SD (d)	4.1±2.6	4.6±2.2	0.487*
Time to canalization, mean±SD (d)	11.0±4.1	11.5±6.1	0.781*
Time to exsufflation, mean±SD (d)	3.5±0.8	4.1±1.1	0.064*
Hospital stay after surgery(d), median (IQR)	14 (10,18)	15 (12,26)	0.232#

*Student t test was used for statistical analysis.
**Chi-square tests was used for statistical analysis.
#Mann-Whitney U was used for statistical analysis.

Table 4. Postoperative complications.

	LRC	ORC	P value**
Early complications 90≤ days (n%)			
Infection[†]	2 (9.6%)	10 (40.0%)	0.019
Ileus[‡]	1 (4.8%)	7 (28.0%)	0.038
Anastomotic leak	1 (4.8%)[a]	2 (8.0%)[b]	1.000
Delirium	1 (4.8%)	3 (12.0%)	0.614
Arrhythmia	2 (9.6%)	2 (8.0%)	1.000
wound dehiscence	0	3 (12.0%)[c]	0.239
Hoarseness	1 (4.8%)	0	0.457
Diarrhea	1 (4.8%)	0	0.457
Late complications >90 days (n%)			
Pyelonephritis	2 (9.6%)	4 (16.0%)	0.673
Ileus	1 (4.8%)	3 (12.0%)	0.614
Ureteral stricture	1 (4.8%)[d]	1 (4.0%)[d]	1.000
Incisional Hernia	0	1 (4.0%)	1.000
Re-operation required	2 (9.6%)	5 (20.0%)	0.436
Mortality (n%)			
≤90 days	0	1 (4.0%)	1.000
>90 days	1 (4.8%)	0	1.000

[†]Patients was diagnosed as infection when they presented continuous fever and antibiotics were considered as the most effective treatment to cure it.
[‡]Ileus was diagnosed when gas- fluid levels were seen in abdominal X-rays.
[a]Treated by fistula resection and Intestinal anastomosis.
[b]One of them treated by fistula resection and Ileostomy, the other one with urine leakage from ileo-ureteral anastomosis healed spontaneously.
[c]All Three treated with primary suture after wound debridement.
[d]Both of them treated by retrograde placement of single J stent with flexible cystoscopy remained indwelling for 8 weeks.
**Chi-square tests was used for statistical analysis.

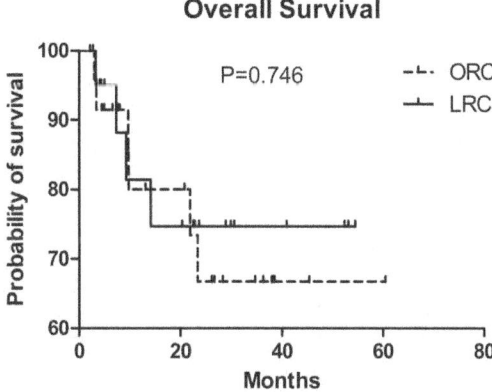

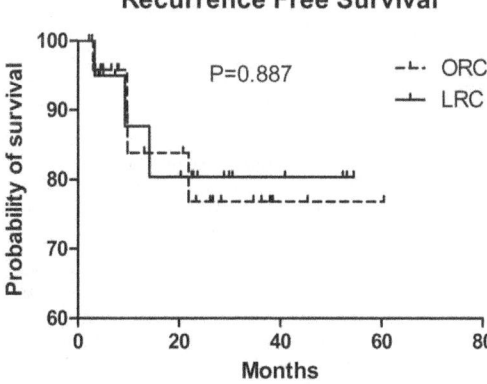

Figure 1. Kaplan-Meier estimate of 3-year survival for overall, cancer-specific, recurrence-free survival. Log-rank test indicates that overall survival, cancer specific survival and recurrence free survival among LRC and ORC groups are not significantly different.

cancer increases distinctly with increasing age, especially those who beyond 70-year-old. [5] Elderly patients with muscle invasive or high risk non-muscle invasive bladder cancer who require major surgery such as cystectomy pose difficult challenges to the operative surgeon. This dilemma is due to the complexity of comorbidities of the elderly patients and great risk of complications and mortality in this subset of patients. [5,9,19] Collectively these considerations have led to delay cystectomy for elderly patients. Prout et al. [20] reported only 25% of patients with muscle-invasive bladder cancer between 70 to 79 years old were

treated with radical cystectomy compared with 55% of those aged 55 to 59 years. Recently, several studies have proved that age is not a limiting factor in selecting radical cystectomy as a treatment method for muscle-invasive bladder cancer. [4,20–23].

Although studies have proved that elderly patients can safely undergo cystectomy, this surgical procedure always associated with high incidence of postoperative complications and morbidity. Patients older than 75-year-old who underwent ORC suffers from 38.6% to 64% early complications and 16.4% to 42% late complications, and a mortality rate ranging from 2% to 6% within 30 days after cystectomy. [22,24–27] Minimally invasive treatments such as laparoscopic surgery has been expanding rapidly, the excellent perioperative and oncological results in the treatment of renal cell cancer and prostate cancer and technical developments have paved the way to LRC. [9,13] It has been reported that LRC could reduce blood loss, analgesic consumption, postoperative complication and promote earlier recovery of bowel function and return to normal activity [9,13,28]. Despite these advantages, ORC has still been considered to be the standard care for muscle-invasive or high-risk non muscle-invasive bladder cancer, especially for elderly patients. [6] Several concerns contribute to this situation such as whether elderly patients can tolerate longer anesthetic period and the steep Trendelenburg position, and whether the older patients with limited renal function reserve can tolerate metabolic acidosis caused by pneumoperitoneum. [9] However, as far as we know, comparative data in terms of morbidity rate and long term survival benefit for LRC and ORC procedures in patients aged older than 75 years are presently lacking.

To the best of our knowledge, we found Richards et al. [9] conducted the first observation to justify the feasibility of robot-assisted radical cystectomy (RRC) compared with ORC in elderly bladder cancer patients. In spite of longer operative time, it was reported that RRC could achieve similar perioperative outcomes without compromising pathologic outcomes, nevertheless, with less blood loss (275 vs. 600 ml), shorter hospital stays (7 vs. 14.5 days) and less major complications (10% vs. 35%) compared with ORC. Richards et al. [9] speculated that RRC was associated with fewer complications than ORC in the elderly was related to less fluid shifts, decreased operative blood loss, and lower rate of transfusions. Although RRC is able to bridge the technical difficulties of conventional LRC, and facilitate a broader diffusion of minimally invasive treatment for muscle-invasive bladder cancer, it is still not available worldwide. In the present study, it was observed that LRC group associated with less EBL, and could significantly reduce the incidence of ileus and perioperative infection within 90 days after surgery in contrast to ORC group. What is more, patients in LRC group recovered more smoothly than ORC group, as was indicated by less multidisciplinary consultation needed after operation (33.3% vs. 64.0%, P = 0.038). Interestingly, it was found that serum albumin both reduced 7.2 to 8.7 g/L in LRC and ORC group respectively. It was thought that serum albumin reflects nutritional status, and strongly associated with 90-day mortality, accounting for a 2.5-fold increase in the risk of 90-day mortality per 7 g/L decrease in serum albumin. [19] So it is necessary that attention should be paid to keep a balanced nutrition after surgery in order to reduce the possibility of delayed recovery.

Despite less complication for LRC group, the hospital stay was similar to ORC group in this study. This was mainly due to the different health-care system compared with the United States or European practice. The mean hospital stay after surgery in our institution was 14 and 15 for LRC and ORC group respectively, which was obviously longer than previous report. [9,13,23,28,29]

The healthcare system is different between China and US, patients in our institution often comes from different provinces, it's not convenient for patients to find an rehabilitation center for medical support after discharging from hospital, so most patients preferred to stay until all the tubes and sutures were removed even if they were fit for discharge in the LRC group. Hemal et al. [30] and Saika et al. [31] considered hospital stay was sometimes a reflection of health-care mode and the prevalent social condition of the patients. Overall survival rate is the golden standard to evaluate the feasibility of a medical intervention, it was observed that the LRC not only achieved less complication but also gained comparable overall survival (81% vs. 76%, P = 0.746) compared with ORC at a median follow-up of 21 months (range 3–61 months).

The limitations of this study should be noted. First of all, the nature of a retrospective study made it impossible to avoid the selection bias and attrition bias. A randomized, prospective study with age, medical comorbidity and urinary diversion stratification, and longtime follow-up would be better to assess the effect of LRC for elderly patients. Secondly, the sample size of this study was small. In most cases, patients more 75-year-old, especially those with worse physical condition, were reluctant to undergo such a major surgery. So the results maybe only reflect the outcome of those elderly patients with better physical condition and more optimistic attitude. Thirdly, although intensive care unit (ICU) monitoring period was a reliable indicator to evaluate the condition of a patient after surgery, all patients underwent cystectomy in our institution routinely stayed in ICU for the first day after surgery. Only if patient underwent a re-operation, he would be sent to ICU again. So the clinical practice of our institution made it less valuable to include this parameter.

Conclusions

The results of this study displays the oncological efficacy of LRC is similar to that of ORC, while with less postoperative complications and blood loss. We suggest that it is promising to accept LRC as the primary intervention to treat muscle invasive or high risk non-muscle invasive bladder cancer in elderly patients with a relative long life expectancy and multidisciplinary cooperation was required to perform a cystectomy for an elderly patient. However, larger sample size and prospective randomized studies are needed to confirm these results.

Author Contributions

Conceived and designed the experiments: CLX SXZ ZSZ. Performed the experiments: CLX SXZ ZSZ XWY JJZ. Analyzed the data: RXS RCW. Contributed reagents/materials/analysis tools: JGH LHW. Wrote the paper: CLX SXZ ZSZ YHS. Performed radical cystectomy surgery: CLX JGH LHW.

References

1. US Department of Health and Human Services (2011) A profile of older Americans: 2011. Available: http://www.aoa.gov/AoAroot/Aging_Statistics/Profile/2011/index.aspx.
2. Siegel R, Naishadham D, Jemal A (2013) Cancer statistics, 2013. CA Cancer J Clin 63: 11–30.
3. Han S, zhang S, Chen W, Li C (2013) Analysis of the status and trends of bladder cancer incidence in China. Oncol Prog 11: 89–95.
4. Farnham SB, Cookson MS, Alberts G, Smith JA Jr, Chang SS (2004) Benefit of radical cystectomy in the elderly patient with significant co-morbidities. Urol Oncol 22: 178–181.
5. Froehner M, Brausi MA, Herr HW, Muto G, Studer UE (2009) Complications following radical cystectomy for bladder cancer in the elderly. Eur Urol 56: 443–454.
6. Gakis G, Efstathiou J, Lerner SP, Cookson MS, Keegan KA, et al. (2013) ICUD-EAU International Consultation on Bladder Cancer 2012: Radical cystectomy and bladder preservation for muscle-invasive urothelial carcinoma of the bladder. Eur Urol 63: 45–57.
7. Mendiola FP, Zorn KC, Gofrit ON, Mikhail AA, Orvieto MA, et al. (2007) Cystectomy in the ninth decade: operative results and long-term survival outcomes. Can J Urol 14: 3628–3634.
8. Bostrom PJ, Kossi J, Laato M, Nurmi M (2009) Risk factors for mortality and morbidity related to radical cystectomy. BJU Int 103: 191–196.
9. Richards KA, Kader AK, Otto R, Pettus JA, Smith JJ, et al. (2012) Is robot-assisted radical cystectomy justified in the elderly? A comparison of robotic versus open radical cystectomy for bladder cancer in elderly >/ = 75 years old. J Endourol 26: 1301–1306.
10. Parra RO, Andrus CH, Jones JP, Boullier JA (1992) Laparoscopic cystectomy: initial report on a new treatment for the retained bladder. J Urol 148: 1140–1144.
11. Haber GP, Gill IS (2007) Laparoscopic radical cystectomy for cancer: oncological outcomes at up to 5 years. BJU Int 100: 137–142.
12. Hemal AK, Kolla SB (2007) Comparison of laparoscopic and open radical cystoprostatectomy for localized bladder cancer with 3-year oncological followup: a single surgeon experience. J Urol 178: 2340–2343.
13. Ha US, Kim SI, Kim SJ, Cho HJ, Hong SH, et al. (2010) Laparoscopic versus open radical cystectomy for the management of bladder cancer: mid-term oncological outcome. Int J Urol 17: 55–61.
14. Springer C, Mohammed N, Alba S, Theil G, Altieri VM, et al. (2013) Laparoscopic radical cystectomy with extracorporeal ileal neobladder for muscle-invasive urothelial carcinoma of the bladder: technique and short-term outcomes. World J Urol, in press.
15. Snow-Lisy DC, Campbell SC, Gill IS, Hernandez AV, Fergany A, et al. (2014) Robotic and Laparoscopic Radical Cystectomy for Bladder Cancer: Long-term Oncologic Outcomes. Eur Urol 65: 193–200.
16. Wein A (2012) Campbell-walsh urology,10th ed, Philadelphia, Elsevier, 2012, 2379–2408.
17. Eble JN, Sauter G, Epstein Jl, Sesterhenn I (2004) WHO classification of classification of tumours of the urinary system and male genital organs. Lyon: IARCC Press, 29–34.
18. Sobin LH, Gospodariwicz M, Wittekind C (2009) TNM classification of malignant tumors. UICC International Union Against Cancer, 7th ed, Wiley-Blackwell, 262–265.
19. Morgan TM, Keegan KA, Barocas DA, Ruhotina N, Phillips SE, et al. (2011) Predicting the probability of 90-day survival of elderly patients with bladder cancer treated with radical cystectomy. J Urol 186: 829–834.
20. Prout GR Jr, Wesley MN, Yancik R, Ries LA, Havlik RJ, et al. (2005) Age and comorbidity impact surgical therapy in older bladder carcinoma patients: a population-based study. Cancer 104: 1638–1647.
21. Chang SS, Alberts G, Cookson MS, Smith JA Jr (2001) Radical cystectomy is safe in elderly patients at high risk. J Urol 166: 938–941.
22. Game X, Soulie M, Seguin P, Vazzoler N, Tollon C, et al. (2001) Radical cystectomy in patients older than 75 years: assessment of morbidity and mortality. Eur Urol 39: 525–529.
23. Guillotreau J, Game X, Mouzin M, Doumerc N, Mallet R, et al. (2009) Radical cystectomy for bladder cancer: morbidity of laparoscopic versus open surgery. J Urol 181: 554–559.
24. May M, Fuhrer S, Braun KP, Brookman-Amissah S, Richter W, et al. (2007) Results from three municipal hospitals regarding radical cystectomy on elderly patients. Int Braz J Urol 33: 764–773.
25. Sogni F, Brausi M, Frea B, Martinengo C, Faggiano F, et al. (2008) Morbidity and quality of life in elderly patients receiving ileal conduit or orthotopic neobladder after radical cystectomy for invasive bladder cancer. Urology 71: 919–923.
26. Soulie M, Straub M, Game X, Seguin P, De Petriconi R, et al. (2002) A multicenter study of the morbidity of radical cystectomy in select elderly patients with bladder cancer. J Urol 167: 1325–1328.
27. Zebic N, Weinknecht S, Kroepfl D (2005) Radical cystectomy in patients aged > or = 75 years: an updated review of patients treated with curative and palliative intent. BJU Int 95: 1211–1214.
28. Guillotreau J, Miocinovic R, Game X, Forest S, Malavaud B, et al. (2012) Outcomes of laparoscopic and robotic radical cystectomy in the elderly patients. Urology 79: 585–590.
29. Kader AK, Richards KA, Krane LS, Pettus JA, Smith JJ, et al. (2013) Robot-assisted laparoscopic vs open radical cystectomy: comparison of complications and perioperative oncological outcomes in 200 patients. BJU Int 112: E290–294.
30. Hemal AK, Kolla SB, Wadhwa P, Dogra PN, Gupta NP (2008) Laparoscopic radical cystectomy and extracorporeal urinary diversion: a single center experience of 48 cases with three years of follow-up. Urology 71: 41–46.
31. Saika T, Suyama B, Murata T, Manabe D, Kurashige T, et al. (2001) Orthotopic neobladder reconstruction in elderly bladder cancer patients. Int J Urol 8: 533–538.

2

Fibroblast Growth Factor Receptors-1 and -3 Play Distinct Roles in the Regulation of Bladder Cancer Growth and Metastasis: Implications for Therapeutic Targeting

Tiewei Cheng[1,2,3], Beat Roth[1], Woonyoung Choi[1,2], Peter C. Black[4], Colin Dinney[1,2], David J. McConkey[1,2,3]*

1 Department of Urology, The University of Texas M.D. Anderson Cancer Center, Houston, Texas, United States of America, 2 Department of Cancer Biology, The University of Texas M.D. Anderson Cancer Center, Houston, Texas, United States of America, 3 Experimental Therapeutics Academic Program, The University of Texas-Graduate School of Biomedical Sciences (GSBS) at Houston, Houston, Texas, United States of America, 4 Department of Urologic Science, The University of British Columbia, Vancouver, British Columbia, Canada

Abstract

Fibroblast growth factor receptors (FGFRs) are activated by mutation and overexpressed in bladder cancers (BCs), and FGFR inhibitors are currently being evaluated in clinical trials in BC patients. However, BC cells display marked heterogeneity in their responses to FGFR inhibitors, and the biological mechanisms underlying this heterogeneity are not well defined. Here we used a novel inhibitor of FGFRs 1–3 and RNAi to determine the effects of inhibiting FGFR1 or FGFR3 in a panel of human BC cell lines. We observed that FGFR1 was expressed in BC cells that also expressed the "mesenchymal" markers ZEB1 and vimentin, whereas FGFR3 expression was restricted to the E-cadherin- and p63-positive "epithelial" subset. Sensitivity to the growth-inhibitory effects of BGJ-398 was also restricted to the "epithelial" BC cells and it correlated directly with FGFR3 mRNA levels but not with the presence of activating FGFR3 mutations. In contrast, BGJ-398 did not strongly inhibit proliferation but did block invasion in the "mesenchymal" BC cells in vitro. Similarly, BGJ-398 did not inhibit primary tumor growth but blocked the production of circulating tumor cells (CTCs) and the formation of lymph node and distant metastases in mice bearing orthotopically implanted "mesenchymal" UM-UC3 cells. Together, our data demonstrate that FGFR1 and FGFR3 have largely non-overlapping roles in regulating invasion/metastasis and proliferation in distinct "mesenchymal" and "epithelial" subsets of human BC cells. The results suggest that the tumor EMT phenotype will be an important determinant of the biological effects of FGFR inhibitors in patients.

Editor: Chih-Hsin Tang, China Medical University, Taiwan

Funding: This study was funded by MD Anderson Bladder SPORE (P50 CA91846), The Baker Foundation, and the MD Anderson CCSG (P30 016672). The funders had no role in study design, data collection and analysis, decision to publish, or preparation of the manuscript.

Competing Interests: The authors have declared no competing interests.

* E-mail: dmcconke@mdanderson.org

Introduction

Bladder cancer (BC) is the fifth most common cancer in Western countries. Bladder cancers can be divided into two major subgroups that possess distinct pathological, clinical, and molecular characteristics [1,2]. Most BCs (70%–80%) are low grade, non-muscle invasive papillary ("superficial") tumors (NMIBCs) that rarely progress, so patients with this form of cancer have a very good prognosis. On the other hand, patients with muscle-invasive bladder cancers (MIBCs) have a much poorer prognosis (<50% 5-year survival) [1,2]. MIBCs often progress to become metastatic, and patients with metastatic disease have a dismal 5-year survival rate of less than 5%. Consequently, identifying the molecular mechanisms involved in BC invasion and metastasis and identifying therapeutic strategies that target these processes are very high priorities in ongoing research.

Fibroblast growth factor receptors (FGFRs) are very attractive candidate targets in both subsets of BCs [3]. At least two thirds of NMIBCs contain activating FGFR3 mutations that result in ligand-independent receptor dimerization and constitutive downstream signal transduction [4,5,6,7], and in vitro studies have established that FGFR inhibitors block proliferation in normal urothelial cells that overexpress these receptors [8,9]. Although the frequency of activating FGFR3 mutations in MIBCs is much lower (<25%), many of them express high levels of FGFR3 and other FGFRs [3,10,11]. In addition to promoting proliferation, FGFRs have been implicated in the regulation of epithelial-to-mesenchymal transition (EMT), invasion, and anchorage-independent growth in BC cells [11].

BGJ-398 is a selective inhibitor of FGFRs 1, 2, and 3 that was synthesized using a novel chemical approach [12]. It exhibits IC_{50}'s of approximately 5 nM against wild-type FGFRs and the most common mutant form of FGFR3 that is expressed in BCs (S249C) [12]. An initial characterization of the compound's growth inhibitory effects in a panel of 8 human BC cell lines revealed marked heterogeneity in responses, where it displayed

IC_{50}'s of 5–30 nM in half of the cell lines and IC_{50}'s of over 1 μM in the other half [12]. The observed heterogeneity is consistent with results obtained using a distinct chemical inhibitor [13], but the molecular basis for this heterogeneity remains unclear. We therefore initiated the present study to obtain a better understanding of the effects of FGFR inhibition in BC cells, with the goal of identifying biological mechanisms and biomarkers that could be used to prospectively identify FGFR-dependent tumors. Our results reveal distinct, EMT-related roles for FGFR3 and FGFR1 in driving proliferation and invasion that have important implications for the development of FGFR inhibitor-based therapies in patients.

Materials and Methods

Chemicals and Reagents

BGJ-398 was generously provided by Novartis. For in vitro studies, BGJ-398 was reconstituted in DMSO at a stock concentration of 10 mmol/L and stored at −20°C. The BGJ-398 stock was diluted in medium just prior to use so that the concentration of DMSO never exceeded 0.1%. For in vivo studies, BGJ-398 was dissolved in 10% Tween-80.

Tumor Cell Lines and Culture Conditions

Cell lines were obtained from the University of Texas MD Anderson Cancer Center Bladder SPORE Tissue Bank, and their identities were confirmed by DNA fingerprinting using the AmpFlSTR® Identifiler® Amplification (Applied Biosystems) or AmpFlSTR® Profiler® PCR Amplification (Applied Biosystems) protocols. All cell lines were maintained as monolayers in modified Eagle's MEM supplemented with 10% fetal bovine serum, vitamins, sodium pyruvate, L-glutamine, penicillin, streptomycin, and nonessential amino acids at 37°C in a 5% CO_2 incubator.

Animals

Female athymic nude mice (NCr-nu) were purchased from the National Cancer Institute. The mice were housed under specific pathogen-free conditions in the Animal Core Facility at The University of Texas M. D. Anderson Cancer Center. The facility has received approval from the American Association for Accreditation of Laboratory Animal Care and in agreement with current regulations and standards of the U.S. Department of Health and Human Services, the U.S. Department of Agriculture, and the NIH. The mice used in these experiments were 6 to 8 weeks old.

FGFR3 Mutation Analyses

DNA was isolated from BC cell lines using a genomic DNA extraction kit (Qiagen). PCR was performed to amplify exons 7 and 10 using AmpliTaq Gold DNA polymerase (Applied Biosystems) and the primers 5′-CGGCAGTGGCGGTGGTG-GTG-3′(sense) and 5′-AGCACCGCCGTCTGGTT GGC-3′ (antisense) for exon 7 (23) and 5′-CCTCAACGCC-CATGTCTTT-3′ (sense) and 5′-AGGCAGCTCA-GAACCTGGTA-3′ (antisense) for exon 10 (purchased from Sigma Genosys). The following cycling variables were used: 95°C for 10 min, then 35 cycles of 95°C for 30 s, 65°C (exon 7) or 58°C (exon 10) for 30 s, and 72°C for 30 s, followed by a final incubation at 72°C for 10 min (23). Unincorporated primers and deoxynucleotides were removed using shrimp alkaline phosphatase and exonuclease I (U.S. Biochemical). Products were analyzed by Big Dye Terminator Cycle Sequencing (Applied Biosystems), and the data were analyzed with Sequencing Analysis 3.0 software (Applied Biosystems).

RNAi-mediated Knockdown of FGFR3, FGFR1 or bFGF

UM-UC14 and RT4 were transfected with small interfering RNAs (siRNAs) targeting FGFR3 and FGFR1 using Oligofec-tamine (Invitrogen) according to the manufacturer's instructions. Targeted oligonucleotides (sequence) and a non-targeting control were purchased from Ambion. Total RNA was collected 48 hours after transfection and analyzed by RT-PCR to confirm target knockdown. In parallel, siRNA transfected cells were harvested at 48 hours and analyzed using the cell proliferation and cell cycle assays described below. UM-UC3 and UM-UC13 were transduced with lentiviral short hairpin RNAs (shRNA-s)(Open Biosystems). Cells were continuously cultured for 5∼7 days in 10% MEM containing puromycin. Total RNA was collected after selection and analyzed by RT-PCR to confirm target knockdown. Stable knockdown cells were maintained in puromycin and used in the MTT and Boyden chamber invasion assays described below.

Immunoblotting Analyses

Cells were harvested at ∼75% to 85% confluence and lysed. Protein concentrations were measured using the Bradford assay (Bio-Rad Laboratories, Hercules, CA). Lysates were boiled in sample buffer (62.5 mmol/L Tris-HCl (pH 6.8), 10% (w/v) glycerol, 100 mmol/L DTT, 2.3% SDS, 0.002% bromophenol blue) for 5 minutes and cooled on ice for 5 minutes. Samples were separated on 8% or 12% SDS-PAGE gels at 110 V in electrophoresis buffer (25 mmol/L Tris-HCl (pH 8.3), 192 mmol/L glycine, 0.1% SDS) and then electrophoretically transferred onto methanol-prewetted polyvinylidene difluoride (PVDF) membranes in transfer buffer (25 mmol/L Tris-HCl, 192 mmol/L glycine, 20% methanol) for 1 hour at 100 mV. The membranes were incubated in blocking buffer (TBS: 10 mmol/L Tris-HCl (pH 8.0), 150 mmol/L NaCl, 5% nonfat milk) for 1 hour at room temperature while shaking and then rinsed once briefly with TBS-T (TBS containing 0.1% Tween-20). The membranes were incubated with primary antibodies diluted 1:1000 in blocking buffer overnight, washed, and then incubated with second antibodies (anti-mouse or anti-rabbit immunoglobulin, horseradish peroxidase–linked F(ab)2 fragment from mouse) diluted 1:8,000 in blocking buffer for 1 hour at room temperature while shaking. Immunoreactive proteins were detected using enhanced chemiluminescence (Amersham Biosciences, Piscataway, NJ) according to the manufacturer's instructions.

Gene Expression Profiling

Gene expression profiling was performed on a panel of 30 human BC cell lines using the Illumina platform. For each cell line, mRNA was generated from a single log-phase culture. RNA purity and integrity were measured using a NanoDrop ND-1000 and an Agilent Bioanalyzer, and only high quality RNA was used for cRNA amplification. Biotin-labeled cRNA was prepared using the Illumina RNA amplification kit (Ambion, Inc, Austin, TX), and amplified cRNA was hybridized to Illumina HT12 V4 chips (Illumina, Inc., San Diego, CA). After they were washed, the slides were scanned with IScan (Illumina, Inc.). Signal intensities were quantified with GenomeStudio (Illumina, Inc.), and quantile normalization was used to normalize the data. BRB ArrayTools version 4.2 developed by National Cancer Institute [14] was used to analyze the data. To observe the expression patterns of differentially expressed genes, specific gene expression values, adjusted to a mean of zero, were used for clustering with Cluster and TreeView [15].

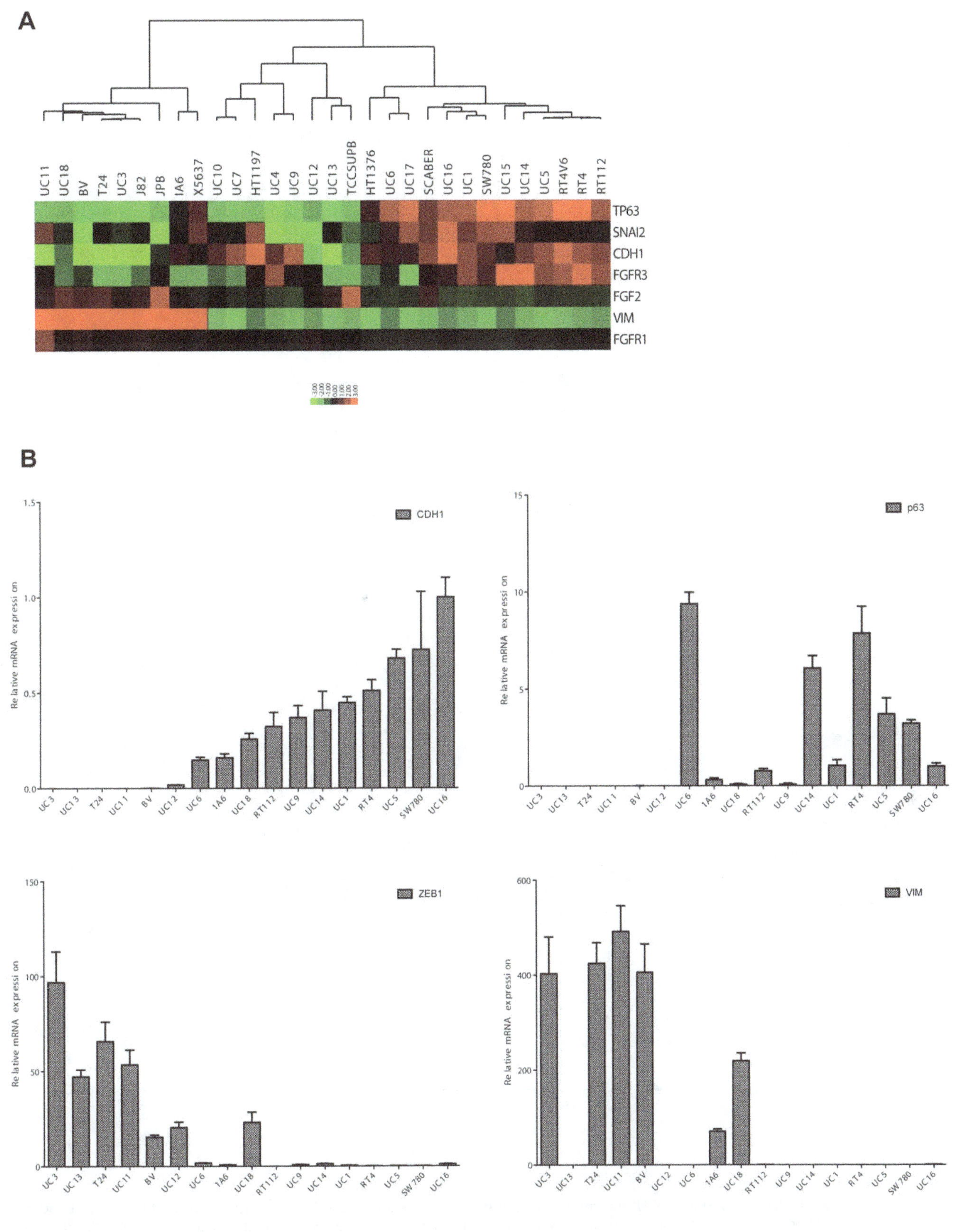

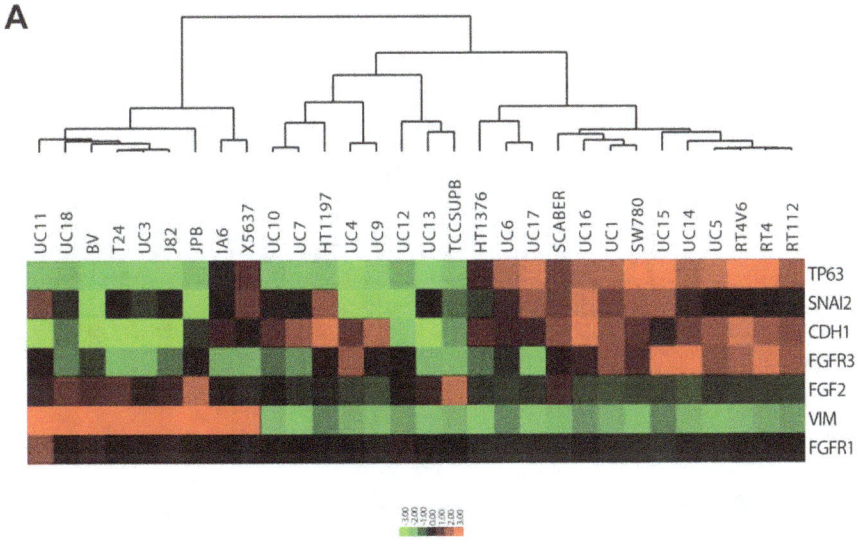

Figure 1. Expression of FGFR1, FGFR3, and bFGF in distinct subsets of human BC cell lines. A. Correlation of FGFR1 and FGFR3 with canonical EMT markers. mRNA levels were measured using whole genome mRNA expression profiling (Illumina platform). The heat map depicts the expression of FGFR1, FGFR3, FGF2 (bFGF), p63 (TP63), E-cadherin (CDH1), Slug (SNAI2), and vimentin. B. Quantitative analysis of EMT marker expression. Relative levels of the "epithelial" markers E-cadherin (CDH1) and p63, and the "mesenchymal" markers ZEB1 and vimentin were measured by quantitative real-time RT-PCR.

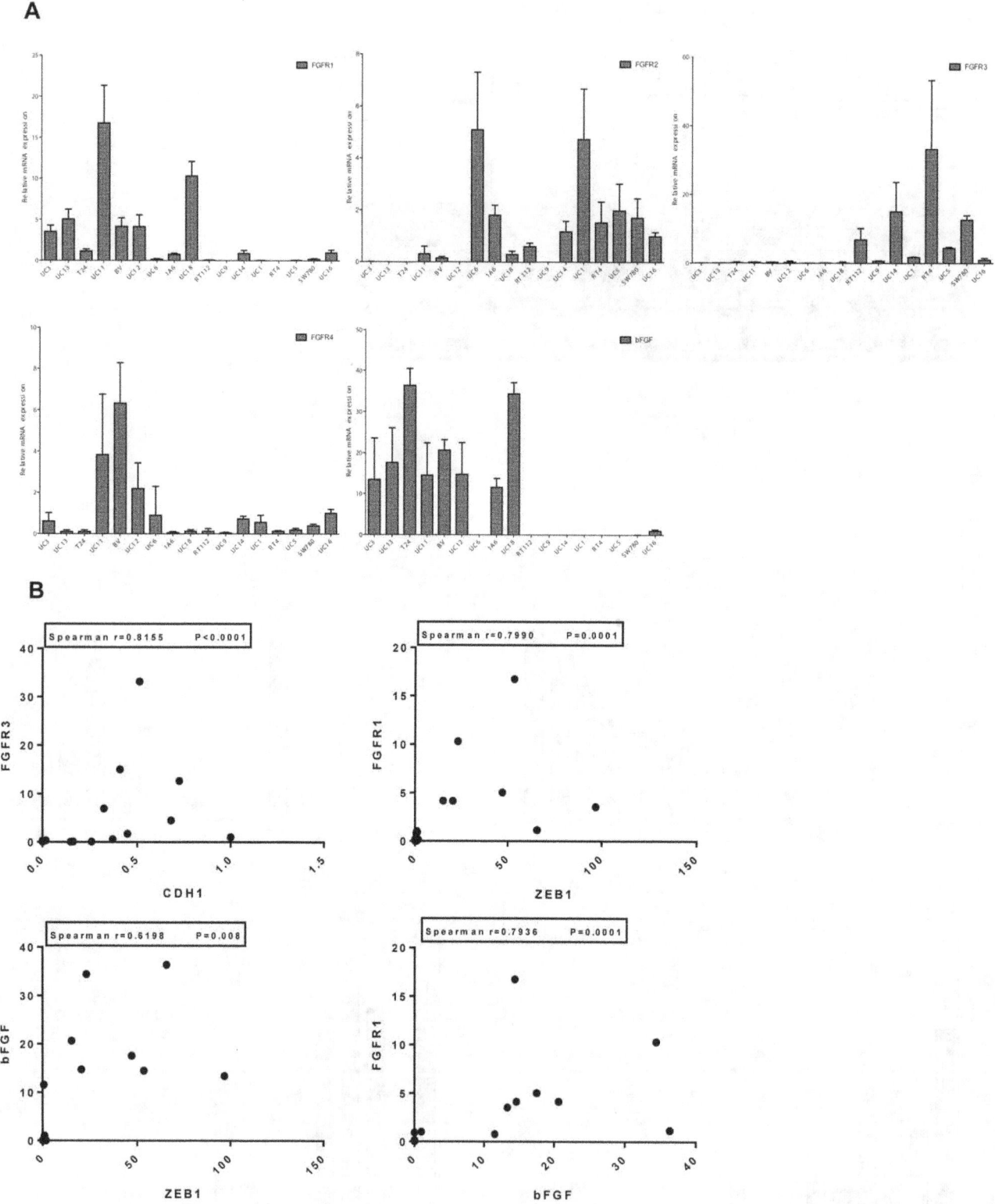

Figure 2. Relationship between FGFR/bFGF expression and EMT. A. Expression of FGFRs 1–4 and bFGF in relationship to E-cadherin expression. The relative mRNA levels were measured by quantitative real-time RT-PCR. The cell lines in each panel are organized by relative E-cadherin expression (low to high, from left to right; see Fig. 1B). B. Scatterplots depicting the relationships between FGFR1, bFGF, FGFR3, and EMT marker expression. Nonparametric correlation analyses were used to evaluate the relationships between FGFR3 and E-cadherin (CDH1) expression, FGFR1 and ZEB1 expression, bFGF and ZEB1 expression, and bFGF and FGFR1 expression. Correlation coefficients and p values are indicated on the figure.

MTT Assays

Cells (5×10^3) were plated in 96-well plates and allowed to adhere for 24 hours before they were incubated with or without increasing concentrations of BGJ-398 for 48 h or 5 days. MTT (3-(4,5-dimethylthiazol-2-yl)-2,5-diphenyltetrazolium bromide) assays were used to measure relative cell numbers based on conversion of MTT to formazan in viable cells. Fifty μl MTT dissolved in PBS (50 μg/ml) was added to each well and plates were incubated for 3 hours. The medium was then removed and 100 μl DMSO was added to each well to lyse cells and solubilize the formazan. A standard micro-plate reader was used to determine the absorbance (600 nm). Each experimental data point represents average values obtained from six replicates and each experiment was performed at least twice.

Real-time Reverse Transcriptase PCR Analyses

Cells were harvested at 75% to 85% confluence and total RNA was isolated using mirVANA^{TM} miRNA Isolation Kit (Ambion, Life Science, CA). FGFRs and other genes of interests were analyzed by Taqman-based real-time PCR (ABI PRISM 7500; Applied Biosystems). The comparative CT method was used to determine relative gene expression for each target gene; the cyclophilin A gene was used as internal control to normalized the amount of amplifiable RNA. Taqman primers was purchased from the manufacture (Applied Biosystem, CA) as follows: E-cadherin; Hs00170423_m1, TP63; Hs00978343_m1, ZEB1; Hs00232783_m1, Vimentin; Hs00185584_m1, FGFR1; Hs00915142_m1, FGFR2; Hs01552926_m1, FGFR3; Hs00179829_m1, FGFR4; Hs01106908_m1, bFGF; Hs00266645_m.

Cell Cycle Analyses

Cells were plated in 6-well plates and maintained in 10% FBS MEM for 24 hours. Cells were then exposed to various concentrations of BGJ-398 for 48 hours or grown another 24 hours (reaching ~75% to 85% confluence) to analyze the effects of FGFR3 or FGFR1 knockdown. Cells were harvested by trypsinization and pelleted by centrifugation. The pellets were then resuspended in PBS containing 50 μg/mL propidium iodide, 0.1% Triton X-100, and 0.1% sodium citrate. Propidium iodide fluorescence was measured by fluorescence-activated cell sorting (FL-3 channel, Becton Dickinson, Mountain View, CA) using the instrument's cycle analysis software.

Boyden Chamber Invasion Assays

Invasion chambers containing Matrigel-coated polyethylene terephthalate membranes with 8 μm pores were purchased from BD Science in a 24-well plate format. Cells (2.5×10^5) were released from tissue culture flasks using EDTA (1 mmol/L), centrifuged, suspended in a serum free medium and placed in the upper compartments of invasion chambers. Thirty percent fetal bovine serum medium was placed in the lower compartments as a chemoattractant and invasion assays were carried out for 48 h. Each cell line was plated in triplicate. To examine cell invasion after exposure to BGJ-398, cells that had not invaded were removed and the cells on the lower surface of the filter were stained with Diff-Quick (American Scientific Products, McGaw Park, IL). Invasive activity was measured by counting the cells that had migrated to the lower side of the filter. To evaluate invasion after silencing FGFR1 or bFGF, membranes were removed after incubation for 48 hours at 37°C and stained in propidium iodide (Sigma-Aldrich) without removing cells from the upper surfaces of the membranes. The filters were mounted on glass slides and

analyzed by confocal microscopy at 100× magnification. The planes of focus were adjusted so that the cells that had not invaded could be distinguished from the invaded cells and counted in 8 independent fields. Invasive activity was measured by calculating ratios of invaded to noninvaded cells.

Archorage Independent Growth Assay

UM-UC3 and UM-UC13 wild type or bFGF/FGFR1 silenced cells were plated at 1×10^4 cells per well in 6-well-plates supplemented with 10% FBS MEM containing 0.6% agar. Cells were allowed to grow for 2 weeks. Images were acquired using an Olympus IX inverted-phase contrast microscope. The total numbers of colonies per random view (100×) and the average diameter of colonies per random view (100×) were determined using a SliderBook image analyzer.

Orthotopic Xenograft Experiments

The human BC cell line UM-UC-3 was transduced with a lentiviral vector encoding luciferase (luc) and red fluorescent protein (RFP; mCherry) as described previously [16]. After stable transduction with the luc-RFP reporter, cells were sorted by Fluorescence Activated Cell Sorting (FACS) using an Influx High-Speed sorter (BD Biosciences). Luciferase activity was quantified in vitro using D-luciferin (150 μg/mL) and the IVIS biolumines-cence system (Xenogen Co.). To produce tumors in nude mice, subconfluent cultures of labeled UM-UC3 were lifted with trypsin, mixed with 10% FBS MEM, centrifuged at 1,200 rpm for 5 min, washed in PBS, and resuspended in HBSS. Cells were then injected orthotopically into the bladder wall at a concentration of $5 \times 10^5/50$ μL using a lower laparotomy. Mice bearing metastases were euthanized 5 to 8 weeks after tumor cell injection, the lymph node and distant metastases were excised, cut into small pieces using scalpels, exposed to 1% trypsin for 20 minutes, centrifuged (1,200 rpm for 5 min), and cultured in 10% supplemented MEM. After FACS sorting, the recycled cells were subconfluently cultured and reinjected at a concentration of $2 \times 10^5/50$ μL HBSS as described above. Thus, tumor cell recycling was performed three times in order to select a highly metastatic UM-UC3 subpopulation which develops metastases in ~75% of mice. For our therapy experiment, we injected the 4th cycle of recycled UM-UC3 at a concentration of $2 \times 10^5/50$ μL. Mice with detectable tumor growth at the time of the first imaging (5 days after injection) were randomized into two groups (n = 7/group).

In vivo Bioluminescence Imaging

Bioluminescence imaging was conducted on an IVIS 100 imaging system with Living Image software (Xenogen) as de-scribed elsewhere [16]. In brief, animals were anesthetized before imaging with a 2.5% isoflurane/air mixture and injected s.c. with 15 mg/mL of luciferin potassium salt in PBS at a dose of 150 mg/kg body weight. A digital gray-scale animal image was acquired and a pseudocolored image was overlaid representing the spatial distribution of detected photons emerging from active luciferase. Signal intensity was quantified as the sum of all detected photons within the region of interest per second, separately counting each primary tumor and each metastatic site.

Collection of Primary Tumors and Circulating Tumor Cells (CTCs)

Forty days after injection, when animals in the control group became moribund, mice were anesthetized with isoflurane as described above. To measure the number of CTCs, the maximal amount of blood (600–1200 μl) was collected by cardiac puncture

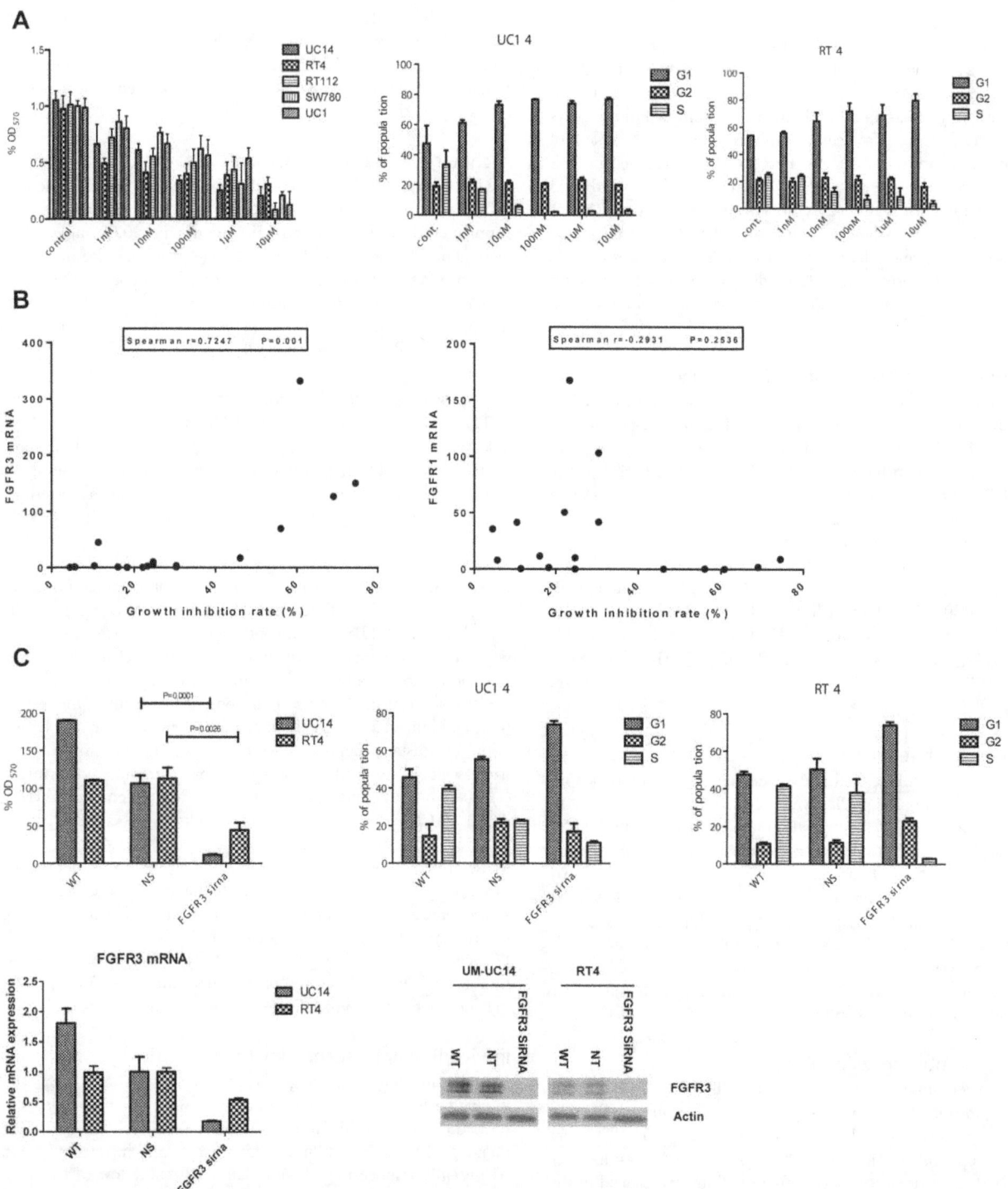

Figure 3. FGFR3 levels predict sensitivity to BGJ-398-induced cell cycle arrest. A. Effects of BGJ-398 on cell proliferation in the drug-sensitive cells. In the left panel, cells were incubated for 48 h in the presence of the indicated concentrations of BGJ-398 and cell growth was measured by MTT reduction. Mean ± SEM, n=6. In the center and right panels, UM-UC14 or RT4 cells were incubated with the indicated concentrations of BGJ-398 and the percentages of cells within each cell cycle quadrant were quantified by propidium iodide staining and FACS analysis. Mean ± SEM, n=3. B. Sensitivity to the anti-proliferative effects of BGJ-398 correlates with FGFR3 expression but not with the presence of activating FGFR3 mutations. The level of growth inhibition observed after 48 h exposure to 1 μM BGJ-398 (as measured in MTT assays) was correlated with the relative level of FGFR3 (left panel) or FGFR1 (right panel) mRNA expression in a panel of 17 human BC cell lines.. C. Effects of FGFR3 knockdown on cell proliferation. Left panel: UM-UC14 or RT4 cells were transiently transfected with either non-targeting (NT) or FGFR3-specific siRNAs and cell growth was measured at 48 h by MTT reduction. Mean ± SEM, n=6. Center and right panels: UM-UC14 or RT4 cells were transiently transfected with either non-targeting (NT) or FGFR3-specific siRNAs and percentages of cells within each phase of the cell cycle were quantified by propidium iodide staining and FACS analysis. Mean ± SEM, n=3. Lower panel: the efficiency of FGFR3 silencing was measured by quantitative RT-PCR and immunoblotting.

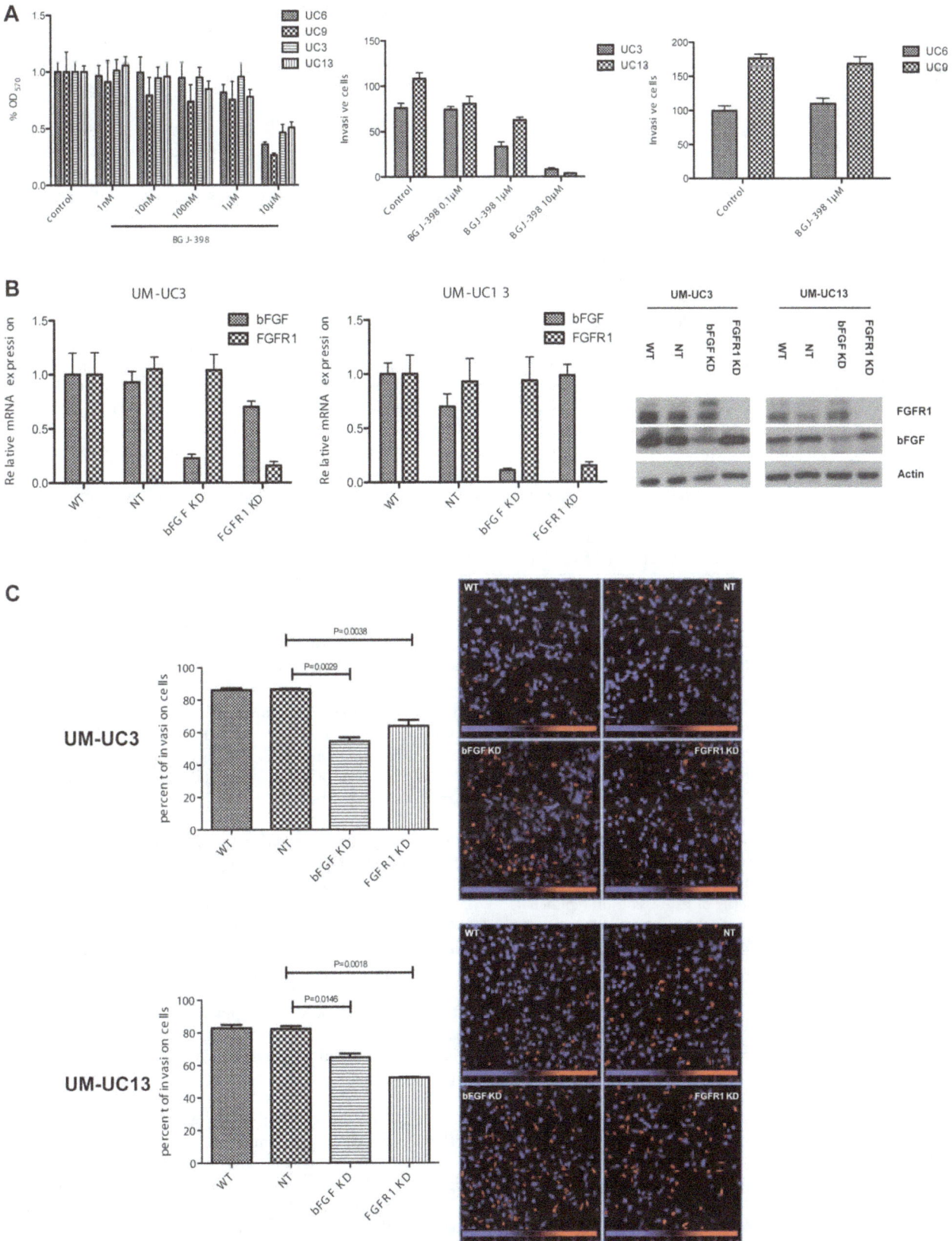

Figure 4. FGFR1 selectively regulates invasion in "mesenchymal" bladder cancer cells. A. Left panel: effects of BGJ-398 on cell growth in two "mesenchymal" (UM-UC3, UM-UC13) and two "epithelial" (UM-UC6, UM-UC9) cell lines that were found to be resistant to the anti-proliferative effects of the drug. Growth inhibition was measured at 48 h by MTT reduction. Mean ± SEM, n = 6. Center panel: concentration-dependent effects of BGJ-398 on invasion in the UM-UC3 and UM-UC13 cells. Invasion was measured using modified Boyden chambers and standard light microscopy as described in Materials and Methods. Mean ± SEM, n = 3. Right panel: effects of BGJ-398 on invasion in the UM-UC6 and UM-UC9 cells. Note that the

drug had no effect on invasion in either cell line. B. Stable knockdown of FGFR1 or bFGF in cells transduced with lentiviral shRNAs. Relative mRNA levels were measured by quantititative real-time RT-PCR and protein levels were measured by immunoblotting. C. Effects of FGFR1 or bFGF knockdown on invasion. Left panels: percentages of cells that invaded through Matrigel in modified Boyden chambers were quantified by propidium iodide staining and confocal microscopy. The right panels display representative confocal images where the nuclei of the cells that invaded are pseudo-colored blue and the cells that did not invade are depicted in red.

using 1 ml syringe, 22 gauge needle, and heparin-coated collection tubes as described previously [17]. Mice were then euthanized with carbon monoxide. Tumors were excised, and samples were either formalin fixed and embedded in paraffin, embedded in OCT (Miles, Inc), or frozen rapidly in liquid nitrogen and stored at $-80°$C for RNA and protein extraction. For further blood processing, red blood cells were lysed twice for 5 min with 1 ml ACK lysis buffer (Invitrogen), and centrifuged for 5 min at 1200 rpm in Eppendorf tubes. The pellet was finally lysed and further processed for total RNA isolation using the mirVANA™ miRNA Isolation kit (Ambion, Life Science). For Real-time PCR analysis, PCR technology (Step One; Applied Biosystems) was used together with TaqMan® Gene Expression Assays (Applied Biosystems). Absolute quantification was used to generate cycle threshold (CT) values for human specific HLA-C primer (Hs00740298_g1) for each sample. RT-PCR analysis of the blood samples (in triplicates) was run together with standard isolates (0, 2, 20, 200, 2000, and 20,000 UM-UC3 cells in 100 μl mouse blood). CT values of the standards were used to create a standard curve for UM-UC3 CTC, and the number of CTCs of each blood sample was calculated accordingly.

Results

Relationship between E-cadherin and bFGF/FGFR Expression in UC Cells

We analyzed the expression of the 4 FGFRs and the dominant cancer-associated ligand (FGF-2/basic FGF) at the mRNA level in a panel of 30 UC cell lines by whole genome expression profiling (Illumina platform). Expression of FGFR3 correlated directly with expression of p63 [18,19] and E-cadherin [20](Fig. 1A), indicating that FGFR3 is expressed by the "epithelial" subset of BC cells. Conversely, the expression of FGFR1 correlated more directly with the "mesenchymal" marker vimentin (Fig. 1A). We used quantitative real-time reverse transcriptase PCR (RT-PCR) to more accurately define the patterns of expression of "epithelial" and "mesenchymal" markers across the panel of cell lines. The results are displayed in Figure 1B, where we organized the BC cell lines in all of the panels according to their relative expression of the canonical "epithelial" marker E-cadherin (Fig. 1B, upper left panel) [20]. The expression of E-cadherin correlated directly with expression of p63 and inversely with expression of ZEB1 and vimentin, demonstrating that the "epithelial" and "mesenchymal" markers are expressed in a largely non-overlapping fashion in the BC lines (Fig. 1B). Only two of the cell lines (1A6 and UM-UC18) co-expressed "epithelial" and "mesenchymal" markers (Fig. 1B).

We then measured expression of FGFRs 1–4 and FGF-2 by quantitative RT-PCR (Fig. 2A). Confirming the gene expression profiling results, FGFR1 was expressed primarily by cells within the "mesenchymal" subset (UM-UC3, UM-UC13, T24, BV and UC12)(Fig. 2A top left), whereas FGFR3 expression was concentrated within the "epithelial" cells, with RT4 having the highest expression followed by UM-UC14, SW780 and RT112 (Fig. 2A, top right). FGFR2 also appeared to be somewhat enriched in the "epithelial" and FGFR4 in the "mesenchymal" cells, respectively, but their levels of expression were much lower than the levels of FGFR3 or FGFR1 (mean of 36 cycles versus 30 cycles of PCR),

consistent with previous findings [10]. Finally, the "mesenchymal" cells expressed higher levels of FGF2 (bFGF) than did the "epithelial" cells (Fig. 2A). We confirmed that FGFR3 expression was enriched in the "epithelial" and FGFR1 and bFGF expression was enriched in the "mesenchymal" cell lines at the protein level by immunoblotting (Figure S1). Using nonparametric correlation analyses, we confirmed that FGFR3 expression correlated strongly and directly with expression of E-cadherin (Spearman r = 0.8155, p<0.0001, Fig. 2B) and inversely with expression of the "mesenchymal" markers (Fig. S2). Conversely, expression of FGFR1 and bFGF strongly and directly correlated with expression of ZEB1 (Spearman r = 0.799, p = 0.0001 for FGFR1 and r = 0.6198, p = 0.008 for bFGF) (Fig. 2B). In addition, bFGF and FGFR1 expression correlated directly with each other as expected (Fig. 2B). We then examined whether the observed differences in mRNA expression translated into differential expression at the protein level in a subset of the cell lines by immunoblotting. We found that FGFR3 but not FGFR1 was expressed in the epithelial UM-UC14, RT4 and RT112 cells, whereas FGFR1 but not FGFR3 was expressed in mesenchymal UM-UC3, UM-UC12 and UM-UC13. FGF-2 was expressed in all 6 cell lines, but the mesenchymal cells expressed more FGF-2 than the epithelial" cells did. Together, these data support the idea that FGFR3 and bFGF/FGFR1 probably function in non-overlapping epithelial and mesenchymal subsets of BC cells.

Effects of BGJ-398 on Cell Proliferation

Previous studies concluded that FGFR inhibitors block proliferation in some human BC cells in vitro [12,13]. We therefore tested the effects of BGJ-398 on proliferation in 17 BC cell lines to characterize the extent of the heterogeneity in drug sensitivity. We incubated the cells with increasing concentrations of BGJ-398 for 48 hours and measured cytotoxicity and growth arrest using MTT assays. We identified 5 cell lines (UM-UC14, SW780, RT4, RT112 and UM-UC1) that were drug-sensitive as defined by ≥50% growth inhibition at drug concentrations of 1 μmol/L or lower (Fig. 3A left panel and data not shown). To determine the relative contributions of growth arrest and cell death to these effects, we exposed the UM-UC14 and RT4 cells to increasing concentrations of BGJ-398 for 48 hours and directly measured cell cycle arrest and apoptosis by propidium iodide staining and FACS analysis. In both cell lines increasing concentrations of BGJ-398 produced increases in the percentages of cells in the G1 phase and parallel decreases in the percentages of cells in S phase. Specifically, the percentages of cells within the G1 phase increased from 47.5% and 54% to 74.2% and 69.1%, while percentages of cells in S phase decreased from 33.5% and 25% to 2.7% and 8.8% in the BGJ-398-exposed UM-UC14 and RT4 cells, respectively (Fig. 3A). On the other hand, BGJ-398 did not induce apoptosis in either cell line at concentrations below 10 μM (data not shown). Therefore, BGJ-398 exerts primarily cytostatic effects on BC cells in vitro.

We then examined the relationship between BGJ-398 sensitivity and the presence of activating FGFR3 mutations. Using exon sequencing we identified 5 cell lines within our panel that contained activating FGFR3 mutations (UM-UC6, UM-UC14, UM-UC15, UM-UC16 and UM-UC17) (Fig. S3). Strikingly, only

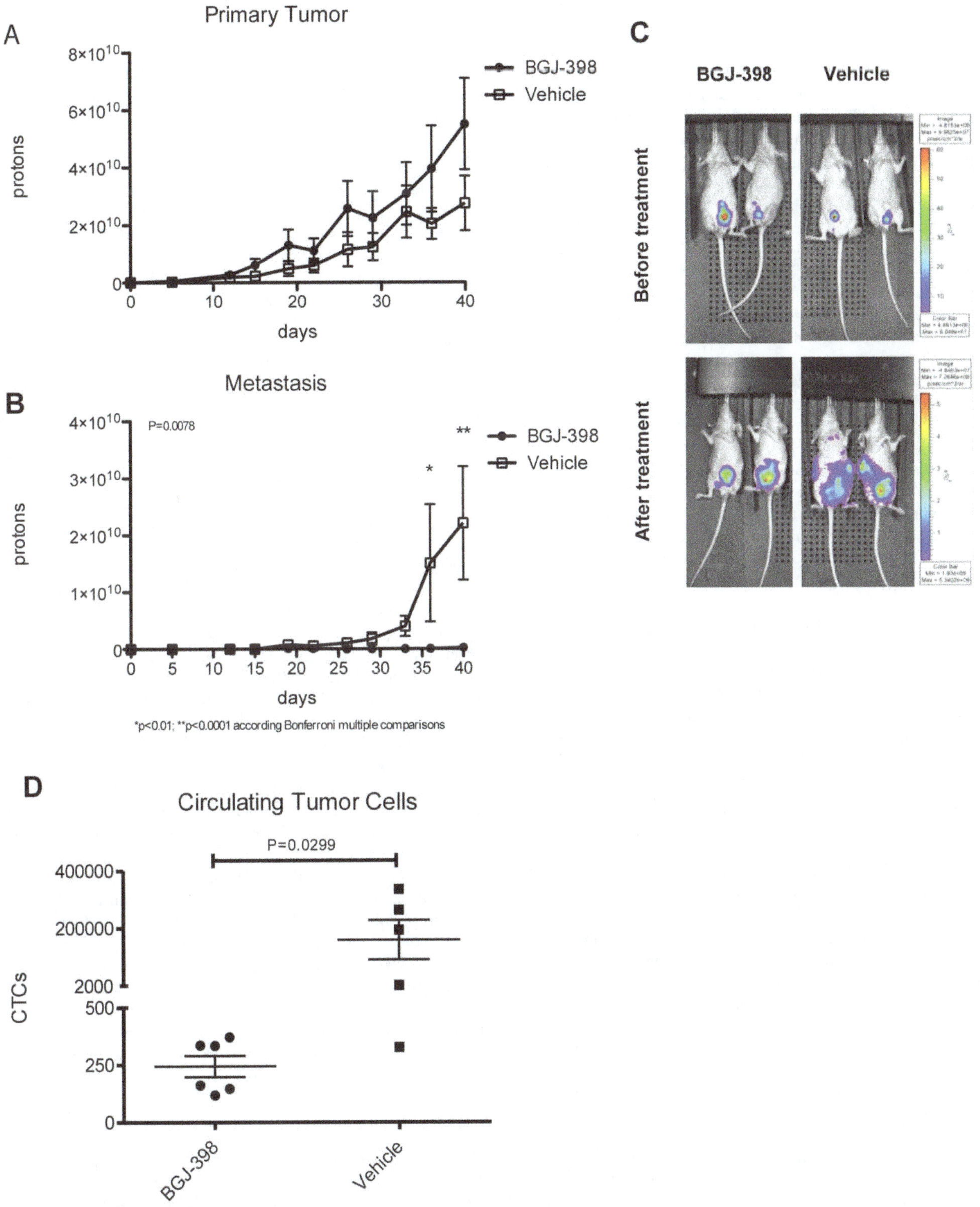

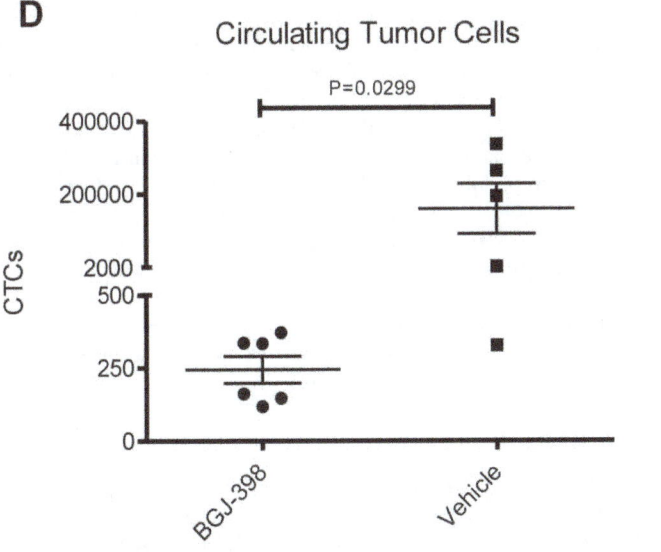

Figure 5. Effects of BGJ-398 on UM-UC3 primary tumor growth and metastasis. A. Effects on primary tumor growth. Luciferase-labelled, orthotopically recycled UM-UC3 cells were implanted into the bladders of nude mice, and tumors were allowed to grow for 8 days prior to initiating therapy with BGJ-398 (daily via oral gavage). Tumor growth was measured biweekly by luciferase imaging. Mean ± SEM from 6 (control) or 7 (treated) mice per group. B. Effects on metastasis. Whole animal metastatic burdens were determined non-invasively by luciferase imaging. Mean ± SEM, n = 6 (control mice) or 7 (treated mice). C. Representative whole body luciferase images taken just prior to the initiation of therapy and at the conclusion of the experiment. D. Effects of BGJ-398 on CTC production. CTC numbers were estimated by measuring human HLA levels in isolated whole blood by quantitative PCR; cell numbers were determined using a UM-UC3 standard curve. The scatterplot displays the results obtained from each animal; the lines denote the mean values for each group.

one of the FGFR3-mutant cell lines (UM-UC14) was also BGJ-398 sensitive. On the other hand, we observed a good correlation between FGFR3 mRNA expression and drug sensitivity (Spearman $r = 0.7247$ $p = 0.01$) (Fig. 3B left panel), whereas there was no correlation between sensitivity to BGJ-398 and FGFR1 expression (Spearman $r = -0.2931$ $p = 0.2536$) (Fig. 3B right panel).

Given the non-overlapping patterns of FGFR1 and FGFR3 expression, the results suggested that FGFR3 plays a more important role than FGFR1 in driving proliferation human BC cells. To more directly test this hypothesis, we used RNAi to knock down FGFR1 or FGFR3 in the BGJ-398-sensitive UM-UC14 and RT4 cells and measured the effects on cell proliferation using MTT assays. Quantitative RT-PCR revealed knockdown efficiencies of 50% and over 80% in the RT4 and UM-UC14 cells transfected with FGFR3-specific siRNAs, respectively compared with cells transfected with the non-specific siRNA control, and these results were also confirmed at the protein level by immunoblotting (Fig. 3C lower panel). The corresponding effects on cell proliferation were very similar, in that proliferation was reduced by almost 50% in the RT4 cells and by over 80% in UM-UC14 transfected with the FGFR3 siRNA (Fig. 3C left panel). Cell cycle analyses confirmed that FGFR3 knockdown increased the percentages of cells in the G1 phase and decreased the fractions of cells in S phase (Fig. 3C center/right panels), consistent with the MTT results and the previously observed effects of BGJ-398 [12]. In contrast, knockdown of FGFR1 had no significant effect on proliferation (Fig. S4).

Effects of BGJ-398 on Invasion

Although the "mesenchymal" UM-UC3 and UM-UC13 cells expressed relatively high levels of FGFR1, they were resistant to the anti-proliferative effects of BGJ-398 (Fig. 4A left panel). Because invasion, migration, and metastasis are characteristic features of "mesenchymal" tumor cells [20], we examined the effects of BGJ-398 on invasion in the UM-UC3 and UM-UC13 cells, using two "epithelial", BGJ-398-resistant cell lines (UM-UC6 and UM-UC9) as controls. We exposed cells to increasing concentrations of BGJ-398 and measured invasion using modified Boyden chambers. BGJ-398 strongly inhibited invasion in the UM-UC3 and UM-UC13 cells in a concentration-dependent manner, whereas it had no effects on invasion in the "epithelial" UM-UC6 and UM-UC9 cells (Fig. 4A center/right panels).

To more directly examine the involvement of FGFR1 and bFGF in the regulation of invasion, we stably silenced their expression in the UM-UC3 and UM-UC13 cells using lentiviral shRNAs, and we used quantitative RT-PCR analyses to confirm that silencing produced over 75% knockdown in all cases, and we confirmed that these effects resulted in reduced protein expression by immunoblotting (Fig. 4B). We then quantified the effects of knockdown on invasion using modified Boyden chambers and confocal microscopy. In the UM-UC3 background the percentage of invading cells was reduced from 85% in the parental cells or cells transduced with a control lentiviral construct to 54.5% in bFGF KD cells (P = 0.0029) and 63.8% in FGFR1 KD cells (P = 0.0038). Similarly, in the UM-UC13 background, the levels of invasion were reduced from 82% in parental cells or cells transduced with the non-targeting lentivirus to 64.8% in the bFGF KD cells (P = 0.0146) and 52.4% in FGFR1 KD cells (P = 0.0018) (Fig. 4C). Together, the data confirm that bFGF and FGFR1 both promote invasion in "mesenchymal" BC cells.

Our observation that FGFR inhibition blocked invasion without affecting proliferation in the cells that express high levels of FGFR1 seemed to contradict previous work implicating FGFR1 in the regulation of cell proliferation [10,11]. We therefore performed additional experiments to determine whether FGFR1 inhibition produced effects on growth that become more obvious in longer-term assays. Consistent with this idea, knockdown of FGFR1 in UM-UC3 or either bFGF or FGFR1 in UM-UC13 partially inhibited cell growth in 5-day MTT assays (Fig. S5A) and assays that measure colony formation in soft agar (Fig. S5B).

Effects of BGJ-398 on Tumor Growth and Metastasis

Although in vitro models are excellent tools for studying molecular mechanisms, the process of cancer metastasis is regulated by tumor-stromal interactions that cannot be modeled well in vitro. Therefore, in order to better define the effects of BGJ-398 on primary tumor growth versus metastasis in "mesenchymal" BC cells, we first isolated a highly metastatic form of UM-UC3 using orthotopic "recycling" in nude mice [21]. We transduced the cells with a lentiviral vector encoding luciferase and red fluorescent protein (RFP), which enabled us to monitor primary tumor growth and metastasis non-invasively by luciferase imaging and to isolate circulating tumor cells (CTCs) by cell sorting. After 3 rounds of recycling, the UM-UC3 cells formed orthotopic tumors in 100% of mice and consistently produced metastases to lymph nodes, lungs, and bone in over 70% of mice. We then implanted 200,000 of the recycled UM-UC3 cells orthotopically in nude mice and initiated therapy with BGJ-398 or vehicle (via oral gavage) once primary tumors were well established (on day 8), monitoring tumor growth and metastasis biweekly by IVIS imaging (Fig. 5). Interestingly, primary tumors in the mice treated with BGJ-398 appeared to grow slightly faster than controls, although the differences in growth rates were not statistically significant (Fig. 5A: P>0.05). In contrast, BGJ-398 strongly inhibited the development of CTCs and metastases. Specifically, 5 out of 7 mice within the control group developed lymph node metastasis by day 15, and two of these subsequently developed bone and lung metastasis at day 36 (Fig. 5C right lower panel). However, we detected only 1 lymph node metastasis in the 7 animals within the BGJ-398 treatment group. When we quantified total metastatic burden using luciferase imaging, the differences between the vehicle and BGJ-398 treatment groups were highly significant (Fig. 5B,C: p = 0.0078). Finally, we quantified the numbers of circulating tumor cells in the mice at the time of sacrifice on day 40 by measuring human HLA-C levels in whole peripheral blood by quantitative PCR. CTC numbers within the control group ranged from 325 to 336,008 cells (mean = 158,977), whereas CTC numbers in the treated group ranged from 160 to 370 (mean = 243.6)(Fig. 5D: p<0.01). Together, the results demonstrate that BGJ-398 had no inhibitory effect on the growth of UM-UC3 primary tumors but did block tumor cell extravasation into the vasculature (as measured by CTC production) and metastasis.

Discussion

The prevalence of activating FGFR3 mutations [5,7,22] and FGFR-1 [10] and -3 [3,23] overexpression in BCs, coupled with the fact that the mutant forms of FGFR3 drive cell proliferation [9,24], makes FGFR inhibitors among the most attractive candidates for clinical development [25]. However, it is clear from the results of the preclinical studies that have been published to date that human BC cells display marked heterogeneity in their sensitivities to selective and non-selective FGFR inhibitors [13,26,27,28], which could pose significant challenges to the identification of the appropriate subset(s) of BC patients who will benefit most from FGFR-directed therapy. Based on previous experience in other solid tumors, it seemed likely that the presence of activating FGFR3 mutations identifies FGFR3-dependent BC cells. It also seemed likely that overexpression of either FGFR-1 or FGFR-3 would be linked to FGFR-1 or -3 dependency, respectively. However, our results demonstrate that the presence of an activating FGFR3 mutation does not predict sensitivity to BGJ-398 in established human BC cell lines. Specifically, although some of the BC cell lines that contain activating FGFR3 mutations were highly sensitive to BGJ-398 and other FGFR inhibitors (UM-UC14, 97-7, and MGHU3) [9,13,24,26,27,28], several other FGFR3-mutant lines were not (UM-UC6, UM-UC15, UM-UC16, UM-UC17, 94-10, 97-18, J82) [13,27], and some FGFR3 wild-type cell lines were just as sensitive to BGJ-398 and the other inhibitors as the most sensitive FGFR3 mutant cells (UM-UC1, RT4, RT112, and SW780) [13,28]. On the other hand, sensitivity to BGJ-398 did correlate closely with FGFR3 mRNA levels (Fig. 3) [13]. Importantly, the cell lines that expressed the highest levels of FGFR1 expressed low levels of FGFR3 and were all relatively resistant to BGJ-398-induced growth arrest when the effects of the drug were measured early (48–72 h), strongly suggesting that FGFR3 is a more important driver of BC cell proliferation than FGFR1. Our data also demonstrate that the effects of BGJ-398 are largely cytostatic (rather than cytotoxic), so clinical "responses" may not be associated with tumor regression, and in future studies we plan to investigate whether FGFR3 inhibition can promote the cytotoxic effects of conventional chemotherapy and/or other investigational agents. Within this context, it is worth noting that all of the available human BC cell lines are derived from muscle-invasive tumors (with the possible exception of RT4), and it seems likely that muscle-invasive BCs that gave rise to the FGFR inhibitor-resistant, FGFR3 mutant cell lines had progressed beyond the point where mutant FGFR3 was essential to maintain proliferation and/or survival. Thus, we suspect that the preclinical data underestimate the potential impact of FGFR3-based therapy in patients with low-grade, non-muscle invasive FGFR3-mutant cancers.

Although our results indicate that FGFR1 plays a less important role than FGFR3 in driving BC tumor cell proliferation, they also strongly suggest that FGFR1 plays crucial roles in invasion and metastasis. Inhibition of FGFR signaling with either BGJ-398 or FGFR1 knockdown resulted in strong suppression of invasion in vitro, and BGJ-398 blocked CTC production and metastasis (without inhibiting primary tumor growth) in mice inoculated with orthotopic, FGFR1-positive UM-UC3 tumors in vivo (Fig. 5). On the surface our conclusions may seem to contradict previous work implicating FGFR1 in tumor cell proliferation in vitro and in primary tumor growth in vivo, especially because some of the experiments employed the same UM-UC3 cell line used here [10]. However, we were able to replicate the effects of FGFR1 knockdown on proliferation in long-term MTT assays and soft agar colony formation, and our conclusion that FGFR1 inhibition does not attenuate primary tumor growth is based on BGJ-398 therapy in established UM-UC3 tumors rather than on experiments with cells stably transduced with an FGFR1 shRNA (where FGFR1 would not be available for tumor establishment), so we are confident that the results of the two studies are consistent with each other. Perhaps a more important question is why inhibition of FGFR3 has stronger effects on proliferation than inhibition of FGFR1, since the effects of both have been clearly linked to inhibition of ERK signaling [10,11,27,28]. We speculate that the differential effects are related to the very distinct epithelial versus mesenchymal biological phenotypes of the FGFR3- versus FGFR1-positive cells and that the "epithelial" cells may be more dependent on autocrine growth factors for proliferation, a conclusion that is consistent with our previous work with inhibitors of the EGF receptor [29,30]. Clinically, some non-muscle invasive tumors progress to become muscle-invasive and metastatic. If appropriate biomarkers (possibly including FGFR1 and EMT marker expression) can be identified, it is conceivable that these potentially lethal non-muscle invasive tumors could be controlled with FGFR1 inhibitor-based chemoprevention strategies.

Finally, our data show that FGFR3 and FGFR1 are expressed by the "epithelial" and "mesenchymal" subsets of bladder cancer cells, respectively. The strong associations suggested to us that direct cause-effect relationships might exist between them, and we performed some preliminary experiments to address this possibility. We did not detect any changes in FGFR1 and FGFR3 mRNA expression in UM-UC3 cells after knockdown of either ZEB1 or SNAIL (data not shown), strongly suggesting that these canonical EMT transcription factors are not involved in regulating their expression. However, we did observe changes in several EMT regulators in the UM-UC3 or UM-UC13 cells following knockdown of FGFR1 (Fig. S6), consistent with the idea that FGFR1 signaling functions upstream to drive EMT. Parallel studies have implicated PLCγ, ERK, and cyclooxygenase-2 in FGFR1-mediated EMT in BC cells [11]. Defining the transcriptional targets of FGFR1 responsible for mediating EMT will be an important area for future research.

Supporting Information

Figure S1 *Baseline expression of FGFR1, FGFR3 and bFGF proteins in subsets of epithelial and mesenchymal human bladder cancer cells.* Protein levels in 3 representative "epithelial" (UM-UC14, RT4 and RT112) and 3 "mesenchymal" (UM-UC3, UM-UC12 and UM-UC13) cell lines were measured by immunoblotting.

Figure S2 *Correlation between FGFR/bFGF expression and EMT markers.* The figure displays the results of the correlation analyses. Correlation coefficients are displayed in red, and corresponding p values are depicted in black. Negative correlation coefficients indicate the presence of an inverse relationship between markers.

Figure S3 *FGFR3 mutation status in human bladder cancer cells.* The presence of activating FGFR3 mutations was determined by exome sequencing. Note that among the 5 cell lines within the panel that contain activating mutations, only one (UM-UC14) is sensitive to BGJ-398.

Figure S4 *Effects of FGFR1 knockdown on FGFR1 expression and proliferation in RT4 and UM-UC14 cells.* A. Left panel: UM-UC14 or RT4 cells were transiently transfected with either non-targeting (NT) or FGFR1-specific siRNAs and cell growth was measured at 48 h using MTT. Mean ± SEM, n = 8. Right Panel: the efficiency of FGFR1 silencing by siRNA was determined by quantitative RT-PCR. B. UM-UC14 or RT4 cells were transiently transfected with either non-targeting (NT) or FGFR1-specific siRNAs and percentages of cells within each phase of the cell cycle were quantified by propidium iodide staining and FACS analysis. Mean ± SEM, n = 3.

Figure S5 *Effects of bFGF or FGFR1 knockdown in long-term assays.* A. MTT results obtained in 5-day assays. Mean ± SEM, n = 6. *p<0.05. B. Results obtained in soft agar colony formation assays. The left panels display the numbers of colonies and the right panels colony diameters as determined by measuring colony growth in soft agar. Mean ± SEM, n = 5.

Figure S6 *Effects of bFGF or FGFR1 knockdown on EMT marker expression.* Mean ± SEM, n = 3.
(TIF)

Author Contributions

Clinical context: CD. Financial support: CD. Conceived and designed the experiments: DJM TC BR WC PB. Performed the experiments: TC BR PB WC. Analyzed the data: DJM TC BR WC PB CD. Contributed reagents/materials/analysis tools: TC BR WC. Wrote the paper: DJM TC.

References

1. Shah JB, McConkey DJ, Dinney CP (2011) New strategies in muscle-invasive bladder cancer: on the road to personalized medicine. Clin Cancer Res 17: 2608–2612.
2. Dinney CP, McConkey DJ, Millikan RE, Wu X, Bar-Eli M, et al. (2004) Focus on bladder cancer. Cancer Cell 6: 111–116.
3. Knowles MA (2008) Novel therapeutic targets in bladder cancer: mutation and expression of FGF receptors. Future Oncol 4: 71–83.
4. Sibley K, Cuthbert-Heavens D, Knowles MA (2001) Loss of heterozygosity at 4p16.3 and mutation of FGFR3 in transitional cell carcinoma. Oncogene 20: 686–691.
5. Billerey C, Chopin D, Aubriot-Lorton MH, Ricol D, Gil Diez de Medina S, et al. (2001) Frequent FGFR3 mutations in papillary non-invasive bladder (pTa) tumors. Am J Pathol 158: 1955–1959.
6. van Rhijn BW, Lurkin I, Radvanyi F, Kirkels WJ, van der Kwast TH, et al. (2001) The fibroblast growth factor receptor 3 (FGFR3) mutation is a strong indicator of superficial bladder cancer with low recurrence rate. Cancer Res 61: 1265–1268.
7. Cappellen D, De Oliveira C, Ricol D, de Medina S, Bourdin J, et al. (1999) Frequent activating mutations of FGFR3 in human bladder and cervix carcinomas. Nat Genet 23: 18–20.
8. di Martino E, L'Hote CG, Kennedy W, Tomlinson DC, Knowles MA (2009) Mutant fibroblast growth factor receptor 3 induces intracellular signaling and cellular transformation in a cell type- and mutation-specific manner. Oncogene 28: 4306–4316.
9. Tomlinson DC, Hurst CD, Knowles MA (2007) Knockdown by shRNA identifies S249C mutant FGFR3 as a potential therapeutic target in bladder cancer. Oncogene 26: 5889–5899.
10. Tomlinson DC, Lamont FR, Shnyder SD, Knowles MA (2009) Fibroblast growth factor receptor 1 promotes proliferation and survival via activation of the mitogen-activated protein kinase pathway in bladder cancer. Cancer Res 69: 4613–4620.
11. Tomlinson DC, Baxter EW, Loadman PM, Hull MA, Knowles MA (2012) FGFR1-induced epithelial to mesenchymal transition through MAPK/PLCgamma/COX-2-mediated mechanisms. PLoS One 7: e38972.
12. Guagnano V, Furet P, Spanka C, Bordas V, Le Douget M, et al. (2011) Discovery of 3-(2,6-dichloro-3,5-dimethoxy-phenyl)-1-{6-[4-(4-ethyl-piperazin-1-yl)-phenylamin o]-pyrimidin-4-yl}-1-methyl-urea (NVP-BGJ398), a potent and selective inhibitor of the fibroblast growth factor receptor family of receptor tyrosine kinase. J Med Chem 54: 7066–7083.
13. Lamont FR, Tomlinson DC, Cooper PA, Shnyder SD, Chester JD, et al. (2012) Small molecule FGF receptor inhibitors block FGFR-dependent urothelial carcinoma growth in vitro and in vivo. Br J Cancer 104: 75–82.
14. Wright GW, Simon RM (2003) A random variance model for detection of differential gene expression in small microarray experiments. Bioinformatics 19: 2448–2455.
15. Eisen MB, Spellman PT, Brown PO, Botstein D (1998) Cluster analysis and display of genome-wide expression patterns. Proc Natl Acad Sci U S A 95: 14863–14868.
16. Lu C, Kamat AA, Lin YG, Merritt WM, Landen CN, et al. (2007) Dual targeting of endothelial cells and pericytes in antivascular therapy for ovarian carcinoma. Clin Cancer Res 13: 4209–4217.
17. Hoff J (2000) Methods of blood collection in the mouse. Lab Animal 29: 47–53.
18. Marquis L, Tran M, Choi W, Lee IL, Huszar D, et al. (2012) p63 expression correlates with sensitivity to the Eg5 inhibitor ZD4877 in bladder cancer cells. Cancer Biol Ther 13: 477–486.
19. Choi W, Shah JB, Tran M, Svatek R, Marquis L, et al. (2012) p63 expression defines a lethal subset of muscle-invasive bladder cancers. PLoS One 7: e30206.
20. Polyak K, Weinberg RA (2009) Transitions between epithelial and mesenchymal states: acquisition of malignant and stem cell traits. Nat Rev Cancer 9: 265–273.
21. Dinney CP, Fishbeck R, Singh RK, Eve B, Pathak S, et al. (1995) Isolation and characterization of metastatic variants from human transitional cell carcinoma passaged by orthotopic implantation in athymic nude mice. J Urol 154: 1532–1538.
22. Sibley K, Stern P, Knowles MA (2001) Frequency of fibroblast growth factor receptor 3 mutations in sporadic tumours. Oncogene 20: 4416–4418.
23. Tomlinson DC, Baldo O, Harnden P, Knowles MA (2007) FGFR3 protein expression and its relationship to mutation status and prognostic variables in bladder cancer. J Pathol 213: 91–98.
24. Bernard-Pierrot I, Brams A, Dunois-Larde C, Caillault A, Diez de Medina SG, et al. (2006) Oncogenic properties of the mutated forms of fibroblast growth factor receptor 3b. Carcinogenesis 27: 740–747.
25. Knowles MA (2007) Role of FGFR3 in urothelial cell carcinoma: biomarker and potential therapeutic target. World J Urol 25: 581–593.
26. Gozgit JM, Wong MJ, Moran L, Wardwell S, Mohemmad QK, et al. (2012) Ponatinib (AP24534), a multitargeted pan-FGFR inhibitor with activity in multiple FGFR-amplified or mutated cancer models. Mol Cancer Ther 11: 690–699.
27. Miyake M, Ishii M, Koyama N, Kawashima K, Kodama T, et al. (2009) 1-tert-butyl-3-[6-(3,5-dimethoxy-phenyl)-2-(4-diethylamino-butylamino)-pyrido[2,3-d]pyrimidin-7-yl]-urea (PD173074), a selective tyrosine kinase inhibitor of fibroblast growth factor receptor-3 (FGFR3), inhibits cell proliferation of bladder cancer carrying the FGFR3 gene mutation along with up-regulation of p27/Kip1 and G1/G0 arrest. J Pharmacol Exp Ther 332: 795–802.
28. Qing J, Du X, Chen Y, Chan P, Li H, et al. (2009) Antibody-based targeting of FGFR3 in bladder carcinoma and t(4;14)-positive multiple myeloma in mice. J Clin Invest 119: 1216–1229.
29. Black PC, Brown GA, Inamoto T, Shrader M, Arora A, et al. (2008) Sensitivity to epidermal growth factor receptor inhibitor requires E-cadherin expression in urothelial carcinoma cells. Clin Cancer Res 14: 1478–1486.
30. Shrader M, Pino MS, Brown G, Black P, Adam L, et al. (2007) Molecular correlates of gefitinib responsiveness in human bladder cancer cells. Mol Cancer Ther 6: 277–285.

3

Diagnosis of Bladder Cancer Recurrence based on Urinary Levels of *EOMES, HOXA9, POU4F2, TWIST1, VIM,* and *ZNF154* Hypermethylation

Thomas Reinert[1]**, Michael Borre**[2]**, Anders Christiansen**[1]**, Gregers G. Hermann**[3]**, Torben F. Ørntoft**[1]**,
Lars Dyrskjøt**[1]*

1 Department of Molecular Medicine, Aarhus University Hospital, Aarhus, Denmark, 2 Department of Urology, Aarhus University Hospital, Aarhus, Denmark, 3 Department of Urology, Frederiksberg Hospital, Copenhagen University, Frederiksberg, Denmark

Abstract

Background: Non muscle invasive bladder cancer (NMIBC) has the highest recurrence rate of any malignancy and as many as 70% of patients experience relapse. Aberrant DNA methylation is present in all bladder tumors and can be detected in urine specimens. Previous studies have identified DNA methylation markers that showed significant diagnostic value. We evaluated the significance of the biomarkers for early detection of tumor recurrence in urine.

Methodology/Principal Findings: The methylation levels of *EOMES, HOXA9, POU4F2, TWIST1, VIM,* and *ZNF154* in urine specimens were measured by real-time PCR (MethyLight). We analyzed 390 urine sediments from 184 patients diagnosed with NMIBC. Urine from 35 age-matched control individuals was used to determine the methylation baseline levels. Recurrence was diagnosed by cystoscopy and verified by histology. Initially, we compared urine from bladder cancer patients and healthy individuals and detected significant hypermethylation of all six markers (P<0.0001) achieving sensitivity in the range 82%–89% and specificity in the range 94%–100%. Following, we validated the urinary hypermethylation for use in recurrence surveillance and found sensitivities of 88–94% and specificities of 43–67%. *EOMES, POU4F2, VIM* and *ZNF154* were more frequently methylated in urine from patients with higher grade tumors (P≤0.08). Univariate Cox regression analysis showed that five markers were significantly associated with disease recurrence; *HOXA9* (HR = 7.8, P = 0.006), *POU4F2* (HR = 8.5, P = 0.001), *TWIST1* (HR = 12.0, P = 0.015), *VIM* (HR = 8.0, P = 0.001), and *ZNF154* (HR = 13.9, P<0.001). Interestingly, for one group of patients (n = 15) we found that hypermethylation was consistently present in the urine samples despite the lack of tumor recurrences, indicating the presence of a field defect.

Conclusion/Significance: Methylation levels of *EOMES, HOXA9, POU4F2, TWIST1, VIM,* and *ZNF154* in urine specimens are promising diagnostic biomarkers for bladder cancer recurrence surveillance.

Editor: Brock C. Christensen, Geisel School of Medicine at Dartmouth, United States of America

Funding: This work was supported by the John and Birthe Meyer Foundation, the Danish Council for Independent Research, the Lundbeck Foundation, the NOVO Nordisk Foundation, an EU grant to UROMOL Consortium no. 201663, the Danish Cancer Society, the University of Aarhus, and the Danish Ministry of the Interior and Health. The funders had no role in study design, data collection and analysis, decision to publish, or preparation of the manuscript.

Competing Interests: The authors have declared that no competing interests exist.

* E-mail: lars@ki.au.dk

Introduction

Cancer of the urinary bladder is the fifth most common neoplasm in the industrialized countries. In approximately 75% of all cases, the patients will present with stage Ta or T1 non-muscle invasive bladder cancer (NMIBC), whereas the remaining 25% of the tumors will be muscle invasive stage T2-4 cancers (MIBC) [1]. About 60%–70% of patients with NMIBC experience tumor recurrences within 3 years after resection [2,3] and patients may develop recurrent tumors annually for many years without disease progression. However, up to 25% will progress to muscle invasive disease [4]. The high recurrence rate and the risk of progression prompt the need for frequent and long surveillance, making bladder cancer the most expensive cancer to treat [5,6]. Following resection of the primary tumor, patients are frequently monitored by cystoscopy and cytology. Biopsies taken during cystoscopy are the gold standard for diagnosing bladder tumors. The sensitivity of cystoscopy for NMIBC is close to 80% for white light cystoscopy, and 96% when using the more costly, fluorescence-guided cystoscopy using hexaminolevulinate (HAL). For detection of dysplasia and carcinoma in situ (CIS), the sensitivity of white light cystoscopy decreases to 48% and 68%, respectively; whereas the sensitivity of cystoscopy using HAL for these lesions remains in the range from 93%–95% [7–9]. Cytology is often used in combination with cystoscopy, owing to a high specificity of 99% (0.83–0.997; 95% CI), but with a low sensitivity of 34% (0.20–0.53; 95% CI). The sensitivity of cytology increases for high-stage and high-grade tumors, especially for primary tumors [10]. It has been proposed that a bladder field defect may be causing the high frequency of tumor recurrences in bladder cancer patients [11]. Several molecular changes have been shown to be present in normal appearing areas of the urothelium in patients with bladder cancer [12,13], and recently an epigenetic field defect was described [14].

Epigenetics is the study of mitotically and/or meiotically heritable changes in gene expression that cannot be explained by changes in DNA sequence [15]. DNA methylation is a well-studied epigenetic mechanism involved in normal processes like development, genomic imprinting, and X-chromosome inactivation [16–18]. Alterations in DNA methylation have been associated with several human pathologic disorders including cancer [19], and transcriptional inactivation by aberrant hyper-methylation is a well-established mechanism for gene silencing in bladder cancers [20–23]. Identification of DNA methylation markers for detection of bladder cancer has been ongoing for some years. Several studies have reported high sensitivities and specificities for these markers, making them potentially useful as diagnostic markers for bladder cancer [24–31]. In a previous study we identified a number of DNA methylation markers (*EOMES*, *HOXA9*, *POU4F2*, and *ZNF154*) that showed potential diagnostic value in urine specimens from BC patients [26].

We now validated the diagnostic and prognostic value of these biomarkers together with earlier reported *TWIST1* [25] and *VIM* [30] in urine samples. Initially, to validate the significance of the selected methylation markers, and to determine of the marker cut-off values, we compared the first urine sample from each patient with NMIBC to urine samples from healthy individuals. Following, we evaluated the diagnostic and prognostic value of the markers for early detection of tumor recurrence using urine samples obtained at later follow-up visits.

Materials and Methods

Ethics Statement

Informed written consent was obtained from all patients, and research protocols were approved by the Central Denmark Region Committees on Biomedical Research Ethics.

Patient Material

A total of 652 voided urine samples were collected at the Department of Urology at Aarhus University Hospital from 390 bladder cancer patients and 47 individuals with benign prostatic hyperplasia or bladder stones, but no history of bladder cancer (control individuals). From these we excluded 227 samples, because the DNA amount was below our threshold (Suppl. Table 1), which left 425 samples (390 samples from 184 BC patients and 35 from control individuals) (Table 1 and Suppl. Figure 1). Ten to fifty mL urine was collected at regular follow-up visits. Urine specimens were collected immediately before cystos-copy; cells were sedimented by centrifugation, and frozen at −80°C. The tumors were staged according to the TNM system [32] and graded according to Bergkvist [33]. Fifteen of the control individuals were stix positive for nitrite in the urine indicating bacterial infection. Patient treatment and follow-up were performed in accordance with the guidelines of the European Association of Urology [34].

DNA Extraction and Bisulfite Modification

DNA was extracted with the QIAsymphony Virus/Bacteria Midi kit (96) (Qiagen) using the QIAsymphony® SP instrument and employing the Complex800_V5_DSP protocol. Five hundred nanograms of DNA was bisulfite modified using EZ-96 DNA methylation D5004 (Zymo Research) according to the manufac-turer's recommendations and eluted in 60 μl of elution buffer and stored at −20°C until use.

Real-time Quantitative Methylation-specific Polymerase Chain Reaction (MethyLight)

Methylation analysis was performed using methyLight [35]. Primers and probes for the six genes of interest were designed to include eight to ten CpG dinucleotides (Suppl. Table 2). For normalization of DNA input material, we used the ALU-C4 repeat element sequence [36]. qPCR amplifications were carried out with the TaqMan Universal PCR Master Mix No AmpErase (Applied Biosystems) according to the manufacturer's instructions in duplicates using 2 μl (5 ng) of bisulfite-modified DNA in a final volume of 5 μl in 384-well plates on an ABI 7900 HT Fast Real Time PCR System (Applied Biosystems). If duplicates were inconsistent, one replicate being positive for methylation and one negative for methylation, the analysis was repeated. The sample was excluded with regard to that specific marker if another inconsistent result was obtained. Amplification protocols are listed in suppl. Table 2. Amplification data were analyzed by sequence detection system (SDS 2.4, Applied Biosystems). Each plate included a serial dilution (25–0.04ng) of fully methylated DNA: CpGenome^{TM} Universal Methylated DNA) (Millipore) with the gene of interest and ALU-C4, several no template controls (NTC) wells, 5 nanograms of a methylated control sample [CpGenome^{TM} Universal Methylated DNA (Millipore)], and unmethylated sample consisting of whole-genome amplified DNA from periph-eral blood DNA. The percentage of methylated reference (PMR) was calculated for each sample according to the equation: $100 \times [$(gene-x copy value) sample/(ALU-C4 copy value) sam-ple]/[(gene-x copy value) Universal Methylated DNA/(ALU-C4copy value) Universal Methylated DNA].

Statistical Analysis

Stata 11 (Statacorp, Texas, USA) was used for all statistical calculations. Two-tailed tests were considered statistically signifi-cant if $P<0.05$. Methylation differences were evaluated by nonparametric Wilcoxon-Mann-Whitney test. Fisher's exact test was used for analyzing dichotomous variables. The exact x^2test was used for analyzing associations between clinic-pathological parameters with two or more categories. Correlations of the methylation levels of the markers were calculated with Spearman correlation coefficients. A ROC curve was made for each marker and combinations of markers by plotting sensitivity against (1-specificity) and the area under the curve (AUC) was calculated. Log-Rank tests were applied to evaluate equality of survival and Kaplan-Meier survival plots were used for visualization. Univar-iate Cox regression analysis was used to analyze associations of age, gender, stage, grade, multiplicity, and CIS with recurrence-free survival.

Results

Our analysis was divided into two parts: 1) to establish the cutoff level of the methylation markers and to demonstrate the significance of the selected markers we analyzed the first urine sample from each patient and compared to control urine samples from healthy individuals; 2) using the determined marker cutoff levels we then validated the diagnostic and prognostic value of the methylation markers in urine samples taken during patient surveillance.

Establishment of Test Cut-off levels and Initial Validation of Marker Significance

Initially, we defined the cut-off levels by the mean methylation level of each marker +2x standard deviation of the methylation level in urine samples from 35 control individuals (only samples

Table 1. Demographic and clinical characteristics of bladder cancer patients and control individuals.

Characteristics	Control individuals
Individuals with no history of BC (controls)	35
Gender, n (%)	
Male	30 (86)
Female	5 (14)
Age, mean (min-max)	70 (35–88)
Nitrite test, n (%)	
Positive	15 (43)
Negative	20 (57)

Characteristics	All patients – first visit	Patients with recurrent tumor at control visit	Patients without tumor at control visit
Bladder cancer patients	184	101[c]	57[c]
Samples collected	184	139	67
Primary cases	44		
Recurrent cases	140	139	
Gender, n (%)			
Male	148 (81)	106 (76)	58 (87)
Female	36(19)	33 (24)	9 (13)
Age, mean (min-max)	69 (33–89)	71 (43–89)	69 (49–86)
Ta	69 (33–85)	70 (43–87)	
T1	70 (42–89)	74 (43–89)	
CIS	71 (67–74)	73 (66–81)	
T2-4	0	71 (43–83)	
Pathological stage, n (%)			
Ta	132 (72)	92 (66)	
T1	50 (27)	29 (21)	
CIS	2 (1)	5 (4)	
T2-4	0	13 (9)	
Grade, n (%)[b]			
I	17 (9)	12 (9)	
II	74 (40)	55 (40)	
III	93 (51)	71 (51)	
Nitrite test, n (%)			
Positive	16 (9)	13 (9)	7 (10)
Negative	163 (89)	121 (87)	57 (85)
N/A[a]	5 (3)	5 (4)	3 (5)
Tumor cells in urine[d], n (%)			
Positive	119 (65)	87 (63)	22 (33)
Negative	28 (15)	25 (18)	24 (36)
N/A	37 (20)	27 (19)	21 (31)

[a]N/A Not available.
[b]Bergkvist.
[c]Of the 184 patients, 26 were lost for follow-up.
[d]The presence of tumor cells in the urine was determined by urine cytology.
Demographic and clinical characteristics of bladder cancer patients and control individuals from whom urine specimens were collected and methylation analysis performed. Histology was used as the gold standard for the diagnosis of bladder tumors.

with methylation values above zero were included). Cut-off levels (PMR values – see materials and methods) used to dichotomize the methylation markers were: $EOMES = 0.348$, $HOXA9 = 0.077$, $POU4F2 = 0.371$, $TWIST1 = 0.405$, $VIM = 0.368$, and $ZNF154 = 1.51$. Other cut-off levels (mean +1xSD and +3xSD) based on methylation levels in control urine samples were initially considered (results not shown). To validate the significance of the markers for bladder cancer diagnosis we compared the first urine sample from 184 patients diagnosed with NMIB to urine samples from 35 control individuals (Table 1). All six markers were highly significantly hyper-methylated in the urine from patients with NMIBC compared to urine from healthy individuals (Mann-Whitney, P<0.0001) (Table 2). Better sensitivities of the markers were observed when analyzing urine samples from patients with an incident tumor compared to urine from patients with a recurrent tumor (Suppl. Table 3). No association was observed between the individual markers and tumor stage, but *EOMES, POU4F2, VIM,* and *ZNF154* were more methylated in grade III lesions compared to grade I lesions (Fisher's exact test, P≤0.048) (Suppl. Table 4). *EOMES, POU4F2,* and *ZNF154* were less methylated in tumors with a size below 3 cm. (Fisher's exact test, P≤0.047) (Suppl. Table 4).

Detection of Recurrences by Methylation Markers

We validated the clinical usefulness of the markers for bladder cancer surveillance. We stratified our analysis to only include patients that initially showed hypermethylation of one or more methylation markers. Depending on the marker studied, 11–18% of patients showed no methylation in the first tumor and was therefore not included. This restricted the analysis to 158 patients and 206 urine samples from the follow-up visits; 139 urine samples were from patients with a recurrent bladder tumor and 67 urine samples were from patients with no tumor recurrence (Table 1). Employing the cut-points determined initially using the urine from healthy individuals; we obtained sensitivities in the range from 87% to 94%, and specificities in the range from 28% to 47% (Table 3). In comparison, the sensitivity of cytology was 77% and the specificity was 60%. We observed no significant associations between methylation levels and clinicopathologic variables for this patient cohort with recurrent tumors (Suppl. Table 5).

The molecular tests may have a higher sensitivity compared to the gold standard cystoscopy. To address this we therefore used cystoscopy results from a 12 months period after the urine was sampled. We found many of the samples formerly classified as false positives to be true positives; they simply had a positive lead time compared to cystoscopy. The sensitivity obtained ranged from 88% to 94%, and the specificity ranged from 43% to 67% (Table 4). Including tumors diagnosed during a 12 month follow-up period and combining two markers with the requirement that both markers were positive for a positive test result the sensitivity decreased (range: 86–93%), while the specificity increased (range:

50–73%). If just one of two markers should be positive, the sensitivity increased (range: 92–98%), while the specificity decreased (range: 29–60%) (Suppl. Table 6 and Suppl. Table 7, respectively). Overall, combinations of markers did not improve both sensitivity and specificity of the tests.

Prognostic Value of Methylation Markers for Predicting Later Recurrences

To address the prognostic value of the methylation markers we analyzed the urine samples from patients at visits where no tumors were diagnosed using cystoscopy. For all markers we found that a positive marker at a tumor-negative visit was significantly associated with later tumor recurrence during 24- and 60-month follow-up periods (Log-Rank test, P≤0.04) (Figure 1 and Suppl. Figure 3). The most significant differences in the 24-month time-frame were observed for *POU4F2* and *ZNF154* (Log-Rank test, P<0.0001) where only 12% (3/25) and 8% (2/26) with no methylation experienced a recurrence within 2 years, respectively. For the methylation-positive samples the percentage of patients with later recurrence was 68% (21/31) for *POU4F2* and 63% (20/32) for *ZNF154*. Univariate Cox regression analysis showed that *HOXA9* (HR (95% CI) = 7.8 (1.8–33.7)), *POU4F2* (HR (95% CI) = 8.5 (2.5–28.5)), *TWIST1* (HR (95% CI) = 12.0 (1.6–88.6)), *VIM* (HR (95% CI) = 8.0 (2.4–26.8)), and *ZNF154* (HR (95% CI) = 13.9 (3.3–59.7)) were significantly associated with recurrence-free survival. Age, gender, previous stage, previous grade, previous multiplicity, and previous CIS were not significantly associated with recurrence-free survival (P>0.05). Consequently, the presence of an altered methylation of DNA in urine seemed to be strongly related to the prognosis.

Identification of Patients with a Possible Epigenetic Field Defect

If the methylation of the biomarkers was confined to malignant cells, we should only detect the markers in urine when a tumor was present, or occurring within a foreseeable future depending on the growth rate of the tumor. However, our results showed that even high urinary levels of methylation could be present at visits without recurrences (Suppl. Figure 2, patients C and D; Suppl. Figure 3). We could identify one group of 15 patients (31%) in which methylation was present in urine at the first visit and continued to be present in the urine samples taken at later follow-up visits,

Table 2. Diagnostic significance of the urinary markers.

Gene	Sensitivity, % (pos./total[a])	Specificity, % (neg./total)	AUC (95% CI)	PPV[b], %	NPV[c], %	P value[d]
EOMES	88 (160/182)	97 (34/35)	0.96 (0.94–0.99)	99	61	**<0.0001**
HOXA9	82 (141/173)	100 (35/35)	0.91 (0.88–0.94)	100	52	**<0.0001**
POU4F2	85 (154/182)	94 (33/35)	0.94 (0.91–0.97)	99	54	**<0.0001**
TWIST1	88 (159/180)	100 (35/35)	0.94 (0.92–0.97)	100	63	**<0.0001**
VIM	89 (159/179)	100 (35/35)	0.97 (0.94–0.99)	100	64	**<0.0001**
ZNF154	87 (160/184)	100 (35/35)	0.95 (0.93–0.97)	100	59	**<0.0001**
Cytology	81 (119/147)	N/A[e]	N/A	100	N/A	N/A

[a]Some urine samples provided inconclusive results for some markers.
[b]Positive predictive value.
[c]Negative predictive value.
[d]Mann-Whitney *U* test.
[e]Not available.
Diagnostic significance of the urinary markers *EOMES, HOXA9, POU4F2, TWIST1, VIM,* and *ZNF154,* when comparing urine samples from 184 patients with NMIBC to urine from healthy individuals.

Table 3. Diagnostic significance of the urinary markers for surveillance of bladder cancer.

Gene	Sensitivity, % (pos./total[a])	Specificity, % (neg./total[a])	AUC (95% CI)	PPV, %	NPV, %	P value[b]
EOMES	94 (116/124)	39 (24/61)	0.78 (0.71–0.85)	76	75	<0.0001
HOXA9	92 (108/117)	38 (18/48)	0.70 (0.61–0.80)	78	67	<0.0001
POU4F2	87 (104/120)	47 (28/60)	0.75 (0.68–0.83)	76	64	<0.0001
TWIST1	89 (113/127)	28 (17/60)	0.71 (0.63–0.80)	72	55	<0.0001
VIM	90 (113/126)	43 (24/56)	0.72 (0.63–0.81)	78	65	<0.0001
ZNF154	93 (115/123)	47 (29/62)	0.78 (0.71–0.86)	78	78	<0.0001
Cytology	77 (88/115)	60 (35/58)	0.68 (0.61–0.76)	79	56	<0.0001

[a]Some urine samples provided inconclusive results for some markers.
[b]Mann-Whitney U test.
Diagnostic significance of the urinary markers EOMES, HOXA9, POU4F2, TWIST1, VIM, and ZNF154, when comparing urine samples from patients with NMIBC to urine samples from bladder cancer patients with no recurrence and using DNA collected at control visits in patients with a methylation positive first tumor. Histology was used as the gold standard for the diagnosis of bladder tumors.

although no tumor occurred. As an example, one methylation-positive patient with the most prolonged follow-up was diagnosed with CIS after 118 months, but had no lesions in between. The 15 patients with a field defect, but no recurrence, have a significant lower number of tumors at previous visits (P = 0.02) compared to patients with disease recurrence.

Discussion

In this study we performed an independent validation of EOMES, HOXA9, POU4F2, TWIST1, VIM, and ZNF154 methylation for the urinary diagnosis in bladder cancer surveillance. We obtained sensitivities in the range 87%–93% and specificities in the range 28%–47%. When including tumors resected in a 12-month follow-up period we obtained sensitivities in the range 88%–94% and specificities in the range 43%–67%. Univariate Cox regression analysis showed that the methylation markers predicted future recurrences with hazard ratios in the range from 7.8 to 13.9 (P≤0.015). Previous stage, grade, multiplicity and CIS were not significantly associated with tumor recurrence. Interestingly, we also observed that some bladder cancer patients without recurrence still maintained aberrant urinary methylation that distinguished them from control individuals. We believe that

this may be caused by a general epigenetic bladder mucosa alteration.

The controls applied in this study were from patients with benign prostatic hyperplasia (BPH) or bladder stones and 43% of the controls were nitrite positive, indicating bladder infections. Some of the cells in the urine of the controls may originate from the hyperplasia, or may be immunological or bacterial cells. Similar control samples were applied when the markers were initially investigated as markers of bladder cancer, suggesting that the methylation frequency of the selected markers is low in these cell types [25,26,30]. Cells from the prostate or from a bladder infection may still bias the obtained results by dilution of the tumor cells. This could lead to false negative test results. Bacterial infections are much less common and in our study infections were not significantly associated with marker methylation, indicating that infections did not influence the marker sensitivity (Suppl. Table 4).

It is noteworthy that only 9% of the recurrences are grade I. Therefore the calculated sensitivities of the markers may be higher compared to sensitivities that would be obtained from a consecutive series of low-risk patients with a much higher number of grade I tumors.

One of the main challenges using urinary markers is getting sufficient tumor cells, and while MethyLight is a very sensitive

Table 4. Diagnostic significance of the urinary markers for surveillance of bladder cancer when including a 12-months follow-up period.

Gene	Sensitivity, % (pos./total[a])	Specificity, % (neg./total[a])	AUC (95% CI)	PPV, %	NPV, %	P value[b]
EOMES	94 (133/141)	55 (24/44)	0.85 (0.77–0.92)	87	75	<0.0001
HOXA9	93 (123/132)	55 (18/33)	0.78 (0.68–0.89)	89	67	<0.0001
POU4F2	88 (120/136)	64 (28/44)	0.80 (0.72–0.89)	88	64	<0.0001
TWIST1	90 (133/147)	43 (17/40)	0.76 (0.66–0.86)	85	55	<0.0001
VIM	90 (129/143)	59 (23/39)	0.78 (0.68–0.89)	89	62	<0.0001
ZNF154	94 (134/142)	67 (29/43)	0.83 (0.74–0.92)	91	78	<0.0001
Cytology	79 (99/126)	74 (35/47)	0.77 (0.69–0.84)	89	56	<0.0001

[a]Some urine samples provided inconclusive results for some markers.
[b]Mann-Whitney U test.
Diagnostic significance of the urinary markers EOMES, HOXA9, POU4F2, TWIST1, VIM, and ZNF154, when comparing urine samples from patients with NMIBC to urine samples from bladder cancer patients with no recurrence and using DNA collected at control visits in patients with a methylation positive first tumor. Tumors diagnosed during a 12 month follow-up period were included. Histology was used as the gold standard for the diagnosis of bladder tumors.

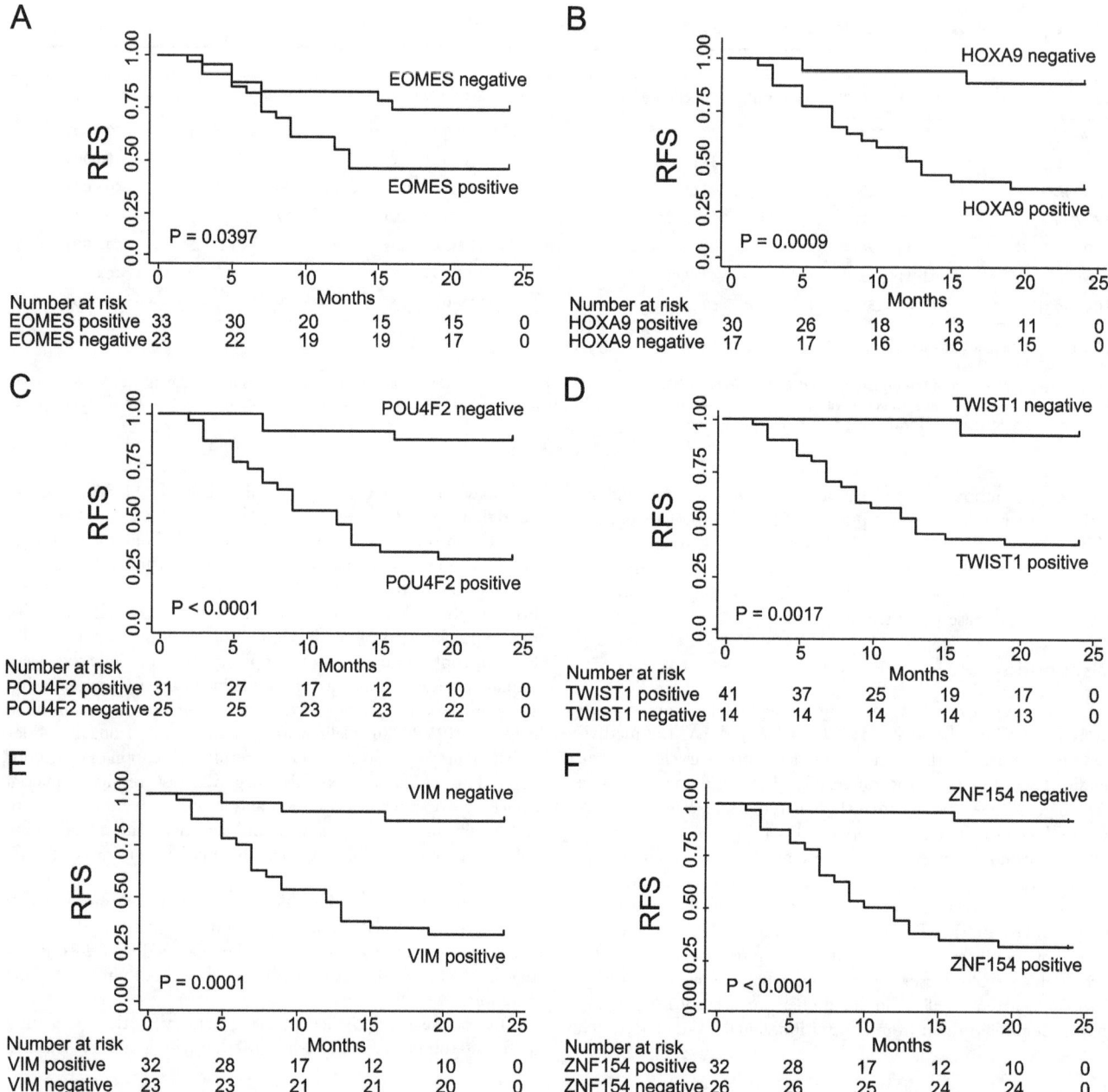

Figure 1. Kaplan-Meier plot of the time to recurrence. DNA methylation is associated with subsequent tumor recurrence within 24 months for patients without tumor but with methylation-positive urine samples. Kaplan-Meier plots of recurrence-free survival as a function of dichotomized methylation levels for *EOMES* (P = 0.0397) (A), *HOXA9* (P = 0.0009) (B), *POU4F2* (P<0.0001) (C), *TWIST1* (P = 0.0017) (D), *VIM* (P = 0.0001) (E), and *ZNF154* (P<0.0001) (F).

method we still had to exclude 227 (35%) samples from the study due to insufficient amounts of DNA. We observed that if we included samples with less than 5 ng of DNA as template in the analysis, the sensitivity decreased, and for patients under surveillance the specificity increased. By excluding patients based on the amount of DNA extracted from the voided urine samples, we maintain the integrity of the MethyLight assay at the cost of introducing a bias where especially patients with stage Ta grade I tumors are excluded, as grade I lesions exfoliate the smallest number of cells [37] (Fisher's exact test, P<0.05) (Suppl. Table 1). Recently, a study by Zuiverloon et al. reported an increase in the sensitivity of the *FGFR3* mutation as a marker for tumor

recurrence from 75% to 100% when the volume of urine used for the test was increased [38]. By increasing the volume of collected urine from the current 10 to 50 mL, fewer samples will have to be excluded [39,40]. Other possibilities to improve the assay for detecting methylation may include analyzing two or more samples separately or to use another technology than Methylight (e.g. Nested PCR).

The methylation marker test may be complemented by *FGFR3* mutation analysis. *FGFR3* mutations are present in about 70%–80% of low-grade NMIBC, and mutations in the *FGFR3* gene have been shown to be detectable in DNA from voided urine [41,42]. Similar to the methylation analysis, the *FGFR3* analysis is

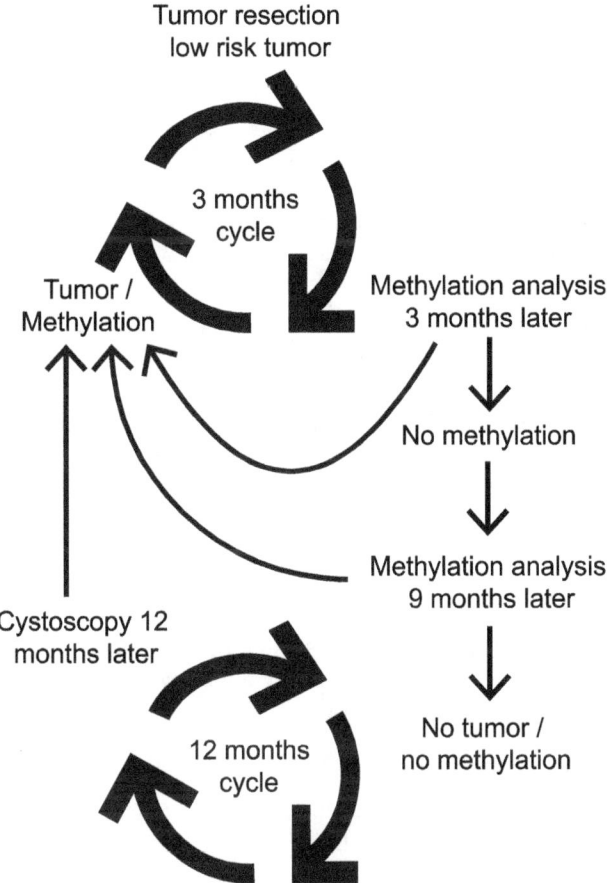

Tumor resection
low risk tumor

3 months
cycle

Tumor /
Methylation

Methylation analysis
3 months later

No methylation

Methylation analysis
9 months later

Cystoscopy 12
months later

12 months
cycle

No tumor /
no methylation

Figure 2. Follow-up model for low-risk NMIBC applying methylation markers. Modified from Hermann GG et al. (http://skejby.net/Webudgaven/DaBlaCa2010.htm.).

based on DNA, and the primary visit can be used to stratify for the presence of the mutation. Recent studies with *FGFR3* mutations alone to detect NMIBC recurrences report a sensitivity of 58% for concomitant recurrences. The sensitivity increased when 12 months of follow-up were included [43]. The combination of *FGFR3* mutations and methylation markers has been tested by Serizawa et al., and they observed an increase in sensitivity of DNA from voided urine when combining methylation markers and *FGFR3* mutations [44]. It is noteworthy that they observed an inverse correlation between hypermethylation and *FGFR3* mutations.

The fact that we find no associations between methylation and clinicopathologic variables when using only urine from patients with recurrent tumors is intriguing, but it may be that the lower sensitivity observed in low-grade tumors is not only caused by few exfoliated tumor cells in the urine, but rather that the hypermethylation is not present in the tumor or in the surrounding urothelium, and by stratifying for methylation at an earlier visit these patients are excluded. It is possible that patients with no methylation are to be considered as a distinct group of bladder tumors. Finally, the lack of association between methylation and clinic-pathologic variables may also be a consequence of the relatively small data set.

The methylation markers have specificity values in the range 43% to 67%, which is low considering that they all have between 94%–100% tumor specificity when compared to control individuals. An equivalent low specificity was observed in a study investigating the mRNA levels of hTERT, SENP1, PPP1CA, and MCM5 in urine obtained from patients during disease surveillance [45]. Low specificity was also observed by Zuiverloon et al. when studying *FGFR3* mutations to detect bladder cancer recurrences [38]. Furthermore, low specificity of methylation markers was previously reported elsewhere by two studies aimed at detecting NMIBC recurrences [46,47].

The methylation observed in urine samples from cystoscopy-negative visits may have several sources, (i) a small tumor not detected by cystoscopy, (ii) residual tumor cells at site of the resection, or (iii) it may be a symptom of epigenetically changed urothelial cells present in the urothelium surrounding the tumor or at other places (field defect) that have no phenotype to distinguish them from normal urothelial cells – an epigenetic urothelial methylator phenotype [14]. Some of the false positive samples with a recurrence within 12 months after cystoscopy are most likely caused by missed tumors or residual tumor cells, but for the rest of the false positive samples this explanation is unlikely and our results correspond well with the presence of a bladder field defect. Recent data support the notion that there is a DNA hypermethylation field defect in bladders from BC patients where the normal-appearing tissue contains widespread DNA methylation [14]. Wolff and co-workers suggest that the aberrant methylation is not due to clonal expansion, but instead is caused by generalized epigenetic alteration in the urothelium across the bladder. It has been suggested that this widespread field of aberrant methylated normal-appearing urothelium may be the origin of the high recurrence rate in bladder cancer [14].

With the discovery of methylation markers with very high sensitivity, implementation of methylation markers in the surveillance of patients with low-grade NMIBC seems likely. At the time of diagnosis, the methylation level of each methylation marker has to be established before the marker can be applied for surveillance. In advance of the next control visit, the patient may supply a urine sample for the analysis, and three possible outcomes exist: i) if the test is positive the patient will have a cystoscopy done, and in 67 patients out of 100 a recurrent tumor will be found, whereas the remaining 33 patients will not have a tumor recurrence. This is not a major problem, as the false positive patients would have had a cystoscopy done in any case; ii) a negative test will allow the patients to skip the current cystoscopy. With the current performance of the analysis, 94 out of 100 BC patients with a tumor recurrence are correctly diagnosed and six patients are wrongly diagnosed as not having a tumor recurrence. This amount of false negatives is comparable with HAL-guided cystoscopy and better than white light cystoscopy, where 20 patients can be expected to be wrongly diagnosed as not having a tumor recurrence [7–9]. However, in this study the *ZNF154* marker failed to diagnose two muscle-invasive bladder cancers that progressed from two T1 grade III tumors. This would not be acceptable in a clinical setting, and indicates that patients with a high risk of progression (e.g. all T1, grade III tumors, or CIS) have to continue with the regular treatment regimen. Another option could be to use a more conservative cut-off. By defining the cut-off values as the mean plus 1x standard deviation of the methylation level, the two muscle invasive tumors would not have been missed; iii) a urine sample with insufficient DNA should lead to continuation of the original treatment regimen. In all three situations the patient will supply a new urine sample before the next control visit that will determine whether or not the patient must have a cystoscopy performed. The methylation markers may also increase the detection rate of CIS lesions, as a positive test with a negative cystoscopy could then be followed by another cystoscopy including HAL.

In conclusion, by applying a very sensitive and semi-quantitative methodology for detecting bladder cancer recurrences and stratifying for methylation status of the initial tumor, we have shown that using a single marker (*ZNF154*) we can detect a concomitant tumor recurrence with a sensitivity of 94% and a specificity of 67%. According to the EAU Guidelines on NMIBC, the current treatment regime for low-risk NMIBC patients is cystoscopy at 3 and 12 months following TUR and then each year for an additional 4 years [48]. This study suggests that methylation markers can be utilized as markers of bladder cancer recurrence to reduce the number of cystoscopies in low-risk patients with no concomitant tumor (Figure 2) and consequently improve the quality of life for the patients as well as decrease health care expenditure.

Supporting Information

Figure S1   Flow chart illustrating the flow of samples during the course of the study.

Figure S2   Examples of methylation levels at first visit and two subsequent visits for 5 patients with or without recurrences. Patients with two subsequent recurrences (A and B). Patient with no recurrences at first control visit, but recurrence at a later control visits (C and D). A patient with no subsequent recurrences (E). PMR is the percentage of relative reference. A value of 0% means no methylation and a value of 100% means fully methylated. A dark bar represents a visit with concomitant tumor and a gray bar represents a visit with no tumor.

Figure S3   Kaplan-Meier plot of the time to recurrence. DNA methylation is associated with subsequent tumor recurrence within 60 months for patients without tumor but with methylation positive urine samples. Kaplan-Meier plots of recurrence-free survival as a function of dichotomized methylation levels for *EOMES* ($P = 0.0254$) (A), *HOXA9* ($P = 0.0024$) (B), *POU4F2* ($P = 0.0001$) (C), *TWIST1* ($P = 0.0034$) (D), and *VIM* ($P = 0.0001$) (E), and *ZNF154* ($P < 0.0001$) (F).

Table S1   Excluded samples.

Table S2   Primer and probe sequences for real-time PCR.

Table S3   Performance of the urinary markers on the first urine samples.

Table S4   Associations between methylation markers and clinicopathologic parameters.

Table S5   Associations between methylation markers and clinicopathologic parameters for patients under surveillance.

Table S6   Diagnostic significance of two markers both positive for methylation for a positive test result.

Table S7   Diagnostic significance of two markers with one positive for methylation for a positive test result.

Acknowledgments

We are grateful to Margaret Gellett and Anette Stenderup for their technical assistance. We thank the staff at the Departments of Urology at Aarhus University Hospital for their skillful assistance.

Author Contributions

Conceived and designed the experiments: TR MB TFØ LD. Performed the experiments: TR. Analyzed the data: TR AC GGH TFØ LD. Contributed reagents/materials/analysis tools: TR MB TFØ LD. Wrote the paper: TR TFØ LD.

References

1. Epstein JI, Amin MB, Reuter VR, Mostofi FK (1998) The World Health Organization/International Society of Urological Pathology consensus classification of urothelial (transitional cell) neoplasms of the urinary bladder. Bladder Consensus Conference Committee. Am J Surg Pathol 22: 1435–1448.
2. Millan-Rodriguez F, Chechile-Toniolo G, Salvador-Bayarri J, Palou J, Algaba F, et al. (2000) Primary superficial bladder cancer risk groups according to progression, mortality and recurrence. J Urol 164: 680–684.
3. Holmang S, Hedelin H, Anderstrom C, Johansson SL (1995) The relationship among multiple recurrences, progression and prognosis of patients with stages Ta and T1 transitional cell cancer of the bladder followed for at least 20 years. J Urol 153: 1823–1826; discussion 1826–1827.
4. Wolf H, Kakizoe T, Smith PH, Brosman SA, Okajima E, et al. (1986) Bladder tumors. Treated natural history. Prog Clin Biol Res 221: 223–255.
5. Botteman MF, Pashos CL, Redaelli A, Laskin B, Hauser R (2003) The health economics of bladder cancer: a comprehensive review of the published literature. Pharmacoeconomics 21: 1315–1330.
6. Avritscher EB, Cooksley CD, Grossman HB, Sabichi AL, Hamblin L, et al. (2006) Clinical model of lifetime cost of treating bladder cancer and associated complications. Urology 68: 549–553.
7. Grossman HB, Gomella L, Fradet Y, Morales A, Presti J, et al. (2007) A phase III, multicenter comparison of hexaminolevulinate fluorescence cystoscopy and white light cystoscopy for the detection of superficial papillary lesions in patients with bladder cancer. J Urol 178: 62–67.
8. Jocham D, Witjes F, Wagner S, Zeylemaker B, van Moorselaar J, et al. (2005) Improved detection and treatment of bladder cancer using hexaminolevulinate imaging: a prospective, phase III multicenter study. J Urol 174: 862–866; discussion 866.
9. Hermann GG, Mogensen K, Carlsson S, Marcussen N, Duun S (2011) Fluorescence-guided transurethral resection of bladder tumours reduces bladder tumour recurrence due to less residual tumour tissue in Ta/T1 patients: a randomized two-centre study. BJU Int 108: E297–303.
10. Lotan Y, Roehrborn CG (2003) Sensitivity and specificity of commonly available bladder tumor markers versus cytology: results of a comprehensive literature review and meta-analyses. Urology 61: 109–118; discussion 118.
11. Dalbagni G, Ren ZP, Herr H, Cordon-Cardo C, Reuter V (2001) Genetic alterations in tp53 in recurrent urothelial cancer: a longitudinal study. Clin Cancer Res 7: 2797–2801.
12. Takahashi T, Habuchi T, Kakehi Y, Mitsumori K, Akao T, et al. (1998) Clonal and chronological genetic analysis of multifocal cancers of the bladder and upper urinary tract. Cancer Res 58: 5835–5841.
13. Hafner C, Knuechel R, Stoehr R, Hartmann A (2002) Clonality of multifocal urothelial carcinomas: 10 years of molecular genetic studies. Int J Cancer 101: 1–6.
14. Wolff EM, Chihara Y, Pan F, Weisenberger DJ, Siegmund KD, et al. (2010) Unique DNA methylation patterns distinguish noninvasive and invasive urothelial cancers and establish an epigenetic field defect in premalignant tissue. Cancer Res 70: 8169–8178.
15. Russo VEA, Martienssen RA, Riggs AD (1996) Epigenetic mechanisms of gene regulation. Cold Spring Harbor Laboratory Press, Plainview, NY.
16. Migeon BR (1992) Concerning the role of X-inactivation and DNA methylation in fragile X syndrome. Am J Med Genet 43: 291–298.
17. Li E, Bestor TH, Jaenisch R (1992) Targeted mutation of the DNA methyltransferase gene results in embryonic lethality. Cell 69: 915–926.
18. Li E, Beard C, Jaenisch R (1993) Role for DNA methylation in genomic imprinting. Nature 366: 362–365.
19. Egger G, Liang G, Aparicio A, Jones PA (2004) Epigenetics in human disease and prospects for epigenetic therapy. Nature 429: 457–463.

20. Veerla S, Panagopoulos I, Jin Y, Lindgren D, Hoglund M (2008) Promoter analysis of epigenetically controlled genes in bladder cancer. Genes Chromosomes Cancer 47: 368–378.

21. Urakami S, Shiina H, Enokida H, Kawakami T, Tokizane T, et al. (2006) Epigenetic inactivation of Wnt inhibitory factor-1 plays an important role in bladder cancer through aberrant canonical Wnt/beta-catenin signaling pathway. Clin Cancer Res 12: 383–391.

22. Lee MG, Kim HY, Byun DS, Lee SJ, Lee CH, et al. (2001) Frequent epigenetic inactivation of RASSF1A in human bladder carcinoma. Cancer Res 61: 6688–6692.

23. Kim WJ, Kim EJ, Jeong P, Quan C, Kim J, et al. (2005) RUNX3 inactivation by point mutations and aberrant DNA methylation in bladder tumors. Cancer Res 65: 9347–9354.

24. Yu J, Zhu T, Wang Z, Zhang H, Qian Z, et al. (2007) A novel set of DNA methylation markers in urine sediments for sensitive/specific detection of bladder cancer. Clin Cancer Res 13: 7296–7304.

25. Renard I, Joniau S, van Cleynenbreugel B, Collette C, Naome C, et al. (2009) Identification and Validation of the Methylated TWIST1 and NID2 Genes through Real-Time Methylation-Specific Polymerase Chain Reaction Assays for the Noninvasive Detection of Primary Bladder Cancer in Urine Samples. Eur Urol.

26. Reinert T, Modin C, Castano FM, Lamy P, Wojdacz TK, et al. (2011) Comprehensive genome methylation analysis in bladder cancer: identification and validation of novel methylated genes and application of these as urinary tumor markers. Clin Cancer Res 17: 5582–5592.

27. Lin HH, Ke HL, Huang SP, Wu WJ, Chen YK, et al. (2009) Increase sensitivity in detecting superficial, low grade bladder cancer by combination analysis of hypermethylation of E-cadherin, p16, p14, RASSF1A genes in urine. Urol Oncol.

28. Hoque MO, Begum S, Topaloglu O, Chatterjee A, Rosenbaum E, et al. (2006) Quantitation of promoter methylation of multiple genes in urine DNA and bladder cancer detection. J Natl Cancer Inst 98: 996–1004.

29. Dulaimi E, Uzzo RG, Greenberg RE, Al-Saleem T, Cairns P (2004) Detection of bladder cancer in urine by a tumor suppressor gene hypermethylation panel. Clin Cancer Res 10: 1887–1893.

30. Costa VL, Henrique R, Danielsen SA, Duarte-Pereira S, Eknaes M, et al. (2010) Three epigenetic biomarkers, GDF15, TMEFF2, and VIM, accurately predict bladder cancer from DNA-based analyses of urine samples. Clin Cancer Res 16: 5842–5851.

31. Chung W, Bondaruk J, Jelinek J, Lotan Y, Liang S, et al. (2011) Detection of bladder cancer using novel DNA methylation biomarkers in urine sediments. Cancer Epidemiol Biomarkers Prev 20: 1483–1491.

32. Sobin LH WC (2002) TNM Classification of Malignant Tumours. International Union Against Cancer Sixth edition.

33. Bergkvist A, Ljungqvist A, Moberger G (1965) Classification of bladder tumours based on the cellular pattern. Preliminary report of a clinical-pathological study of 300 cases with a minimum follow-up of eight years. Acta Chir Scand 130: 371–378.

34. Babjuk M, Oosterlinck W, Sylvester R, Kaasinen E, Bohle A, et al. (2008) EAU guidelines on non-muscle-invasive urothelial carcinoma of the bladder. Eur Urol 54: 303–314.

35. Campan M, Weisenberger DJ, Trinh B, Laird PW (2009) MethyLight. Methods Mol Biol 507: 325 337.

36. Weisenberger DJ, Campan M, Long TI, Kim M, Woods C, et al. (2005) Analysis of repetitive element DNA methylation by MethyLight. Nucleic Acids Res 33: 6823–6836.

37. Steineck G (2001) Demographic and epidemiologic aspects of bladder cancer. Bladder Cancer Current Diagnosis and Treatment, Droller MJ (Ed), Humana Press Inc, Totowa, NJ 2001.: p.1.

38. Zuiverloon TC, Tjin SS, Busstra M, Bangma CH, Boeve ER, et al. (2011) Optimization of nonmuscle invasive bladder cancer recurrence detection using a urine based FGFR3 mutation assay. J Urol 186: 707–712.

39. Mowatt G, Zhu S, Kilonzo M, Boachie C, Fraser C, et al. (2010) Systematic review of the clinical effectiveness and cost-effectiveness of photodynamic diagnosis and urine biomarkers (FISH, ImmunoCyt, NMP22) and cytology for the detection and follow-up of bladder cancer. Health Technol Assess 14: 1–331, iii-iv.

40. Gazdar AF, Czerniak B (2001) Filling the void: urinary markers for bladder cancer risk and diagnosis. J Natl Cancer Inst 93: 413–415.

41. van Rhijn BW, Lurkin I, Chopin DK, Kirkels WJ, Thiery JP, et al. (2003) Combined microsatellite and FGFR3 mutation analysis enables a highly sensitive detection of urothelial cell carcinoma in voided urine. Clin Cancer Res 9: 257–263.

42. Rieger-Christ KM, Mourtzinos A, Lee PJ, Zagha RM, Cain J, et al. (2003) Identification of fibroblast growth factor receptor 3 mutations in urine sediment DNA samples complements cytology in bladder tumor detection. Cancer 98: 737–744.

43. Zuiverloon TC, van der Aa MN, van der Kwast TH, Steyerberg EW, Lingsma HF, et al. (2010) Fibroblast growth factor receptor 3 mutation analysis on voided urine for surveillance of patients with low-grade non-muscle-invasive bladder cancer. Clin Cancer Res 16: 3011–3018.

44. Serizawa RR, Ralfkiaer U, Steven K, Lam GW, Schmiedel S, et al. (2010) Integrated genetic and epigenetic analysis of bladder cancer reveals an additive diagnostic value of FGFR3 mutations and hypermethylation events. Int J Cancer.

45. Brems-Eskildsen AS, Zieger K, Toldbod H, Holcomb C, Higuchi R, et al. (2010) Prediction and diagnosis of bladder cancer recurrence based on urinary content of hTERT, SENP1, PPP1CA, and MCM5 transcripts. BMC Cancer 10: 646.

46. Zuiverloon TC, Beukers W, van der Keur KA, Munoz JR, Bangma CH, et al. (2011) A methylation assay for the detection of non-muscle-invasive bladder cancer (NMIBC) recurrences in voided urine. BJU Int.

47. Roupret M, Hupertan V, Yates DR, Comperat E, Catto JW, et al. (2008) A comparison of the performance of microsatellite and methylation urine analysis for predicting the recurrence of urothelial cell carcinoma, and definition of a set of markers by Bayesian network analysis. BJU Int 101: 1448–1453.

48. Babjuk M, Oosterlinck W, Sylvester R, Kaasinen E, Bohle A, et al. (2011) EAU guidelines on non-muscle-invasive urothelial carcinoma of the bladder, the 2011 update. Eur Urol 59: 997–1008.

4

Side Population in Human Non-Muscle Invasive Bladder Cancer Enriches for Cancer Stem Cells that are Maintained by MAPK Signalling

Anastasia C. Hepburn[1], Rajan Veeratterapillay[2], Stuart C. Williamson[1], Amira El-Sherif[3], Neha Sahay[1], Huw D. Thomas[1], Alejandra Mantilla[1], Robert S. Pickard[2,4], Craig N. Robson[1], Rakesh Heer[1,2]*

1 Northern Institute for Cancer Research, Newcastle University, Framlington Place, Newcastle upon Tyne, United Kingdom, 2 Department of Urology, Freeman Hospital, The Newcastle upon Tyne Hospitals NHS Foundation Trust, Newcastle upon Tyne, United Kingdom, 3 Department of Pathology, Royal Victoria Infirmary, The Newcastle upon Tyne Hospitals NHS Foundation Trust, Newcastle upon Tyne, United Kingdom, 4 Institute of Cellular Medicine, Medical School, Newcastle University, Framlington Place, Newcastle upon Tyne, United Kingdom

Abstract

Side population (SP) and ABC transporter expression enrich for stem cells in numerous tissues. We explored if this phenotype characterised human bladder cancer stem cells (CSCs) and attempted to identify regulatory mechanisms. Focusing on non-muscle invasive bladder cancer (NMIBC), multiple human cell lines were used to characterise SP and ABC transporter expression. In vitro and in vivo phenotypic and functional assessments of CSC behaviour were undertaken. Expression of putative CSC marker ABCG2 was assessed in clinical NMIBC samples (n = 148), and a role for MAPK signalling, a central mechanism of bladder tumourigenesis, was investigated. Results showed that the ABCG2 transporter was predominantly expressed and was up-regulated in the SP fraction by 3-fold (ABCG2^{hi}) relative to the non-SP (NSP) fraction (ABCG2^{low}). ABCG2^{hi} SP cells displayed enrichment of stem cell markers (Nanog, Notch1 and SOX2) and a three-fold increase in colony forming efficiency (CFE) in comparison to ABCG2^{low} NSP cells. In vivo, ABCG2^{hi} SP cells enriched for tumour growth compared with ABCG2^{low} NSP cells, consistent with CSCs. pERK was constitutively active in ABCG2^{hi} SP cells and MEK inhibition also inhibited the ABCG2^{hi} SP phenotype and significantly suppressed CFE. Furthermore, on examining clinical NMIBC samples, ABCG2 expression correlated with increased recurrence and decreased progression free survival. Additionally, pERK expression also correlated with decreased progression free survival, whilst a positive correlation was further demonstrated between ABCG2 and pERK expression. In conclusion, we confirm ABCG2^{hi} SP enriches for CSCs in human NMIBC and MAPK/ERK pathway is a suitable therapeutic target.

Editor: Dean G. Tang, The University of Texas M.D Anderson Cancer Center, United States of America

Funding: This work was funded by JGW Patterson Foundation and NHS Trustees. The funders had no role in study design, data collection and analysis, decision to publish, or preparation of the manuscript.

Competing Interests: The authors have declared that no competing interests exist.

* E-mail: rakesh.heer@ncl.ac.uk

Introduction

Transitional cell carcinoma (TCC) of the urinary bladder has a worldwide annual incidence of over 350,000 new cases and 145,000 deaths [1]. In the US, it is the fifth most common malignancy accounting for over 70,000 new cases a year and an estimated annual spend of $3.5 billion on cancer treatment [2,3]. Although 85% of patients present with less aggressive non-muscle invasive bladder cancer (NMIBC), they have a high risk of recurrence and those with unfavourable characteristics such as multifocal disease, high grade tumours, with or without concomitant carcinoma in situ (CIS), are at particular risk of disease progression. Intravesical Bacille Calmette-Guérin (BCG) can reduce the risk of progression by 27% in patients with high risk NMIBC [4] but those that fail to respond typically undergo morbid surgery to remove the bladder. For patients that present with, or progress to, muscle invasive bladder cancer (MIBC), the chance of surviving more than 5 years following treatment is approximately 50–60% [5,6]. This background indicates that novel therapeutic approaches against NMIBC are urgently needed to eradicate disease before an invasive phenotype develops [7].

Recent advances in cancer biology have included the characterisation of cancer stem cells (CSCs), a small subpopulation of tumour cells that are tumour initiating and drive the production of the rest of the cancer. CSCs have been described in an increasing number of tumour sites including haematopoetic, breast, colon, melanoma and prostate [8–12]. It is becoming clear that it is essential to target these cells as they determine response to treatment [13]. The categorisation and selection of a side population (SP) phenotype by flow cytometry [14] enriches for CSCs in numerous tumours [15–18]. Recent demonstration of SP in bladder cancer necessitates further investigation of its potential role in characterising CSCs [19].

The pathogenesis of bladder cancer appears closely linked to distinct molecular pathways [20,21]. Over 70% of NMIBCs harbour activating mutations of fibroblast growth factor receptor 3 (FGFR3) leading to constitutive activation of MAPK signalling [22,23]. Furthermore, up-regulation of EGFR/ErbB family receptors is associated with increasing grade and stages of bladder cancer [24,25]. Of relevance, SP phenotype is mediated by the ATP-binding cassette (ABC) family of transporter proteins [14], and the breast cancer-resistant protein-1 (BCRP1)/ABCG2 transporter has been shown to be the main mediator of this phenotype [26]. In particular, ABCG2 is in turn regulated by MAPK [27] and a role for MAPK/ERK signalling pathway in the regulation of SP has been suggested (Tsichuda et al 2008).

As a first step in informing the design of novel therapies for NIMBC, we aimed to characterise CSCs in human bladder cancer using SP selection and explore regulation through the MAPK/ERK signalling axis.

Materials and Methods

Reagents and Cell culture

Human bladder cancer cell RT4, RT112 and J82 were obtained from the American Type Culture Collection (ATCC) and cultured in RPMI 1640 (Sigma) supplemented with 10% fetal bovine serum (FBS) and 1% L-glutamine - referred to as full media (FM). The highly metastatic human TCC cell line 253JB-V was generously provided by Prof Colin Dinney [28] and cultured in MEMalpha media supplemented with 5% FBS. All cells were grown at 37°C in the presence of 5% CO_2. MEK1/2 specific inhibitor, U0126 (Cell Signalling Technology), and rEGF (Sigma) were utilised in studies to modulate MAPK signalling. Control cells for comparison included cultures in basal media (BM) lacking FBS and FM.

Hoechst Dye Efflux Assay

Cells were stained with Hoechst 33342 dye using modification of a previously described protocol [14]. Briefly, Hoechst 33342 dye (2.5 µg/ml) was added alone or in the presence of reserpine (50 µM), verapamil (50 µM) or fumitremorgin C (10 µM) and cells were incubated at 37°C for 90 min and shaken every 30 min. Cell surface marker analyses following Hoechst 33342 dye staining

were performed with anti-ABCG2-FITC (clone 5D3, Millipore) co-labelling on ice for 20 min. Normal mouse IgG-FITC was used as isotype control (Upstate). Propidium iodide (PI) (2 µg/ml) gated viable cells. Analysis and sorting were carried out on a FACSDIVA flow cytometer (Becton Dickinson).

RNA Extraction and Real-time PCR Analysis

Total RNA was extracted using the High Pure RNA kit (Roche) and reversed transcribed using random primers (Promega) and Superscript III reverse transcriptase enzyme (Invitrogen). Real time PCR was carried out with SYBR Green mastermix containing Rox[TM] and UDG (Invitrogen) using the ABI Prism 7900HT Sequence Detection System (Applied Biosystems). For primer sequences see Table S1. Levels of expression were normalised to GAPDH housekeeping gene.

Colony Forming Assay

FACS sorted cells were seeded into six-well plates at a density of 100 cells/well. After 14 days colonies were fixed with Carnoy's fixative and stained with 0.4% crystal violet (w/v) for colony counting using ColCounter (Oxford Optronix), omitting <64 cell colonies as they represent early abortive colonies. Colony forming efficiency (CFE, %) was calculated as [(no. colonies counted/no. cells seeded) × 100].

Cell Cycle

FACS sorted cells were stained with DAPI for cell cycle analysis using CyStain DNA 2step kit (Partec). Propidium iodide (2 µg/ml) gated viable cells. To discriminate against nuclear debris and doublets, cells were gated on FSC and SSC. Flow cytometry cell cycle software (CellQuest Pro, BD Biosciences) was used to calculate DNA content and calculate subG1, G1, S-phase and G2M phase statistics.

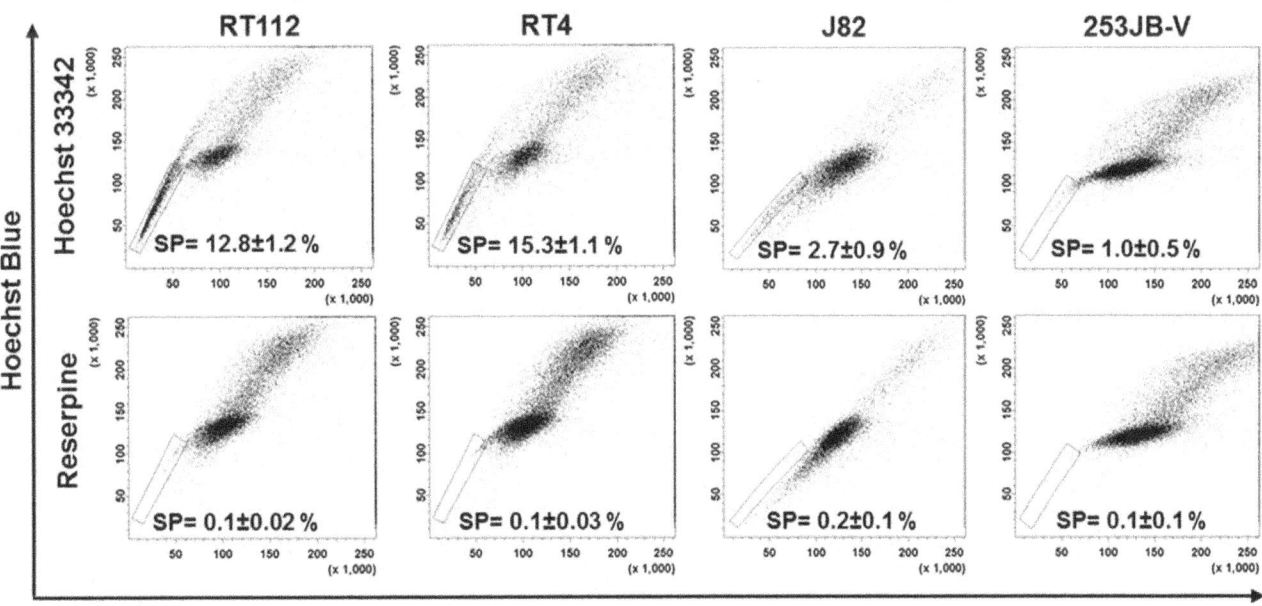

Figure 1. Identification of SP phenotype in bladder cancer cell lines. RT112, RT4, J82 and 253JB-V cells were stained with Hoechst 33342 dye alone or in the presence of reserpine and analysed by flow cytometry measuring Hoechst blue vs Hoechst red fluorescence. The SP was gated and represented as a percentage of the whole viable cell population following PI exclusion (mean ±SE).

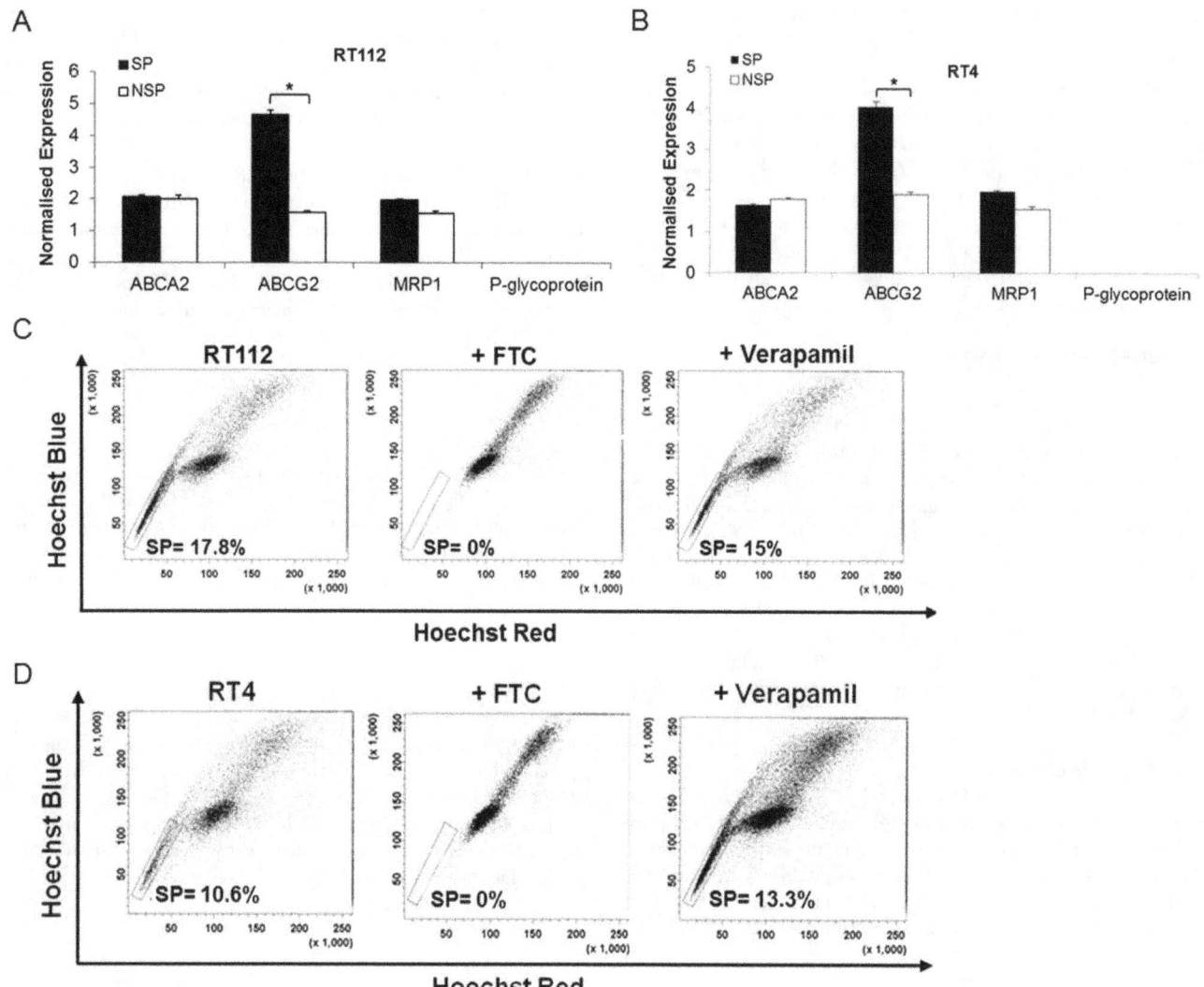

Figure 2. NMIBC SP cells show elevated ABCG2 transporter expression. Relative mRNA expression of ABCA2, ABCG2, MRP1 and P-glycoprotein was determined in SP and NSP fractions of RT112 (A) and RT4 (B) cells using real time PCR. Data shown are the mean of three independent experiments each performed in triplicate (mean ±SE). *P<0.05 (Student's two-tailed t-test). Inhibition studies were performed on RT112 (C) and RT4 (D) cells using ABCG2-specific inhibitor fumitremorgin C (FTC) and P-glycoprotein inhibitor verapamil.

In vivo Tumourigenicity

Animal experiments were performed and conducted in accordance to regulatory guidelines. Twenty three female athymic CD1 nude mice (Charles River, UK) were injected with RT112 SP and NSP sorted cells into the right flank subcutaneous tissue. Tumour growth was monitored by two dimensional measurement with electronic callipers with tumour volume calculated using the formula $a^2 \times b/2$, where a is the smallest measurement and b the largest. The mice experiments were terminated when tumours grew to a maximum of 750 mm^3. The tumours were removed and halved for immunohistochemical studies and real time PCR studies.

Immunohistochemitry

Formalin fixed paraffin embedded archival material from patients undergoing endoscopic resection of bladder tumour or radical cystectomy was accessed for immunohistochemical studies with appropriate informed consent and ethical regulatory approval. In total, 148 NMIBC cases were stained with anti-ABCG2 (1:250; clone BXP-21, Millipore) and anti-p-ERK (1:100, E-4, Santa Cruz Biotechnology) before incubation with secondary biotinylated goat anti-mouse IgG antibody (DAKO). Immunoreactivity was visualised using Vectastain Avidin Biotin Complex Kit (Vector Laboratories) and 3'3'-diaminobenzidetetrahydrochloride. Scoring was initially assessed by percentage and stain intensity. However, the vast majority of cores expressed uniform epithelial staining with a single intensity, with heterogeneous staining present in only a few cases. In these cores, the intensity with >50% area of staining was taken as the score. The immunostaining was reviewed and scored independently by three assessors that were blinded to the clinical data to give average scores of staining intensity of absent (0), weak (1), moderate (2) or strong (3). Xenografts were also stained with anti-Nanog (1:5000, Cell Signalling), anti-Notch 1 (1:500, C-20, Santa Cruz Biotechnology) and anti-SOX2 (1:500, Millipore).

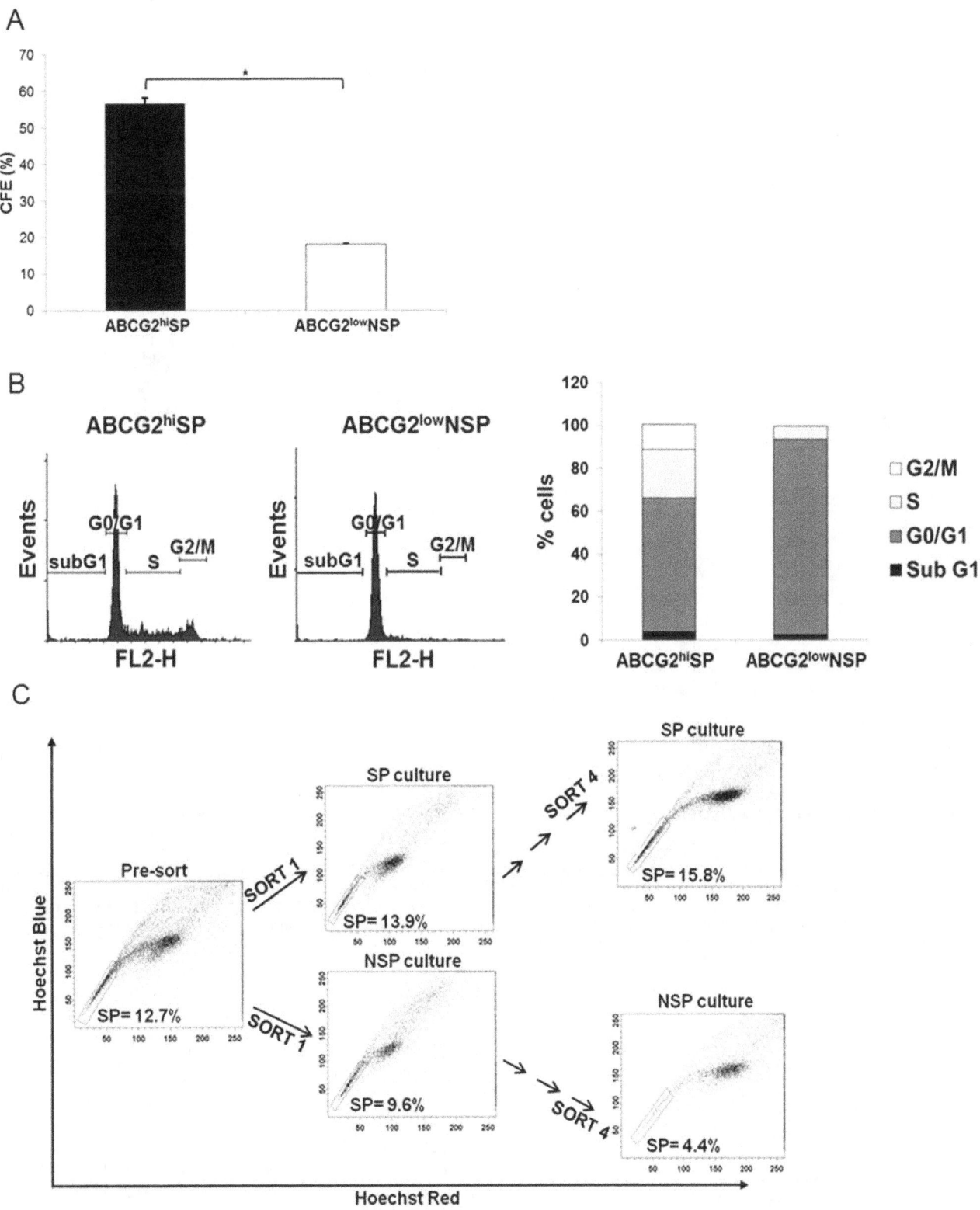

Figure 3. ABCG2^{hi} SP cells have a higher clonogenic ability in comparison to ABCG2^{low} NSP cells. (A) FACS sorted cells were seeded in 6-well plates at a density of 1×10^2 cells/well and colonies were counted after 2 weeks. Colony forming efficiency (CFE) was calculated as described in Materials and Methods. Data shown are the mean ($\pm$SE) of three independent experiments each done in triplicate. *P<0.05 (Student's two-tailed *t*-test). (B) Cell cycle profiles of RT112 ABCG2^{hi} SP and ABCG2^{low} NSP cells showing an increase in S-phase in the ABCG2^{hi} SP fraction. (C) Serial selection, sub-culture and cytometric fractioning between RT112 SP and NSP cells. SP and NSP cells sorted from RT112 were cultured for two weeks, restained with Hoechst 33342 dye and reanalysed by flow cytometry. This process was repeated 4 times.

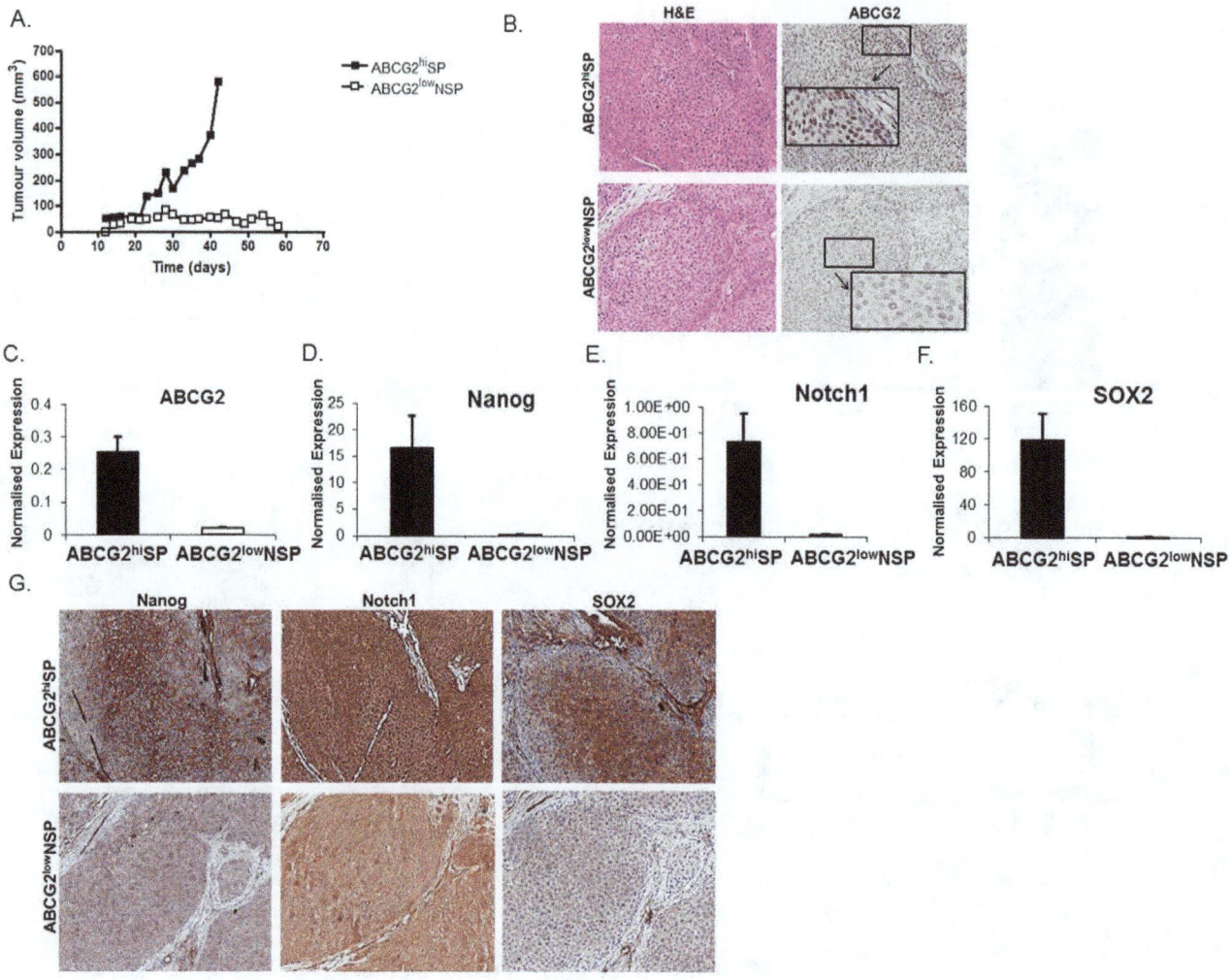

Figure 4. SP cells are more tumourigenic. (A) 1×10^3 ABCG2^{hi} SP and ABCG2^{low} NSP sorted RT112 cells were subcutaneously injected into nude mice and monitored for tumour growth. (B) Immunohistochemical staining of serial sections, of tumours derived from mice injected with 1×10^3 ABCG2^{hi} SP and residual cell pellets from mice injected with 1×10^3 ABCG2^{low} NSP sorted RT112 cells, with H&E and ABCG2 and at higher magnification (20x). Markedly increased immunoreactivity for ABCG2 is seen in the ABCG2^{hi}SP derived tumours. (C) Relative mRNA expression of ABCG2 in tumours formed following injection of 1×10^3 ABCG2^{hi} SP and ABCG2^{low} NSP sorted RT112 cells was determined using real time PCR. (D–F) Relative mRNA expression of Nanog, Notch1 and SOX2 in tumours formed following injection of 1×10^3 ABCG2^{hi} SP and ABCG2^{low} NSP sorted RT112 cells was determined using real time PCR. (G) Immunohistochemical staining of serial sections, of tumours formed following injection of 1×10^3 ABCG2^{hi} SP and ABCG2^{low} NSP sorted RT112 cells, with Nanog, Notch1 and SOX2.

Western Blotting

Cells were lysed in SDS sample buffer (0.125 M Tris pH 6.8, 2% SDS, 10% glycerol, 10% β-mercaptoethanol and 0.01% bromophenol blue) and analysed by SDS-PAGE on 12% polyacrylamide gels, followed by transfer to nitrocellulose Hybond^{TM} membrane (Fisher Scientific). Antibodies were used

at the following dilutions: anti-ERK 1:500 (K-23, Santa Cruz Biotechnology) and anti-phospho-ERK 1:500 (E-4, Santa Cruz Biotechnology). Horseradish peroxidase-conjugated secondary antibodies (DAKO) were used at 1:500 and detected using the enhanced chemiluminescence detection kit (Fisher Scientific).

Statistical Analysis

For real time PCR studies, the two-tailed paired t-test was used to determine statistical significance at a level of $P<0.05$. For immunohistochemistry, differences in the frequency and expression of ABCG2 were examined using Mann-Whitney U test to assess correlations with pathological cancer grade and stage. Patient survival was analysed using the Kaplan-Meier method with log-rank testing, and multivariate analysis was performed using the Cox proportional hazards model. Pearson's correlation was used to correlate ABCG2 and pERK expression. All tests were undertaken using SPSS version 11.0 computer software (SPSS,

Table 1. Tumourigenesis of ABCG2^{hi}SP and ABCG2^{low}NSP cells in nude mice at 30 days.

Cell Number Injected	ABCG2^{hi}SP	ABCG2^{low}NSP
100,000	3/3	–
10,000	5/5	5/5
1,000	5/5	0/5

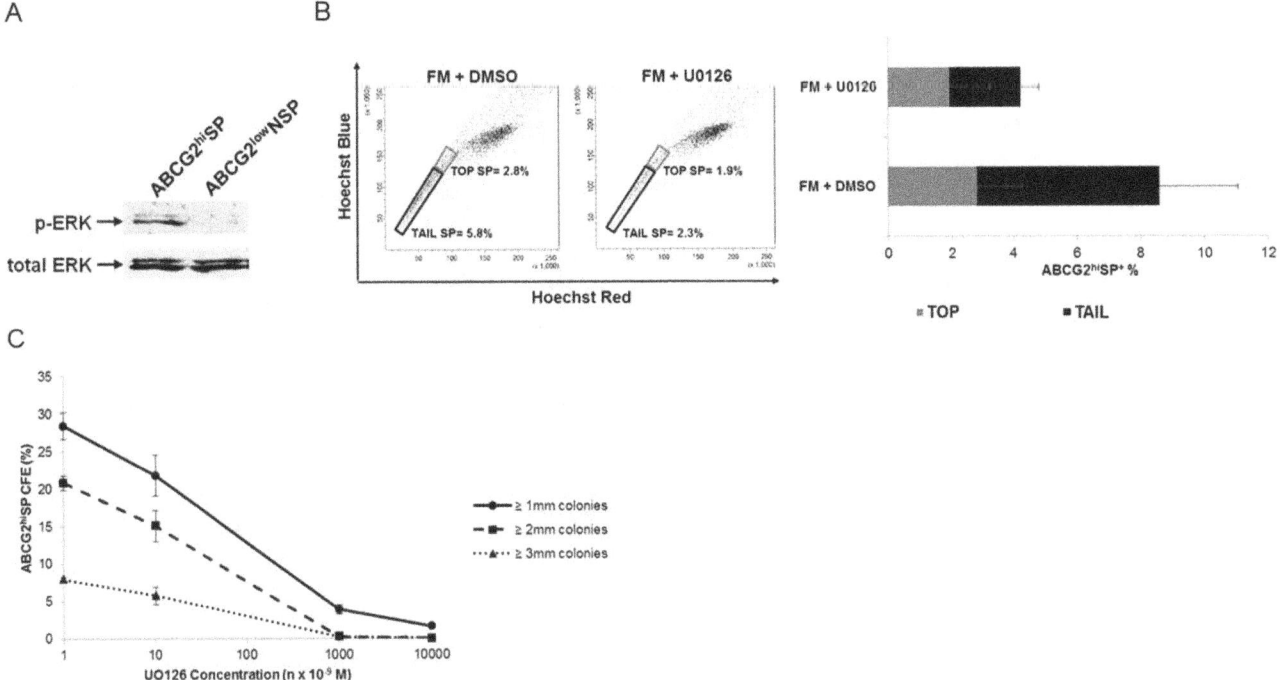

Figure 5. Inhibition of ERK signalling attenuates the fraction of ABCG2^{hi} SP RT112 cells. (A) Western blot analysis was performed with phospho-ERK1/2 and ERK1/2 antibodies. (B) RT112 cells were placed in FM alone or in the presence of U0126 (10 μM) for 30 min prior to staining with Hoechst 33342. The effect of U0126 on the 'tail' and 'top' end compartments of ABCG2^{hi}SP^{+} was investigated. (C) CFE of ABCG2^{hi} SP cells with increasing concentrations of U0126 and different sized colonies (≥1 mm, ≥2 mm and ≥3 mm in diameter).

Inc.). All tests were two-sided and a *P* value of <0.05 was taken to indicate statistical significance.

Results

SP Cells and ABC Transporter Expression can be Identified in Human Bladder Cancer Cells

We investigated the presence of SP in two NMIBC cell lines (RT112 and RT4) and two MIBC cell lines (J82 and 253JB-V). Following staining with Hoechst 33342, a SP was identified in all four cell lines as a distinct tail extending from the main population with the characteristic low fluorescent profile in dual wavelength analysis (Figure 1). The gating strategy undertaken was followed as described by Golebiewska et. al. [29] (Figure S1). Appropriate discrimination of single and viable cells is crucial for adequate SP characterisation. The median (±SE) proportion of each total cell population accounted for by the SP was 12.8% (±1.2%) in RT112, 15.3% (±1.1%) in RT4, 2.7% (±0.9%) in J82, and 1.0% (±0.5%) in 253JB-V. The pan-ABC transporter inhibitor reserpine verified SP phenotype by blocking Hoechst efflux and inhibiting low red/blue staining phenotype that characterises SP cells.

We assessed ABC transporter expression patterns of bladder cancer cell lines using real time PCR. Heterogeneous expressions of multiple multidrug resistant genes were demonstrated in the MIBC cell lines J82 and 253JB-V. However, in the NMIBC cell lines RT4 and RT112 higher expressions of ABCG2 were seen (Figure S2).

ABCG2 is Significantly Enriched within NMIBC SP Cells and Maintains this Phenotype

We next focused on NMIBC disease and examined the relative mRNA expression of four ABC transporters (ABCA2, ABCG2, MRP1 and P-glycoprotein) in RT112 and RT4 SP and NSP fractions using real time PCR (Figure 2A and 2B).The results demonstrated that, in addition to ABCG2 being the major ABC transporter in NMIBC, its expression was higher in SP cells compared to NSP cells. The key role of ABCG2 in generating the SP phenotype was confirmed by complete loss of SP population following treatment with the ABCG2-specific inhibitor fumitremorgin C (FTC) compared to the lack of effect of treatment with the P-glycoprotein inhibitor verapamil (Figure 2C and 2D). In contrast, P-glycoprotein was the most differentially expressed and functionally relevant ABC transporter in the MIBC cell line J82 (Figure S3). Furthermore, we confirmed that in NMIBC cells the SP fraction was associated with only highest levels of ABCG2 (ABCG2^{hi}) expression (Figure S4).

SP Cells Enrich for Stem Cell Function *in vitro*

We next compared the clonogenic potential of RT112 ABCG2^{hi} SP and ABCG2^{low} NSP cells. ABCG2^{hi} SP cells displayed a three-fold increase in mean (±SE) colony forming enrichment to 56.7% (±1.6%) from 18.2% (±0.2%) in ABCG2^{low} NSP cells (Figure 3A). Similar increase in ABCG2^{hi} SP clonogenicity compared with ABCG2^{low} NSP cells was demonstrated in the additional NMIBC cell line RT4 (Figure S5). Following the gating of non-viable cells using propidium iodide, cell cycle analysis revealed that a greater proportion of ABCG2^{hi} SP cells were in S-phase in comparison to ABCG2^{low} NSP cells, with mean (±SE) values of 19% (±5%) versus 5.5% (±1) for S-

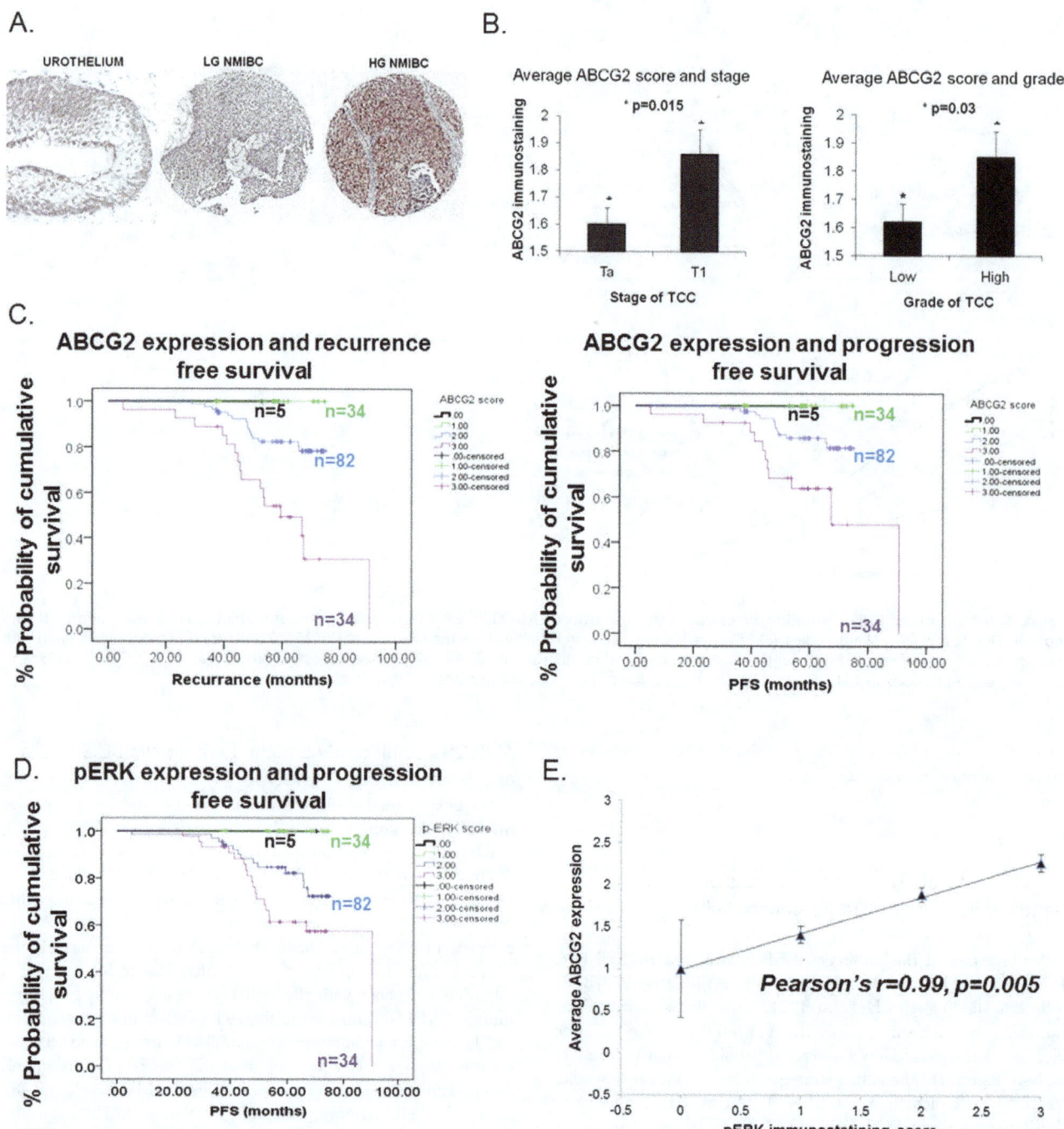

Figure 6. Immunohistochemical expression of ABCG2 in clinical bladder cancer. (A) ABCG2 expression in normal urothelium, low grade (LG) and high grade (HG) NMIBC is typically non-specific and can be seen nuclear and cytoplasmic. (B) Correlation of ABCG2 immunostaining intensity with grade and stage in NMIBC. (C) Kaplan-Meier curves illustrating outcomes of ABCG2 intensity (0, 1, 2 and 3) with recurrence and progression free survival (p<0.001, Log Rank analyses). (D) Kaplan-Meier curves illustrating outcomes of pERK intensity (0, 1, 2 and 3) with progression free survival (p<0.001, Log Rank analyses). (E) Correlation of ABCG2 and pERK expression (p = 0.005, Pearson's r = 0.99).

phase and 68% (±8%) versus 94% (±1%) for G1-phase, respectively (Figure 3B).

To consider the ability of ABCG2^{hi} SP cells to repopulate the original phenotypic spectrum of the parent RT112 cell line, we performed serial cultures and selections of SP and NSP fractions before re-staining with Hoechst 33342 and reanalysing by flow cytometry (Figure 3C). The results showed that following the first round of selection, culture and flow cytometry, cultures derived

from both SP and NSP cells each gave rise again to a similar distribution of SP and NSP cells. If this process was then continued with repeated cycles of selection, separate culture and flow cytometric sorting, the proportion of cells from SP sub-cultures that were located in the SP fraction increased with each round, whilst there was a marked decrease in the SP fraction of cells derived from NSP sub-cultures.

We assessed stem cell marker expression in RT112 ABCG2^{hi} SP and ABCG2^{low} NSP cells by real time PCR (Figure S6A). ABCG2^{hi} SP cells showed increased expression of Nanog, Notch1 and SOX2 compared to ABCG2^{low} NSP cells. Additionally, expression of bladder basal cell markers, including CK14, CD44, CD49f (α6 integrin) and CD104 (β4 integrin) also associated with enrichment of CSCs, was investigated (Figure S6B). All basal cell markers were expressed in ABCG2^{hi} SP cells but similar levels of expression were also seen in ABCG2^{low} NSP cells.

SP Cells Enrich for Greater Tumour Initiating Ability
in vivo

To investigate the comparative ability of ABCG2^{hi} SP and ABCG2^{low} NSP cells to form viable tumours *in vivo*, sorted cells from each sub-population were separately injected subcutaneously into CD1 nude mice and the implant sites monitored for growth. Rapid tumour growth was observed in 5 of 5, 5 of 5, and 3 of 3 animals following implantation of 10^3, 10^4, and 10^5 ABCG2^{hi} SP cells respectively. However, ABCG2^{low}NSP tumour growth was exhausted by dilution of seeding numbers to 10^3 cells whilst 5 of 5 mice engrafted with 10^3 ABCCG2^{hi} SP cells grew tumours (Table 1). Examining median tumour volume over time revealed exponential growth within the ABCG2^{hi} SP cell inoculum group in contrast to those receiving ABCG2^{low} NSP cells (Figure 4A).

Immunohistochemical analysis of ABCG2 expression in tumours, formed following the injection of 1×10^3 ABCG2^{hi} SP cells in comparison to the residual cell pellets (which were not associated with any active growth) harvested from mice injected with ABCG2^{low} NSP sorted RT112 cells, showed increased expression in ABCG2^{hi}SP compared with ABCG2^{low}NSP derived tumours (Figure 4B).

We subsequently demonstrated increased expression of ABCG2 (Figure 4C) and recognised embryonic/pluripotent stem cell markers Nanog, Notch1 and SOX2 (Figure 4D–F), which have been associated with tumorigenesis [30], using real time PCR in the tumours formed following the injection of ABCG2^{hi} SP cells compared with the residual cell pellets harvested from mice injected with ABCG2^{low} NSP cells. These *in vivo* results were consistent with those obtained with the parent *in vitro* cultured cells (Figure S6A) with high expression of stem cell markers maintained in tumours originating from ABCG2^{hi} SP cells contrasting with low expression in residual ABCG2^{low} NSP. Of note, the selection of tumour initiating cells by this *in vivo* assay resulted in enrichment of these stem cell markers, over baseline levels *in vitro*, where differences were 11-fold, 80-fold, 44-fold and 140-fold for ABCG2, Nanog, Notch1 and SOX2 expression, respectively (p<0.05). Furthermore, increased Nanog, Notch1 and SOX2 expression by the ABCG2^{hi} SP mouse xenografts was also observed by immunohistochemical analysis (Figure 4G).

Inhibition of ERK Signalling Attenuates the SP Cancer Stem Cell Function

We investigated the potential role of MAPK in the regulation of the SP phenotype in NMIBC RT112 cells. Expression of ERK, JNK and p38 as well as the PI3K/Akt and STAT signalling pathways was determined by real time PCR (Figure S7A). EGFR, ERK1 and ERK2 expression by both ABCG2^{hi} SP and ABCG2^{low} NSP cells was documented at much higher levels than the other signalling components, suggesting that these enzymes were likely to play a significant role in the MAPK signalling in RT112 cells. Enzymatic activation was subsequently explored and pERK was confirmed to be constitutively expressed at a higher level in ABCG2^{hi} SP cells (Figure 5A). Furthermore, elevated

pERK expression was also seen in the ABCG2^{hi} SP xenografts (Figure S7B). To further test the relevance of the MAPK/ERK pathway as a potential target in RT112 ABCG2^{hi} SP, the functional effects of U0126, a specific inhibitor for MEK1 and MEK2, were assessed. Cells pre-treated with U0126 for 30, 60 or 120 minutes had no detectable phosphorylated ERK expression, thus confirming the inhibition of ERK activation even in the presence of EGF stimulation (Figure S7C). Additionally, there was no significant change in PI positive cells with treatment of U0126 (p = 0.38) following staining with Hoechst 33342 (Figure S7D). We subdivided the ABCG2^{hi}SP fraction into cells located at the top of the tail and cells located at the end of the tail (Figure 5B), as it has been reported that cells at the tip of the SP tail, which have the highest Hoechst 33342 efflux capacity (Hoechst^{low}), highly enriched the stem cell population [31]. Treatment with the MEK inhibitor had a marked inhibitory effect on the cells located in the tail end of the ABCG2^{hi}SP, reducing the ABCG2^{hi}SP by 2.5-fold (5.8% to 2.3%). In contrast, the inhibitor only reduced the ABCG2^{hi}SP in the non-tail end by 1.5-fold (2.8% to 1.9%). These data show that U0126 is also exerting its effect on ABCG2^{hi} Hoechst^{low} cells. Treatment with U0126 also caused a dose-dependent inhibition of CFE in RT112 ABCG2^{hi} SP and ABCG2^{low} NSP cells (Figure S7E). As we have shown that ABCG2^{hi} SP cells can give rise to both SP and NSP cells (Figure S7F) and ABCG2^{low} NSP cells have very low levels of pERK, the suppression of ABCG2^{low} NSP cell CFE appears to be indirect through the effects of U0126 on ABCG2^{hi} SP cells. Of note, preferential inhibition of larger colonies, more indicative of CSC growth, was seen as the presence of colonies $\geq$3mm was inhibited altogether at 10^{-6} M (Figure 5C). These data show that the ABCG2^{hi} SP fraction is, at least in part, maintained by the MAPK/ERK pathway which in turn we have shown to maintain the ABCG2^{low} NSP cells.

Expression of ABCG2 in Clinical Bladder Cancer Correlates with Grade, Stage, Recurrence and Progression Free Survival and pERK Expression

To determine the clinical significance of our *in vitro* and *in vivo* cell line findings, we investigated the expression of ABCG2 in sections of human bladder cancer. Tissue sections from a panel of 148 NMIBC (Table S2– illustrates clinical features) were processed for immunoreactivity to ABCG2 (Figure 6A). ABCG2 positivity was detected in 143 (97%) cases, and for comparison a section of normal urothelium is included which demonstrates a greater intensity of basal ABCG2 expression, which is in keeping with the emerging evidence for a basal stem cell [32]. Average immuno-staining intensity scores for ABCG2 were shown to be associated with early invasive stage, pTa (n = 87) versus pT1 (n = 61), and increasing tumour grade, low grade (n = 93) versus high grade (n = 55) (p<0.05) (Figure 6B). Median follow up was for 59 months (inter-quartile range = 48.3–96.3 months), and 31 cases (21%) showed disease recurrence and 23 cases (16%) showed disease progression. Correlations with time to recurrence and progression free survival (PFS) revealed worse outcomes associated with increasing ABCG2 expression as illustrated with Kaplan-Meier curves and Log-Rank analyses (p<0.001) (Figure 6C). These correlations remained statistically significant when stratified for grade, stage and presence of CIS (p<0.001). Using Cox multivariate analysis, which included the variables of grade, stage and intensity of ABCG2 immunostaining, revealed that ABCG2 expression remained an independent predictor of disease progression (p<0.001; RR = 5.1; 95%CI = 2.6–9.9). Additionally, increasing pERK expression was also associated with worse outcomes (Log-Rank p = 0.001) (Figure 6D). Furthermore, a positive correlation was demonstrated between ABCG2 and pERK expression (p = 0.005, Pearson's r = 0.99) (Figure 6E).

Discussion

Recent advances in the isolation and characterisation of putative CSCs have provided exciting insights into the basis of carcinogenesis and led to increasing optimism for the development of more effectively targeted cancer therapy. Studies have presented compelling data demonstrating that a number of human cancers follow the CSC model, whereby a small subpopulation of cells within a tumour is capable of tumour initiation and responsible for tumour growth and recurrence [8,9]. The existence of cells with increased tumour initiating potential has recently been described in human bladder cancer [33–35] and SP has been demonstrated in bladder cancer patient samples [19]. In this study, we characterised bladder CSCs using SP and explored their modulation by the MAPK/ERK signalling pathway.

In search of a CSC hierarchy in human bladder cancer, our *in vitro* studies showed ABCG2^{hi} SP cells displayed a three-fold increase in colony forming efficiency. These data were further supported by our *in vivo* studies whereby ABCG2^{hi} SP cells were tumour initiating in comparison to ABCG2^{low} NSP cells which displayed loss of tumour growth at 1×10^3 cell dilution. These observations highlight enrichment of CSCs within the ABCG2^{hi} SP selections. Subsequent serial transplantations would further support a hierarchical CSC relationship in these tumours. However, we have taken an analogous approach by performing serial selections and *in vitro* cultures of ABCG2^{hi} SP and ABCG2^{low} NSP cultures demonstrated the ability of ABCG2^{hi} SP cells to repopulate the original phenotypic spectrum of the parent RT112 cell line. Serial selections of ABCG2^{low} NSP cells showed weakening in the potential to regenerate both populations indicating dilution of the ability to select or generate CSCs.

ABCG2 has been shown to be the main molecular determinant of the SP phenotype [26]. Indeed, we found the SP of NMIBC RT112 and RT4 cells had higher ABCG2 mRNA expression, was completely abrogated by ABCG2-specific inhibitor FTC and contained the top 5% of ABCG2^{hi} expressing cells. Correlation to clinical NMIBC outcomes revealed ABCG2^{hi} immunostaining to be associated with worse clinical outcomes of cancer recurrence and progression, indicating a role for CSCs in bladder cancer development. Interestingly, the SP of MIBC J82 cell line had higher P-glycoprotein expression and was inhibited by verapamil, a P-glycoprotein-specific inhibitor. P-glycoprotein mRNA levels have been found to be elevated in high grade bladder tumours [36]. Additionally, the molecular pathology of NMIBC is distinct from MIBC [20]. These findings may account for the differences seen in the % of SP cells in the NMIBC and MIBC cell lines and suggest a possible switch of CSC phenotype in MIBC.

The existence of CSCs in human bladder cancer has been reported based on the use of SP, aldehyde dehydrogenase activity assay, cell surface and cytokeratin markers generally suggesting basal markers as CSC markers [19,33–35,37,38]. Transcripts of bladder basal cell markers CK14, CD44, CD49f and CD104 were all expressed in ABCG2^{hi} SP cells but similar levels of expression were also seen in ABCG2^{low} NSP cells. Further investigation of protein expression is required. Of note, we showed protein expression of ABCG2, the main mediator of SP, is basal consistent with published data pointing towards basal markers as CSC markers. Embryonic/pluripotent stem cell-like signatures are found to be over-expressed in poorly differentiated human cancers, including bladder cancers [30]. We show that ABCG2^{hi} SP cells exhibited higher expression levels of Nanog, Notch1 and

SOX2 in comparison to ABCG2^{low} NSP cells. The expression of these pluripotent stem cell factors may contribute to greater multipotency in generating SP and NSP from the ABCG2^{hi} SP cells. Interestingly, increased expression of Nanog in NMIBC CSCs has also been shown to correlate with overexpression of self-renewing marker Bmi-1 and a larger population of SP cells [39]. Furthermore, our cell cycle studies showed a greater proportion of ABCG2^{hi} SP cells were in S-phase in contrast to the G1 positioning of ABCG2^{low} NSP cells, which is consistent with Nanog, SOX2 and Oct4 in inducing longer S-phase and a shorter G1 [40,41]. The data presented highlights a potential mechanism for the ESC-like signatures in promoting tumorigenicity and the function of these genes in bladder cancer represents an important area for further study.

Similarly to observations reported in colon cancer cells, we found inhibition of the MAPK/ERK signalling pathway by MEK1/2-specific inhibitor U0126 to reduce SP, possibly through altering ABCG2 expression or localisation [42]. MEK inhibition has also been shown to down-regulate ABCG2 expression by promoting its degradation [27] as well as downregulating a cisplatin-induced SP that is highly tumorigenic and overexpresses Nanog [43].Additionally, our data showed that inhibition of MAPK/ERK signalling pathway targeted both bladder CSCs and non-CSCs as demonstrated by reduced colony forming ability of ABCG2^{hi} SP and ABCG2^{low} NSP cells. However, the effect of U0126 on ABCG2^{low} NSP cells appears to be indirect as ABCG2^{low} NSP cells have very low levels of active ERK but are hierarchically dependent on ABCG2^{hi} SP cells with high ERK activity that would be more susceptible to U0126 inhibition. We show that ABCG2 expression correlated with NMIBC recurrence and progression, and that ABCG2 expression is, in part, regulated by MAPK activity and this correlates with ours and published findings of activated ERK predicting poor prognosis in bladder cancer [44]. Additionally, we demonstrate ABCG2 expression to positively correlate with pERK expression. Indeed, the MAPK/ERK signalling pathway has been distinctively shown to have a role in CSC self-renewal and tumourigenicity in a number of cancers [45,46]. Our data therefore goes some way to support the MAPK pathway being central to maintenance of bladder CSC phenotype and potentially highlights strategies to usefully modulate CSCs; this approach being already a focus of preclinical and clinical studies for a number of malignancies [47–49]. There are encouraging results from clinical trials with MEK inhibitors [50], and our data validates the therapeutic targeting of MEK or its upstream regulators (e.g. clinical trials of erlotinib) in bladder cancer [7,51].

In conclusion, we confirm that ABCG2^{hi} SP enriches for CSCs in human bladder cancer and provide evidence for the importance of the MAPK pathway as a suitable therapeutic target for NMIBC CSCs.

Supporting Information

Figure S1 Gating strategy for SP data analysis. An example of the step-by-step gating strategy and the resulting percentage of cell populations is shown for RT112. (A) Gating strategy. Cells are distinguished from debris on the flow cytometric profile based on Forward Scatter (FSC) and Side Scatter (SSC) (A, 1). The Hoechst 3342 dye is excited with the UV laser at 350 nm and its fluorescence is measured with a 2-355/450/50 filter (Hoechst Blue) and a 2-355/675lp filter (Hoechst Red). Doublets and aggregates are gated out based on Hoechst Blue area versus height to ensure that a detected signal arises from single cells. PI, having been excited at 350 nm, is also measured through the 2-355/675lp filter but is much brighter than the Hoechst red signal so the dead cells line up on a vertical line to the far right (A, 2). SP cells are recognised as a distinct tail extending from the main population with the characteristic low fluorescent profile based on Hoechst Red versus Hoechst Blue (A, 3). (B) The gating tree illustrates the sequential procedure applied to select out the SP population and the percentage of cells resulting from each gating step. '% Parent' indicates the percentage of gated events relative to the preceding gate. '% Total' indicates the percentage of gated events relative to all events recorded.

Figure S2 ABC transporter expression in bladder cancer cell lines. Real time PCR was used to determine relative expression of ABC transporter mRNA in bladder cancer cell lines. Expression levels were normalised to the housekeeping gene GAPDH. Data shown are the mean of three independent experiments each done in triplicate (mean ± SE).

Figure S3 P-glycoprotein transporter mediates SP phenotype in J82 bladder cancer cells. (A) Real time PCR analysis of ABC transporter expression in J82 SP and NSP cell. Data shown are the mean of three independent experiments each done in triplicate (mean ± SE). *P<0.05 (Student's two-tailed t-test). (B) Inhibition studies were performed on J82 cells using ABCG2-specific inhibitor fumitremorgin C (FTC) and P-glycoprotein inhibitor verapamil.

Figure S4 ABCG2 transporter mediates SP phenotype in RT112 and RT4 bladder cancer cells. Following staining with Hoechst 33342, cells were labelled with anti-ABCG2-FITC and normal mouse IgG-FITC was used as isotype control. (A) The 5% of cells showing the highest intensity immunofluorescence (population P2 for SP fraction and population P4 for NSP fraction) were categorised as ABCG2^{hi} population whilst the 5% of cells showing the lowest intensity of immunofluorescence (population P1 for SP fraction and population P3 for NSP fraction) were categorised as ABCG2^{low} population (representative dot plot). (B) The gating tree illustrates the sequential procedure applied to select out the ABCG2^{hi} and ABCG2^{low} populations and the percentage of cells resulting from each gating step. RT112 (C) and RT4 (D) cells labelled with anti-ABCG2-FITC and resulting ABCG2^{hi} and ABCG2^{low} populations for SP and NSP fractions. These data show that SP cells equate to ABCG2^{hi} expressing cells and the NSP equate to ABCG2^{low} expressing cells.

Figure S5 RT4 SP cells have a higher clonogenic ability in comparison to RT4 NSP cells. RT4 FACS sorted cells were

seeded in 6-well plates at a density of 1×10^2 cells/well and colonies were counted after 2 weeks. Data shown are the mean (± SE) of three independent experiments each done in triplicate. *P<0.05 (Student's two-tailed t-test).

Figure S6 Stem and basal cell marker expression in ABCG2^{hi} SP and ABCG2^{low} NSP fractions of RT112 cells. Relative mRNA expression of stem (A) and basal (B) cell markers was determined in ABCG2^{hi} SP and ABCG2^{low} NSP fractions of RT112 cells using real time PCR. Data shown are the mean of three independent experiments each done in triplicate (mean ± SE). *P<0.05 (Student's two-tailed t-test).

Figure S7 Inhibition of ERK signalling attenuates the fraction of ABCG2^{hi} SP RT112 cells. (A) Real time PCR analysis of MAPK pathway component gene expression was carried out in ABCG2^{hi} SP and ABCG2^{low} NSP sorted RT112 cells. Data shown are the mean (±SE) of three independent experiments each done in triplicate. (B) ABCG2^{hi} SP and ABCG2^{low} NSP xenografts were stained for pERK. (C) RT112 cells were starved overnight in basal media (BM) and pretreated with MEK inhibitor U0126 (10μM) for 30, 60 and 120 mins before being stimulated with recombinant EGF (r-EGF, 10 and 100 ng/ml) for 5 mins. Western blotting demonstrating pERK levels. Total ERK levels were used as loading control. (D) Cell viability using propidium iodide (PI, 2μg/ml) following staining with Hoechst 33342 in the absence or presence of U0126 (10μM) (p = 0.38, Student's two-tailed t-test). (E) U0126 decreases the CFE of both ABCG2^{hi} SP and ABCG2^{low} NSP. (F) SP cells sorted from RT112 were cultured for two weeks, restained with Hoechst 33342 dye and reanalysed by flow cytometry.

Table S1 Primer sequences for real time PCR.

Table S2 Characteristics of 148 patients with non muscle invasive bladder cancer. Table shows number of patients (%) according to age and sex, in addition to grade and stage stratified for ABCG2 immunostaining score.

Author Contributions

Conceived and designed the experiments: RH CNR. Performed the experiments: ACH SCW NS HDT. Analyzed the data: ACH RV SCW AE-S AM NS HDT RSP CNR RH. Contributed reagents/materials/analysis tools:. Wrote the paper: ACH RH.

References

1. Ploeg M, Aben KK, Kiemeney LA (2009) The present and future burden of urinary bladder cancer in the world. World J Urol 27: 289–293.
2. SEER (2010) Surveillance, Epidemiology, and End Results (SEER) Program and the National Center for Health Statistics. Available: http://seercancergov/.
3. NIH (2010) US National Institute of Heath; National Cancer Institute: Cancer Trends Progress Report. Available: http://progressreportcancergov.
4. Sylvester RJ, van der MA, Lamm DL (2002) Intravesical bacillus Calmette-Guerin reduces the risk of progression in patients with superficial bladder cancer: a meta-analysis of the published results of randomized clinical trials. J Urol 168: 1964–1970.
5. Shelley MD, Barber J, Mason MD (2001) Surgery versus radiotherapy for muscle invasive bladder cancer. Cochrane Database Syst Rev: CD002079.
6. Shariat SF, Karakiewicz PI, Palapattu GS, Lotan Y, Rogers CG, et al. (2006) Outcomes of radical cystectomy for transitional cell carcinoma of the bladder: a contemporary series from the Bladder Cancer Research Consortium. J Urol 176: 2414–2422.

7. Shah JB, McConkey DJ, Dinney CP (2011) New strategies in muscle-invasive bladder cancer: on the road to personalized medicine. Clin Cancer Res 17: 2608–2612.
8. Al-Hajj M, Wicha MS, Benito-Hernandez A, Morrison SJ, Clarke MF (2003) Prospective identification of tumorigenic breast cancer cells. Proc Natl Acad Sci U S A 100: 3983–3988.
9. Lapidot T, Sirard C, Vormoor J, Murdoch B, Hoang T, et al. (1994) A cell initiating human acute myeloid leukaemia after transplantation into SCID mice. Nature 367: 645–648.
10. Vermeulen L, De Sousa EMF, van der Heijden M, Cameron K, de Jong JH, et al. (2010) Wnt activity defines colon cancer stem cells and is regulated by the microenvironment. Nat Cell Biol 12: 468–476.
11. Ricci-Vitiani L, Lombardi DG, Pilozzi E, Biffoni M, Todaro M, et al. (2007) Identification and expansion of human colon-cancer-initiating cells. Nature 445: 111–115.
12. Schatton T, Murphy GF, Frank NY, Yamaura K, Waaga-Gasser AM, et al. (2008) Identification of cells initiating human melanomas. Nature 451: 345–349.

13. Clarke MF, Dick JE, Dirks PB, Eaves CJ, Jamieson CH, et al. (2006) Cancer stem cells–perspectives on current status and future directions: AACR Workshop on cancer stem cells. Cancer Res 66: 9339–9344.

14. Goodell MA, Brose K, Paradis G, Conner AS, Mulligan RC (1996) Isolation and functional properties of murine hematopoietic stem cells that are replicating in vivo. J Exp Med 183: 1797–1806.

15. Ho MM, Ng AV, Lam S, Hung JY (2007) Side population in human lung cancer cell lines and tumors is enriched with stem-like cancer cells. Cancer Res 67: 4827–4833.

16. Brown MD, Gilmore PE, Hart CA, Samuel JD, Ramani VA, et al. (2007) Characterization of benign and malignant prostate epithelial Hoechst 33342 side populations. Prostate 67: 1384–1396.

17. Bleau AM, Hambardzumyan D, Ozawa T, Fomchenko EI, Huse JT, et al. (2009) PTEN/PI3K/Akt pathway regulates the side population phenotype and ABCG2 activity in glioma tumor stem-like cells. Cell Stem Cell 4: 226–235.

18. Patrawala L, Calhoun T, Schneider-Broussard R, Zhou J, Claypool K, et al. (2005) Side population is enriched in tumorigenic, stem-like cancer cells, whereas ABCG2+ and ABCG2- cancer cells are similarly tumorigenic. Cancer Res 65: 6207–6219.

19. Oates JE, Grey BR, Addla SK, Samuel JD, Hart CA, et al. (2009) Hoechst 33342 side population identification is a conserved and unified mechanism in urological cancers. Stem Cells Dev 18: 1515–1522.

20. Knowles MA (2008) Molecular pathogenesis of bladder cancer. Int J Clin Oncol 13: 287–297.

21. Dinney CP, McConkey DJ, Millikan RE, Wu X, Bar-Eli M, et al. (2004) Focus on bladder cancer. Cancer Cell 6: 111–116.

22. Kassouf W, Dinney CP, Brown G, McConkey DJ, Diehl AJ, et al. (2005) Uncoupling between epidermal growth factor receptor and downstream signals defines resistance to the antiproliferative effect of Gefitinib in bladder cancer cells. Cancer Res 65: 10524–10535.

23. van Rhijn BW, Lurkin I, Radvanyi F, Kirkels WJ, van der Kwast TH, et al. (2001) The fibroblast growth factor receptor 3 (FGFR3) mutation is a strong indicator of superficial bladder cancer with low recurrence rate. Cancer Res 61: 1265–1268.

24. Kassouf W, Black PC, Tuziak T, Bondaruk J, Lee S, et al. (2008) Distinctive expression pattern of ErbB family receptors signifies an aggressive variant of bladder cancer. J Urol 179: 353–358.

25. Forster JA, Paul AB, Harnden P, Knowles MA (2011) Expression of NRG1 and its receptors in human bladder cancer. Br J Cancer 104: 1135–1143.

26. Zhou S, Schuetz JD, Bunting KD, Colapietro AM, Sampath J, et al. (2001) The ABC transporter Bcrp1/ABCG2 is expressed in a wide variety of stem cells and is a molecular determinant of the side-population phenotype. Nat Med 7: 1028–1034.

27. Imai Y, Ohmori K, Yasuda S, Wada M, Suzuki T, et al. (2009) Breast cancer resistance protein/ABCG2 is differentially regulated downstream of extracellular signal-regulated kinase. Cancer Sci 100: 1118–1127.

28. Dinney CP, Fishbeck R, Singh RK, Eve B, Pathak S, et al. (1995) Isolation and characterization of metastatic variants from human transitional cell carcinoma passaged by orthotopic implantation in athymic nude mice. J Urol 154: 1532–1538.

29. Golebiewska A, Brons NH, Bjerkvig R, Niclou SP (2011) Critical appraisal of the side population assay in stem cell and cancer stem cell research. Cell Stem Cell 8: 136–147.

30. Ben-Porath I, Thomson MW, Carey VJ, Ge R, Bell GW, et al. (2008) An embryonic stem cell-like gene expression signature in poorly differentiated aggressive human tumors. Nat Genet 40: 499–507.

31. Camargo FD, Chambers SM, Drew E, McNagny KM, Goodell MA (2006) Hematopoietic stem cells do not engraft with absolute efficiencies. Blood 107: 501–507.

32. Shin K, Lee J, Guo N, Kim J, Lim A, et al. (2011) Hedgehog/Wnt feedback supports regenerative proliferation of epithelial stem cells in bladder. Nature 472: 110–114.

33. Bentivegna A, Conconi D, Panzeri E, Sala E, Bovo G, et al. (2010) Biological heterogeneity of putative bladder cancer stem-like cell populations from human bladder transitional cell carcinoma samples. Cancer Sci 101: 416–424.

34. Chan KS, Espinosa I, Chao M, Wong D, Ailles L, et al. (2009) Identification, molecular characterization, clinical prognosis, and therapeutic targeting of human bladder tumor-initiating cells. Proc Natl Acad Sci U S A 106: 14016–14021.

35. He X, Marchionni L, Hansel DE, Yu W, Sood A, et al. (2009) Differentiation of a highly tumorigenic basal cell compartment in urothelial carcinoma. Stem Cells 27: 1487–1495.

36. Clifford SC, Neal DE, Lunec J (1996) High level expression of the multidrug resistance (MDR1) gene in the normal bladder urothelium: a potential involvement in protection against carcinogens? Carcinogenesis 17: 601–604.

37. Falso MJ, Buchholz BA, White RW (2012) Stem-like cells in bladder cancer cell lines with differential sensitivity to cisplatin. Anticancer Res 32: 733–738.

38. Volkmer JP, Sahoo D, Chin RK, Ho PL, Tang C, et al. (2012) Three differentiation states risk-stratify bladder cancer into distinct subtypes. Proc Natl Acad Sci U S A 109: 2078–2083.

39. Zhang Y, Wang Z, Yu J, Shi J, Wang C, et al. (2012) Cancer stem-like cells contribute to cisplatin resistance and progression in bladder cancer. Cancer Lett 322: 70–77.

40. Becker KA, Ghule PN, Therrien JA, Lian JB, Stein JL, et al. (2006) Self-renewal of human embryonic stem cells is supported by a shortened G1 cell cycle phase. J Cell Physiol 209: 883–893.

41. Zhang X, Neganova I, Przyborski S, Yang C, Cooke M, et al. (2009) A role for NANOG in G1 to S transition in human embryonic stem cells through direct binding of CDK6 and CDC25A. J Cell Biol 184: 67–82.

42. Tabu K, Kimura T, Sasai K, Wang L, Bizen N, et al. (2010) Analysis of an alternative human CD133 promoter reveals the implication of Ras/ERK pathway in tumor stem-like hallmarks. Mol Cancer 9: 39.

43. Tsuchida R, Das B, Yeger H, Koren G, Shibuya M, et al. (2008) Cisplatin treatment increases survival and expansion of a highly tumorigenic side-population fraction by upregulating VEGF/Flt1 autocrine signaling. Oncogene 27: 3923–3934.

44. Karlou M, Saetta AA, Korkolopoulou P, Levidou G, Papanastasiou P, et al. (2009) Activation of extracellular regulated kinases (ERK1/2) predicts poor prognosis in urothelial bladder carcinoma and is not associated with B-Raf gene mutations. Pathology 41: 327–334.

45. Sunayama J, Matsuda K, Sato A, Tachibana K, Suzuki K, et al. (2010) Crosstalk between the PI3K/mTOR and MEK/ERK pathways involved in the maintenance of self-renewal and tumorigenicity of glioblastoma stem-like cells. Stem Cells 28: 1930–1939.

46. Wang YK, Zhu YL, Qiu FM, Zhang T, Chen ZG, et al. (2010) Activation of Akt and MAPK pathways enhances the tumorigenicity of CD133+ primary colon cancer cells. Carcinogenesis 31: 1376–1380.

47. Dubrovska A, Elliott J, Salamone RJ, Kim S, Aimone LJ, et al. (2010) Combination therapy targeting both tumor-initiating and differentiated cell populations in prostate carcinoma. Clin Cancer Res 16: 5692–5702.

48. Gupta PB, Onder TT, Jiang G, Tao K, Kuperwasser C, et al. (2009) Identification of selective inhibitors of cancer stem cells by high-throughput screening. Cell 138: 645–659.

49. Yilmaz OH, Valdez R, Theisen BK, Guo W, Ferguson DO, et al. (2006) Pten dependence distinguishes haematopoietic stem cells from leukaemia-initiating cells. Nature 441: 475–482.

50. Yeh TC, Marsh V, Bernat BA, Ballard J, Colwell H, et al. (2007) Biological characterization of ARRY-142886 (AZD6244), a potent, highly selective mitogen-activated protein kinase kinase 1/2 inhibitor. Clin Cancer Res 13: 1576–1583.

51. Pruthi RS, Nielsen M, Heathcote S, Wallen EM, Rathmell WK, et al. (2010) A phase II trial of neoadjuvant erlotinib in patients with muscle-invasive bladder cancer undergoing radical cystectomy: clinical and pathological results. BJU Int 106: 349–354.

5

Diabetes Mellitus and Risk of Bladder Cancer

Zhaowei Zhu[1]⦾, Xiaohua Zhang[1]⦾, Zhoujun Shen[1]*, Shan Zhong[1], Xianjin Wang[1], Yingli Lu[2]*, Chen Xu[3,4]

1 Department of Urology, Ruijin Hospital, Shanghai Jiaotong University School of Medicine, Shanghai, China, 2 Institute and Department of Endocrinology and Metabolism, Shanghai Ninth People's Hospital, Shanghai Jiaotong University School of Medicine, Shanghai, China, 3 Department of Embryology and Histology, Shanghai Jiaotong University School of Medicine, Shanghai, China, 4 Shanghai Key Laboratory of Reproductive Medicine, Shanghai Jiaotong University School of Medicine, Shanghai, China

Abstract

Background: Increasing evidence suggests that diabetes mellitus (DM) may be associated with an increased risk of bladder cancer. To provide a quantitative assessment of this association, we evaluated the relation between DM and incidence and mortality of bladder cancer in an updated meta-analysis of cohort studies. **Methods** We identified cohort studies by searching the EMBASE and MEDLINE databases, through 31 March 2012. Summary relative risks (RRs) with 95% confidence intervals (CIs) were calculated with random-effects models.

Results: A total of 29 cohort studies (27 articles) were included in this meta-analysis. DM was associated with an increased incidence of bladder cancer (RR 1.29, 95% CI: 1.08–1.54), with significant evidence of heterogeneity among these studies (p<0.001, $I^2 = 94.9\%$). In stratified analysis, the RRs of bladder cancer were 1.36 (1.05–1.77) for diabetic men and 1.28 (0.75–2.19) for diabetic women, respectively. DM was also positively associated with bladder cancer mortality (RR 1.33, 95% CI: 1.14–1.55), with evident heterogeneity between studies (p = 0.002, $I^2 = 63.3\%$). The positive association was observed for both men (RR 1.54, 95% CI: 1.30–1.82) and women (RR 1.50, 95% CI: 1.05–2.14).

Conclusion: These findings suggest that compared to non-diabetic individuals, diabetic individuals have an increased incidence and mortality of bladder cancer.

Editor: Hamid Reza Baradaran, Tehran University of Medical Sciences, Iran (Republic of Islamic)

Funding: This work was supported by The National Natural Science Foundation of China (No. 81072098), Science and Technology Commission of Shanghai Municipality (No. 10DZ2270600), Shanghai Leading Academic Discipline Project (No. S30201) and Shanghai Basic Research Project (No. 09DJ1400400). The funders had no role in study design, data collection and analysis, decision to publish, or preparation of the manuscript.

Competing Interests: The authors have declared that no competing interests exist.

* E-mail: shenzj6@sina.com (ZS); luy662003@yahoo.com.cn (YL)

⦾ These authors contributed equally to this work.

Introduction

Bladder cancer is one of the most common malignancies of the urinary tract. Based on incidence and mortality data from several agencies, the American Cancer Society estimates that 73,510 new bladder cancer cases and 14,880 deaths from bladder cancer are projected to occur in the United States in 2012 [1]. To explore the effective tools for prevention of bladder cancer, great investment has been made to gain new insight into how environmental and genetic factors influence the development of bladder cancer. The chemical and environmental exposures include aromatic amines [2], aniline dyes [3], bitumen [4], nitrites and nitrates [5], paint [6] and arsenic [7], but the most important environmental factor is cigarette smoking [8].

Diabetes mellitus (DM) is considered to be one of the major public health challenges in both industrialized and developing countries [9]. A number of studies have found that diabetes may be associated with increased risk of a variety of cancers, including cancers of the pancreas [10], liver [11], kidney [12], colon and rectal [13]. A previous meta-analysis of 16 studies (seven case-control studies, three cohort studies and six cohort

studies of diabetic patients) conducted in 2006 showed that diabetes was associated with an increased risk of bladder cancer in case-control studies and cohort studies, but not in cohort studies of diabetic patients [14]. However, the association between diabetes and mortality from bladder cancer remains unclear. Since the meta-analysis was published, a variety of relevant studies on such association have yielded inconsistent results [15,16,17,18,19,20,21,22,23,24,25,26,27,28,29,30]. Currently, we aim to analyze the relation between DM and incidence and mortality of bladder cancer in an updated meta-analysis of cohort studies. This updated analysis of 29 cohort studies will allow us to provide more precise risk estimates than the previous analysis. We also evaluated whether the association varied by sex, and assessed potential confounders including smoking and obesity.

Methods

Data Sources and Searches

A computerized literature search was conducted using MEDLINE (from 1 January 1966) and EMBASE (from 1 January 1974) through 31 March 2012 by two independent investigators. The search strategy used medical subject heading (MeSH) terms and keywords: diabetes or diabetes mellitus; bladder; neoplasm(s) or cancer; mortality; and epidemiologic studies. Diabetes mellitus was determined through medical records, fasting plasma glucose, hospital discharge register or self-reported history of diabetes. Bladder cancer was assessed by cancer registries, medical records, death certificates and ambulatory and inpatient claims. We also manually reviewed the reference lists to identify additional relevant studies. No language restrictions were imposed. Our systematic review was conducted according to the meta-analysis of observational studies in epidemiology (MOOSE) guidelines [31].

Study Selection

We included those studies that met all of the following criteria: (1) they had a prospective or retrospective cohort design; (2) one of the exposure of interest was DM; (3) one of the outcome of interest was bladder cancer; and (4) reported rate ratio, hazard ratio, or standardized incidence/mortality rate (SIR/SMR) with their 95% confidence intervals (CIs), or provided sufficient information to calculate them. We summarized results from cohort studies because they are less prone to selection bias compared to case-control studies.

Studies were excluded if (1) case–control design was used; or (2) they provided only an effect estimate with no means to calculate a CI. To evaluate studies' eligibility for inclusion, titles, abstracts, and articles were reviewed independently by two authors; discrepancies were resolved by a third reviewer or by consensus. Articles or reports from non-peer-reviewed sources were not included in this meta-analysis. In the event of multiple publications from the same study population, the most recent publication with the largest number of bladder cancer cases was included in the meta-analysis. We did not consider studies in which the exposure of interest was mainly or solely type 1 diabetes, defined as diagnosis before 30 years of age.

Data Extraction

Two investigators independently performed the data extraction. When discrepancies were found, a third investigator would make the definitive decision for data extraction. The extracted information included: the first author's last name, publication year, study location, participant characteristics (age and sex), sample size, measure of association, length of follow-up (if applicable), variables adjusted in the analysis, and the risk estimates with corresponding 95% CIs. From each study, we extracted the RR estimate that was adjusted for the greatest number of potential confounders.

Statistical Analysis

We divided epidemiologic studies of the relationship between diabetes and risk of bladder cancer into two general types according to the measure of relative risks (RRs): cohort studies (rate ratio or hazard ratio), and cohort studies of diabetic patients using external population comparisons (SIR/SMR). In practice, these four measures of effect yield similar estimates of RR because the absolute risk of bladder cancer is low. We conducted separate meta-analyses of bladder cancer incidence and mortality.

For incidence and mortality of bladder cancer, the study quality was assessed according to the following: evaluation of diabetes, outcome ascertainment, duration of follow-up, loss to follow-up, and number of adjustments [32]. In this meta-analysis, the maximum quality score was 10 points, and studies with quality score greater than or equal to 5 points were considered high quality (Supporting Information **Figure S1 and S2**).

The variance of the log RR from each study was calculated by converting the 95% CI to its natural logarithm by taking the width of the CI and dividing by 3.92 [10,32]. Summary relative risk estimates with corresponding 95% CIs were derived using the method of DerSimonian and Laird with the assumptions of a random-effects model, which considers both within-study and between-study variations [33]. When sex-specific estimates were available, we first analyzed together (as RR estimates for bladder cancer) and then separately (as RR estimates for bladder cancer in different gender groups).

To investigate the sources of heterogeneity in relative risk, we performed heterogeneity tests and sensitivity analysis. In assessing heterogeneity among studies, we used the Cochran Q test and I^2 statistics [34]. This was used to test whether the differences obtained between studies were due to chance. For the Q test, a p value of less than 0.05 was used as an indication of the presence of heterogeneity; for I^2, a value >50% is considered a measure of severe heterogeneity. To explore the potential heterogeneity between studies, we conducted analyses stratified by study design, geographic region, publication year, gender, and we also evaluated the impact of adjustment for smoking and body mass index (BMI) on the association between diabetes and the risk of bladder cancer. Sensitivity analysis was performed by excluding each study individually to assess its influence on the overall result of the meta-analysis.

Publication bias was evaluated using a funnel plot of a trial's effect size against the SE. Because funnel plots have several limitations and represent only an informal approach to detect publication bias, we further carried out formal testing using the test proposed by the Begg's adjusted rank correlation test and by the Egger's regression test [35,36]. All statistical analyses were performed using STATA version 11.0 (STATA, College Station, TX, USA). A two-tailed P value of less than 0.05 was considered to be statistically significant.

Results

Characteristics in Selected Studies

The search strategy generated 258 citations, of which 72 were considered of potential value and the full text was retrieved for detailed evaluation (**Figure 1**). Fifty-three of these 72 articles were subsequently excluded from the systematic review. 50 studies did not satisfy inclusion criteria. Two cohort studies were excluded because they presented a relationship between bladder cancer and type 1 DM [37,38]. Another one study was also excluded because it presented results on an association of DM and mortality of urinary system diseases, but not specific for the association between diabetes and risk of bladder cancer [39]. Additional eight articles were included from reference review. Thus, a total of 27 articles (29 studies), which met the inclusion and exclusion criteria, were used in this meta-analysis.

Of these 29 cohort studies which reported an association between diabetes and risk of bladder cancer, 20 studies employed incidence and/or mortality rates as the measurement of RR (**Table S1**) [40,41,42,16,18,19,20,21,23,43,15,17,22,44,25,26,27,28,29], and nine studies used SIR/SMR as the measurement of RR (**Table S2**) [45,46,47,24,48,49,50,30]. Eight studies were conducted in North America, 11 in Europe, eight in Asia, and two in multiple countries. The study population in 24 studies consisted of men and women, four studies consisted entirely of men and one study included women only.

DM was determined mainly on the basis of blood glucose levels, medical records, hospital discharge diagnosis in most studies and in four studies, the criteria for DM diagnosis was not indicated clearly [20,21,49,30]. Bladder cancer diagnosis was made by

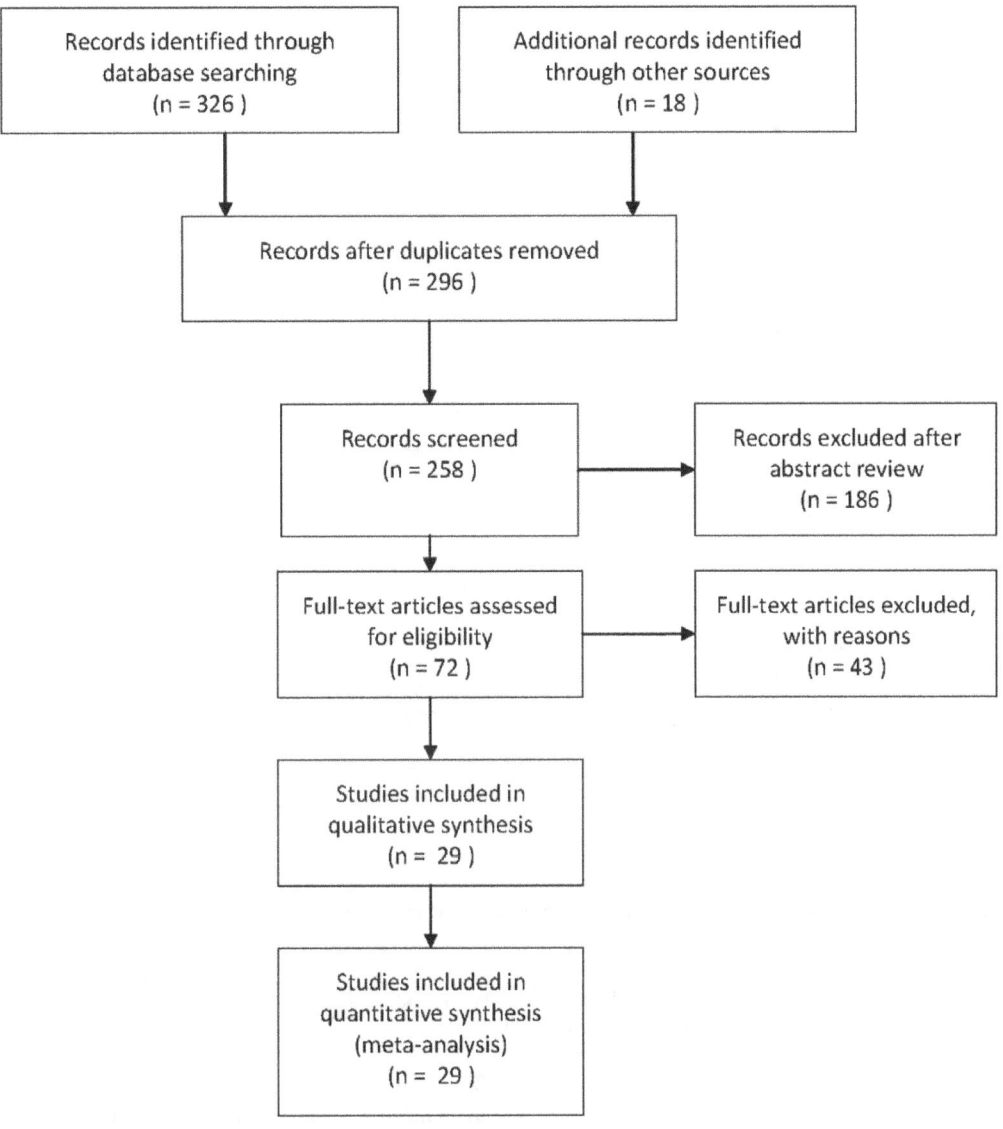

Figure 1. Flow chart on the articles selection process.

cancer registry or death certificate, except for three studies in which the method of outcome ascertainment was not available [21,27,49]. Potential confounders were controlled in most of the studies, except in 10 studies [17,45,46,47,24,48,49,50,48,30], the confounders adjusted for were not indicated clearly.

DM and Bladder Cancer Incidence

We identified 18 cohort studies that reported results on diabetes and bladder cancer incidence (**Tables S1, S2**). As shown in **Figure 2**, the summary RR was 1.29 (95% CI 1.08–1.54) in a random-effects model for diabetic patients, compared with individuals without DM. There was significant heterogeneity among these studies (Q = 331.00, P<0.001, I^2 = 94.9%).

In a sensitivity analysis in which we removed one study at a time and analyzed the rest, the RRs ranged from 1.32 (95% CI 1.09–1.60) after excluding the study by Atchison et al. [15] (the study which carried the most weight) to 1.30 (95% CI 1.08–1.56) after excluding the study by Khan et al. [42] (the study which carried the least weight).

In analysis stratified by study design, the summary RR was 1.36 (95% CI 1.04–1.78) in cohort studies. However, diabetes was not associated with bladder cancer incidence in cohort studies of diabetic patients (RR 1.12, 95% CI 0.91–1.37). The summary estimates were significantly higher for studies conducted in Asia and North America than in Europe, and for studies published in 2006 or later than for studies published before 2006. The positive association between diabetes and bladder cancer incidence was observed in the men (RR 1.36, 95% CI 1.05–1.77), but not in the women (RR 1.28, 95% CI 0.75–2.19) (**Table 1**).

We also investigated the impact of confounding factors on the estimates of relative risk. When we restricted the meta-analysis to those studies controlled for smoking, the positive association between diabetes and bladder cancer incidence remained (RR 1.33, 95% CI 1.19–1.47). The summary estimates were similar for studies that adjusted for BMI and for studies that did not. There was statistically significant heterogeneity within most subgroups.

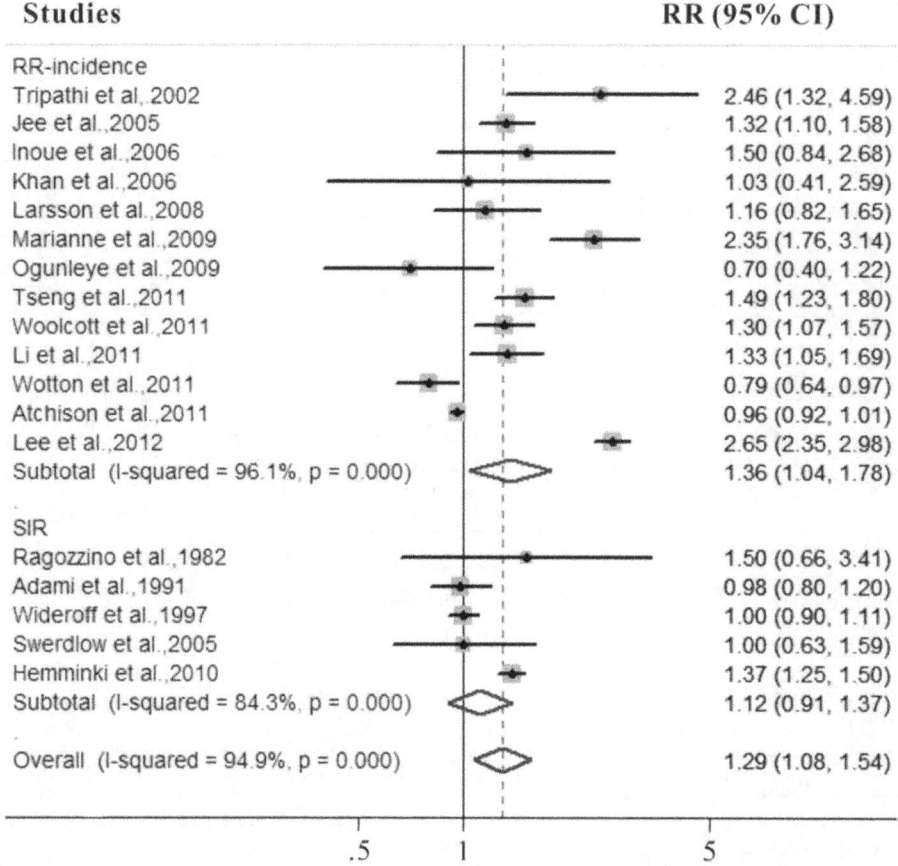

Figure 2. Forest plots of bladder cancer incidence/standard incidence rate associated with diabetes.

DM and Bladder Cancer Mortality

We identified 11 cohort studies that presented results on diabetes and mortality from bladder cancer (**Tables S1, S2**). As shown in **Figure 3**, the summary RR was 1.33 (95% CI 1.14–1.55) in a random-effects model for diabetic patients, compared with individuals without DM. There was significant heterogeneity among these studies (Q = 27.26, $P = 0.002$, $I^2 = 63.3\%$).

In the sensitivity analysis, our analysis confirmed the stability of the positive association between DM and mortality from bladder cancer. For example, when we excluded the study of Liu et al. [28] from the analysis (this was the study that clearly carried the most weight), the estimated pooled RR was similar (RR 1.33, 95% CI 1.09–1.63), with significant heterogeneity ($P = 0.001$, $I^2 = 66.5\%$).

In analysis stratified by study design, the summary RR was 1.29 (95% CI 1.20–1.39) in cohort studies. However, diabetes was not associated with mortality from bladder cancer in cohort studies of diabetic patients (RR 1.19, 95% CI 0.58–2.43). The summary estimates were higher for studies conducted in Asia than in other region and for studies published in 2006 or later than for studies published before 2006. Three studies provided results on cancer mortality specific for gender; additional two studies consisted entirely of men. Diabetes was associated with an increased mortality from bladder cancer in both males and females (RR = 1.54, 95% CI 1.30–1.82 in males, and RR = 1.50, 95% CI 1.05–2.14 in females, respectively) (**Table 2**).

When we restricted the meta-analysis to those studies controlled for smoking, a significant positive association was found between diabetes and mortality from bladder cancer (RR 1.29, 95% CI 1.19–1.39). The summary estimates were also significantly higher

for studies that reported BMI-adjusted RRs than for those which did not [RR (95% CI): 1.35 (1.23–1.49) versus 1.31 (0.97–1.76)].

Publication Bias

There was no funnel plot asymmetry for the association between DM and risk of bladder cancer. P values for Begg's adjusted rank correlation test was 0.268 and the Egger's regression asymmetry test was 0.139, suggesting a low probability of publication bias (**Figure 4**).

Discussion

Findings of this meta-analysis of cohort studies indicated that compared with non-diabetics or general population, individuals with diabetes may have more than 29% increased incidence of bladder cancer. However, the positive association was only observed in men. Of note, diabetes is associated with an increased mortality from bladder cancer in both males and females.

The previous meta-analysis has evaluated the association of diabetes and risk of bladder cancer. Most studies included in the meta-analysis were performed in Western countries, and only one study was conducted in the Asian population in Korea [14]. Moreover, the association in different gender groups is worthy of investigation, but has not been looked at. On account of the dismal prognosis, this meta-analysis extracted mortality rate as a substitution for incidence rate in several studies. However, the association between diabetes and mortality from bladder cancer is unclear.

Table 1. Summary relative risks for the association between diabetes and bladder cancer incidence/SIR.

Subgroup	No. of studies	RR (95% CI)	Tests	for	heterogeneity
			Q	P	I^2 (%)
Study design					
DM-free as controls	13	1.36 (1.04–1.78)	304.98	0.000	96.1
Population as controls	5	1.12 (0.91–1.37)	25.53	0.000	84.3
Geographical region					
Europe	7	1.01 (0.84–1.22)	40.61	0.000	85.2
North America	6	1.49 (1.08–2.05)	57.41	0.000	91.3
Asia	5	1.61 (1.09–2.38)	54.40	0.000	92.6
Publication year					
1970–2005	6	1.16 (0.96–1.40)	15.41	0.009	67.6
2006–2012	12	1.32 (1.03–1.69)	311.80	0.000	96.5
Gender					
Male	10	1.36 (1.05–1.77)	190.22	0.000	95.3
Female	6	1.28 (0.75–2.19)	78.04	0.000	93.6
Adjustment for smoking					
Yes	7	1.33 (1.19–1.47)	4.83	0.565	0.0
No	11	1.24 (0.98–1.58)	318.26	0.000	96.9
Adjustment for BMI, yes					
Yes	5	1.30 (0.95–1.77)	17.52	0.002	77.2
No	13	1.28 (1.03–1.59)	216.39	0.000	94.5

RR relative risk, CI confidence interval, DM diabetes mellitus, BMI body mass index.

Our study extends previous meta-analysis by providing a more precise estimate of the association between diabetes and risk of bladder cancer risk (based on 29 cohort studies). Case-control studies are susceptible to recall and selection biases which might inflate the RRs. Most of the included original studies were prospective, which probably do not reduce so much the possibility of reverse causation if a rather long time interval (at least 1 year) between inclusion and cancer diagnosis is not required. Moreover, we also investigated the impact of confounding factors, including smoking and BMI, on the estimates of relative risk.

Studies investigating the association between diabetes mellitus and cancer have reported inconsistent findings. Ogunleye and colleagues found that significantly increased risks were only observed for pancreatic, liver and colon cancer [20]. Wotton et al. demonstrated that diabetes mellitus was associated with an elevated risk of cancers of the liver, pancreas and uterus [23]. It has also been suggested that DM is a cancer preventive agent in some studies. There were significantly low rate ratios for cancer of the prostate and non-melanoma skin cancer in people admitted to hospital for diabetes mellitus when aged 30 or older [23]. Zhang et al. also observed that diabetes mellitus was associated with decreased incidence of prostate cancer, specifically in the population of the United States [51]. In overweight and obese patients with type 2 diabetes, lower androgen levels could explain a potentially protective effect against prostate cancer [52].

These inconsistent results may be due to different study population and follow-up periods. Furthermore, therapeutic agents used in the treatment have been also implicated in altering cancer risk [53,54]. Metformin therapy in diabetic patients appears to be associated with a significantly lower risk of cancer incidence and mortality [55,56,57]. Colmers et al. found that use of thiazolidinediones (TZDs) was associated with a modest but

significantly decreased risk of lung, colorectal and breast cancers [58]. However, TZDs were associated with an increased risk of bladder cancer among adults with type 2 diabetes [59]. The important outstanding prognostic question is whether diabetes mellitus is associated with an increased or a reduced risk of certain cancer. Noteworthy, it is possible to draw more accurate conclusions in a larger cohort of diabetic patients by conducting meta-analysis of the studies published on the subject.

This study has several limitations which should be recognized. First, cohort studies, which may not be prone to recall bias but are prone to selection bias because patients with diabetes are under increased medical surveillance. This bias may distort the true effects.

Second, diabetes in some studies was based on self-report, which may result in misclassification of diabetic persons as non-diabetic persons. This underestimation would tend to attenuate any true association between diabetes and risk of bladder cancer.

Third, great heterogeneity exists in terms of study design, geographical region, publication year, gender and adjustment for confounding factors. Despite the use of appropriate meta-analytic techniques with random-effect models, we could not account for these differences.

Fourth, most studies included in this meta-analysis did not consider the role of anti-diabetic drugs in bladder cancer. For example, increasing studies have suggested that use of pioglitazone (a common anti-diabetic drug) was associated with an increased incidence of bladder cancer [60,61]. In our meta-analysis, the association between diabetes and incidence of bladder cancer was weaker in women than in men. Neumann observed a significant association between pioglitazone and bladder cancer for men but not women [62]. Noteworthy, pioglitazone use might be also involved in such a sex discrepancy. However, only a few studies

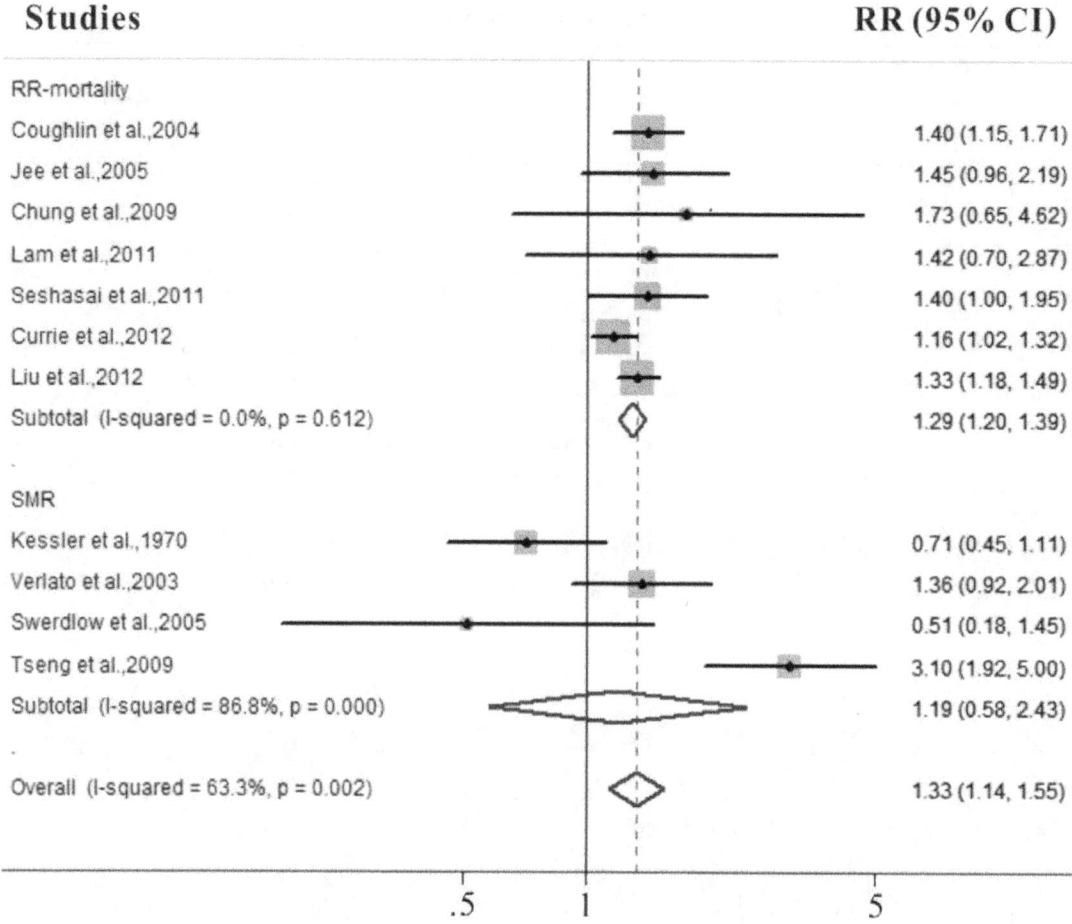

Studies   **RR (95% CI)**

RR-mortality

Coughlin et al.,2004   1.40 (1.15, 1.71)

Jee et al.,2005   1.45 (0.96, 2.19)

Chung et al.,2009   1.73 (0.65, 4.62)

Lam et al.,2011   1.42 (0.70, 2.87)

Seshasai et al.,2011   1.40 (1.00, 1.95)

Currie et al.,2012   1.16 (1.02, 1.32)

Liu et al.,2012   1.33 (1.18, 1.49)

Subtotal (I-squared = 0.0%, p = 0.612)   1.29 (1.20, 1.39)

SMR

Kessler et al.,1970   0.71 (0.45, 1.11)

Verlato et al.,2003   1.36 (0.92, 2.01)

Swerdlow et al.,2005   0.51 (0.18, 1.45)

Tseng et al.,2009   3.10 (1.92, 5.00)

Subtotal (I-squared = 86.8%, p = 0.000)   1.19 (0.58, 2.43)

Overall (I-squared = 63.3%, p = 0.002)   1.33 (1.14, 1.55)

.5   1   5

Figure 3. Forest plots of bladder cancer mortality/standard mortality rate associated with diabetes.

adjusted for anti-diabetic drugs. Fifth, confounding cannot be fully excluded as a potential explanation for the observed association, because these two diseases share several risk factors, such as smoking and obesity. In our meta-analysis, adjustment for smoking and BMI significantly alter the relationship between diabetes and risk of bladder cancer.

Finally, inherent in any meta-analysis of published data is the possibility of publication bias, that is small studies with null results tend not to be published. Publication bias may have resulted in an overestimate of the relationship between DM and risk of bladder cancer. However, the results obtained from funnel plot analysis and formal statistical tests did not provide evidence for such bias.

The possible mechanisms underlying the association of diabetes with bladder cancer risk are still uncertain. Insulin has been hypothesized to be a cancer growth promoter which could explain an increased cancer risk in adults with type 2 diabetes [63,64]. Elevated insulin concentrations would lower concentrations of IGF-binding proteins (IGFBPs), which in turn contribute to an up-regulated level of IGFs. In the circulation, IGF-I binds mainly to IGFBP-3 and stimulates cell proliferation and inhibits apoptosis [65]. Emerging evidence indicates that IGF-I and IGFBP-3 may also play a role in the development of bladder cancer. In a US case-control study, patients with bladder cancer have higher plasma levels of IGF-1 and lower levels of IGFBP-3 than controls [66]. Dunn and colleagues demonstrated that IGF-I could contribute to bladder carcinogenesis in animal studies [67]. Moreover, a lower preoperative plasma IGFBP-3 level was

associated with metastases to regional lymph nodes, bladder cancer progression, and survival [68].

Although the absolute risk of bladder cancer is low among diabetic individuals, our results have important clinical and public health significance. As a serious and growing health problem in USA, DM affects nearly 25.8 million children and adults in the United States, 8.3% of the U.S.population in 2010 (http://www. diabetes.org/diabetes-basics/diabetes-statistics/). In China, the age-standardized prevalences of total diabetes and prediabetes among Chinese adults (20 years of age or older) are 9.7 and 15.5%, respectively [69]. Due to growing obesity epidemic, the prevalence of diabetes will probably increase and contribute to the risk of bladder cancer among diabetic patients. In patients with non-muscle invasive bladder cancer, DM was found to be an independent factor for recurrence- and progression-free survival [70]. For diabetic patients undergoing radical cystoprostatectomy and ileal orthotopic bladder substitution, it takes longer to regain daytime and nighttime continence than nondiabetic patients [71]. In clinical practice, the diabetic patients should be informed of the potential negative impact of DM on disease recurrence, progression, survival and the recovery of urinary continence after an ileal orthotopic bladder substitution.

In conclusion, this meta-analysis supports the hypothesis that diabetic individuals have an increased incidence of bladder cancer. Further analysis indicates that the positive relation is observed only in the men, but not in the women. However, diabetes is associated with an increased mortality from bladder cancer in both males and

Table 2. Summary relative risks for the association between diabetes and bladder cancer mortality/SMR.

Subgroup	No. of studies	RR (95% CI)	Tests	for	heterogeneity
			Q	P	I^2 (%)
Study design					
DM-free as controls	7	1.29 (1.20–1.39)	4.48	0.612	0.0
Population as controls	4	1.19 (0.58–2.43)	22.75	0.000	86.8
Geographical region					
North America	4	1.03 (0.53–2.00)	7.35	0.007	86.4
Europe	2	1.25 (1.15–1.36)	5.38	0.146	44.2
Asia	3	1.98 (1.47–2.66)	5.64	0.060	64.5
Other[a]	2	1.40 (1.04–1.89)	0.00	0.971	0.0
Publication year					
1970–2005	5	1.15 (0.85–1.55)	10.81	0.029	63.0
2006–2012	6	1.45 (1.18–1.78)	16.39	0.006	69.5
Gender					
Men	5	1.54 (1.30–1.82)	7.34	0.119	45.5
Women	3	1.50 (1.05–2.14)	2.44	0.296	17.9
Adjustment for smoking					
Yes	5	1.29 (1.19–1.39)	4.06	0.398	1.5
No	6	1.30 (0.77–2.18)	23.05	0.000	78.3
Adjustment for BMI					
Yes	3	1.35 (1.23–1.49)	0.24	0.888	0.0
No	8	1.31 (0.97–1.76)	25.1	0.001	72.1

RR relative risk, CI confidence interval, DM diabetes mellitus, BMI body mass index.
[a]One study conducted in Asia-Pacific region, the other study conducted in North America, Europe, Japan and other region.

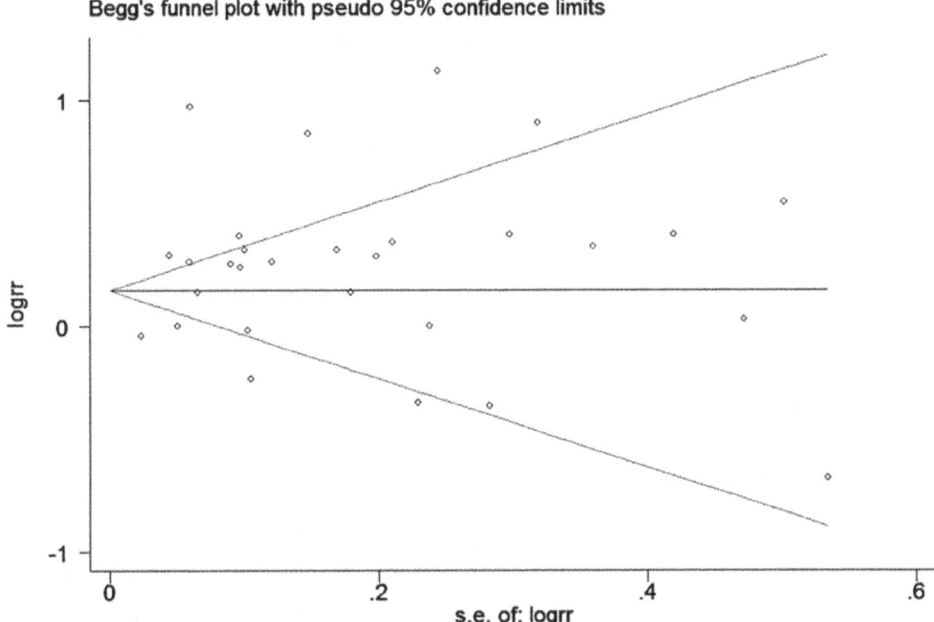

Figure 4. Funnel plot of cohort studies evaluating the association between diabetes and bladder cancer risk.

females. More research, both epidemiological and mechanistic, is warranted to clarify the association between diabetes and risk of bladder cancer.

Supporting Information

Figure S1 Quality scores of cohort studies of diabetes and bladder cancer risk based on rate/hazard ratio.

Figure S2 Quality scores of cohort studies of diabetes and bladder cancer risk based on standardized incidence/mortality ratio.

Table S1 Characteristics of 20 cohort studies of diabetes and bladder cancer risk based on rate/hazard ratio.

Table S2 Characteristics of 9 cohort studies of diabetes and bladder cancer risk based on standardized incidence/mortality ratio.

Diagram S1 PRISMA (Preferred Reporting Items for Systematic Reviews and Meta-Analyses) flow diagram.

Checklist S1 PRISMA (Preferred Reporting Items for Systematic Reviews and Meta-Analyses) checklist.

Author Contributions

Conceived and designed the experiments: ZS YL CX. Performed the experiments: ZZ XZ. Analyzed the data: ZZ XZ. Contributed reagents/materials/analysis tools: XZ SZ. Wrote the paper: ZZ XZ XW.

References

1. Siegel R, Naishadham D, Jemal A (2012) Cancer statistics, 2012. CA Cancer J Clin 62: 10–29.
2. Pira E, Piolatto G, Negri E, Romano C, Boffetta P, et al. (2010) Bladder cancer mortality of workers exposed to aromatic amines: a 58-year follow-up. J Natl Cancer Inst 102: 1096–1099.
3. Bulbulyan MA, Figgs LW, Zahm SH, Savitskaya T, Goldfarb A, et al. (1995) Cancer incidence and mortality among beta-naphthylamine and benzidine dye workers in Moscow. Int J Epidemiol 24: 266–275.
4. Behrens T, Schill W, Ahrens W (2009) Elevated cancer mortality in a German cohort of bitumen workers: extended follow-up through 2004. J Occup Environ Hyg 6: 555–561.
5. Ferrucci LM, Sinha R, Ward MH, Graubard BI, Hollenbeck AR, et al. (2010) Meat and components of meat and the risk of bladder cancer in the NIH-AARP Diet and Health Study. Cancer 116: 4345–4353.
6. Guha N, Steenland NK, Merletti F, Altieri A, Cogliano V, et al. (2010) Bladder cancer risk in painters: a meta-analysis. Occup Environ Med 67: 568–573.
7. Fernandez MI, Lopez JF, Vivaldi B, Coz F (2012) Long-term impact of arsenic in drinking water on bladder cancer health care and mortality rates 20 years after end of exposure. J Urol 187: 856–861.
8. Freedman ND, Silverman DT, Hollenbeck AR, Schatzkin A, Abnet CC (2011) Association between smoking and risk of bladder cancer among men and women. JAMA 306: 737–745.
9. Zimmet P, Alberti KG, Shaw J (2001) Global and societal implications of the diabetes epidemic. Nature 414: 782–787.
10. Ben Q, Xu M, Ning X, Liu J, Hong S, et al. (2011) Diabetes mellitus and risk of pancreatic cancer: A meta-analysis of cohort studies. Eur J Cancer 47: 1928–1937.
11. Wang C, Wang X, Gong G, Ben Q, Qiu W, et al. (2012) Increased risk of hepatocellular carcinoma in patients with diabetes mellitus: a systematic review and meta-analysis of cohort studies. Int J Cancer 130: 1639–1648.
12. Larsson SC, Wolk A (2011) Diabetes mellitus and incidence of kidney cancer: a meta-analysis of cohort studies. Diabetologia 54: 1013–1018.
13. Yuhara H, Steinmaus C, Cohen SE, Corley DA, Tei Y, et al. (2011) Is diabetes mellitus an independent risk factor for colon cancer and rectal cancer. Am J Gastroenterol 106: 1911–1921; quiz 1922.
14. Larsson SC, Orsini N, Brismar K, Wolk A (2006) Diabetes mellitus and risk of bladder cancer: a meta-analysis. Diabetologia 49: 2819–2823.
15. Atchison EA, Gridley G, Carreon JD, Leitzmann MF, McGlynn KA (2011) Risk of cancer in a large cohort of U.S. veterans with diabetes. Int J Cancer 128: 635–643.
16. Larsson SC, Andersson SO, Johansson JE, Wolk A (2008) Diabetes mellitus, body size and bladder cancer risk in a prospective study of Swedish men. Eur J Cancer 44: 2655–2660.
17. Lee MY, Lin KD, Hsiao PJ, Shin SJ (2012) The association of diabetes mellitus with liver, colon, lung, and prostate cancer is independent of hypertension, hyperlipidemia, and gout in Taiwanese patients. Metabolism 61: 242–249.
18. Li C, Balluz LS, Ford ES, Okoro CA, Tsai J, et al. (2011) Association between diagnosed diabetes and self-reported cancer among U.S. adults: findings from the 2009 Behavioral Risk Factor Surveillance System. Diabetes Care 34: 1365–1368.
19. Marianne UY, Susan AO, Ulka BC, Carol EK (2009) Incidence of cancer in a population-based cohort of patients with type 2 diabetes. Diabetes Metabolic Syndrome 3: 12–16.
20. Ogunleye AA, Ogston SA, Morris AD, Evans JM (2009) A cohort study of the risk of cancer associated with type 2 diabetes. Br J Cancer 101: 1199–1201.
21. Tseng CH (2011) Diabetes and risk of bladder cancer: a study using the National Health Insurance database in Taiwan. Diabetologia 54: 2009–2015.
22. Woolcott CG, Maskarinec G, Haiman CA, Henderson BE, Kolonel LN (2011) Diabetes and urothelial cancer risk: the Multiethnic Cohort Study. Cancer Epidemiol 35: 551–554.
23. Wotton CJ, Yeates DG, Goldacre MJ (2011) Cancer in patients admitted to hospital with diabetes mellitus aged 30 years and over: record linkage studies. Diabetologia 54: 527–534.
24. Hemminki K, Li X, Sundquist J, Sundquist K (2010) Risk of cancer following hospitalization for type 2 diabetes. Oncologist 15: 548–555.
25. Chung H (2009) Diabetes and risk of death from cancer of the prostate, kidney, and urinary bladder. Urology 74: S36–S37.
26. Currie CJ, Poole CD, Jenkins-Jones S, Gale EA, Johnson JA, et al. (2012) Mortality After Incident Cancer in People With and Without Type 2 Diabetes:Impact of metformin on survival. Diabetes Care 35: 299–304.
27. Lam EK, Batty GD, Huxley RR, Martiniuk AL, Barzi F, et al. (2011) Associations of diabetes mellitus with site-specific cancer mortality in the Asia-Pacific region. Ann Oncol 22: 730–738.
28. Liu X, Ji J, Sundquist K, Sundquist J, Hemminki K (2012) The impact of type 2 diabetes mellitus on cancer-specific survival: A follow-up study in sweden. Cancer 118: 1353–1361.
29. Seshasai SR, Kaptoge S, Thompson A, Di AE, Gao P, et al. (2011) Diabetes mellitus, fasting glucose, and risk of cause-specific death. N Engl J Med 364: 829–841.
30. Tseng CH, Chong CK, Tseng CP, Chan TT (2009) Age-related risk of mortality from bladder cancer in diabetic patients: a 12-year follow-up of a national cohort in Taiwan. Ann Med 41: 371–379.
31. Stroup DF, Berlin JA, Morton SC, Olkin I, Williamson GD, et al. (2000) Meta-analysis of observational studies in epidemiology: a proposal for reporting.Meta-analysis Of Observational Studies in Epidemiology (MOOSE) group. JAMA 283: 2008–2012.
32. Jiang Y, Ben Q, Shen H, Lu W, Zhang Y, et al. (2011) Diabetes mellitus and incidence and mortality of colorectal cancer: a systematic review and meta-analysis of cohort studies. Eur J Epidemiol 26: 863–876.
33. DerSimonian R, Laird N (1986) Meta-analysis in clinical trials. Control Clin Trials 7: 177–188.
34. Higgins JP, Thompson SG (2002) Quantifying heterogeneity in a meta-analysis. Stat Med 21: 1539–1558.
35. Begg CB, Mazumdar M (1994) Operating characteristics of a rank correlation test for publication bias. Biometrics 50: 1088–1101.
36. Egger M, Davey SG, Schneider M, Minder C (1997) Bias in meta-analysis detected by a simple, graphical test. BMJ 315: 629–634.
37. Zendehdel K, Nyren O, Ostenson CG, Adami HO, Ekbom A, et al. (2003) Cancer incidence in patients with type 1 diabetes mellitus: a population-basedcohort study in Sweden. J Natl Cancer Inst 95: 1797–1800.
38. Shu X, Ji J, Li X, Sundquist J, Sundquist K, et al. (2010) Cancer risk among patients hospitalized for Type 1 diabetes mellitus: a population-based cohort study in Sweden. Diabet Med 27: 791–797.
39. Liu X, Ji J, Sundquist K, Sundquist J, Hemminki K (2012) Mortality causes in cancer patients with type 2 diabetes mellitus. Eur J Cancer Prev 21: 300–306.
40. Tripathi A, Folsom AR, Anderson KE (2002) Risk factors for urinary bladder carcinoma in postmenopausal women. The Iowa Women's Health Study. Cancer 95: 2316–2323.
41. Inoue M, Iwasaki M, Otani T, Sasazuki S, Noda M, et al. (2006) Diabetes mellitus and the risk of cancer: results from a large-scale population-based cohort study in Japan. Arch Intern Med 166: 1871–1877.
42. Khan M, Mori M, Fujino Y, Shibata A, Sakauchi F, et al. (2006) Site-specific cancer risk due to diabetes mellitus history: evidence from the Japan Collaborative Cohort (JACC) Study. Asian Pac J Cancer Prev 7: 253–259.
43. Jee SH, Ohrr H, Sull JW, Yun JE, Ji M, et al. (2005) Fasting serum glucose level and cancer risk in Korean men and women. JAMA 293: 194–202.

44. Coughlin SS, Calle EE, Teras LR, Petrelli J, Thun MJ (2004) Diabetes mellitus as a predictor of cancer mortality in a large cohort of US adults. Am J Epidemiol 159: 1160–1167.

45. Ragozzino M, Melton LJ 3rd, Chu CP, Palumbo PJ (1982) Subsequent cancer risk in the incidence cohort of Rochester, Minnesota, residents with diabetes mellitus. J Chronic Dis 35: 13–19.

46. Adami HO, McLaughlin J, Ekbom A, Berne C, Silverman D, et al. (1991) Cancer risk in patients with diabetes mellitus. Cancer Causes Control 2: 307–314.

47. Wideroff L, Gridley G, Mellemkjaer L, Chow WH, Linet M, et al. (1997) Cancer incidence in a population-based cohort of patients hospitalized with diabetes mellitus in Denmark. J Natl Cancer Inst 89: 1360–1365.

48. Swerdlow AJ, Laing SP, Qiao Z, Slater SD, Burden AC, et al. (2005) Cancer incidence and mortality in patients with insulin-treated diabetes: a UK cohort study. Br J Cancer 92: 2070–2075.

49. Kessler II (1970) Cancer mortality among diabetics. J Natl Cancer Inst 44: 673–686.

50. Verlato G, Zoppini G, Bonora E, Muggeo M (2003) Mortality from site-specific malignancies in type 2 diabetic patients from Verona(Italy). Diabetes Care 26: 1047–1051.

51. Zhang F, Yang Y, Skrip L, Hu D, Wang Y, et al. (2012) Diabetes mellitus and risk of prostate cancer: an updated meta-analysis based on 12 case-control and 25 cohort studies. Acta Diabetol 49 Suppl 1: 235–246.

52. Corona G, Monami M, Rastrelli G, Aversa A, Sforza A, et al. (2011) Type 2 diabetes mellitus and testosterone: a meta-analysis study. Int J Androl 34: 528–540.

53. Libby G, Donnelly LA, Donnan PT, Alessi DR, Morris AD, et al. (2009) New users of metformin are at low risk of incident cancer: a cohort study among people with type 2 diabetes. Diabetes Care 32: 1620–1625.

54. Colhoun HM (2009) Use of insulin glargine and cancer incidence in Scotland: a study from the Scottish Diabetes Research Network Epidemiology Group. Diabetologia 52: 1755–1765.

55. Zhang ZJ, Zheng ZJ, Kan H, Song Y, Cui W, et al. (2011) Reduced risk of colorectal cancer with metformin therapy in patients with type 2 diabetes: a meta-analysis. Diabetes Care 34: 2323–2328.

56. Noto H, Goto A, Tsujimoto T, Noda M (2012) Cancer risk in diabetic patients treated with metformin: a systematic review and meta-analysis. PLOS ONE 7: e33411.

57. Soranna D, Scotti L, Zambon A, Bosetti C, Grassi G, et al. (2012) Cancer risk associated with use of metformin and sulfonylurea in type 2 diabetes: a meta-analysis. Oncologist 17: 813–822.

58. Colmers IN, Bowker SL, Johnson JA (2012) Thiazolidinedione use and cancer incidence in type 2 diabetes: A systematic review and meta-analysis. Diabetes Metab 38: 475–484.

59. Colmers IN, Bowker SL, Majumdar SR, Johnson JA (2012) Use of thiazolidinediones and the risk of bladder cancer among people with type 2 diabetes: a meta-analysis. CMAJ 184: E675–683.

60. Lewis JD, Ferrara A, Peng T, Hedderson M, Bilker WB, et al. (2011) Risk of bladder cancer among diabetic patients treated with pioglitazone: interim report of a longitudinal cohort study. Diabetes Care 34: 916–922.

61. Piccinni C, Motola D, Marchesini G, Poluzzi E (2011) Assessing the association of pioglitazone use and bladder cancer through drug adverse event reporting. Diabetes Care 34: 1369–1371.

62. Neumann A, Weill A, Ricordeau P, Fagot JP, Alla F, et al. (2012) Pioglitazone and risk of bladder cancer among diabetic patients in France: a population-based cohort study. Diabetologia 55: 1953–1962.

63. Vigneri P, Frasca F, Sciacca L, Pandini G, Vigneri R (2009) Diabetes and cancer. Endocr Relat Cancer 16: 1103–1123.

64. Vigneri R (2009) Diabetes: diabetes therapy and cancer risk. Nat Rev Endocrinol 5: 651–652.

65. Jones JI, Clemmons DR (1995) Insulin-like growth factors and their binding proteins: biological actions. Endocr Rev 16: 3–34.

66. Zhao H, Grossman HB, Spitz MR, Lerner SP, Zhang K, et al. (2003) Plasma levels of insulin-like growth factor-1 and binding protein-3, and their association with bladder cancer risk. J Urol 169: 714–717.

67. Dunn SE, Kari FW, French J, Leininger JR, Travlos G, et al. (1997) Dietary restriction reduces insulin-like growth factor I levels, which modulates apoptosis, cell proliferation, and tumor progression in p53-deficient mice. Cancer Res 57: 4667–4672.

68. Shariat SF, Kim J, Nguyen C, Wheeler TM, Lerner SP, et al. (2003) Correlation of preoperative levels of IGF-I and IGFBP-3 with pathologic parameters and clinical outcome in patients with bladder cancer. Urology 61: 359–364.

69. Yang W, Lu J, Weng J, Jia W, Ji L, et al. (2010) Prevalence of diabetes among men and women in China. N Engl J Med 362: 1090–1101.

70. Hwang EC, Kim YJ, Hwang IS, Hwang JE, Jung SI, et al. (2011) Impact of diabetes mellitus on recurrence and progression in patients with non-muscle invasive bladder carcinoma: a retrospective cohort study. Int J Urol 18: 769–776.

71. Kessler TM, Ochsner K, Studer UE, Thalmann GN (2008) Diabetes mellitus: does it impair urinary continence after radical cystoprostatectomy and ileal orthotopic bladder substitution. Eur Urol 53: 1040–1046.

6

Multifactorial, Site-Specific Recurrence Models after Radical Cystectomy for Urothelial Carcinoma: External Validation in a Cohort of Korean Patients

Hyung Suk Kim, Myong Kim, Chang Wook Jeong, Cheol Kwak, Hyeon Hoe Kim, Ja Hyeon Ku*

Department of Urology, Seoul National University College of Medicine, Seoul, Korea

Abstract

Purpose: The aim of this study was to evaluate the accuracy of site-specific recurrence models after radical cystectomy in the Korean population.

Materials and Methods: We conducted a review of an electronic medical record of 572 patients who underwent radical cystectomy for urothelial carcinoma of the bladder. Primary end point was the site-specific recurrence after radical cystectomy.

Results: The median follow-up in the validation cohort was 42.3 months (interquartile range: 23.0–89.3 months). During the follow-up period, there were 165 patients (28.8%), 85 (14.9%), 31 (5.4%), and 78 (13.6%) who recurred in abdomen/pelvis, thoracic region, upper urinary tract, and bone, respectively. The c-indices of abdomen/pelvis, thoracic region, upper urinary tract, and bone models 3 years after radical cystectomy were 0.69 (95% confidence interval [CI], 0.65–0.73), 0.69 (95% CI, 0.64–0.75), 0.61 (95% CI, 0.52–0.69), and 0.65 (95% CI, 0.59–0.71), respectively. Kaplan-Meier curves demonstrated that models discriminated well and log-rank test were all highly significant (all $p < 0.001$), except upper urinary tract model ($p = 0.366$). Decision curve analysis revealed that the use of prediction models for abdomen/pelvis, thoracic region, and bone recurrence was associated with net benefit gains relative to the treat-all strategy, but not the model for upper urinary tract recurrence.

Conclusions: Abdomen/pelvis, thoracic region, and bone models demonstrate moderate discrimination, adequate calibration, and meaningful net benefit gains, whereas upper urinary tract model does not seem applicable to patients from Asia because it has suboptimal accuracy.

Editor: Bart O. Williams, Van Andel Institute, United States of America

Funding: The authors have no support or funding to report.

Competing Interests: The authors have declared that no competing interests exist.

* E-mail: kuuro70@snu.ac.kr

Introduction

It is estimated that 72,570 new cases of bladder cancer will be diagnosed and 15,210 patients will die of their disease in the United States in 2013 [1]. In Korea, 3,415 new cases of bladder cancer, which consist of 2,752 males and 663 females, was diagnosed and 1,100 bladder cancer related deaths occurred during 2010 [2]. At the time of diagnosis, 25–30% of bladder tumors are found to be muscle-invasive [3]. Radical cystectomy is the standard care treatment for patients with muscle-invasive and some patients with high-risk non-muscle invasive bladder cancer. Nevertheless, up to 50% of patients experience disease recurrence after radical cystectomy [4,5]. The aggressive natural behavior of disease recurrences after radical cystectomy results in poor prognosis [6]. Characterizing recurrence patterns after radical cystectomy is critical for patient counseling and developing evidence-based surveillance guidelines [7].

For tailoring patient-specific disease surveillance, scoring algorithms of site-specific disease recurrence after radical cystectomy have been designed [8]. Sites of disease recurrence in the study were classified into four locations; abdomen/pelvis, thoracic region, upper urinary tract, and bone. To our knowledge, no validation of models has been published to date in the literature to improve the decision-making ability of clinicians caring for patients. Furthermore, since the research of developing the models were entirely based on American population, the generalization of the models to external cohorts of patients with different characteristics is questionable.

The aim of this study was to evaluate the accuracy of site-specific recurrence models after radical cystectomy in the Korean population and to explore the applicability of the models in different clinical environment.

Table 1. Patient characteristics.

Characteristics	Development cohort	Validation cohort
Total	1388 (100)	572 (100)
Macroscopic hematuria	856 (62)	471 (82)
Occupational radiation exposure	26 (2)	0 (0)
Sex		
Men	1117 (80)	502 (88)
Women	271 (20)	70 (12)
Body mass index		
<20	39 (3)	74 (13)
20–25	418 (30)	335 (59)
25–30	644 (46)	147 (26)
30–35	225 (16)	9 (2)
>35	62 (5)	1 (0)
Unknown	0 (0)	6 (1)
Preoperative intravesical therapy	417 (30)	136 (24)
Pathologic tumor classification		
pT0	9 (1)	56 (10)
pTa	14 (1)	26 (5)
pTis	111 (8)	55 (10)
pT1	303 (22)	109 (19)
pT2	519 (37)	126 (22)
pT3	312 (22)	160 (28)
pT4	119 (9)	40 (7)
Lymph node status		
pNx	169 (12)	177 (31)
pN0, 1–10 lymph nodes	430 (31)	121 (21)
pN0, ≥11 lymph nodes	621 (45)	190 (33)
pN1/pN2	165 (12)	84 (15)
Synchronous carcinoma in situ	309 (22)	148 (26)
Multifocality	709 (51)	328 (57)
Urethral, ductal, or stromal prostatic involvement	133 (10)	75 (13)
Margin status		
Positive radical surgical margin	15 (1)	10 (2)
Positive urethral margin	37 (3)	17 (3)
Positive ureteral margin	30 (2)	23 (4)
Neoadjuvant chemotherapy	28 (2)	60 (11)
Adjuvant chemotherapy	72 (5)	139 (24)

Data presented are number of patients (%).

Materials and Methods

Ethics Statement

This study design and the use of patients' information stored in the hospital database were approved by the Institutional Review Board (IRB) at the Seoul National University Hospital. The approval number is H-1403-032-563. We were given exemption from getting informed consents by the IRB because the present study is a retrospective study and personal identifiers were completely removed and the data were analyzed anonymously. Our study was conducted according to the ethical standards laid down in the 1964 Declaration of Helsinki and its later amendments.

Study cohort

We conducted a review of an electronic medical record of all 622 patients who underwent radical cystectomy for bladder cancer at Seoul National University Hospital from January 2001 through December 2001. Our methods for surgery, pathology review, and follow-up have previously been described in detail [9]. Our exclusion criteria were non-urothelial carcinoma, presentation as distant metastasis, and no documentation of all variables as required by each model and/or unavailable pathology. Patients with detectable disease within 30 days of cystectomy were also excluded from the study because this was likely present at the time of cystectomy [8]. Therefore, the validation cohort comprised 572 patients. The demographic data for model development cohort in comparison to external validation cohort is shown in Table 1. Pathologic stage was determined according to the 2009 American Joint Committee on Cancer (AJCC) staging system. Therefore, we re-reviewed the pathologic stage of patients with pT4 in the 2002 AJCC staging system. Consistent with the 2009 AJCC staging system, tumors invading directly into the prostate from the bladder were defined as pT4a, whereas prostate urethra, ducts, and/or stromal involvement with urothelial carcinoma independent of the primary bladder tumor were evaluated separately [8].

Assessed outcomes

Primary end point was the site-specific recurrence after radical cystectomy. Disease recurrence to the abdomen/pelvis included local recurrence in the pelvis and distant metastasis within the abdomen. Disease recurrence to the thoracic region was defined as distant metastatic to the lungs, heart, and thoracic lymph nodes, including the mediastinal and paratracheal lymph nodes. The first recurrence to each location after cystectomy was analyzes [8].

Development of site-specific recurrence models

Abdomen/pelvis model provides a risk estimate of abdomen/pelvis recurrence based on four histopathological variables: primary tumor stage, regional lymph node and extent of lymph node dissection, multifocality, and prostatic invasion. Thoracic region model requires three histopathological variables: primary tumor stage, regional lymph node and extent of lymph node dissection, and multifocality. Upper urinary tract model is developed based on four clinicopathological variables: primary tumor stage, multifocality, positive ureteral margin, and gross hematuria. Bone model included five clinopathological variables: primary tumor stage, regional lymph node and extent of lymph node dissection, positive urethral margin, occupational radiation exposure, and body mass index. Scoring algorithms to predict the likelihood of disease recurrence in the abdomen/pelvis, thoracic region, upper urinary tract, and bone were applied. The scores assigned each predictor are shown in Table 2.

Statistical analysis

The predicted risk of site-specific recurrence was compared with the actual site-specific recurrence in the current study population at 3 years. We quantified the discrimination ability of each model by calculating the c-index, which is identical to the nonparametric area under the receiver operating characteristics curve [10]. A c-index of 1 indicates perfect concordance, whereas a c-index of 0.5 indicates a result equal to chance. The 95% confidence interval [CI] for each c-index was determined using a 1000-replicate bootstrap procedure. The performance of each model was also evaluated by drawing a time-dependent receiver operating characteristics curve and calculating the integrated area under the curve [11]. We plotted the Kaplan-Meier curves for freedom from site-specific recurrence, stratified by each model prediction. We conducted a decision curve analysis that was proposed by Vickers et al. [12] to assess the clinical usefulness of each model by quantifying the net benefits when different threshold probabilities were considered. Although the primary endpoint of this analysis was site-specific recurrence, overall survival also was evaluated as the secondary endpoints to better characterize the behavior of each model.

All test were two-sided and p values <0.05 were considered statically significant. Statistical analysis was performed using SPSS v.18.0 (SPSS, Chicago, IL, USA) and R, version 2.13.2 (R Foundation for Statistical Computing, Vienna, Austria).

Results

The median follow-up in the validation cohort for site-specific recurrence model was 42.3 months (interquartile range: 23.0–89.3 months). During the follow-up period, there were 165 patients (28.8%), 85 (14.9%), 31 (5.4%), and 78 (13.6%) who recurred in abdomen/pelvis, thoracic region, upper urinary tract, and bone, respectively. The 3-, 5-, and 8-year recurrence-free survival rates in abdomen/pelvis were 74.1%, 70.7%, and 67.3%, respectively. The 3-, 5-, and 8-year recurrence-free survival rates in thoracic region were 86.4%, 82.5%, and 80.8%, respectively. The 3-, 5-, and 8-year upper urinary tract recurrence-free survival rates were 95.8%, 92.2%, and 91.3%, respectively. The 3-, 5-, and 8-year bone recurrence-free survival rates were 87.8%, 83.9%, and 82.3%, respectively. Overall survival rates for the same time points were 70.8%, 61.2%, and 57.2%, respectively.

Discrimination estimates of each model are shown in Table 3. The c-indices of abdomen/pelvis, thoracic region, upper urinary tract, and bone models 3 years after radical cystectomy were 0.69 (95% CI, 0.65–0.73), 0.69 (95% CI, 0.64–0.75), 0.61 (95% CI, 0.52–0.69), and 0.65 (95% CI, 0.59–0.71), respectively. The c-indices of each model for 5-year overall survival were also <70%. In particular, the c-index of the upper urinary tract model was 0.56.

To determine the accuracy of the models over the course of a follow-up period, we completed a concordance summary (integrated area under the curve). For time to recurrence for patients, integrated area under the curve values of all models were less than 70%. In particular, those of the upper urinary tract model for 3-year site-specific recurrence and 5-year overall survival were 0.61 and 0.57, respectively.

In Kaplan-Meier curves for patients stratified into groups from each model, patients were clustered into three or five groups according to their model-predicted recurrence. As depicted,

Table 2. Site-specific risk stratification.

	Risk score	Risk stratification
Abdomen/pelvis	pT3 (3), pT4 (4), pNx (2), pN0 and 1–10 LN (1), pN+ (2), multifocality (2), prostatic invasion (1)	0/1–2/3/4–5/6+
Thoracic region	pT3 (4), pT4 (5), pNx (3), pN0 and 1–10 LN (2), pN+ (4), multifocality (2)	0–3/4/5–7/8–9/10+
Upper tract	pT4 (3), multifocality (2), positive ureteral margin (5), gross hematuria (−2)	−2–0/1–2/3+
Bone	pT3 (4), pT4 (4), pN+ (2), positive urethral margin (3), occupational radiation exposure (4), BMI >30 (−2)	−2/0/1–3/4–5/6+

Table 3. Discrimination estimates (c-indices) of risk prediction models for site-specific recurrence.

	Discrimination (95% confidence interval)	
	3-year site-specific recurrence	**5-year overall suvival**
Abdomen/pelvis	0.690 (0.650–0.730)	0.698 (0.666–0.730)
Thoracic region	0.692 (0.636–0.748)	0.698 (0.665–0.731)
Upper tract	0.605 (0.522–0.689)	0.556 (0.518–0.593)
Bone	0.650 (0.589–0.711)	0.660 (0.626–0.694)

models discriminated well and log-rank test were all highly significant (all p<0.001), except upper urinary tract model (p = 0.366) (Fig. 1C). Figure 2 presents the results of the decision curve analysis of site-specific recurrence at 3 years (2A-2D) and overall survival at 5 years (2E) for each model. Decision curve analysis revealed that the use of prediction models for abdomen/ pelvis, thoracic region, and bone recurrence was associated with net benefit gains relative to the treat-all strategy (2A, 2B, and 2D), but not the model for upper urinary tract recurrence (2C). Also, the upper urinary tract model had a lesser net benefit for prediction of overall survival compared with other models (2E).

Discussion

The goal of surveillance after radical cystectomy is to detect recurrence of disease as well as to identify complications. Patient

performance status and the extent of visceral metastatic disease are independent prognostic factors for survival in patients with metastatic bladder cancer [13]. Therefore, surveillance to detect asymptomatic recurrent disease may improve the response to treatment by minimizing tumor burden and maximizing patient performance status at therapy. Volkmer et al. [14] failed to demonstrate a survival benefit for detecting tumor recurrence early by regular follow-up examinations. However, Giannarini et al. [5] noted that patients diagnosed with recurrence during routine follow-up had significantly improved cancer-specific and overall survival compared to patients diagnosed after symptomatic relapse. A recent study from the Mayo clinic also showed that patients who were symptomatic at recurrence had a 60% increased risk of death than those who were asymptomatic [4]. Differences in patient numbers, follow-up and exclusion of

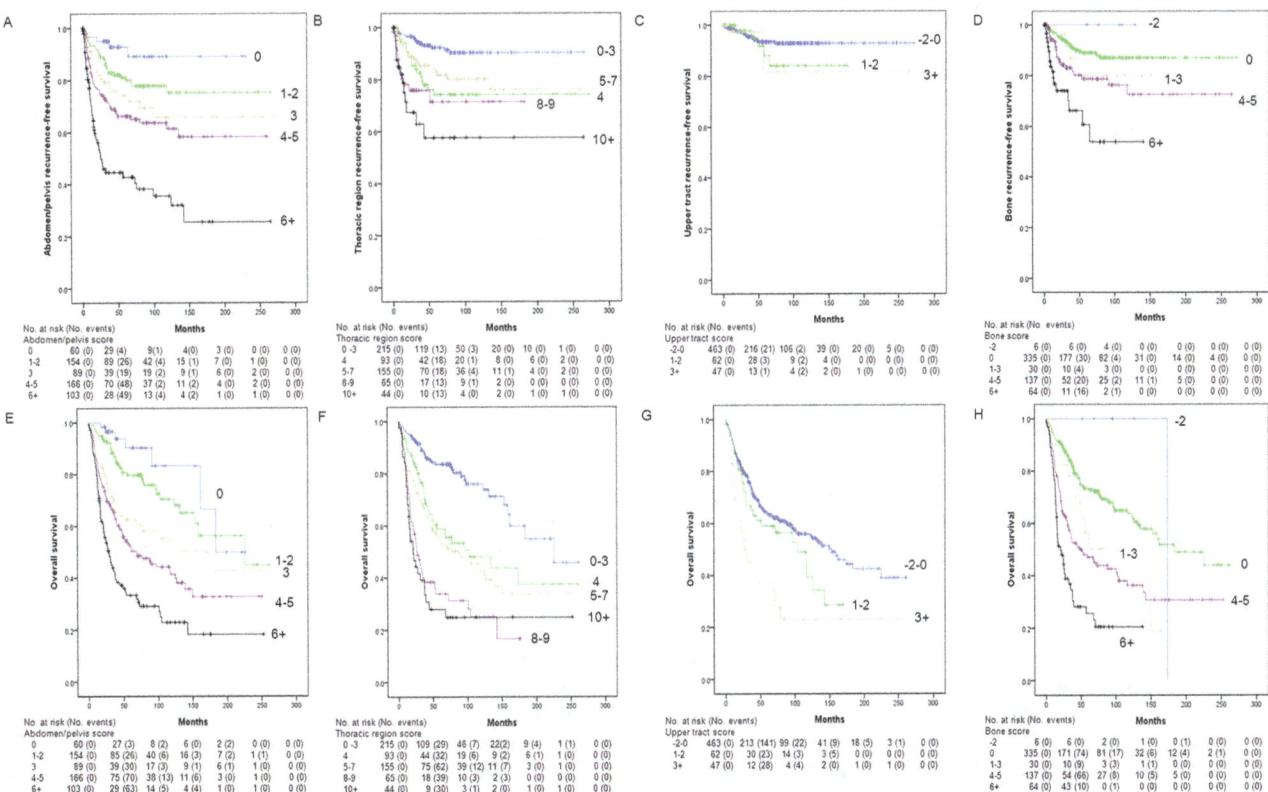

Figure 1. Kaplan-Meier plots. Three-year site-specific recurrence-free survival of abdomen/pelvis model (A), thoracic region model (B), upper urinary tract model (C), and bone model (D). Five-year overall survival of abdomen/pelvis model (E), thoracic region model (F), upper urinary tract model (G), and bone model (H).

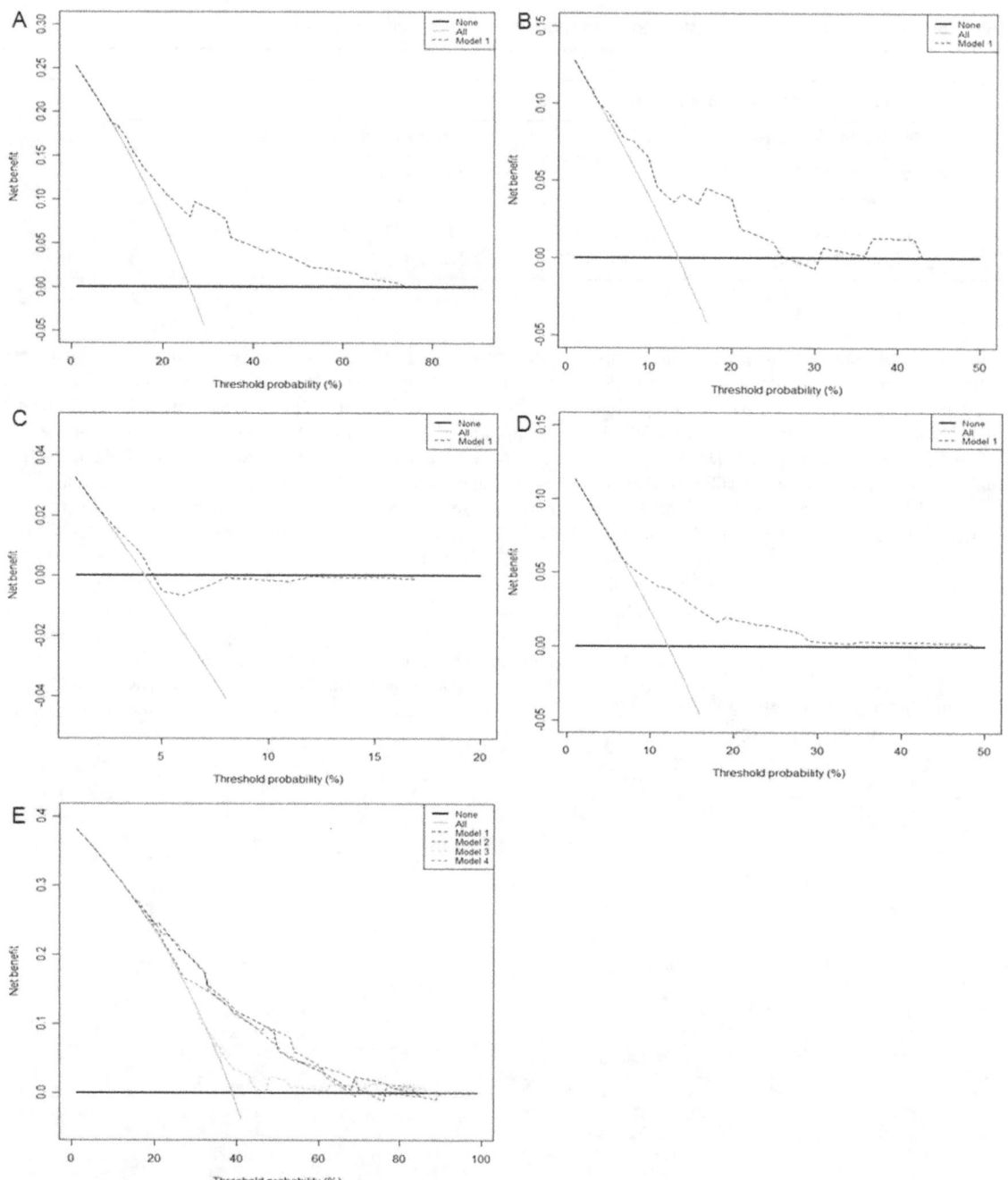

Figure 2. Decision curve analysis. Three-year site-specific recurrence-free survival of abdomen/pelvis model (A), thoracic region model (B), upper urinary tract model (C), and bone model (D). Five-year overall survival (E); model 1– abdomen/pelvis mode; model 2– thoracic region model; model 3– upper urinary tract model; and model 4– bone model. In decision curve analysis, the y-axis measures net benefit, calculated by summing the benefits (true positives) and subtracting the harms (false positives).

secondary urothelial tumors in the study of Volkmer et al [14] may in part account for the disparate findings.

Although modest objective response rates have been observed with cisplatin-based chemotherapy following recurrence, subsequent survival is generally highly attenuated. Previous studies suggested that aggressive surveillance following radical cystectomy is indicated since bladder cancer recurs in an unpredictable pattern [15]. On the contrary, Yafi et al. [16] proposed a stage-based protocol for surveillance of patients with bladder cancer treated with radical cystectomy that captured most recurrences

while limiting over-investigation. They strongly advocated earlier surveillance in patients with extravesical and node-positive disease. However, as seen in other malignancies, recurrence and survival prediction models based on stage alone may be inadequate. An ideal surveillance schedule should rely on the natural history on the disease [17]. Post-recurrence survival course varies in patients depending on when and where their disease recurs [18]. Therefore, characterization of the patterns of recurrence following radical cystectomy is critical for patient counseling and for the development of evidence-based surveillance guidelines [19].

Because no randomized trials have compared follow-up schedules, there is no definitive data guiding follow-up post-radical cystectomy. Models for site-specific disease recurrence may be useful in generating individual patient surveillance protocols based on risk factors present at the time of cystectomy. Recently, Umbret et al. [8] examined the site-specific pattern of disease recurrence and created multifactorial scoring system to predict site-specific recurrence. In their study, site-specific disease recurrences were classified into four locations to correspond to the most commonly used diagnostic modalities in postoperative surveillance. The authors demonstrated that patients with higher scores experiences the majority of recurrences early, and few recurrences were noted after the first 3 years, suggesting that patients with higher scores should be followed closely within the first 2 to 3 years and require less vigorous follow-up thereafter [8]. Therefore, these models lend support to the use of risk-stratified follow-up and emphasize the need for earlier strict surveillance in patients with high-risk site-specific recurrence. However, these models must be externally validated in a variety of data sets, preferably from different continents in order to introduce predictive tools into the daily patient care outside of North America.

The aim of the present study was to externally validate site-specific recurrence models in Asian cohort of patients who had undergone radical cystectomy for urothelial carcinoma. First, these models were constructed with the appropriate selection of variables for inclusion in the analysis. However, discrimination accuracy of models was moderate in our cohort although all currently available predictive tools in bladder cancer are not perfectly accurate. Risk groupings for calculating clinical risk are simple and convenient, but they do pose some problems. The misconception related to this approach is that it assumes that all patients within a risk group are equal despite risk group comprise a heterogeneous group of patients. The individual heterogeneity within a risk group leads to lower predictive accuracy when applying risk classifications to a particular patient. Risk groupings present additional statistical limitations by categorizing data points. When compared to nomogram, risk grouping is an inefficient use of the data and tends to reduce the predictive accuracy of a prognostic model (spectrum bias) [20]. Second, in our validation study, the bone model did not provide sufficient accuracy. Patient factors might influence outcomes. In the development cohort, patients with a history of occupational radiation exposure had an increased risk of osseous recurrence. In the validation cohort, we could not find patients with a history of radiation exposure. Third, the c-index for predicting 3-year upper tract recurrence-free survival using upper urinary tract model was 0.61 (95% CI, 0.52–0.69). The imperfection of upper urinary tract model may have been a reflection of a different biological process of upper urinary tract recurrence since upper urinary tract recurrences represent a different biological process of recurrence, and treatment and prognosis differ greatly from those of true recurrences [6]. While most local and distant failures were observed in the first 2 years following radical cystectomy, the risk of upper urinary tract recurrence is only a problem in the long term. The finding that c-indices were relatively similar for each site except for upper urinary tract might be attributed to the relatively

adequate number of actual recurrence at each site (more than 10% of the validation cohort patients, respectively) during the study follow-up period, unlike small number of patients (5.4%) showing upper urinary tract recurrence. Finally, in the second part of the study, we used site-specific recurrence models to assess their predictive accuracy for overall survival in our patient cohort. As a result, except for upper urinary tract recurrence model, the patients with higher scores were likely to show a worse recurrence-free survival and overall survival in the remaining site-specific recurrence models. Site-specific models except upper urinary tract model identified subgroups that also have significantly different overall survival, confirming the clinical importance of the stratification. Our finding suggests that upper urinary tract recurrence after radical cystectomy is not associated with patient's subsequent risk of death. However, these survival findings related to the site-specific recurrence models were not main focus of our study. The site-specific recurrence and evaluation with regard to the accuracy of site-specific recurrence models were the primary end point and main focus of our study.

The present study is limited because of its retrospective character with inherent biases. Another limitation is that this study comes from a single institution. However, despite the tertiary referral nature of our practice, most patients received postoperative follow-up at our institute. Since neoadjuvant and adjuvant chemotherapy was offered to a subset of patients (11% and 28%, respectively) in the present cohort, this may have potentially altered the recurrence patterns and influenced our surveillance strategies. Moreover, patients were not randomized to neoadjuvant or adjuvant chemotherapy, thereby introducing a selection bias. The fact that only 31 patients had upper urinary tract recurrence is a very limited number of samples for statistical analysis, and perhaps this could be the contributing factor of non-significant c-indices for this site. The different types of follow-up and sensitivity of methods to detect recurrent disease may also influence the result. Finally, 31% of patients in the validation dataset did not undergo pelvic lymph node dissection, whereas 12% in the development cohort did not. Therefore, it is possible that their application to cohorts with different clinical or pathological characteristics might result in the different performance characteristics.

Conclusions

Our study may be meaningful in that it offers a comprehensive validation of site-specific recurrence models in a different cohort. Abdomen/pelvis, thoracic region, and bone models demonstrate moderate discrimination, adequate calibration, and meaningful net benefit gains, whereas upper urinary tract model does not seem applicable to patients from Asia because it has suboptimal accuracy.

Author Contributions

Conceived and designed the experiments: HHK CK JHK CWJ. Performed the experiments: HSK MK JHK. Analyzed the data: HSK MK JHK. Contributed reagents/materials/analysis tools: HHK CK JHK CWJ. Contributed to the writing of the manuscript: HSK JHK.

References

1. Siegel R, Naishadham D, Jemal A (2013) Cancer statistics. CA Cancer J Clin 63: 11–30.
2. Jung KW, Won YJ, Kong HJ, Oh CM, Seo HG, et al. (2013) Cancer Statistics in Korea: Incidence, Mortality, Survival and Prevalence in 2010. Cancer Res Treat 45: 1–14.
3. Burger M, Catto JW, Dalbagni G, Grossman HB, Herr H, et al. (2013) Epidemiology and risk factors of urothelial bladder cancer. Eur Urol 63: 234–41.
4. Boorjian SA, Tollefson MK, Cheville JC, Costello BA, Thapa P, et al. (2011) Detection of asymptomatic recurrence during routine oncological followup after radical cystectomy is associated with improved patient survival. J Urol 186: 1796–802.

5. Giannarini G, Kessler TM, Thoeny HC, Nguyen DP, Meissner C, et al. (2010) Do patients benefit from routine follow-up to detect recurrences after radical cystectomy and ileal orthotopic bladder substitution? Eur Urol 58: 486–94.

6. Visser O, Nieuwenhuijzen JA, Horenblas S (2005) Members of the Urological Oncology Working Group of the Comprehensive Cancer Centre Amsterdam. Local recurrence after cystectomy and survival of patients with bladder cancer: a population based study in greater amsterdam. J Urol 174: 97–102.

7. International Bladder Cancer Nomogram Consortium, Bochner BH, Kattan MW, Vora KC (2006) Postoperative nomogram predicting risk of recurrence after radical cystectomy for bladder cancer. J Clin Oncol 24: 3967–72.

8. Umbreit EC, Crispen PL, Shimko MS, Farmer SA, Blute ML, et al. (2010) Multifactorial, site-specific recurrence model after radical cystectomy for urothelial carcinoma. Cancer. 116: 3399–407.

9. Ku JH, Kim HH, Kwak C (2013) Nodal staging score: a tool for survival prediction of node-negative bladder cancer. Urol Oncol 31: 1731–6.

10. Harrell FE Jr, Lee KL, Mark DB (1996) Multivariable prognostic models: issues in developing models, evaluating assumptions and adequacy, and measuring and reducing errors. Stat Med 15: 361–87.

11. Heagerty PJ, Lumley T, Pepe MS (2000) Time-dependent ROC curves for censored survival data and a diagnostic marker. Biometrics 56: 337–44.

12. Vickers AJ, Elkin EB (2006) Decision curve analysis: a novel method for evaluating prediction models. Med Decis Making 26: 565–74.

13. Bajorin DF, Dodd PM, Mazumdar M, Fazzari M, McCaffrey JA, et al. (1999) Long-term survival in metastatic transitional-cell carcinoma and prognostic factors predicting outcome of therapy. J Clin Oncol 17: 3173–81.

14. Volkmer BG, Kuefer R, Bartsch GC Jr, Gust K, Hautmann RE (2009) Oncological followup after radical cystectomy for bladder cancer-is there any benefit? J Urol 181: 1587–93.

15. Hassan JM, Cookson MS, Smith JA Jr, Chang SS (2006) Patterns of initial transitional cell recurrence in patients after cystectomy. J Urol 175: 2054–7.

16. Yafi FA, Aprikian AG, Fradet Y, Chin JL, Izawa J, et al. (2012) Surveillance guidelines based on recurrence patterns after radical cystectomy for bladder cancer: the Canadian Bladder Cancer Network experience. BJU Int 110: 1317–23.

17. Nieuwenhuijzen JA, de Vries RR, van Tinteren H, Bex A, Van der Poel H, et al. (2014) Follow-up after cystectomy: Regularly scheduled, risk adjusted, or symptom guided?: Patterns of recurrence, relapse presentation, and survival after cystectomy. Eur J Surg Oncol doi: 10.1016/j.ejso.2013.12.017.

18. Mitra AP, Quinn DI, Dorff TB, Skinner EC, Schuckman AK, et al. (2012) Factors influencing post-recurrence survival in bladder cancer following radical cystectomy. BJU Int 109: 846–54.

19. Linder BJ, Boorjian SA, Hudolin T, Cheville JC, Thapa P, et al. (2014) Late Recurrence Following Radical Cystectomy: Patterns, Risk Factors, and Outcomes. J Urol doi: 10.1016/j.juro.2013.11.103.

20. Shariat SF, Karakiewicz PI, Suardi N, Kattan MW (2008) Comparison of nomograms with other methods for predicting outcomes in prostate cancer: a critical analysis of the literature. Clin Cancer Res 14: 4400–7.

7

Identification of Nine Genomic Regions of Amplification in Urothelial Carcinoma, Correlation with Stage, and Potential Prognostic and Therapeutic Value

Yvonne Chekaluk[1], Chin-Lee Wu[2], Jonathan Rosenberg[3], Markus Riester[4], Qishan Dai[2], Sharron Lin[2], Yanan Guo[1], W. Scott McDougal[5]*, David J. Kwiatkowski[1]*

1 Division of Translational Medicine, Brigham and Women's Hospital, Boston, Massachusetts, United States of America, 2 Department of Pathology, Massachusetts General Hospital, Boston, Massachusetts, United States of America, 3 Division of Genitourinary Oncology, Memorial Sloan-Kettering Cancer Center, New York, New York, United States of America, 4 Department of Biostatistics and Computational Biology, Dana-Farber Cancer Institute, and Department of Biostatistics, Harvard School of Public Health, Boston, Massachusetts, United States of America, 5 Department of Urology, Massachusetts General Hospital, Boston, Massachusetts, United States of America

Abstract

We performed a genome wide analysis of 164 urothelial carcinoma samples and 27 bladder cancer cell lines to identify copy number changes associated with disease characteristics, and examined the association of amplification events with stage and grade of disease. Multiplex inversion probe (MIP) analysis, a recently developed genomic technique, was used to study 80 urothelial carcinomas to identify mutations and copy number changes. Selected amplification events were then analyzed in a validation cohort of 84 bladder cancers by multiplex ligation-dependent probe assay (MLPA). In the MIP analysis, 44 regions of significant copy number change were identified using GISTIC. Nine gene-containing regions of amplification were selected for validation in the second cohort by MLPA. Amplification events at these 9 genomic regions were found to correlate strongly with stage, being seen in only 2 of 23 (9%) Ta grade 1 or 1–2 cancers, in contrast to 31 of 61 (51%) Ta grade 3 and T2 grade 2 cancers, p<0.001. These observations suggest that analysis of genomic amplification of these 9 regions might help distinguish non-invasive from invasive urothelial carcinoma, although further study is required. Both MIP and MLPA methods perform well on formalin-fixed paraffin-embedded DNA, enhancing their potential clinical use. Furthermore several of the amplified genes identified here (ERBB2, MDM2, CCND1) are potential therapeutic targets.

Editor: Francisco X. Real, Centro Nacional de Investigaciones Oncológicas (CNIO), Spain

Funding: This work was supported by National Institutes of Health (NIH), National Cancer Institute (NCI) 1P01CA120964. The funders had no role in study design, data collection and analysis, decision to publish, or preparation of the manuscript.

Competing Interests: The authors have declared that no competing interests exist.

* E-mail: dk@rics.bwh.harvard.edu (DJK); WMCDOUGAL@PARTNERS.ORG (WSM)

⑨ These authors contributed equally to this work.

Introduction

Bladder cancer is the fourth most common cancer among men in the USA, accounting for 73,510 cases and 14,880 deaths in the US in 2011 [1]. Bladder cancer develops from the transitional cells of the mucosal urothelium and is found pathologically and clinically to occur in two mostly separate forms [2]. The first form is a non muscle-invasive tumor (stages Ta, Tis and T1), which generally has a good prognosis, but is also characterized by frequent local recurrences, requiring repeated cystoscopic evaluations. The second form is a solid, non-papillary tumor (stages T2–T4) that invades into at least the smooth muscle layer (muscularis propria), and has a high risk for metastasis. Non muscle-invasive papillary tumors growing in the lumen of the bladder constitute 70–80% of new cases each year, while invasive cases make up the remaining 20–30% at initial diagnosis [2]. Although the distinction between papillary and invasive disease is often clear on initial biopsy, the subsequent clinical behavior of each bladder cancer is uncertain, and remains a major problem in clinical management [3]. A variety of histopathologic markers have been assessed and provide some information on prognosis. However, they do not provide accurate prediction for individual patients [3]. The differences in clinical behavior as well as pathologic features suggest that there are separate oncogenic pathways for non-muscle-invasive vs. muscle-invasive bladder cancer. The vast majority of bladder cancers are urothelial carcinoma, and the same histologic type of cancer can arise throughout the urinary tract including the renal pelvis and ureters.

In patients with muscle-invasive disease, complete removal of the bladder with or without cisplatin-based neoadjuvant chemotherapy is the most commonly employed treatment approach [2]. Even with radical treatment, approximately 50% of patients develop metastatic disease, and for such patients no curative treatment exists. Furthermore, no treatment has been shown to extend survival in patients with progression following platinum-based combination chemotherapy. Thus, novel therapeutic and preventive approaches are needed for this relatively common and lethal disease.

Genetic studies of bladder cancer have a rich history, including the identification of the first oncogene, HRAS, in a bladder carcinoma cell line [4]. Subsequently, TP53 mutations were identified [5], the CDKN2A gene was shown to be a consistent target of deletion [6], and mutations were found in both the TSC1 and FGFR3 genes in bladder cancer [7,8], as well as many other genetic changes. In addition, comparative genomic hybridization has been used extensively to identify regions of chromosomal gain and loss in bladder cancer with identification of many consistent changes of potential importance in tumor development although the resolution of these technologies was limited [6,9–13].

Here, we report genomic analysis of 164 urothelial carcinoma samples and 27 bladder cancer cell lines. To assess genomic copy number changes genome-wide, we performed molecular inversion probe (MIP) analysis, which works well on formalin-fixed paraffin-embedded (FFPE) tumor specimens. We identified 44 regions of copy number change in a discovery cohort of 80 urothelial carcinoma samples, and then focused on 9 genomic regions showing significant and relatively common amplification of genes that may function as 'driver' events for urothelial carcinoma development. We validated these regions in a replication design by analysis of a set of bladder cancer cell lines, on nearly half of the original samples, and on a validation cohort of 84 FFPE bladder cancer samples. We found that genomic copy number changes were significantly more common in Ta grade 3 and higher stage/grade tumors than in stage Ta grades 1 and 1–2 tumors. These observations suggest that analysis of these genomic regions might be a useful diagnostic tool to determine the invasive potential of bladder cancer. In addition, the genes in some of these amplified regions are potential therapeutic targets.

Materials and Methods

Human urothelial carcinoma specimens and cell lines

Urothelial carcinoma specimens that had been formalin fixed and embedded in paraffin using standard techniques were obtained from the Pathology archives of the Massachusetts General Hospital (Table S1). Forty of these samples had portions that were rapidly frozen at -80°C as well. Written consent was obtained from each patient for this study on a protocol that was approved by the hospital's institutional review board, "Partners Human Research Committee". Bladder cancer staging was performed according to the current AJCC guidelines [14]. Grade was determined according to the 1973 WHO bladder cancer guidelines [2].

Twenty-four bladder cancer cell lines were obtained from the stocks of the Translational Urology Research Lab at Massachusetts General Hospital, MA. Two other bladder cancer cell lines were generously provided by Margaret A. Knowles (St James's University Hospital, UK) [15], and one was obtained from a German cancer cell line bank. These 27 bladder cancer cell lines were maintained in Dulbecco's Modified Eagle Medium (Cellgro, Manassas, VA) supplemented with 10% Fetal Bovine Serum and 1% penicillin-streptomycin-amphotericin B (Life Technologies, Carlsbad, CA), in an incubator at 37°C in 5% CO2. All 27 cell lines were subject to microsatellite fingerprinting which confirmed that they were unique.

Anonymized discard normal human blood samples were obtained from the clinical laboratory at Brigham and Women's Hospital on a protocol that was approved by the hospital's institutional review board, "Partners Human Research Committee". These were used to prepare control normal DNA.

DNA extraction

DNA was extracted from formalin-fixed paraffin embedded (FFPE) samples using the BiOstic FFPE Tissue DNA isolation Kit (MO BIO Laboratories, Inc., Carlsbad, CA). DNA was extracted from blood using the QIAGEN DNeasy Blood and Tissue kit.

DNA was extracted from cell lines and frozen cancer specimens using the Puregene DNA Purification kit following the protocol for 1–2 million cultured cells. DNA concentrations were determined by nanodrop and confirmed by agarose gel electrophoresis.

Molecular Inversion Probe (MIP) Assay

A molecular inversion probe (MIP) assay examining 330,000 single nucleotide polymorphisms (SNPs) and 412 cancer gene mutations in 46 cancer-related genes (OncoScan) was performed with the assistance of Affymetrix in Santa Clara, California [16]. The SNPs had an average intermarker distance of 3 kb for the 150,000 genic probes, and 9 kb for the non-genic probes. The 412 cancer gene mutations are listed in Table S2. The raw data from this analysis (CEL files) has been put in the GEO archive (GSE44323).

Biostatistical Software Tools

The raw MIP intensity data provided by Affymetrix was loaded and analyzed using Nexus Copy Number v6.0 (BioDiscovery Inc., El Sequendo, CA). Data was normalized using the SNP-FASST2 segmentation algorithm. Normalized probe intensity and allele ratio data were visualized in Nexus v6.0. The quality of the copy number data from each sample was assessed by measuring the Median of Absolute Pairwise Distribution (MAPD). The absolute pairwise difference (APD) is calculated as the $\log_2$ value of the ratio of CN intensity values for each adjacent pair of probes, across the entire set of 330,000 probes.

Normalized copy number data was then segmented using the GLAD algorithm available in GenePattern 3.3.3 [17]. Recurrent copy number alterations were identified using Genomic Identification of Significant Targets in Cancer (GISTIC) [18], implemented in both GenePattern 3.3.3 and in Nexus v6.0. GISTIC identifies regions of the genome that are significantly amplified or deleted across a set of cancer samples. Each amplification or deletion event is assigned a G-score that considers the amplitude as well as the frequency of occurrence among the sample set. False Discovery Rate q-values are then calculated for each region of gain or loss. Regions with q-values <0.1 were considered significant. Genomic coordinates used in the Tables are all from human build hg18.

Multiplex Ligation-Dependent Probe Amplification (MLPA)

MLPA probe sets targeting 16 genes in 9 genomic regions were designed following methods we have used previously [19] (Table S4). Individual probe oligonucleotides (size range 45–84 nt) were synthesized by Integrated Device Technology (IDT, Coralville, IA). MLPA assays were performed on 100–150 ng genomic DNA samples using the MRC Holland Salsa MLPA EK5 reagent kit (MRC Holland, Amsterdam, the Netherlands). MLPA products were separated by capillary electrophoresis on the ABI 3130, and light intensity reflecting fluorescence was captured according size of the fragment, in comparison to Rox 500 size standards. Ten to 24 DNA samples were subject to MLPA analysis in each run. For analysis of control blood DNA and bladder cancer cell line DNAs, the blood DNA samples were used as controls for normalization, as described [19]. Because the amplification patterns of FFPE DNA by MLPA were different from those seen with blood or cell line DNA, a different method was used for normalization of FFPE DNA samples. Within each run, peak heights were initially normalized using all samples analyzed. Samples with no amplification were then identified and used as normalization controls for that particular MLPA run. In practice, several FFPE DNA samples for which there was a large amount of DNA were run repeatedly on different runs and typically served as the controls for several runs. To determine the reproducibility of the assay, replicate analyses of samples in different MLPA runs were compared for each probe value by calculating the coefficient of variation. The coefficient of variation was calculated as the standard deviation of a pair of measurements divided by the mean of those two measurements. A coefficient of variation of <10% was considered a robust assay.

Sanger Sequencing

Sanger sequencing was performed on PCR products by standard methods in the BWH DNA Sequencing Core Facility. Sequencing traces were viewed and analyzed using FinchTV v1.4.0.

Statistical methods

The Fisher exact test was used for analysis of categorical data, and computed in Prism (v4.0a, GraphPad Software, Inc.).

Results

Urothelial carcinoma patient characteristics

One hundred sixty-four urothelial carcinoma specimens prepared in paraffin were used to obtain FFPE DNA for this analysis, and were divided into two cohorts (Table 1, S1). The discovery cohort of 80 samples included cystectomy, nephroureterectomy, and transurethral resection specimens, and had tumor stages ranging from Ta to T4 (Table 1), but were nearly all T1 or higher stage to permit robust detection of mutations associated with invasive urothelial carcinoma. The validation cohort of 84 samples were obtained exclusively by transurethral resection, were a sequential series and consisted of tumor stages Ta–T2 (Table 1).

Table 1. Stage and grade information for 164 urothelial carcinoma samples.

Discovery cohort		
stage grade	#	%
Ta g1,2	3	4%
T1 g2	3	4%
T1 g3	36	49%
T2 g2	1	1%
T2 g3	6	8%
T3 g3	17	23%
T4 g2	2	3%
T4 g3	12	16%
total	80	
Validation cohort		
stage grade	#	%
Ta g1	13	15%
Ta g1–2	10	12%
Ta g3	20	24%
T2 g3	41	49%
total	84	

Upper, 80 samples in the discovery cohort analyzed by MIP. Bottom, 84 samples in the validation cohort analyzed by MLPA.

Full clinical and demographic information on these patients and cancers is given in Table S1.

Molecular Inversion Probe (MIP) genetic mutational analysis

We used MIP analysis [16], to examine both genomic copy number and mutation at 412 potential sites in 46 cancer-related genes (Table S2) on the discovery cohort of 80 urothelial carcinoma FFPE samples. The wide range of grades and stages in this cohort were selected by design to permit analysis of the broad spectrum of urothelial carcinoma. First, we analyzed the mutations identified by the MIP analysis.

Thirty-two mutations in 7 genes were identified in 28 urothelial carcinoma samples by Affymetrix criteria (scores ≥9.0, and <50) as being probable mutations in the 80 urothelial carcinoma FFPE samples. To validate these findings, we performed Sanger sequencing for each mutation-sample pair, and confirmed 20 of the 28 mutations that were called in the MIP analysis (Table 2). Of those that failed to validate, the majority had Affymetrix mutation scores <10.0 or >25. Twenty of 22 (91%) mutation calls with scores between 10.0 and 25 validated by Sanger sequencing.

Molecular Inversion Probe (MIP) genomic copy number variation analysis

We then focused on analysis of the genomic copy number information provided by the MIP analysis. Seven (9%) urothelial carcinoma MIP results were excluded from genomic copy number analysis due to having a MAPD score >1.5, reflecting a high variance in probe to probe measurement (see Methods for details). The median MAPD for the remaining 73 samples was 0.50. Nexus v6.0 (Bio-Discovery) was used to visualize both copy number and allele ratio information for the 330,000 SNPs across the genome (Figure S1).

GISTIC [18] was used to identify regions of significant CN gain or loss in the 73 urothelial carcinoma samples (Figure 1). Forty-four chromosomal regions showed a statistically significant CN loss or gain, with q-value <0.1 (Table S3). These 44 chromosomal regions were compared with a large set of similar CN gain and loss regions available at the tumorscape web-site for other cancers (http://www.broadinstitute.org/tumorscape), and also examined using the Integrated Genome Viewer (IGV, see Methods). Fourteen regions of gain or loss which did not contain protein-

Table 2. Mutations in the discovery cohort of 80 urothelial carcinoma samples identified by MIP analysis and validated by Sanger sequencing.

Gene	Nucleotide	Amino acid	#[1]	Stages[2]
ATM	2572T>C	F858L	3	T1, T1, T4
FBXW7	1393C>T	R465C	1	T1
FGFR3	1118A>G	Y373C	4	T1, T1, T1, T1
HRAS	34G>A	G12S	1	T1
KRAS	35G>A	G12D	1	T1
PIK3CA	1624G>A	E542K	4	T1, T1, T3, T4
TP53	742C>T	R248W	1	T1
TP53	853G>A	E285K	4	T1, T3, T3, T3
TP53	818G>A	R273H	1	T3

[1]Number of different samples with this mutation.
[2]Stage of the urothelial carcinoma samples with mutation.

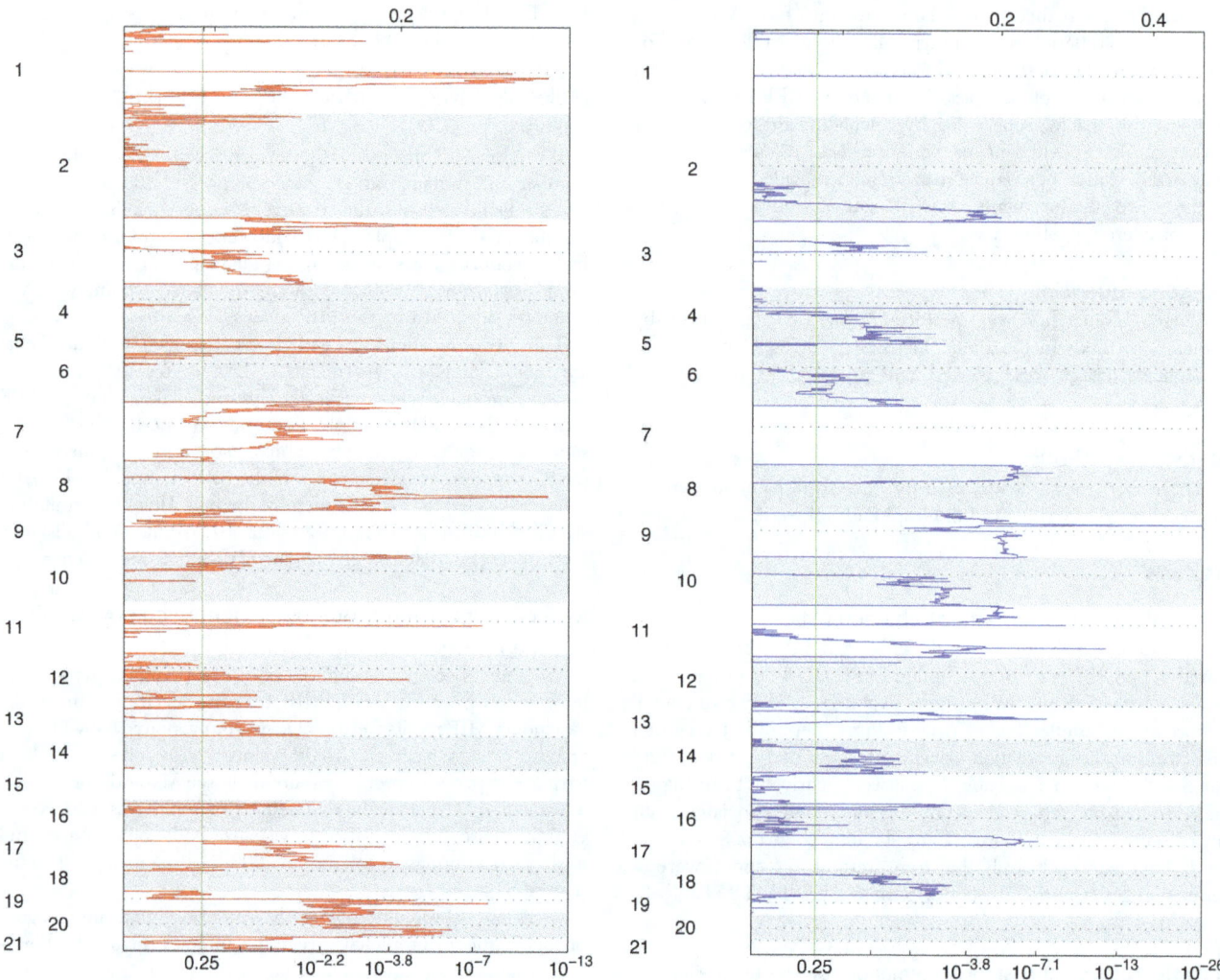

Figure 1. GISTIC plot of genomic regions with CN gain or loss from the MIP analysis on 73 urothelial carcinoma specimens. The 21 autosomes are shown on the y axis, and q values indicating statistical significance from the GISTIC analysis are plotted on the x axis for regions of copy number gain (red at left) and loss (blue at right).

coding genes were not considered further, reducing the number of regions to 16 regions of gain and 14 regions of loss.

We then chose to focus on the 16 regions of amplification since such regions often contain genes that are 'drivers' of cancer development, and may be amenable to specific therapeutic targeting. Manual review of high resolution copy number and allele frequency graphs was performed in both Nexus (Figure S2) and IGV, and nine regions were identified in which there was high level amplification with at least 3 of the 73 urothelial carcinoma samples showing a copy number >5 in the region (Table 3). (Note that these values are not corrected for stromal cell contamination in these samples, so that there are likely more samples with true cancer amplification to >5 copies.) For many of these regions, the amplification target was known from previous studies in bladder and other cancers. However, the identity of the gene on chromosome 1q23.3 was not well-defined from previous work, and for chromosome 6p22.3, there were two candidate genes, *E2F3* and *SOX4*. Hence we chose to analyze 16 distinct genes (Table 4) in a replication study to validate the MIP findings, and examine the possible association of amplification of these regions with bladder cancer stage and grade.

Multiplex Ligation-dependent Probe Assay (MLPA) in bladder cancer cell lines

To replicate these findings, and to generate an assay more easily applied to routine clinical samples, we generated a set of MLPA probes for each of the 16 genes in Table 3 (Table S4). The MLPA assay appeared to work robustly, with the exception of a single control probe set which was subsequently dropped from consideration, and was applied to a set of control blood DNA samples and a set of bladder cancer cell lines (Figure S3). Replicate analyses performed on four blood DNA samples indicated that the coefficient of variation for copy number determined by MLPA analysis was a median of 3.64% and a mean of 4.40%, indicating a relatively low level of variation in this assay. Replicate analyses of copy number performed on 25 bladder cancer cell line DNA preparations indicated that the coefficient of variation was a median of 6.57% and a mean of 7.77% (two samples could not be replicated due to insufficient DNA). This is still a relatively low level of variation, but is higher than blood DNA samples, likely due to the presence of amplified regions in many of the bladder cancer cell lines, which diminishes the size of non-amplified products, increasing the variance in duplicate measurements.

Table 3. Identification of nine genomic regions with high level amplification seen in at least 3 of 73 urothelial carcinoma samples in the discovery cohort by MIP analysis.

chromosome	1p34.2	1q23.3	3p25.2	6p22.3	8p11.2	8q22.2	11q13.2	12q15	17q12
q value	6.47E-04	2.29E-12	3.02E-12	5.26E-14	5.28E-02	2.29E-12	3.01E-08	3.57E-05	1.89E-04
chr region	chr1:39.5–41.0 Mb	chr1:159.1–159.7 Mb	chr3:12.2–12.5 Mb	chr6:21.6–22.0 Mb	chr8:42.34–42.36 Mb	chr8:101.2–103.1 Mb	chr11:68.6–69.6 Mb	chr12:67.3–68.3 Mb	chr17:34.9–35.2 Mb
*copy number	16.0, 6.5, 6.1	12.1, 9.2, 8.6	18.0, 8.0, 7.0	17.2, 15.6, 9.1	10.3, 7.7, 5.2	10.5, 7.6, 5.7	17.5, 9.8, 8.7	16.0, 12.8, 10.8	16.0, 5.5, 5.5
genes	MYCL1	TSTD1	PPARG	SOX4	POLB	YWHAZ	CCND1	MDM2	ERBB2
	hsa-mir-30c-1	PVRL4	SYN2	E2F3	MYST3	POLR2K	FGF3	CPM	GRB7
	BMP8B	NIT1	TSEN2		AP3M2	SPAG1	FGF4	LYZ	NEUROD2
	COL9A2	DEDD			PLAT	RNF19A	FGF19	YEATS4	PNMT
	NFYC	UHMK1			IKBKB	PABPC1	MYEOV	CCT2	TCAP
	PPT1	DDR2				ZNF706	TMEM16A	FRS2	STARD3
	RLF	NUF2				GRHL2	ORAOV1	CPSF6	IKZF3
	PABPC4	APOA2				NCALD		SLC35E3	PPP1R1B
	RIMS3	FCER1G				ANKRD46		NUP107	C17orf37
	ZMPSTE24	FCGR2A				SNX31		BEST3	PERLC1
	PPIE	MPZ				FBXO43		LRRC10	
	CAP1	NDUFS2							
	MACF1	PFDN2							
	HEYL	PPOX							
	HPCAL4	SDHC							
	TRIT1	USF1							
	OXCT2	B4GALT3							
	SMAP2	ADAMTS4							
	C1orf176	NR1I3							
	ZNF643	USP21							
	NT5C1A	F11R							
	MFSD2	UFC1							
	TMCO2	ITLN1							
	ZNF684	TOMM40L							
	ZNF642	KLHDC9							
	BMP8A	ITLN2							
	KIAA0754	ARHGAP30							
		C1orf192							
		LOC642502							
		PCP4L1							
		LOC100134860							

*copy number values of the 3 urothelial carcinoma samples with the largest amplification of the region (largest to smallest).

Table 4. Chromosomal regions and genes analyzed by MLPA.

chromosome	1p34.2	1q23.3	3p25.2	6p22.3	8p11.2	8q22.2	11q13.2	12q15	17q12
q value	6.47E-04	2.29E-12	3.02E-12	5.26E-14	5.28E-02	2.29E-12	3.01E-08	3.57E-05	1.89E-04
chr region	chr1:39.5-41.0 Mb	chr1:159.1-159.7 Mb	chr3:12.2-12.5 Mb	chr6:21.6-22.0 Mb	chr8:42.34-42.36 Mb	chr8:101.2-103.1 Mb	chr11:68.6-69.6 Mb	chr12:67.3-68.3 Mb	chr17:34.9-35.2 Mb
genes	MYCL1	TSTD1	PPARG	SOX4	POLB	YWHAZ	CCND1	MDM2	ERBB2
		PVRL4		E2F3					
		NIT1							
		DEDD							
		UHMK1							
		DDR2							
		NUF2							

Eleven of 27 (41%) bladder cancer cell lines analyzed by the MLPA assay had amplification of one or more of the 16 genes assayed (Table 5), while the remainder had no amplification among the tested genes, considering amplification to be 4 or more copies. Six (22%) cell lines showed amplification of CCND1, while 5 each showed amplification of some or all of the genes on 1q23.3 and of E2F3-SOX4. No cell line had amplification of POLB or ERBB2. These findings validate the original MIP analysis as 7 of the 9 genomic regions of amplification seen by MIP analysis were also seen in these bladder cancer cell lines.

MLPA validation of MIP analysis

To further validate the copy number findings made in the MIP analysis, we performed MLPA analysis of DNA prepared from parallel fresh frozen samples from 39 of the cancers analyzed in the first cohort of 80 FFPE samples. We found that 343 of 351 (98%) of the chromosomal regions analyzed on the paired samples by the two methods showed concordance in detection of amplification or lack of amplification, assessed as $CN > 4$. Furthermore of the 27 chromosomal regions of amplification detected by either MIP or MLPA analysis in individual samples, 19 (70%) showed concordance by the two methods of analysis. Concordant results were seen for amplification in 8 of the 9 genomic regions analyzed for one or more cancers. We suspect that the lack of concordance seen for some samples may reflect tumor heterogeneity with significant differences in gene amplification events seen in different samples of the same cancer, or possibly differences in tumor content in the two samples. Overall, we take these findings as strong validation of the MIP analysis method.

MLPA analysis of the validation cohort and comparison with stage

We then performed a replication analysis assessing amplification of these 9 genomic regions and 16 genes on the validation cohort of 84 FFPE bladder cancer DNA samples. Furthermore, we examined the possibility that genomic amplification of these regions would be associated with stage of disease, and thus might provide a potential prognostic measure for clinical use. Since most clinical bladder cancer specimens on which initial treatment decisions are based are derived from transurethral resection, we analyzed FFPE samples obtained only by that means, and that ranged in stage from Ta grade 1 through T2 grade 3.

To demonstrate the reproducibility of the MLPA assay on FFPE DNA samples, replicate analyses were performed on 26 of the 84 FFPE samples, all of those for which DNA was available. On these samples the coefficient of variation for replicate analyses had a median of 5.66% and an average of 6.75%, indicating that the MLPA assay was reproducible and robust.

Considering amplification to be 4 or more copies, 33 of 84 (39%) samples analyzed showed amplification of one or more genomic regions (Table 6). Similar to the findings with the bladder cancer cell lines, CCND1, the chromosome 1q23.3 region, and E2F3-SOX4 were the most commonly amplified, seen in 11 (13%), 8 (10%), and 12 (14%) samples, respectively.

The frequency of any amplification event was strongly correlated with tumor stage and grade (Table 7). Amplification events were seen in only 2 of 23 (9%) Ta grade 1 or 1–2 cancers. In contrast, amplifications were seen in 11 of 20 (55%) Ta grade 3 cancers, and in 20 of 41 (49%) T2 grade 2 cancers. Comparison of the frequency of amplification among these three groups is highly significant with $p = 0.0020$ and 0.0011, comparing the first group with each of the second two groups (Fisher's exact test). SOX4 was the only individual marker which showed amplification at a

Table 5. MLPA analysis of amplification in bladder cancer cell lines.

Chromosome:	1p34.2	1q23.3	1q23.3	1q23.3	1q23.3	1q23.3	1q23.3	1q23.3	3p25.2	6p22.3	6p22.3	8p11.2	8q22.3	11q13.3	12q15	17q12
	MYCL1	TSTD1	PVRL4	NIT1	DEDD	UHMK1	DDR2	NUF2	PPARG	E2F3	SOX4	POLB	YWHAZ	CCND1	MDM2	ERBB2
UMUC1														10.1		
UMUC7	11.2	6.9	7.4	6.7	7.3	8.2	7.3	7.3			5.2					
UMUC10		5.7	6.1	5.7	5.8					8.9	14.5					
UMUC11														10.3	6.6	
UMUC17														4.2		
HT1376	5.1	5.1	5.8	5.1	5.6	5.4	4.5	4.6		4.9	9.3					
SCABER		4.3	4.9	4.4	4.6	4.6							5.6	5.7		
HT1197											4.1					
5637									10.0	11.3	22.4			4.2		
BL13															16.0	
BL138		4.4	4.8	4.6	4.6	4.6	4.3	4.4						12.7	4.1	

Genomic copy number is shown only when values are ≥4.0. bladder cancer cell lines had no amplification and are not listed above: J82, 639V, MGH-U1, MGH-U3, MGH-U4, MGH-U5, RT4, T24, 253J, 647V, UMUC15, BL17, UMUC3, UMUC6, HCV29, 97-1.

significantly higher rate in Ta grade 3+T2 grade 2 cancers (11 of 61) than in Ta grade 1 or 1–2 cancers (0 of 23, p = 0.03). Examination of the frequency of amplification of these 9 genomic regions in the discovery cohort of 73 samples analyzed by MIP assay showed a similar trend, but the results were not statistically significant due to the small number of Ta tumors in that cohort. None of 3 Ta grade 1 or 2 samples showed amplification, and 31 (44%) of 70 T1–T4 samples showed amplification of one or more of the 9 genomic regions. Since the low frequency of copy number variation in the Ta grade 1 and 1–2 samples might be explained by presence of normal tissue rather than bladder cancer in those specimens, we examined them for mutations in FGFR3. Ten of 11 samples examined (4 grade 1 and 7 grade 1–2) had mutations in FGFR3: 1 had R248C, 8 had S249C, and 1 had Y373C, consistent with previous studies of early stage bladder cancer [20,21].

Discussion

In this study, we used an innovative methodology, MIP analysis, to examine both a set of 412 mutations and to perform copy number analysis across the genome using 330,000 SNP probes. The MIP procedure enables analysis of FFPE DNA, the most commonly available clinical material. Most mutations identified here were in the 12 most commonly mutated genes reported by the Catalogue of Somatic Mutations in Cancer (COSMIC) in bladder cancer [22]. However, we also identified mutations in two other genes not reported in COSMIC for bladder cancer, ATM and FBXW7. Relatively few mutations in FGFR3 were seen in this cohort, four Y373C (5%), likely due to the inclusion of only three Ta samples, two of which arose in the renal pelvis. MIP screening for mutation and copy number change has recently been reported for multiple other cancer types [23–27].

We choose to focus on copy number amplifications, and identified 9 genomic regions of common amplification in an initial cohort of 80 urothelial carcinoma specimens, of which 73 gave reliable copy number information by MIP analysis. We then generated a set of MLPA probes to interrogate those nine regions in a validation cohort of 84 samples. We demonstrated that the performance of the MLPA analysis was robust on control blood DNAs, bladder cancer cell line DNAs, and frozen DNA samples from a subset (39) of the cancers initially evaluated by MIP analysis of FFPE DNA. We then performed the MLPA analysis on a separate validation cohort of 84 bladder cancer FFPE DNA samples. In the validation cohort, we found that all genomic regions showed evidence of amplification in two or more samples, with the highest levels of amplification seen for CCND1 and MDM2 (Table 6). The regions with the most frequent amplification were chromosome 1q23.3, E2F3-SOX4, and CCND1 (Table 6). Amplification was seen significantly more frequently in advanced stage tumors (Ta grade 3, or higher stage) than in early stage tumors (Ta grade 1 or 1–2).

Many previous studies have analyzed genomic copy number changes in bladder cancer using comparative genomic hybridization (CGH) or array CGH [3,9,10,12,13,28–40]. All of the 9 genomic regions with amplification identified in our MIP analysis that contained genes, were highly statistically significant, and were identified in multiple samples, had been identified in these previous studies. However, MYCL1 and POLB have been identified previously in only one or two studies [9–11,13,38,41]. In our validation cohort, we identified MYCL1 and POLB amplification in 3 and 4 samples, respectively. The validation we performed using MLPA analysis of the original MIP samples, and the consistency of these findings strongly support both the value of

Table 6. MLPA analysis of amplification in the validation cohort of 84 bladder cancer FFPE samples.

Chromosome:	1p34.2	1q23.3	1q23.3	1q23.3	1q23.3	1q23.3	1q23.3	1q23.3	3p25.2	6p22.3	6p22.3	8p11.2	8q22.3	11q13.3	12q15	17q12
	MYCL1	TSTD1	PVRL4	NIT1	DEDD	UHMK1	DDR2	NUF2	PPARG	E2F3	SOX4	POLB	YWHAZ	CCND1	MDM2	ERBB2
Ta/grade 1–2														6.9		
Ta/grade 1–2	4.3		4.2											5.2		5.1
Ta/grade 3	4.3										4.6			4.4		
Ta/grade 3		4.6	4.7	4.5	4.6		4.4	4.3					4.5	34.7	14.8	
Ta/grade 3											4.2			26.0	7.7	
Ta/grade 3														4.2		
Ta/grade 3										5.3	6.5					
Ta/grade 3										10.9	4.6				4.8	
Ta/grade 3		4.0	4.5	4.2	5.2	4.4	4.3	7.2								
Ta/grade 3												5.1				
Ta/grade 3		4.1										5.4				
Ta/grade 3									8.0	5.0						
T2/grade 3		7.7	5.9	6.3	5.9		5.0	4.2	5.1				5.0	21.9	10.8	
T2/grade3		4.1	4.2	4.5			6.3	5.3				6.1				
T2/grade 3													5.0			
T2/grade 3											7.4					
T2/grade 3		5.6	4.9	4.4	4.9			4.2								
T2/grade 3										6.7	10.6			40.7	12.0	
T2/grade 3											5.7		4.4			
T2/grade 3		5.3	4.8	4.5	4.2									19.8		
T2/grade 3										7.3	11.1		7.3			
T2/grade 3	4.1															
T2/grade 3												4.7				
T2/grade 3										6.6	5.0					
T2/grade 3														4.1		
T2/grade 3																4.5
T2/grade 3											10.1			4.2	16.4	

Table 6. Cont.

Chromosome:	1p34.2	1q23.3	1q23.3	1q23.3	1q23.3	1q23.3	3p25.2	6p22.3	6p22.3	8p11.2	8q22.3	11q13.3	12q15	17q12
T2/grade 3								5.1	7.8				26.5	

Genomic copy number is shown only when values were ≥4.0.
51 samples are not listed, as they had no amplification events detected (all CN<4.0). The stage and grade distribution of these samples was: 13 Ta grade 1; 8 Ta grade 1–2; 9 Ta grade 3; 21 T2 grade 3.

Table 7. Summary of MLPA findings in FFPE bladder cancer samples according to stage.

		total #	any CN≥4.0	%
group 1	Ta grade 1	13	0	0%
	Ta grade1–2	10	2	20%
group 2	Ta grade 3	20	11	55%
group 3	T2 grade 3	41	20	49%
	total	84	33	39%

Groups 1, 2, and 3 have a statistically significant difference in the frequency of any amplification event, with p = 0.0020 comparing groups 1 and 2, and p = 0.0011 comparing groups 1 and 3. P is not significant comparing group 2 with group 3. Fisher exact test.

MIP analysis as a technology for copy number alteration detection, and provide further validation for the importance of these amplification events in bladder cancer development.

Many previous studies have also found that there is a major difference in genomic events seen in superficial papillary bladder cancer (Ta), in comparison to more advanced stages of disease. Non-invasive Ta papillary tumors commonly have activating mutations in FGFR3 (as seen here), or mutation in one of the RAS genes (mutually exclusive with FGFR3 mutation), and loss of one chromosome 9 [41]. However, few other genomic alterations have been seen by past CGH, array-CGH, or SNP analyses [11,13,41]. Amplification events are generally rare [41], but have recently been identified at a low level in Ta disease [36]. In contrast, many genetic events have been identified in muscle-invasive bladder cancer, including common deletion and mutations in TSC1, PTEN, RB1, and particularly TP53. In addition, recent studies have emphasized the common involvement of the PI3K–mTOR pathway in this disease [15,42], and common mutation in chromatin remodeling genes in invasive bladder cancer [43]. Further investigation of FBXW7 in bladder cancer pathogenesis given its reported involvement in this pathway [44] is of interest.

In aggregate, these observations suggest that a relatively simple assay for amplification of these 9 genomic regions might provide useful clinical information. This might be achieved by the MLPA technique as shown here which can be performed on FFPE tissues. There are also other efficient approaches that could be used for this purpose, including digital droplet PCR [45]. However, prior to clinical use of this analysis, a similar copy number analysis will need to be performed on a large set of stage 1 bladder cancer patients in whom there is good follow-up data to assess the potential prognostic value of this assay.

Most previous genomic studies on bladder cancer have used fresh frozen tissue obtained by cystectomy. In contrast, FFPE samples are the common pathologic resource available in routine clinical practice at the time of critical decision-making. Therefore, molecular tests that can use FFPE DNA are essential. In our study, we demonstrated that MIP technology can be used to study routine FFPE cancer specimens, providing a great deal of mutational and copy number information. We also demonstrated that the simpler MLPA technique also works well on FFPE DNA.

Several of the genes included in our MLPA assay represent potential druggable targets. CCND1 amplified bladder cancers may be sensitive to CDK4 inhibitors [46]; ERBB2 amplified tumors may be sensitive to lapatinib, trastuzumab, or T-DM1 [47]; and MDM2 inhibitors are in current clinical development [48]. The specific clinical importance of each of these alterations in bladder cancer has yet to be determined, but clearly there is promise. Hence detection of amplification in these genes in bladder cancer might also lead to targeted therapy.

Supporting Information

Figure S1 Visualization of copy number and allele specific intensity for 330,000 SNPs using Nexus v6.0. In each quadrant of this figure there are graphs of the intensity of signal for each pair of SNP probes (upper), and each allele (lower). Graphs are shown for four samples: a normal bladder FFPE sample in the upper left; and three different urothelial cancer FFPE samples in the other 3 quadrants. Note that the copy number graph has been normalized such that a y axis value of 0 corresponds to the normal two copies, and other values reflect either copy number loss (negative) or gain (positive). The allele fraction graph shows the relative signal intensity for each of the two alleles, and SNPs for which one allele has no signal have been screened out. The normal control bladder sample is diploid across the entire genome, and has a uniform 50% intensity value for all heterozygous SNPs. The urothelial carcinoma specimens show a variety of copy number changes and allele ratio distortions. Note region of major amplification seen on chromosomes 16p, 18p, and 21 in sample 30 at lower left, indicated by red stars.

Figure S2 Amplified genomic regions in urothelial carcinoma visualized using Nexus v6.0. In each quadrant of this figure, graphs are shown for four different urothelial carcinoma samples and for three different genomic regions. In each quadrant, chromosome cytoband is shown at top, followed by a graph of the total SNP probe intensity, then a graph of the allele specific SNP probe intensity, and then information about the nt start and end position of the amplification, the number of SNP probes in the amplification, and the probe mean and median signals within the amplification. Each dot represents a different SNP analyzed.

Figure S3 MLPA analysis on control, bladder cancer cell line, and urothelial carcinoma DNA samples. Elution

intensity curves are shown for MLPA products analyzed on the ABI 3130. Y axis is light intensity in arbitrary units, reflecting fluorescence; X axis is the size of the DNA fragment being eluted from the capillary. Boxed labels indicate the gene or genomic locus for each elution peak. Note the relatively even size of all probe peaks in the control sample. Note that there is selective increase in the relative signals for the SOX4 and E2F3 probes in the bladder cancer cell line sample. Note that other regions of relative increase are seen in the lower two urothelial carcinoma samples, E2F3 and POLB, respectively.

Table S1 List of all urothelial carcinoma samples analyzed.

Table S2 List of all mutations assessed in the MIP analysis.

Table S3 Chromosomal regions identified by GISTIC analysis of MIP data with significant CN gains or losses, with q<0.1. The chromosomal region, CN change, q value, and G-score (GISTIC) are shown for each region.

Table S4 MLPA probe sequences used in this study.

Acknowledgments

We thank Yuker Wang of Affymetrix for assistance with interpretation of the MIP analysis results, and Soheil Shams for assistance with use of Nexus software.

Author Contributions

Conceived and designed the experiments: CW DJK. Performed the experiments: YC QD SL YG. Analyzed the data: YC CW JR MR DJK. Contributed reagents/materials/analysis tools: CW JR MR WSM. Wrote the paper: YC CW JR MR WSM DJK.

References

1. Siegel R, Naishadham D, Jemal A (2012) Cancer statistics, 2012. CA Cancer J Clin 62: 10–29.
2. National Comprehensive Cancer Network I (2012) NCCN Clinical Practice Guidelines in Oncology for Bladder Cancer.
3. Goebell PJ, Knowles MA (2010) Bladder cancer or bladder cancers? Genetically distinct malignant conditions of the urothelium. Urol Oncol 28: 409–428.
4. Parada LF, Tabin CJ, Shih C, Weinberg RA (1982) Human EJ bladder carcinoma oncogene is homologue of Harvey sarcoma virus ras gene. Nature 297: 474–478.
5. Sidransky D, Von Eschenbach A, Tsai YC, Jones P, Summerhayes I, et al. (1991) Identification of p53 gene mutations in bladder cancers and urine samples. Science 252: 706–709.
6. Williamson MP, Elder PA, Shaw ME, Devlin J, Knowles MA (1995) p16 (CDKN2) is a major deletion target at 9p21 in bladder cancer. Hum Mol Genet 4: 1569–1577.
7. Hornigold N, Devlin J, Davies AM, Aveyard JS, Habuchi T, et al. (1999) Mutation of the 9q34 gene TSC1 in sporadic bladder cancer. Oncogene 18: 2657–2661.
8. Cappellen D, De Oliveira C, Ricol D, de Medina S, Bourdin J, et al. (1999) Frequent activating mutations of FGFR3 in human bladder and cervix carcinomas. Nat Genet 23: 18–20.
9. Kallioniemi A, Kallioniemi OP, Citro G, Sauter G, DeVries S, et al. (1995) Identification of gains and losses of DNA sequences in primary bladder cancer by comparative genomic hybridization. Genes Chromosomes Cancer 12: 213–219.
10. Voorter C, Joos S, Bringuier PP, Vallinga M, Poddighe P, et al. (1995) Detection of chromosomal imbalances in transitional cell carcinoma of the bladder by comparative genomic hybridization. Am J Pathol 146: 1341–1354.
11. Richter J, Jiang F, Gorog JP, Sartorius G, Egenter C, et al. (1997) Marked genetic differences between stage pTa and stage pT1 papillary bladder cancer detected by comparative genomic hybridization. Cancer Res 57: 2860–2864.
12. Simon R, Burger H, Brinkschmidt C, Bocker W, Hertle L, et al. (1998) Chromosomal aberrations associated with invasion in papillary superficial bladder cancer. J Pathol 185: 345–351.
13. Blaveri E, Brewer JL, Roydasgupta R, Fridlyand J, DeVries S, et al. (2005) Bladder cancer stage and outcome by array-based comparative genomic hybridization. Clin Cancer Res 11: 7012–7022.
14. Edge SB, Byrd DR, Compton CC, Fritz AG, Greene FL, et al. (2010) AJCC Cancer Staging Manual: Springer.
15. Platt FM, Hurst CD, Taylor CF, Gregory WM, Harnden P, et al. (2009) Spectrum of phosphatidylinositol 3-kinase pathway gene alterations in bladder cancer. Clin Cancer Res 15: 6008–6017.
16. Wang Y, Carlton VE, Karlin-Neumann G, Sapolsky R, Zhang L, et al. (2009) High quality copy number and genotype data from FFPE samples using Molecular Inversion Probe (MIP) microarrays. BMC Med Genomics 2: 8.
17. Reich M, Liefeld T, Gould J, Lerner J, Tamayo P, et al. (2006) GenePattern 2.0. Nat Genet 38: 500–501.
18. Beroukhim R, Getz G, Nghiemphu L, Barretina J, Hsueh T, et al. (2007) Assessing the significance of chromosomal aberrations in cancer: methodology and application to glioma. Proc Natl Acad Sci U S A 104: 20007–20012.
19. Kozlowski P, Roberts P, Dabora S, Franz D, Bissler J, et al. (2007) Identification of 54 large deletions/duplications in TSC1 and TSC2 using MLPA, and genotype-phenotype correlations. Hum Genet 121: 389–400.
20. van Rhijn BW, van der Kwast TH, Vis AN, Kirkels WJ, Boeve ER, et al. (2004) FGFR3 and P53 characterize alternative genetic pathways in the pathogenesis of urothelial cell carcinoma. Cancer Res 64: 1911–1914.

21. Bakkar AA, Wallerand H, Radvanyi F, Lahaye JB, Pissard S, et al. (2003) FGFR3 and TP53 gene mutations define two distinct pathways in urothelial cell carcinoma of the bladder. Cancer Res 63: 8108–8112.

22. Forbes SA, Tang G, Bindal N, Bamford S, Dawson E, et al. (2010) COSMIC (the Catalogue of Somatic Mutations in Cancer): a resource to investigate acquired mutations in human cancer. Nucleic Acids Res 38: D652–657.

23. Lee HW, Seol HJ, Choi YL, Ju HJ, Joo KM, et al. (2012) Genomic copy number alterations associated with the early brain metastasis of non-small cell lung cancer. Int J Oncol 41: 2013–20.

24. Hasselblatt M, Isken S, Linge A, Eikmeier K, Jeibmann A, et al. (2013) High-resolution genomic analysis suggests the absence of recurrent genomic alterations other than SMARCB1 aberrations in atypical teratoid/rhabdoid tumors. Genes Chrom Cancer 52: 185–90.

25. Jahromi MS, Putnam AR, Druzgal C, Wright J, Spraker-Perlman H, et al. (2012) Molecular inversion probe analysis detects novel copy number alterations in Ewing sarcoma. Cancer Genet 205: 391–404.

26. Johnson CE, Gorringe KL, Thompson ER, Opeskin K, Boyle SE, et al. (2012) Identification of copy number alterations associated with the progression of DCIS to invasive ductal carcinoma. Breast Cancer Res Treat 133: 889–98.

27. Thompson PA, Brewster AM, Kim-Anh D, Baladandayuthapani V, Broom BM, et al. (2011) Selective genomic copy number imbalances and probability of recurrence in early-stage breast cancer. PLoS One 6: e23543.

28. Cheng L, Zhang S, MacLennan GT, Williamson SR, Lopez-Beltran A, et al. (2011) Bladder cancer: translating molecular genetic insights into clinical practice. Hum Pathol 42: 455–481.

29. Feber A, Clark J, Goodwin G, Dodson AR, Smith PH, et al. (2004) Amplification and overexpression of E2F3 in human bladder cancer. Oncogene 23: 1627–1630.

30. Fleischmann A, Rotzer D, Seiler R, Studer UE, Thalmann GN (2011) Her2 amplification is significantly more frequent in lymph node metastases from urothelial bladder cancer than in the primary tumours. Eur Urol 60: 350–357.

31. Hurst CD, Tomlinson DC, Williams SV, Platt FM, Knowles MA (2008) Inactivation of the Rb pathway and overexpression of both isoforms of E2F3 are obligate events in bladder tumours with 6p22 amplification. Oncogene 27: 2716–2727.

32. Kompier LC, Lurkin I, van der Aa MN, van Rhijn BW, van der Kwast TH, et al. (2010) FGFR3, HRAS, KRAS, NRAS and PIK3CA mutations in bladder cancer and their potential as biomarkers for surveillance and therapy. PLoS One 5: e13821.

33. Lae M, Couturier J, Oudard S, Radvanyi F, Beuzeboc P, et al. (2010) Assessing HER2 gene amplification as a potential target for therapy in invasive urothelial bladder cancer with a standardized methodology: results in 1005 patients. Ann Oncol 21: 815–819.

34. Lopez-Beltran A, Ordonez JL, Otero AP, Blanca A, Sevillano V, et al. (2010) Cyclin D3 gene amplification in bladder carcinoma in situ. Virchows Arch 457: 555–561.

35. Mhawech-Fauceglia P, Cheney RT, Schwaller J (2006) Genetic alterations in urothelial bladder carcinoma: an updated review. Cancer 106: 1205–1216.

36. Nord H, Segersten U, Sandgren J, Wester K, Busch C, et al. (2010) Focal amplifications are associated with high grade and recurrences in stage Ta bladder carcinoma. Int J Cancer 126: 1390–1402.

37. Prat E, del Rey J, Ponsa I, Nadal M, Camps J, et al. (2010) Comparative genomic hybridization analysis reveals new different subgroups in early-stage bladder tumors. Urology 75: 347–355.

38. Richter J, Beffa L, Wagner U, Schraml P, Gasser TC, et al. (1998) Patterns of chromosomal imbalances in advanced urinary bladder cancer detected by comparative genomic hybridization. Am J Pathol 153: 1615–1621.

39. Veerakumarasivam A, Scott HE, Chin SF, Warren A, Wallard MJ, et al. (2008) High-resolution array-based comparative genomic hybridization of bladder cancers identifies mouse double minute 4 (MDM4) as an amplification target exclusive of MDM2 and TP53. Clin Cancer Res 14: 2527–2534.

40. Obermann EC, Junker K, Stoehr R, Dietmaier W, Zaak D, et al. (2003) Frequent genetic alterations in flat urothelial hyperplasias and concomitant papillary bladder cancer as detected by CGH, LOH, and FISH analyses. J Pathol 199: 50–57.

41. Knowles MA (2008) Bladder cancer subtypes defined by genomic alterations. Scand J Urol Nephrol Suppl: 116–130.

42. Sjodahl G, Lauss M, Gudjonsson S, Liedberg F, Hallden C, et al. (2011) A systematic study of gene mutations in urothelial carcinoma; inactivating mutations in TSC2 and PIK3R1. PLoS One 6: e18583.

43. Gui Y, Guo G, Huang Y, Hu X, Tang A, et al. (2011) Frequent mutations of chromatin remodeling genes in transitional cell carcinoma of the bladder. Nat Genet 43: 875–878.

44. Mao JH, Kim IJ, Wu D, Climent J, Kang HC, et al. (2008) FBXW7 targets mTOR for degradation and cooperates with PTEN in tumor suppression. Science 321: 1499–1502.

45. Hindson BJ, Ness KD, Masquelier DA, Belgrader P, Heredia NJ, et al. (2011) High-throughput droplet digital PCR system for absolute quantitation of DNA copy number. Anal Chem 83: 8604–8610.

46. Kim JK, Diehl JA (2009) Nuclear cyclin D1: an oncogenic driver in human cancer. J Cell Physiol 220: 292–296.

47. Baselga J, Swain SM (2009) Novel anticancer targets: revisiting ERBB2 and discovering ERBB3. Nat Rev Cancer 9: 463–475.

48. Yuan Y, Liao YM, Hsueh CT, Mirshahidi HR (2011) Novel targeted therapeutics: inhibitors of MDM2, ALK and PARP. J Hematol Oncol 4: 16.

8

Distinct SNP Combinations Confer Susceptibility to Urinary Bladder Cancer in Smokers and Non-Smokers

Holger Schwender[1][*][9], **Silvia Selinski**[2][9], **Meinolf Blaszkewicz**[2], **Rosemarie Marchan**[2], **Katja Ickstadt**[3], **Klaus Golka**[2][¶], **Jan G. Hengstler**[2][¶]

1 Mathematical Institute, Heinrich Heine University Düsseldorf, Düsseldorf, Germany, **2** Leibniz Research Centre for Working Environment and Human Factors (IfADo), Dortmund, Germany, **3** Faculty of Statistics, TU Dortmund University, Dortmund, Germany

Abstract

Recently, genome-wide association studies have identified and validated genetic variations associated with urinary bladder cancer (UBC). However, it is still unknown whether the high-risk alleles of several SNPs interact with one another, leading to an even higher disease risk. Additionally, there is no information available on how the UBC risk due to these SNPs compare to the risk of cigarette smoking and to occupational exposure to urinary bladder carcinogens, and whether the same or different SNP combinations are relevant in smokers and non-smokers. To address these questions, we analyzed the genotypes of six SNPs, previously found to be associated with UBC, together with the *GSTM1* deletion, in 1,595 UBC cases and 1,760 controls, stratified for smoking habits. We identified the strongest interactions of different orders and tested the stability of their effect by bootstrapping. We found that different SNP combinations were relevant in smokers and non-smokers. In smokers, polymorphisms involved in detoxification of cigarette smoke carcinogens were most relevant (*GSTM1*, rs11892031), in contrast to those in non-smokers with *MYC* and *APOBEC3A* near polymorphisms (rs9642880, rs1014971) being the most influential. Stable combinations of up to three high-risk alleles resulted in higher odds ratios (OR) than the individual SNPs, although the interaction effect was less than additive. The highest stable combination effects resulted in an OR of about 2.0, which is still lower than the ORs of cigarette smoking (here, current smokers' OR: 3.28) and comparable to occupational carcinogen exposure risks which, depending on the workplace, show mostly ORs up to 2.0.

Editor: Mohammad O. Hoque, Johns Hopkins University, United States of America

Funding: This work was supported by the Deutsche Forschungsgemeinschaft (Project C4 of the SFB 876 "Providing Information by Resource-Constrained Data Analysis" to KI and grant SCHW 1508/3-1 to HS). The funders had no role in study design, data collection and analysis, decision to publish, or preparation of the manuscript.

Competing Interests: The authors have declared that no competing interests exist.

* E-mail: schwender@math.uni-duesseldorf.de

9 These authors contributed equally to this work.

¶ These authors also contributed equally to this work.

Introduction

Urinary bladder cancer (UBC) is the ninth most common cancer worldwide [1]. The strongest known risk factors include cigarette smoking, occupational exposure to urinary bladder carcinogens, and male gender. It is well established that a deletion variant of the detoxifying phase II metabolizing enzyme glutathione S-transferase M1 (*GSTM1*), in addition to N-acetyltransferase 2 (*NAT2*) slow acetylation are associated with increased urinary bladder cancer risk [2–6]. Recently, further genetic variants have been identified and validated in several genome-wide association studies [7–12] and were extended to occupational exposure [13–15].

The recently discovered SNPs and the corresponding genes have already been comprehensively discussed [1]. Briefly, rs1014971 maps to a non-genic region of chromosome 22q13.1 [9] close to *CBX6* and *APOBEC3A*. Chromobox homolog 7 (*CBX7*) positively regulates E-cadherin expression by interacting with histone deacetylase 2 [16]. This possibly explains why loss of *CBX7* expression is associated with a highly malignant phenotype of carcinomas. Overexpression of *APOBEC3* genes may lead to

genetic instability [17]. Rs11892031 is located on chromosome 2q37 in an intronic region of the UDP-glucuronosyltransferase 1A (*UGT1A*) locus. UGT1A is a phase II metabolizing enzyme that catalyzes the glucuronidation and elimination of numerous xenobiotics [18,19]. Rs1495741 (on chromosome 8p22) is known as a tagging SNP of N-acetyltransferase 2 (*NAT2*) that distinguishes between fast and slow acetylators [20,21]. Compared to fast acetylators, slow acetylators have an increased bladder cancer risk, probably because of their decreased ability to efficiently detoxify aromatic amines. Rs710521[A] on chromosome 3q28 close to *TP63* is associated with urinary bladder cancer risk [7,14]. *TP63* shows strong homology to the tumour suppressor P53 [22,23; review: 1]. Rs8102137 on 19q12 maps to Cyclin E (*CCNE1*) which controls cell cycle progression at the G1/S transition [24; review: 1]. Rs9642889, 30 kb upstream of the *MYC* gene on chromosome 8q24.21, confers susceptibility to bladder cancer and influences expression of *MYC* [7,13]. The well-known proto oncogene *MYC* is involved in the control of proliferation and cell cycle progression [25]. Deletion of the detoxifying phase II enzyme glutathione S-transferase M1 (*GSTM1*) on chromosome 1q13.3 leads to a decreased detoxification of numerous xenobiotics, including polycyclic aromatic hydrocarbons that are known bladder carcinogens [13,26]. Although the association of each of these SNPs with urinary bladder cancer risk has been validated and confirmed in several independent cohorts, it is still not known if there is an interaction among the high-risk alleles, and if their influence differs between smokers and non-smokers. Therefore, we determined the most influential genetic variants (rs1014971, rs11892031, rs1495741, rs710521, rs8102137, rs9642880, and GSTM1) in 1,595 bladder cancer cases and 1,760 controls. We performed interaction analyses addressing the following questions: Are there specific and stable SNP interactions resulting in higher odds ratios than individual SNPs? If so, are these SNP combinations identical or distinct between smokers and non-smokers? Finally, how high is the combined genetic (SNP-based) risk compared to that of cigarette smoking and occupational exposure? We report that specific SNP combinations show a higher UBC risk than individual SNPs, where distinct SNP combinations confer susceptibility in smokers and non-smokers. These risks are, however, still small when compared to that of cigarette smoking.

Materials and Methods

Ethics Statement

The sample collection by the Leibniz Research Centre for Working Environment and Human Factors (IfADo) was approved by the ethics commission of the Leibniz Research Centre for Working Environment and Human Factors (Ethikkommission des Leibniz-Instituts für Arbeitsforschung an der TU Dortmund) and the institutional review board of the Leibniz Research Centre for Working Environment and Human Factors (Wissenschaftlicher Beirat des Leibniz-Instituts für Arbeitsforschung an der TU Dortmund). All participants provided their written informed consent.

Patients

To investigate whether there is a combined effect of SNPs associated with UBC, a total of 1,595 UBC cases of European descent and 1,760 controls of European descent from four case-control series collected by the Leibniz Research Centre for Working Environment and Human Factors (IfADo) were genotyped at the glutathione S-transferase M1 (GSTM1) and six SNPs (rs1014971, rs11892031, rs1495741, rs710521, rs8102137, rs9642880) previously identified in genome-wide association studies to be associated with UBC [7,9].

This data set comprised confirmed urinary bladder cancer cases and controls without malignant disease from the Department of Urology, Semmelweis University, Budapest, Hungary ("Hungary"; 246 cases and 78 controls), the Department of Urology, Paul Gerhardt Foundation, Lutherstadt Wittenberg, Germany ("East Germany"; 218 cases and 213 controls), the "West Germany – Ongoing" case-control series conducted at five hospitals (in total, 646 cases and 525 controls), and the "West Germany – Industrial" burdened case-control series (in total, 485 cases –111 UBC cases from the Department of Urology, Klinikum Dortmund, Germany, and 374 UBC cases surveyed for recognition of an occupational disease – and 944 controls). Information on profession obtained by questionnaire was available for the "East Germany" case-control series only (information on profession: 216 cases and 211 controls) [27,28]. Detailed descriptions of these four case-control series can be found in [15].

Patients' characteristics, such as distribution of gender, age at diagnosis for cases and age at examination for controls, as well as numbers of cases and controls in the individual case-control series,

are summarized in Tables S1, S2, and S3. 101 cases and 37 controls with unknown smoking habits were excluded from the interaction analysis in the study groups, leading to a total of 1,494 cases and 1,723 controls that were finally considered to determine the impact of SNP combinations on the UBC risk.

Polymorphisms

Isolation of genomic DNA of leucocytes was performed according to standard procedures. Genotypes of the SNPs rs1014971, rs11892031, rs1495741, rs710521, rs8102137, and rs9642880 were detected via TaqMan® Assay. Details of the SNPs are given in Appendix S1 and Table S4.

The homozygous GSTM1 deletion was detected by the amplification of the GSTM1 DNA sequence segment with 218 base pairs by means of PCR [29,30]. After gel-electrophoresis using ethidium bromide, the DNA product was detected using UV light. This method helped determine whether at least one copy of the GSTM1 gene was present or totally missing.

Statistical Analysis

Cigarette smoking was defined as non-smokers, former smokers, i.e. smokers that quit smoking at least one year before diagnosis (cases) or examination (controls), and current smokers. Former and current smokers were pooled together as "ever smokers". Analyses were performed stratified for non-smokers, former smokers and current smokers as well as for ever smokers. Analyses on the combined ever smokers groups reflect the past exposure to bladder carcinogens accounting for the latency time of bladder cancer of several decades. Age was defined as "age at diagnosis" for the cases and "age at examination" for the control persons.

Deviations from Hardy-Weinberg equilibrium (HWE) were checked in each study group and separately for cases and controls using χ^2 tests (for the results, see Table S5). Associations of polymorphisms and smoking habits with UBC were evaluated applying χ^2 tests, odds ratios (OR), and 95% confidence intervals (95% CI). Moreover, ORs and 95% CIs adjusted for age, gender, smoking habits, and study site were estimated using logistic regression.

The ORs of the individual polymorphisms, and combinations of these polymorphisms in the total cohort as well as in subgroups defined by the smoking status of the subjects, were determined by considering the dominant and recessive effects of the SNPs. For each interaction of p polymorphisms ($p = 2, ..., 7$), the ten combinations showing the OR with the lowest p-values were identified in each of the subgroups. To check whether it is appropriate to compute p-values for higher-order SNP interactions based on a χ^2 distribution with one degree of freedom, we also determined permutation p-values and compared these with the parametric p-values. Additionally, a bootstrap strategy was used to investigate the stability of the ORs of the SNP combinations of different sizes in the subgroups. To achieve this, 500 bootstrap samples were drawn from the respective subgroup and counted to determine how often the top 10 SNP combinations from the original analysis appeared among the top 10, top 20, and top 50 SNP combinations (of the same number of SNPs) from the analyses of the corresponding 500 bootstrap samples.

To test whether the OR of a certain SNP combination differs between the ever smokers and the non-smokers, logistic regression models were fitted containing parameters for the respective SNP combination, smoking status, and the interaction between these two factors. The standard test for the interaction parameter in this logistic regression model was used to test whether the ORs differ significantly between smokers and non-smokers. Details on this and other statistical analyses can be found in Appendix S2.

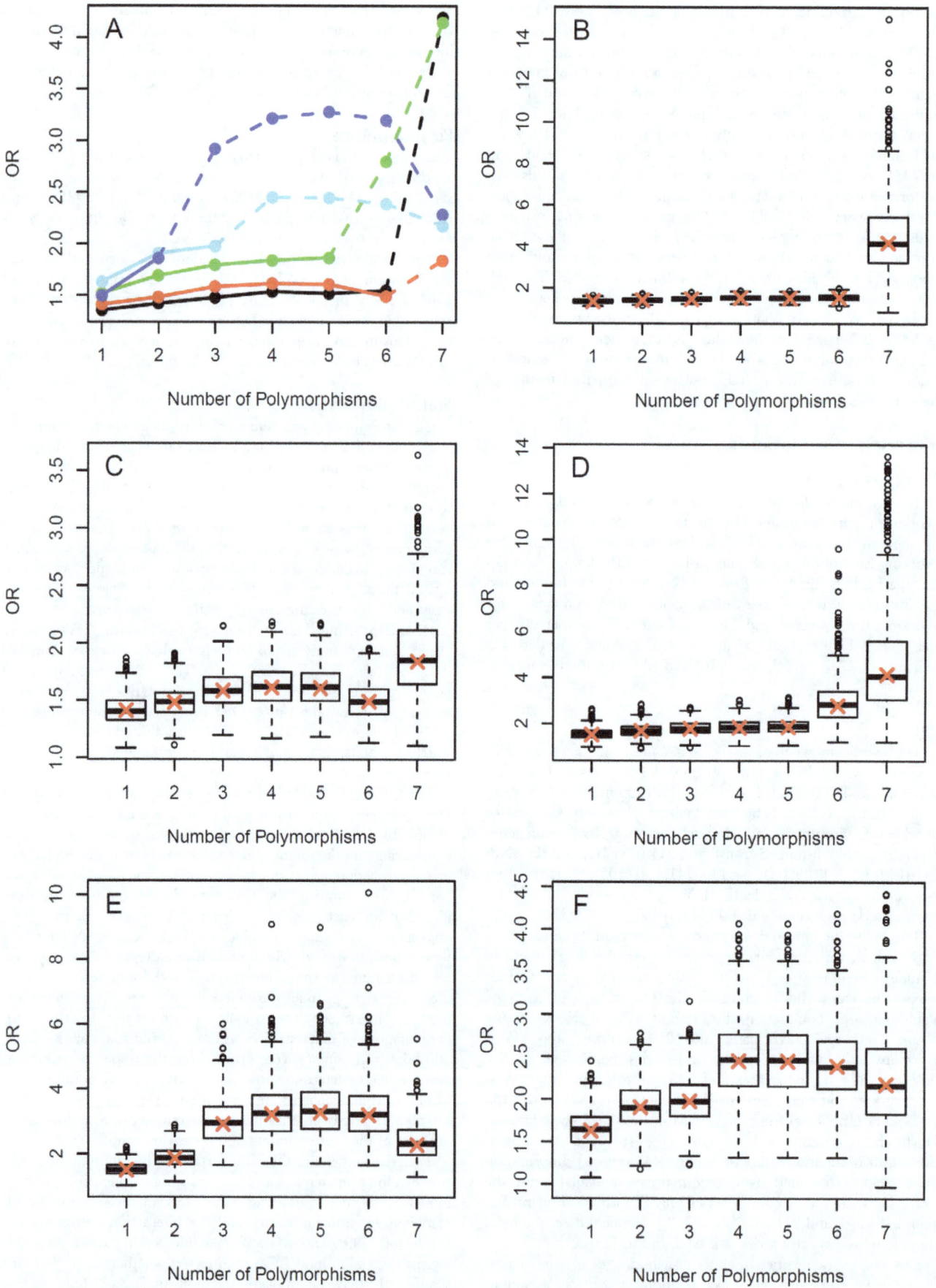

Figure 1. Optimal odds ratios for combinations of one to seven polymorphisms. For the computation of the optimal odds ratios (OR), all possible combinations of one to seven of the polymorphisms rs1014971, rs9642880, rs710521, rs8102137, rs11892031, rs1495741 and *GSTM1* were considered. (A) Profile plots for the odds ratios in the total group (black line) and the subgroups of ever smokers (red line), current smokers (green), former smokers (blue) and non-smokers (cyan). The lines were included for clarity of information and not to suggest a continuous development. Dashed lines indicate when number of cases and/or number of controls fall below 100. In these situations, the corresponding odds ratios should be interpreted with caution. (B)–(F): For the optimal combinations shown in (A), box plots of odds ratios computed in 500 bootstrap samples from (B) the total group, (C) the ever smokers, (D) the current smokers, (E) the former smokers and (F) the non-smokers. In twelve of the bootstrap samples (all but one in the analyses of the seven-way interactions in the total and the smoker group), the odds ratios were larger than 15. For a better presentation, these odds ratios are not displayed in the corresponding box plots. The crosses mark the odds ratios of the optimal combinations in the original analysis. The corresponding plots of the test statistics are shown in Figure S1.

Population attributable risks (PAR) indicating the proportion of cases that could be attributed to a certain risk factor, and combined PARs for two or more independent risk factors were calculated according to [31]. The PARs of the individual polymorphism were calculated based on adjusted and unadjusted ORs. Combined PARs were determined based on the adjusted ORs of the homozygous and heterozygous vs. the reference genotypes of each SNP. ORs were adjusted for age, gender, smoking habits, study site (in case of combined study groups) and all measured polymorphisms but rs11892031, as this SNP has a rather protective effect in about 16% of the population of European descent [32]. All four study groups were used to determine the PAR due to smoking habits and genetic risk factors in the present study, whereas the PAR for certain professions was based on the "East Germany" case-control series only.

For an overview of UBC risk factors from the literature, we performed an extensive literature search using PubMed. We included the relevant papers on UBC causes in populations of European descent. If possible, we used the given adjusted ORs to determine the PAR from published studies. Otherwise, unadjusted ORs or ORs calculated from the published frequencies were used. Estimation of ORs of combined genetic risk factors was done for varying frequencies assuming a PAR of 30%.

Results

Analysis of ORs of SNP Combinations

Currently, it is unknown whether genetic variants associated with increased UBC risk interact with one another resulting in higher odds ratios (OR) for combinations than for individual

SNPs. Therefore, we analyzed the ORs from combinations of up to seven polymorphisms that were previously found to be individually associated with UBC [2,7,9,20]. The ORs as well as the corresponding 95% confidence intervals (95% CI) and p-values for the individual SNPs, determined in the analysis of our total study group and subgroups defined by the smoking habits, are summarized in Table S6.

Analyzing the SNP combinations, the ORs of the optimal SNP combinations, in general, increased with the numbers of combined SNPs (Figure 1A). However, case numbers of the high-risk alleles decreased rapidly when several SNPs were combined, thus leading to relatively high variability of the odds ratios in the bootstrap sample (Figure 1B–F). Here the variation typically increased with decreasing number of subjects. In contrast to the ORs, the Wald statistics corresponding to the ORs increased from individual SNPs to combinations of three polymorphisms. However, no further increase was observed (Figure S1), which is again due to high variances and small sample sizes.

In Tables 1, 2, 3 and 4, the ORs with 95% CIs and the p-values of the ten combinations of two and three polymorphisms with the smallest p-values found in the analysis of the ever smokers and the non-smokers are shown. The ORs of the top ten individual effects as well as the top ten two-way and three-way interactions in the total group and in the smoker subgroups are presented in Tables S7, S8, S9, S10, S11, S12, S13, S14, S15, S16, S17, S18, S19 S20 and S21. Additionally, we summarized how often the seven polymorphisms occur in the top ten two-way and three-way interactions in the different subgroups (Table 5).

Table 1. Top ten two-way interactions found in the analysis of the ever smokers.

SNP combination	OR (95% CI)	P-value
rs11892031 [A/A] × *GSTM1* null	1.48 (1.25–1.76)	0.0024
rs8102137 [C/T, T/T] × *GSTM1* null	1.51 (1.25–1.82)	0.0040
rs710521 [A/A, A/G] × *GSTM1* null	1.46 (1.22–1.73)	0.0062
rs710521 [A/A, A/G] × *GSTM1* present	0.69 (0.58–0.83)	0.0105
rs9642880 [G/G, G/T] × *GSTM1* present	0.69 (0.57–0.82)	0.0113
rs11892031 [A/A, A/C] × *GSTM1* present	0.70 (0.59–0.84)	0.0185
rs11892031 [A/A, A/C] × *GSTM1* null	1.42 (1.19–1.69)	0.0204
rs1014971 [C/C, C/T] × *GSTM1* present	0.71 (0.60–0.84)	0.0303
rs1495741 [A/A, A/G] × *GSTM1* null	1.40 (1.18–1.66)	0.0398
rs1014971 [C/C, C/T] × *GSTM1* null	1.38 (1.16–1.64)	0.0703

The top ten of the 288 possible two-way interactions comprised of the six SNPs and *GSTM1* as well as their odds ratios (OR) with 95% confidence intervals (CI) are listed in order of their p-values, where the p-values were adjusted for multiple comparisons by the Bonferroni correction.

Table 2. Top ten two-way interactions found in the analysis of the non-smokers.

SNP combination	OR (95% CI)	P-value
rs9642880 [G/T, T/T] × rs1014971 [C/C]	1.91 (1.44–2.51)	0.0015
rs9642880 [G/G, G/T] × rs1014971 [C/T, T/T]	0.56 (0.43–0.74)	0.0112
rs710521 [A/A, A/G] × rs1014971 [C/C]	1.68 (1.28–2.20)	0.0458
rs1014971 [C/C] × rs1495741 [A/A, A/G]	1.66 (1.27–2.16)	0.0524
rs1014971 [C/C] × rs11892031 [A/A, A/C]	1.65 (1.27–2.16)	0.0564
rs1014971 [C/T, T/T] × rs8102137 [C/C, C/T]	0.61 (0.46–0.79)	0.0640
rs1014971 [C/C] × rs11892031 [A/A]	1.65 (1.26–2.15)	0.0761
rs9642880 [T/T] × rs710521 [A/A, A/G]	1.75 (1.29–2.37)	0.0827
rs1014971 [C/T, T/T] × rs1495741 [A/A, A/G]	0.62 (0.47–0.81)	0.1051
rs1014971 [C/C] × *GSTM1* null	1.73 (1.28–2.35)	0.1111

The top ten of the 288 possible two-way interactions comprised of the six SNPs and *GSTM1* as well as their odds ratios (OR) with 95% confidence intervals (CI) are listed in order of their p-values, where the p-values were adjusted for multiple comparisons by the Bonferroni correction.

Table 3. Top ten three-way interactions found in the analysis of the ever smokers.

SNP combination	OR (95% CI)	P-value
rs8102137 [C/T, T/T] × rs11892031 [A/A] × GSTM1 null	1.58 (1.30–1.92)	0.0059
rs710521 [A/A, A/G] × rs11892031 [A/A] × GSTM1 null	1.51 (1.26–1.80)	0.0080
rs710521 [A/A, A/G] × rs8102137 [C/T, T/T] × GSTM1 null	1.55 (1.28–1.88)	0.0135
rs9642880 [G/G, G/T] × rs710521 [A/A, A/G] × GSTM1 present	0.66 (0.55–0.79)	0.0171
rs8102137 [C/T, T/T] × rs1495741 [A/A, A/G] × GSTM1 null	1.52 (1.26–1.84)	0.0248
rs8102137 [C/T, T/T] × rs11892031 [A/A, A/C] × GSTM1 null	1.50 (1.25–1.81)	0.0315
rs1014971 [C/C, C/T] × rs11892031 [A/A] × GSTM1 null	1.46 (1.22–1.74)	0.0419
rs9642880 [G/G, G/T] × rs11892031 [A/A, A/C] × GSTM1 present	0.68 (0.57–0.82)	0.0520
rs710521 [A/A, A/G] × rs11892031 [A/A, A/C] × GSTM1 null	1.45 (1.22–1.72)	0.0552
rs710521 [A/A, A/G] × rs1014971 [C/C, C/T] × GSTM1 present	0.69 (0.57–0.82)	0.0582

The top ten of the 1,760 possible three-way interactions comprised of the six SNPs and GSTM1, as well as their odds ratios (OR) with 95% confidence intervals (CI) are listed in order of their p-values, where the p-values were adjusted for multiple comparisons by the Bonferroni correction.

Appropriateness of Parametric p-values

Since the p-values were determined using a χ^2 distribution with one degree of freedom, we examined the suitability of employing such parametric p-values for combinations of several SNPs by comparing these p-values with the corresponding permutation-based p-values. In addition, we computed both the mean and the variance of the test statistics determined in the 100,000 permutations used in the derivation of the latter p-values. The results of these computations are displayed in the supporting information. Figures S2, S3 and S4 indicate that the χ^2 approximation worked well for most of the combinations of two or three SNPs, and in particular, for the respective top ten combinations. However, the χ^2 approximation became worse as the number of SNPs forming an interaction increased. Surprisingly, the most extreme differences in p-values for the combinations of two SNPs were larger than the ones for, for example, three-way interactions. This, however, was only relevant for a few combinations.

Stability of the Estimated ORs

The above results, together with the relatively small case numbers in the subgroups of current, former and non-smoker for combinations of more than three SNPs, led us to focus on the interaction of two and three polymorphisms when we analyzed the stability of the ranks of the SNP combinations in the bootstrap samples (Tables S12, S13, S14, S15, S16 and Tables S17, S18, S19, S20 and S21, respectively). The ranks were very stable considering the individual variables coding for the polymorphisms (Tables S7, S8, S9, S10 and S11). In addition, the top two-way interactions occurred among the top ten interactions in a large majority of the bootstrap samples (Tables S12, S13, S14, S15 and S16). However, the instability of the ranks increased with the number of polymorphisms forming a combination (for example, the ranks for three-way SNP combinations in Tables S17, S18, S19, S20 and S21).

Differences in relevant SNP interactions between smokers and non-smokers. Interestingly, different SNP combinations were obtained for non-smokers and smokers. The optimal three-way SNP combinations (resulting in maximal odds ratios) for non-smokers consisted of (i) rs1014971, (ii) rs9642880, and (iii) one of the three SNPs: rs11892031, rs1495741, or rs710521 (Tables 2 and 4 as well as Table 5). In contrast, the optimal combinations for the current smokers were composed of GSTM1, rs1014971, and one of the three SNPs: rs11892031,

Table 4. Top ten three-way interactions found in the analysis of the non-smokers.

SNP combination	OR (95% CI)	P-value
rs9642880 [G/T, T/T] × rs710521 [A/A, A/G] × rs1014971 [C/C]	1.98 (1.49–2.63)	0.0044
rs9642880 [G/T, T/T] × rs1014971 [C/C] × rs1495741 [A/A, A/G]	1.95 (1.47–2.58)	0.0054
rs9642880 [G/T, T/T] × rs1014971 [C/C] × rs11892031 [A/A, A/C]	1.93 (1.46–2.55)	0.0061
rs9642880 [G/T, T/T] × rs1014971 [C/C] × GSTM1 null	2.21 (1.58–3.10)	0.0070
rs9642880 [G/G, G/T] × rs1014971 [C/T, T/T] × rs8102137 [C/C, C/T]	0.54 (0.40–0.71)	0.0318
rs9642880 [G/G, G/T] × rs710521 [A/A, A/G] × rs1014971 [C/T, T/T]	0.54 (0.40–0.71)	0.0325
rs9642880 [G/G, G/T] × rs1014971 [C/T, T/T] × rs1495741 [A/A, A/G]	0.56 (0.42–0.74)	0.0735
rs710521 [A/A, A/G] × rs1014971 [C/C] × GSTM1 null	1.93 (1.41–2.64)	0.0773
rs9642880 [G/T, T/T] × rs1014971 [C/C] × rs11892031 [A/A]	1.80 (1.35–2.40)	0.0954
rs710521 [A/A, A/G] × rs1014971 [C/C] × rs11892031 [A/A]	1.74 (1.33–2.29)	0.1142

The top ten of the 1,760 possible three-way interactions comprised of the six SNPs and GSTM1, as well as their odds ratios (OR) with 95% confidence intervals (CI) are listed in order of their p-values, where the p-values were adjusted for multiple comparisons by the Bonferroni correction.

Table 5. Number of times the considered polymorphisms appear in the ten top two- and three-way interactions when analyzing the different smoker groups.

Polymorphism	Total	Ever	Current	Former	Never
GSTM1	10 (9)	10 (10)	10 (10)	7 (4)	2 (1)
rs11892031	6 (3)	6 (3)	4 (3)	3 (2)	3 (2)
rs710521	5 (4)	5 (2)	4 (2)	5 (3)	4 (2)
rs9642880	5 (3)	2 (1)	3 (1)	8 (7)	8 (3)
rs8102137	3 (1)	4 (1)	2 (1)	5 (2)	1 (1)
rs1495741	1 (0)	1 (1)	0 (0)	2 (1)	2 (2)
rs1014971	0 (0)	2 (2)	7 (3)	0 (1)	10 (9)

Numbers in brackets are from the analysis of the two-way interactions. Numbers outside the brackets are from the analysis of the three-way interactions. The corresponding groupwise top ten two-way interactions are listed in Tables S12, S13, S14, S15 and S16, and the top ten three-way interactions are presented in Tables S17, S18, S19, S20 and S21.

rs710521, and rs9642880 (Table 5 as well as Tables S14 and S19). A similar result was obtained for the ever smokers in which, however, rs1014971 was only rarely present in the top SNP combinations (Table 5 as well as Tables 1 and 3). This SNP also did not appear in any of the top ten three-way interactions in the former smokers (Table 4 as well as Tables S15 and S20). Interestingly, the former smokers showed a mixed SNP pattern of smokers and non-smokers, including GSTM1 (the top "smoker SNP"), rs9642880 (the second-best scoring "non-smoker SNP"), rs710521 (present in both the smoker and non-smoker SNP combination), as well as rs8102137 (the least or second least important SNP when considering the three-way interactions in non-smokers and current smokers, respectively).

Comparison with Published Results

Considering the genetic risks due to single well-known and novel polymorphisms, ORs range between null and 1.34 in the present study in accordance with the published results from case-controls studies, meta-analyses and GWAS that did not exceed 1.81 (Table 6). Particularly, UBC risks attributed to GSTM1 and

NAT2 show a remarkable variation in the literature ranging from 1.28 to 1.70 in case of GSTM1, and no considerable effect to mild risks of 1.43 due to slow NAT2 genotypes not stratified by smoking habits. In terms of relevance for the populations – depending on relative risks and frequency of the risk factors – a considerable fraction of the UBC cases can be attributed to overall genetic risks (30%) or single polymorphisms, in particular GSTM1 with population attributable risks (PAR) ranging from 13% to 26% (Table 6).

Comparison of Interaction Effects with Occupational and Environmental Risk

The situation is less clear for risks due to occupational exposure to bladder carcinogens. The risk depends strongly on the population under investigation and time of recruitment, both of which reflects the structure of the local industry and changes in exposure (Table 7). Estimates of overall PARs range from 2–5% for women and 7–10% for men [33,34] to 20–26% [35–37] for highly industrialized areas. Strongly increased risks due to exposure to bladder carcinogens, in particular β-naphthylamine, 4-aminobiphenyl and 4-chloro-o-toluidine, can be found in old studies on highly exposed workers whereas clearly and moderately increased risks are still present but do not exceed ORs of two [38]. Determination of PARs for single professions is hampered by their different frequencies in different regions, though common occupations as painters or hairdressers contribute to 0.2–0.9% of the UBC cases.

Most UBC cases can clearly be attributed to cigarette smoking (Table 8; present study PAR: 46%; other studies PAR: 50–56%). While current smokers have an approximately 3-fold risk (present study OR = 3.28, other studies OR = 2.77–4.95) of developing UBC – increasing with amount and time – the UBC risk of former smokers decreases to an OR of about two (present study OR = 2.12, other studies OR = 1.74–2.34). Both subgroups contribute almost equally to the UBC cases in the present study (former smokers PAR = 29%, current smokers PAR = 30%), whereas in published studies estimates of the PAR range from 28–40% for former smokers to 39% in current smokers. Interestingly, among men more UBC cases are attributable to smoking (former 41%, current 55%, ever 66%) than among women (former 17%, current 32%, ever 30%).

Table 6. Population attributable risks and odds ratios due to genetic factors.

Genetic Factors	Present study		Published	
	PAR	OR	PAR	OR
All	–	–	30% [47,51]	1.04–1.81 [1,9,31,48]
GSTM1	13%[a]	1.28	14–26% [47,48,54,55]	1.28–1.70 [47,48,54,55]
NAT2	1%[b]	1.02[b]	8.2%[c] [54]	1.04–1.43 [47,48,54,56]
"wimp" SNPs	33%[d]	1.02–1.34[e]	–	1.11–1.81 [1,9,32]
Top 3-way interaction	16%	1.48	–	–

Population attributable risks (PARs) and odds ratios (ORs) were calculated from the data of the present study and summarized from previously published studies for different genetic factors. Numbers in brackets refer to the publications in which the PARs and ORs were published.
[a]Adjusted for age, gender, smoking habits, all measured SNPs and study site; crude PAR/OR: 16%/1.39; adjusted for age and gender: 16%/1.37; adjusted for all measured SNPs: 15%/1.36.
[b]Adjusted for age, gender, smoking habits, all measured SNPs and study site; crude PAR/OR: 5%/1.09; adjusted for age and gender: 3%/1.05; adjusted for all measured SNPs: 5%/1.10.
[c]Data from Moore et al. [48] and Garcia-Closas et al.[47] result in PARs of 2–18%.
[d]Combined PAR, individual SNP OR and PAR adjusted for age, gender, smoking habits and all measured SNPs.
[e]Range of individual SNP OR adjusted for age, gender, smoking habits, all measured SNPs and study site depending on the mode of inheritance.

Table 7. Population attributable risks and odds ratios for different occupational exposures.

Increased risk	Occupation/Exposure	Present study		Published	
		PAR	OR	PAR	OR
	All	–	–	20–26% [35–37]	–
				M: 7–10% [33,34]	
				F: 2–5% [33,34]	
Moderately	Painter	0.89%	1.38	0.7% [33,34]	1.17–1.98 [36,38,57–59][a]
	Hairdresser	–	–	0.2% [33,34]	1.23–2.10 [36,38,63]
	Coal miner	2.81%	1.47	–	1.31–2.40 [38,58,64,65]
Clearly	Aluminium Worker[b]	–	–	–	1.50–2.34 [36,66]
	Rubber Industry	2.80%	1.76	–	1.29–1.30 [36,38]
	Roofer and Slater	–	–	–	1.70 [36]
Strongly	Benzidine/β-Naphthylamine	–	–	–	1.60 [37]
	Benzidine[c]	–	–	–	30–75 [67,68]
	β-Naphthylamine[c]	–	–	–	5–200 [68]
	4-Aminobiphenyl[c]	–	–	–	11%[d] [68]
	4-Chloro-o-toluidine	–	–	–	38–90 [68]

Population attributable risks (PARs) and odds ratios (ORs) were calculated from the data of the present study and summarized from previously published studies for different occupations and occupational exposures, partly stratified by gender (M: Male, F: Female). Numbers in brackets refer to the publications in which the PARs and ORs were published.
[a]Painters before 1960 had a clearly increased risk: OR = 2.42–2.78 [60–62].
[b]More exactly, Aluminium Workers (Soderberg Processing).
[c]Results from historical studies.
[d]Prevalence in exposed workers.

Table 8. Population attributable risks and odds ratios in the different smoker groups.

Smoking habits	Present study		Published	
	PAR	OR	PAR	OR
Former smokers	30%[a]	2.12[a]	28–40% [48,53]	1.74–2.34 [48,53,71]
			M: 41% [69]	M: 2.74 [69]
			F: 17% [70]	F: 1.42 [70]
Current smokers	29%[b]	3.28[b]	39% [48,53]	2.77–4.95 [48,53,71]
			M: 55% [69]	M: 4.72 [69]
			F: 32% [70]	F: 1.89 [70]
Ever smokers	46%[c]	2.47[c]	50–56% [48,52,53]	2.61–2.89 [48,53]
			M: 66% [69]	M: 3.65 [69]
			F: 30% [70]	F: 1.69 [70]

Population attributable risks (PARs) and odds ratios (ORs) were calculated from the data of the present study and summarized from previously published studies for the different smoker groups, partly stratified by gender (M: Male, F: Female), where non-smokers were used as a reference group having no additional risk. Numbers in brackets refer to the publications in which the PARs and ORs were published.
[a]Adjusted for age and gender; crude PAR/OR: 39%/2.65; adjusted for age, gender, SNPs: 30%/2.15.
[b]Adjusted for age and gender; crude PAR/OR: 29%/3.21; adjusted for age, gender, SNPs: 28%/3.17.
[c]Adjusted for age and gender; crude PAR/OR: 51%/2.83; adjusted for age, gender, SNPs: 46%/2.47.

Discussion

Comparison of the Results from Analyzing Non-smokers and Smokers

The distinct SNP patterns for smokers and non-smokers found in our analysis are remarkable, since the genes closest to the top scoring "smoker variants" are involved in the detoxification of carcinogens in cigarette smoke, whereas the top scoring "non-smoker SNPs" are associated with cell cycle control and DNA stability. The deletion variant of GSTM1, the polymorphism found in our analysis to be the most important in smokers, results in loss of activity of the phase II metabolizing enzyme glutathione S-transferase M1, which is involved in detoxification of numerous polycyclic aromatic hydrocarbons [39,40]. The second scoring "smoker variant" rs11892031 is located closest to the UGT1A cluster [9]. UDP-glucuronosyltransferase is also a phase II metabolizing enzyme responsible for the conjugation and detoxification of several urinary bladder carcinogens present in cigarette smoke [27,41–45].

In contrast, the two top scoring "non-smoker SNPs" are not involved in carcinogen detoxification. Rs1014971 is located approximately 25 kb centromeric of APOBEC3A, which deaminates cytosine to uracil, thereby playing a role in endogenous mutagenesis [1,9]. The second, rs9642880 is known to influence the expression of the proto oncogene MYC, which controls transcription of numerous genes involved in proliferation [7,13]. This scenario suggests that control factors of proliferation and DNA integrity are critical for susceptibility to bladder cancer in non-smokers. In contrast, enzymes detoxifying cigarette smoke carcinogens seem to be of highest relevance in smokers.

Another striking observation is that the three SNPs forming the optimal three-way SNP combination in non-smokers, i.e. rs9642880[G/T, T/T] x rs710521[A/A, A/G] x rs1014971[C/

Table 9. Distribution of smoking habits and UBC risk in the present case-control study.

Smoking Habit (n_{Ca}/n_{Co})	Cases	Controls	OR (95% CI)	OR adj (95% CI adj)
Non-smokers (321/752)	21%	44%	(reference)	(reference)
Former smokers (742/656)	50%	38%	2.65 (2.24–3.31)	2.12 (1.78–2.53)
Current smokers (431/315)	29%	18%	3.21 (2.64–3.90)	3.28 (2.67–4.03)
Ever smokers (1173/971)	79%	56%	2.83 (2.42–3.31)	2.47 (2.10–2.90)

For each of the smoker subgroups containing n_{Ca} cases and n_{Co} controls, the odds ratios (OR) and their corresponding 95% confidence intervals (95% CI) were computed, both not adjusted and adjusted for age and gender. The latter odds ratios are abbreviated by OR adj.

C], differ from the three polymorphisms composing the optimal three-way interaction in ever smokers, i.e. rs8102137[C/T, T/T] x rs11892031[A/A] x *GSTM1* null. Moreover, the optimal three-SNP combination in non-smokers results in an OR of 1.98 (95% CI: 1.49–2.63) that is significantly higher (p-value: 1.78×10^{-4}) than the OR of this combination in the ever smokers (OR: 1.03, 95% CI: 0.86–1.24). Conversely, the optimal three-SNP combination in ever smokers exhibits an OR of 1.58 (95% CI: 1.30–1.92), which is substantially, but not significantly (p-value: 0.143) higher than the OR of this three-SNP combination in non-smokers (OR: 1.21; 95% CI: 0.90–1.64). However, cigarette smoking is already associated with an OR of 3.28 (95% CI: 2.67–4.03) when current smokers are compared to non-smokers in our study population (Table 9). This high OR suggests that under conditions of continuous exposure to cigarette smoke carcinogens, the contribution of the "non-smoker SNPs" with their relatively small influence on cell cycle and DNA integrity control, is of minor relevance.

Comparison with Published Results

To study the consistency of this observation, we re-visited the data of the genome-wide association study on UBC of Rothman et al. [9] who validated rs9642880 and rs710521 in 3,532 UBC cases and 5,120 controls, and confirmed the impact of the *GSTM1* deletion in 2,480 cases and 3,222 controls. Assuming a multiplicative model, they also obtained higher ORs for non-smokers compared to ever smokers for rs9642880 (1.24 for non-smokers versus 1.16 for smokers) and rs11892031 (1.49 versus 1.31). The higher OR for rs9642880 contradicts the study of Kiemeney et al. [7] who reported no association of rs9642880 with smoking habits. Also, the findings of a higher OR for rs11892031 in non-smokers is

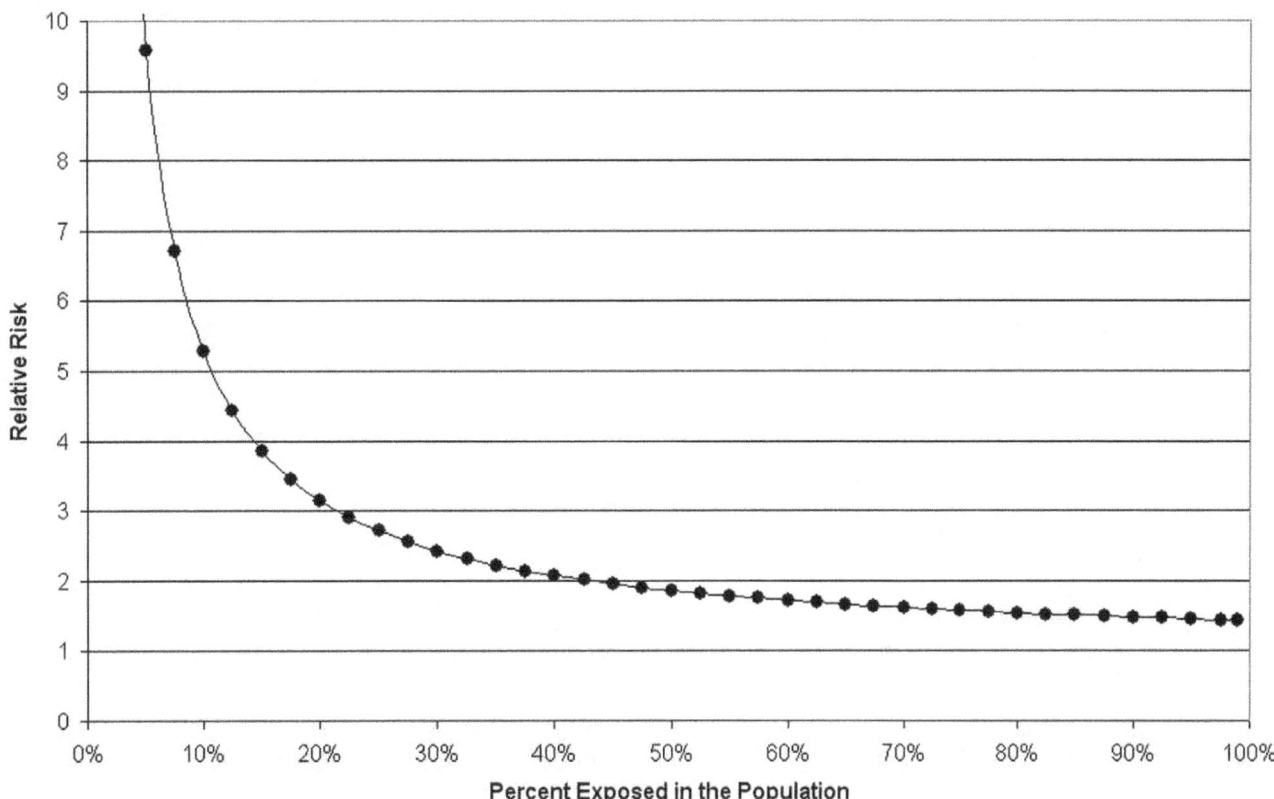

Figure 2. Relative risks and frequency of risk factors assuming a PAR of 30%. Relative risks are calculated depending on the frequency of the risk factor in the population assuming a population attributable risk (PAR) of 30%, corresponding to the supposed PAR of genetic risk factors for UBC. Given a PAR of 30%, the relative risk does not fall below 1.43 if the frequency of the risk factor is present in almost the entire population.

in contrast to Tang et al. [32] who found a higher risk in ever smokers (OR = 1.28) than in non-smokers (OR = 1.23) based on a subset of study groups from Rothman et al. (GWAS stage 1 [9]). However, no difference was found for rs710521 (1.13 vs. 1.14) in accordance with the discovery GWAS [7], and an opposite trend was shown for rs1014971 (1.11 vs. 1.16) and the *NAT2* tagging SNP rs1495741 (1.00 vs. 1.18) in accordance with the assumed higher risk of slow acetylators in smokers. Therefore, the difference should still be interpreted with caution until independent confirmatory data are available.

The association among the *GSTM1* null genotype, smoking habits and bladder cancer has been controversial since the first study by Bell et al. in 1993 [2]. In their study, smokers had an OR of 1.8 and non-smokers an OR of 1.3, indicating higher risks in smokers due to the lack of *GSTM1*. However, recent meta analyses and large or pooled studies found no or only weak evidence for an association between *GSTM1* and smoking habits [9,46–48], whereas Rothman et al. [9] reported an even higher OR for non-smokers than for ever smokers (1.71 vs. 1.47). In this context, it should be mentioned that our study groups present a higher proportion of occupationally exposed bladder cancer cases. This may be particularly important for *GSTM1*. For example, it was shown that bladder cancer patients with occupational histories in coal, iron, and steel industries, i.e. exposure to polycyclic aromatic hydrocarbons, presented with high percentages of *GSTM1* null genotypes [49]. Decades after the closure of these industries, the *GSTM1* genotypes were equal in both cases and controls (*GSTM1* null: 52%) [50].

Gain of Considering SNP Interactions

We have shown that SNP combinations result in less than additive ORs compared to the influence of the individual SNPs. For example, the ORs of the "non-smoker SNPs" rs1014971 and rs9642880 are 1.63 = 1/0.61 and 1.48, respectively, in non-smokers (for all ORs of individual SNPs, see Table S6). In comparison, the combination of both SNPs results in an OR of 1.91 in this subgroup (Table S16), which is larger than the individual effects, but smaller than 1.63+1.48 = 3.11. Adding a third SNP to the rs1014971 × rs9642880 combination results in an increase of only 0.07 (Table S21). The less than additive effect is not surprising considering the relatively high frequencies of the high-risk alleles (rs1014971 [C/C]: 40%; rs9642880 [G/T, T/T]: 71%; rs710521 [A/A, A/G]: 93%) in non-smoking controls and their overlap between individual SNPs (two-way interaction: 27%; three-way interaction 24%). Therefore, it seems unlikely that the addition of further "low impact" or "wimp SNPs" [1] would lead to a relevant increase in the combined ORs in populations of European descent.

Analysis of Population Attributable Risks

Altogether, it is estimated that up to 30% of bladder cancer cases can be explained by genetic risk factors [47,51] (see also Table 6), whereas about half of all UBC cases are caused by cigarette smoking [48,52,53] (see also Table 8). Estimates of the population attributable risk (PAR) for occupations vary widely, ranging from 7.1% in men and 1.9% in women [34] to 20–26% in both genders [35–37] (see also Table 7). The PAR – as a measure of the proportion of cases that could be explained by a certain risk factor – depends on and increases with both the frequency of the risk factor in the population and the relative risk (which is often approximated by the OR). Thus, assuming that the PAR of the genetic risk factors is limited to about 30% in the general population, the OR of the frequent combinations of these polymorphisms must be limited to modest ORs of about two

(Figure 2). For instance, a PAR of 30% results from a risk factor present in 40% of the population and a relative risk of 2.1, whereas a risk factor present in 10% of the population requires a relative risk of 5.3 to obtain the same PAR. However, in subgroups different impacts of the genetic risk factors can be observed, not only in terms of relevance of single SNPs and their combinations, but also with respect to their combined attributable risks. In our study, combined PARs for the "wimp SNPs" range from 28% in ever smokers to 43% in non-smokers and also reflect the different impact of genetic risk factors in subpopulations with higher or lower exposure to bladder carcinogens from tobacco smoke.

Conclusion

In conclusion, we have shown that different types of genetic variants confer different susceptibility to smokers and non-smokers. In addition, the present work fuels the debate regarding the degree to which genetic disposition or environmental exposure contributes to carcinogenesis. Whereas the odds ratio of cigarette smoking is approximately 3.5 for current smokers in most studies, the combined high-risk alleles of the SNPs recently discovered in genome-wide association studies add up to ORs of approximately 2.0. Therefore, the environmental factors seem to have a higher impact on the UBC risk than genetic disposition based on the SNPs derived from recent genome-wide association studies.

Supporting Information

Figure S1 Test statistics for the optimal combinations consisting of one to seven SNPs in the bootstrap samples. Data are shown for (A) the total group, (B) the ever smokers, (C) the current smokers, (D) the former smokers, and (E) the non-smokers. For each of the optimal combinations from in Figure 1A, box plots of the test statistics in the 500 bootstrap samples drawn from the respective subgroups are displayed. The plots correspond to the odds ratios shown in Figure 1B–F. The crosses mark the test statistics for the respective optimal combinations.

Figure S2 Mean test statistic over 100,000 permutations of the case-control status. For the top 100 SNP combinations of each size and in each subgroup, the means over the Wald statistics in 100,000 permutations of the case-control status were computed. The subgroup-wise distributions of these means are shown as box plots, and the subgroup-wise means of the top 10 combinations are marked by red crosses. For a better representation, six outliers (with means smaller than 0.9) were removed from the box plots for the two-way interactions. For reference, the minimum and maximum of the sample means from 100 samples consisting of 100,000 random draws from a χ^2-distribution with 1 degree of freedom are marked by dashed blue lines. If the χ^2-approximation is reasonable, the mean test statistic over the 100,000 permutations should be approximately 1, i.e. close to the solid blue lines marking the mean of the χ^2-distribution with 1 degree of freedom.

Figure S3 Variance of the test statistic over 100,000 permutations of the case-control status. In addition to the mean test statistic displayed in Figure S2, the variances of the test statistics for the top 100 interactions in the different subgroups were computed. The subgroup-wise distributions of these variances are shown as box plots, and the variances of the top ten combinations in the subgroups are marked by red crosses. For a better representation, six outliers (with variances smaller than

1.3) were removed from the box plots for the two-way interactions. For reference, the minimum and maximum of the sample variances from 100 samples consisting of 100,000 random draws from a χ^2-distribution with 1 degree of freedom are marked by dashed blue lines. If the χ^2-approximation is reasonable, the variance of the test statistic over the 100,000 permutations should be approximately 2, i.e. close to the solid blue lines marking the variance of the χ^2-distribution with 1 degree of freedom.

Figure S4 Differences between parametric and permutation-based p-values. Box plots of the differences between the parametric p-values of the top 100 SNP combinations of each size from the analysis of each subgroup and the corresponding p-values computed based on 100,000 permutations of the case-control status. The differences of the respective top ten SNPs are additionally marked by red crosses. Ideally, this difference is zero (which is marked by a dashed blue line). The six outliers removed from Figures S2 and S3 (with means smaller than 0.9 and variances smaller than 1.3) were also removed before constructing the box plots.

Table S1   Distribution of gender in the study groups.

Table S2   Distribution of age at diagnosis (cases) or examination (controls) in the study groups.

Table S3   Frequency of non-smokers, former smokers and current smokers in the study groups.

Table S4   Chromosomal and data base information on the six analyzed SNPs.

Table S5   Testing for Hardy-Weinberg equilibrium.

Table S6   Maximum odds ratios of the seven polymorphisms in the subgroups.

Table S7   Stability of the ranks of the top ten individual effects in the total study group.

Table S8   Stability of the ranks of the top ten individual effects in the ever smoker group.

Table S9   Stability of the ranks of the top ten individual effects in the current smoker group.

Table S10   Stability of the ranks of the top ten individual effects in the former smoker group.

Table S11   Stability of the ranks of the top ten individual effects in the non-smoker group.

Table S12   Stability of the ranks of the top ten two-way interactions in the total study group.

Table S13   Stability of the ranks of the top ten two-way interactions in the ever smoker group.

Table S14   Stability of the ranks of the top ten two-way interactions in the current smoker group.

Table S15   Stability of the ranks of the top ten two-way interactions in the former smoker group.

Table S16   Stability of the ranks of the top ten two-way interactions in the non-smoker group.

Table S17   Stability of the ranks of the top ten three-way interactions in the total study group.

Table S18   Stability of the ranks of the top ten three-way interactions in the ever smoker group.

Table S19   Stability of the ranks of the top ten three-way interactions in the current smoker group.

Table S20   Stability of the ranks of the top ten three-way interactions in the former smoker group.

Table S21   Stability of the ranks of the top ten three-way interactions in the non-smoker group.

Appendix S1   Details on the polymorphisms.

Appendix S2   Details on the statistical analysis.

Acknowledgments

The authors thank Ms. Kirsten Liesenhoff-Henze, Ms. Marion Page, and Ms. Claudia Schulte-Dahmann for excellent technical support. We also wish to acknowledge the contribution of our collaborating partners from the Department of Urology, St.-Josefs-Hospital, Dortmund, Germany; Department of Urology and Department of Surgery, Klinikum Dortmund gGmbH, Dortmund, Germany; Department of Urology, Lukaskrankenhaus Neuss, Germany; Department of Urology, Heinrich Heine University Düsseldorf, Germany; Department of Urology, Johannes Gutenberg University Mainz, Germany; Department of Urology, Paul Gerhardt Foundation, Lutherstadt Wittenberg, Germany; Institute for Occupational, Social and Environmental Medicine, Castrop-Rauxel, Germany; Department of Anaesthesia and Critical Care, St. Vincenz Hospital, Menden, Germany; Institute and Outpatient Clinic of Occupational, Social and Environmental Medicine (IPASUM), University of Erlangen-Nuremberg, Erlangen, Germany; Department of Urology, Semmelweis University Budapest, Budapest, Hungary; Practice for Urology, St. Augustin, Germany; Institute for General Medicine, University Hospital of Essen, Essen, Germany.

Author Contributions

Conceived and designed the experiments: JGH KG HS SS KI RM. Performed the experiments: MB. Analyzed the data: HS SS. Wrote the paper: JGH KG HS SS RM MB KI.

References

1. Golka K, Selinski S, Lehmann ML, Blaszkewicz M, Marchan R, et al. (2011) Genetic variants in urinary bladder cancer: collective power of the "wimp SNPs". Arch Toxicol 85: 539–554.

2. Bell DA, Taylor JA, Paulson DF, Robertson CN, Mohler JL, Lucier GW (1993) Genetic risk and carcinogen exposure: a common inherited defect of the carcinogen-metabolism gene glutathione S-transferase M1 (GSTM1) that increases susceptibility to bladder cancer. J Natl Cancer Inst 85: 1159–1164.

3. Cartwright RA, Glashan RW, Rogers HJ, Ahmad RA, Barham-Hall D, et al. (1984) Role of N-acetyltransferase phenotypes in bladder carcinogenesis: a pharmacogenetic epidemiological approach to bladder cancer. Lancet 2: 842–845.

4. Golka K, Prior V, Blaszkewicz M, Cascorbi I, Schöps W, et al. (1996) Occupational history and genetic N-acetyltransferase polymorphism in urothelial cancer patients of Leverkusen, Germany. Scand J Work Environ Health 22: 332–338.

5. Kempkes M, Golka K, Reich S, Reckwitz T, Bolt HM (1996) Glutathione S-transferase GSTM1 and GSTT1 null genotypes as potential risk factors for urothelial cancer of the bladder. Arch Toxicol 71: 123–126.

6. Hengstler JG, Arand M, Herrero ME, Oesch F (1998) Polymorphisms of N-acetyltransferases, glutathione S-transferases, microsomal epoxide hydrolase and sulfotransferases: influence on cancer susceptibility. Recent Results Cancer Res 154: 47–85.

7. Kiemeney LA, Thorlacius S, Sulem P, Geller F, Aben KK, et al. (2008) Sequence variant on 8q24 confers susceptibility to urinary bladder cancer. Nat Genet 40: 1307–1312.

8. Kiemeney LA, Sulem P, Besenbacher S, Vermeulen SH, Sigurdsson A, et al. (2010) A sequence variant at 4p16.3 confers susceptibility to urinary bladder cancer. Nat Genet 42: 415–419.

9. Rothman N, Garcia-Closas M, Chatterjee N, Malats N, Wu X, et al. (2010) A multi-stage genome-wide association study of bladder cancer identifies multiple susceptibility loci. Nat Genet 42: 978–984.

10. Rafnar T, Sulem P, Stacey SN, Geller F, Gudmundsson J, et al. (2009) Sequence variants at the TERT-CLPTM1L locus associate with many cancer types. Nat Genet 41: 221–227.

11. Rafnar T, Vermeulen SH, Sulem P, Thorleifsson G, Aben KK, et al. (2011) European genome-wide association study identifies SLC14A1 as a new urinary bladder cancer susceptibility gene. Hum Mol Genet 20: 4268–4281.

12. Wu X, Ye Y, Kiemeney LA, Sulem P, Rafnar T, et al. (2009) Genetic variation in the prostate stem cell antigen gene PSCA confers susceptibility to urinary bladder cancer. Nat Genet 41, 991–995. Erratum in: Nat Genet 41: 1156.

13. Golka K, Hermes M, Selinski S, Blaszkewicz M, Bolt HM, et al. (2009) Susceptibility to urinary bladder cancer: relevance of rs9642880[T], GSTM1 0/0 and occupational exposure. Pharmacogenet Genomics 19: 903–906.

14. Lehmann ML, Selinski S, Blaszkewicz M, Orlich M, Ovsiannikov D, et al. (2010) Rs710521[A] on chromosome 3q28 close to TP63 is associated with increased urinary bladder cancer risk. Arch Toxicol 84: 967–978.

15. Selinski S, Lehmann ML, Blaszkewicz M, Ovsiannikov D, Moormann O, et al. (2012) Rs11892031[A] on chromosome 2q37 in an intronic region of the UGT1A locus is associated with urinary bladder cancer risk. Arch Toxicol 86: 1369–1378.

16. Federico A, Pallante P, Bianco M, Ferraro A, Esposito F, et al. (2009) Chromobox protein homologue 7 protein, with decreased expression in human carcinomas, positively regulates E-cadherin expression by interacting with the histone deacetylase 2 protein. Cancer Res 69: 7079–7087.

17. Vartanian J-P, Guetard D, Henry M, Wain-Hobson S (2008) Evidence for editing of human papillomavirus DNA by APOBEC3 in benign and precancerous lesions. Science 320: 230–233.

18. Hengstler JG, Utesch D, Steinberg P, Platt KL, Diener B, et al. (2000) Cryopreserved primary hepatocytes as a constantly available in vitro model for the evaluation of human and animal drug metabolism and enzyme induction. Drug Metab Rev 32: 81–118.

19. Strassburg CP, Lankisch TO, Manns MP, Ehmer U (2008) Family 1 uridine-5-diphosphate glucuronosyltransferases (UGT1A): from Gilbert's syndrome to genetic organization and variability. Arch Toxicol 82: 415–433.

20. García-Closas M, Hein DW, Silverman D, Malats N, Yeager M, et al. (2011) A single nucleotide polymorphism tags variation in the arylamine N-acetyltransferase 2 phenotype in populations of European background. Pharmacogenet Genomics 21: 231–236.

21. Selinski S, Blaszkewicz M, Lehmann ML, Ovsiannikov D, Moormann O, et al. (2011) Genotyping NAT2 with only two SNPs (rs1041983 and rs1801280) outperforms the tagging SNP rs1495741 and is equivalent to the conventional 7-SNP NAT2 genotype. Pharmacogenet Genomics 21: 673–678.

22. Lefkimmiatis K, Caratozzolo MF, Merlo P, D'Erchia AM, Navarro B, et al. (2009) p73 and p63 sustain cellular growth by transcriptional activation of cell cycle progression genes. Cancer Res 69: 8563–8571.

23. Sayan BS, Sayan AE, Yang AL, Aqeilan RI, Candi E, et al. (2007) Cleavage of the transactivation-inhibitory domain of p63 by caspases enhances apoptosis. Proc Natl Acad Sci USA 104: 10871–10876.

24. Koff A, Cross F, Fisher A, Schumacher J, Leguellec K, et al. (1991) Human cyclin E, a new cyclin that interacts with two members of the CDC2 gene family. Cell 66: 1217–1228.

25. Dominguez-Sola D, Ying CY, Grandori C, Ruggiero L, Chen B, et al. (2007) Non-transcriptional control of DNA replication by c-Myc. Nature 448: 445–451.

26. Bolt HM, Thier R (2006) Relevance of the deletion polymorphisms of the glutathione S-transferases GSTT1 and GSTM1 in pharmacology and toxicology. Curr Drug Metab 7: 613–628.

27. Zimmermann A, Blaszkewicz M, Roth G, Seidel T, Dietrich H, et al. (2008) UDP-glucuronosyltransferase 2B7 C802T (His268Tyr) polymorphism in bladder cancer cases. J Toxicol Environ Health A 71: 911–914.

28. Golka K, Abreu-Villaca Y, Anbari Attar R, Angeli-Greaves M, Aslam M, et al. (2012) Bladder cancer documentation of causes: multilingual questionnaire "Bladder Cancer Doc". Front Biosci E4: 2709–2722.

29. Arand M, Mühlbauer R, Hengstler J, Jäger E, Fuchs J, et al. (1996) A multiplex polymerase chain reaction protocol for the simultaneous analysis of the glutathione S-transferase GSTM1 and GSTT1 polymorphisms. Anal Biochem 236: 184–186.

30. Krause G, Müller M, Lewalter J, Schulz T (2004) Glutathione S-transferase T1 and M1 (GSTT1, GSTM1) (genotyping). In: Angerer J, Müller, M, editors. Analyses of hazardous substances in biological materials, Vol 9, Special issue: Marker of susceptibility. Weinheim, Germany: Wiley-VCH Verlag GmbH. 183–210.

31. Steenland K, Armstrong B (2006) An overview of methods for calculating the burden of disease due to specific risk factors. Epidemiology 17: 512–519.

32. Tang W, Fu YP, Figueroa JD, Malats N, Garcia-Closas M, et al. (2012) Mapping of the UGT1A locus identifies an uncommon coding variant that affects mRNA expression and protects from bladder cancer. Hum Mol Genet 21: 1918–1930.

33. Doll R, Peto R (1981) The causes of cancer: Quantitative estimates of avoidable risks of cancer in the United States today. J Natl Cancer Inst 66: 1191–1308.

34. Rushton L, Bagga S, Bevan R, Brown TP, Cherrie JW, et al. (2010) Occupation and cancer in Britain. Br J Cancer 102: 1428–1437.

35. Delclos GL, Lerner SP (2008) Occupational risk factors. Scand J Urol Nephrol 42 (Suppl 218): 58–63.

36. Silverman DT, Levin LI, Hoover RN, Hartge P (1989) Occupational risks of bladder cancer in the United States: I. White men. J Natl Cancer Inst 81: 1472–1480.

37. Vineis P, Pirastu R (1997) Aromatic amines and cancer. Cancer Causes Control 8: 346–355.

38. Reulen RC, Kellen E, Buntinx F, Brinkman M, Zeegers MP (2008) A meta-analysis on the association between bladder cancer and occupation. Scand J Urol Nephrol 42 (Suppl 218): 64–78.

39. Ketterer B, Harris JM, Talaska G, Meyer DJ, Pemble SE, et al. (1992) The human glutathione S-transferase supergene family, its polymorphism, and its effects on susceptibility to lung cancer. Environ Health Perspect 98: 87–94.

40. Lee KH, Lee J, Ha M, Choi JW, Cho SH, et al. (2002) Influence of polymorphism of GSTM1 gene on association between glycophorin a mutant frequency and urinary PAH metabolites in incineration workers. J Toxicol Environ Health A 65: 355–363.

41. Carreón T, LeMasters GK, Ruder AM, Schulte PA (2006) The genetic and environmental factors involved in benzidine metabolism and bladder carcinogenesis in exposed workers. Front Biosci 11: 2889–2902.

42. Giuliani L, Ciotti M, Stoppacciaro A, Pasquini A, Silvestri I, et al. (2005) UDP-glucuronosyltransferases 1A expression in human urinary bladder and colon cancer by immunohistochemistry. Oncol Rep 13: 185–191.

43. Giuliani L, Gazzaniga P, Caporuscio F, Ciotti M, Frati L, Aglianò AM (2001) Can down-regulation of UDP-glucuronosyltransferases in the urinary bladder tissue impact the risk of chemical carcinogenesis? Int J Cancer 91: 141–143.

44. Lin GF, Guo WC, Chen JG, Qin YQ, Golka K, et al. (2005) An association of UDP-glucuronosyltransferase 2B7 C802T (His268Tyr) polymorphism with bladder cancer in benzidine-exposed workers in China. Toxicol Sci 85: 502–506.

45. Zenser TV, Lakshmi VM, Hsu FF, Davis BB (2002) Metabolism of N-acetylbenzidine and initiation of bladder cancer. Mutat Res 506–507: 29–40.

46. Engel LS, Taioli E, Pfeiffer R, Garcia-Closas M, Marcus PM, et al. (2002) Pooled analysis and meta-analysis of glutathione S-transferase M1 and bladder cancer: a HuGE review. Am J Epidemiol 156: 95–109.

47. García-Closas M, Malats N, Silverman D, Dosemeci M, Kogevinas M, et al. (2005) NAT2 slow acetylation, GSTM1 null genotype, and risk of bladder cancer: results from the Spanish Bladder Cancer Study and meta-analyses. Lancet 366: 649–659.

48. Moore LE, Baris DR, Figueroa JD, Garcia-Closas M, Karagas MR, et al. (2011) GSTM1 null and NAT2 slow acetylation genotypes, smoking intensity and bladder cancer risk: results from the New England bladder cancer study and NAT2 meta-analysis. Carcinogenesis 32: 182–189.

49. Golka K, Reckwitz T, Kempkes M, Cascorbi II, Blaskewicz M, et al. (1997) N-Acetyltransferase 2 (NAT2) and glutathione S-transferase μ (GSTM1) in bladder-cancer patients in a highly industrialized area. Int J Occup Environ Health 3: 105–110.

50. Ovsiannikov D, Selinski S, Lehmann ML, Blaszkewicz M, Moormann O, et al. (2012) Polymorphic enzymes, urinary bladder cancer risk, and structural change in the local industry. J Toxicol Environ Health A 75: 557–565.

51. Lichtenstein P, Holm NV, Verkasalo PK, Iliadou A, Kaprio J, et al. (2000) Environmental and heritable factors in the causation of cancer – analyses of

cohorts of twins from Sweden, Denmark, and Finland. N Engl J Med 343: 78–85.

52. Yu MC, Skipper PL, Tannenbaum SR, Chan KK, Ross RK (2002) Arylamine exposures and bladder cancer risk. Mutat Res 506–507: 21–28.

53. Puente D, Hartge P, Greiser E, Cantor KP, King WD, et al. (2006) A pooled analysis of bladder cancer case-control studies evaluating smoking in men and women. Cancer Causes Control 17: 71–79.

54. Vineis P (2002) The relationship between polymorphisms of xenobiotic metabolizing enzymes and susceptibility to cancer. Toxicology 181–182: 457–462.

55. Zhang R, Xu G, Chen W, Zhang W (2011) Genetic polymorphisms of glutathione S-transferase M1 and bladder cancer risk: a meta-analysis of 26 studies. Mol Biol Rep 38: 2491–2497.

56. Vineis P, Marinelli D, Autrup H, Brockmoller J, Cascorbi I, et al. (2001) Current smoking, occupation, N-acetyltransferase-2 and bladder cancer: a pooled analysis of genotype-based studies. Cancer Epidemiol Biomarkers Prev 10: 1249–1252.

57. Bolm-Audorff U, Jöckel KH, Kilguss B, Pohlabeln H, Siepenkothen T (1993). Bösartige Tumoren der ableitenden Harnwege und Risiken am Arbeitsplatz. Scientific report Fb 697 from the report series of the Federal Institute for Occupational Safety and Health, Dortmund, Germany. Bremerhaven, Germany: Wissenschaftsverlag NW. In German.

58. Golka K, Bandel T, Reckwitz T, Urfer W, Bolt HM, et al. (1999) Occupational risk factors for bladder carcinoma. A case control study. Urologe A 38: 358–363. In German.

59. Guha N, Steenland NK, Merletti F, Altieri A, Cogliano V, Straif K (2010) Bladder cancer risk in painters: a meta-analysis. Occup Environ Med 67: 568–573.

60. Golka K, Bandel T, Schlaefke S, Reich SE, Reckwitz T, et al. (1998) Urothelial cancer of the bladder in an area of former coal, iron, and steel industries in Germany: a case-control study. Int J Occup Environ Health 4: 79–84.

61. Golka K, Goebell PJ, Rettenmeier AW (2007) Bladder cancer: etiology and prevention. Dtsch Arztebl 104: A 719–723.

62. Myslak ZW, Bolt HM, Brockmann W (1991) Tumors of the urinary bladder in painters: a case-control study. Am J Ind Med 19: 705–713.

63. Colt JS, Baris D, Stewart P, Schned AR, Heaney JA, et al. (2004) Occupation and bladder cancer risk in a population-based case-control study in New Hampshire. Cancer Causes Control 15: 759–769.

64. Cordier S, Clavel J, Limasset JC, Boccon-Gibod L, Le Moual N, et al. (1993) Occupational risks of bladder cancer in France: a multicentre case-control study. Int J Epidemiol 22: 403–411.

65. Schifflers E, Jamart J, Renard V (1987) Tobacco and occupation as risk factors in bladder cancer: a case-control study in southern Belgium. Int J Cancer 39: 287–292.

66. Thériault G, Tremblay C, Cordier S, Gingras S (1984) Bladder cancer in the aluminium industry. Lancet 1: 947–950.

67. Golka K, Prior V, Blaszkewicz M, Bolt HM (2002) The enhanced bladder cancer susceptibility of NAT2 slow acetylators towards aromatic amines: a review considering ethnic differences. Toxicol Lett 128: 229–241.

68. Golka K, Wiese A, Assennato G, Bolt HM (2004) Occupational exposure and urological cancer. World J Urol 21: 382–391.

69. Brennan P, Bogillot O, Cordier S, Greiser E, Schill W, et al. (2000) Cigarette smoking and bladder cancer in men: a pooled analysis of 11 case-control studies. Int J Cancer 86: 289–294.

70. Brennan P, Bogillot O, Greiser E, Chang-Claude J, Wahrendorf J, et al. (2001) The contribution of cigarette smoking to bladder cancer in women (pooled European data). Cancer Causes Control 12: 411–417.

71. Gandini S, Botteri E, Iodice S, Boniol M, Lowenfels AB, et al. (2008) Tobacco smoking and cancer: a meta-analysis. Int J Cancer 122: 155–164.

9

IL-6 Expression Regulates Tumorigenicity and Correlates with Prognosis in Bladder Cancer

Miao-Fen Chen[1,2], Paul-Yang Lin[2,3], Ching-Fang Wu[2,4], Wen-Cheng Chen[1,2], Chun-Te Wu[2,5]*

1 Department of Radiation Oncology, Chang Gung Memorial Hospital, Chiayi, Taiwan, 2 Chang Gung University, College of Medicine, Taoyuan, Taiwan, 3 Department of Pathology, Chang Gung Memorial Hospital, Chiayi, Taiwan, 4 Department of Urology, Chang Gung Memorial Hospital, Chiayi, Taiwan, 5 Department of Urology, Chang Gung Memorial Hospital, Keelung, Taiwan

Abstract

Identification of potential tumor markers will help stratify and identify a tumor's malignant potential and its response to specific therapies. IL-6 has been reported to be a predictor in various cancers. Therefore, the present study was performed to highlight the role of IL-6 in improving treatment and determining prognosis of bladder cancer. The human bladder cancer cell lines HT1376 and HT1197 were selected for cell and animal experiments, in which biological changes after experimental manipulation of IL-6 were explored, including tumor behavior and related signaling in bladder cancer. In addition, clinical specimens from 85 patients with muscle-invasive, and 50 with non-muscle invasive bladder cancers were selected for immunohistochemical staining to evaluate the predictive capacity of IL-6 in relation to clinical outcome. The data revealed that IL-6 was overexpressed in the bladder cancer specimens compared with non-malignant tissues at both mRNA and protein levels. Positive staining of IL-6 was significantly correlated with higher clinical stage, higher recurrence rate after curative treatment, and reduced survival rate. Tumor growth and invasive capability were attenuated when IL-6 was blocked. The underlying changes included decreased cell proliferation, less epithelial-mesenchymal transition (EMT), decreased DNA methyltransferase 1 expression and attenuated angiogenesis. In conclusion, our findings showed that IL-6 could be a significant predictor for clinical stage and prognosis of bladder cancer. Moreover, targeting IL-6 may be a promising strategy for treating bladder cancer.

Editor: Peter Canoll, Columbia University, United States of America

Funding: The work was supported by Chang Gung Memorial Hospital, Taiwan, grant CMRPG690332-3. The funder had no role in study design, data collection and analysis, decision to publish, or preparation of the manuscript.

Competing Interests: The authors have declared that no competing interests exist.

* E-mail: wucgmh@gmail.com

Introduction

Urinary bladder cancer represents a spectrum of neoplasms, including non-muscle invasive (NMIBC), muscle invasive, and metastatic lesions. Transitional cell carcinoma (TCC) of the bladder is the most common form of bladder cancer and is manifested in two distinct forms with different clinical and biological behaviors. Approximately 70% of patients present with non-muscle invasive tumors, while the remaining 30% present with muscle-invasive tumors. Despite good prognosis for patients with superficial disease, recurrence is common and is associated with development of muscle-invasive disease [1]. Nearly half of all patients presenting with muscle-invasive disease or those who have already progressed to this state harbor occult distant metastasis and have poor 5-year survival rate [2]. Unlike other urological cancers, bladder cancer lacks clinical useful biomarkers for predicting disease stage and clinical outcome. Therefore, molecular markers that can be used to stratify and identify a tumor's true malignant potential and its response to specific therapies are required.

Chronic inflammation often precedes or accompanies a substantial number of cancers [3–5]. An increase in inflammatory mediators has been shown to lead to tumor promotion, invasion, and angiogenesis [6–7]. Although the role of chronic inflammation in the etiology of TCC of the bladder has not been well established, there is mounting evidence that proinflammatory cytokines play critical roles in the pathogenesis of bladder cancer, such as IL-6, IL-8 and TNF- α [8]. Moreover, persistently STAT3 activation was shown to maintain constitutive NF-κB activity, thus providing evidence for the relation between oncology signaling pathways within the inflammatory microenvironment [9]. IL-6 is a major activator of STAT3 signaling pathways, and the main cytokine influencing the inflammatory response in humans [10,11]. IL-6 signaling has been implicated in regulation of tumor growth and metastatic spread, and its level could be correlated with poor prognosis in different cancers [11,12]. Furthermore, increased IL-6 serum levels were reported to be associated with metastasis and poor prognosis of prostate, ovarian, and bladder cancers [13–15]. Although there is evidence suggesting that IL-6 may be a critical factor in various malignancies, its role in bladder cancer remains unclear. Therefore, in the present study, we focused on the underlying mechanisms of IL-6 and its possible usefulness for addressing the need of aggressive treatment for bladder cancer.

Materials and Methods

Patient characteristics

The Institutional Review Board of Chang Gung Memorial Hospital approved the present study (Permit Number: 99-0207B).

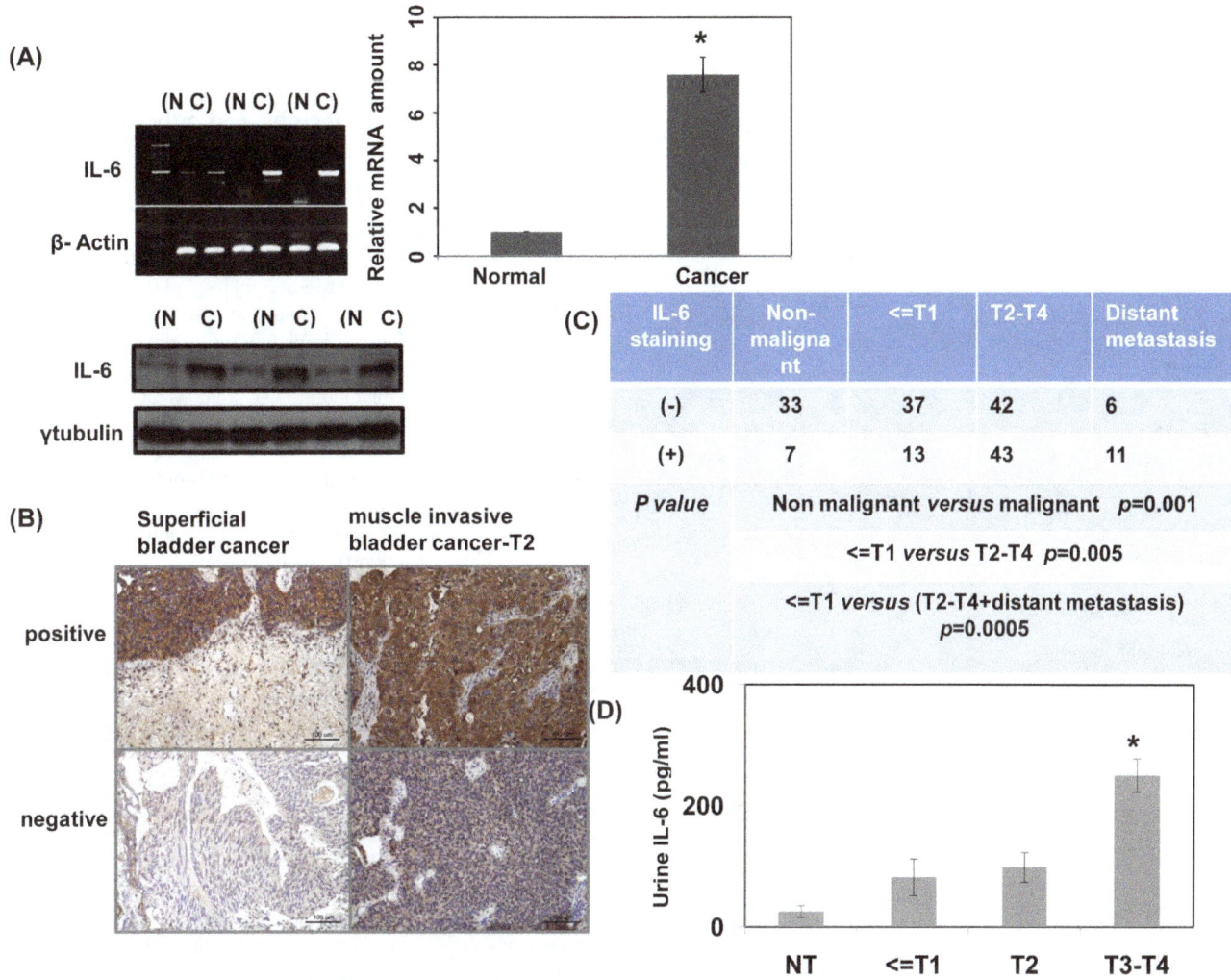

Figure 1. Levels of IL-6 in bladder cancer. A. Levels of IL-6 were examined in six specimens (paired cancer (C) and adjacent non-malignant tissue (N); two specimens in a lane) by RT-PCR and Western blotting analysis. For real-time RT-PCR analysis, the y-axis shows the ratio of IL-6 in cancer tissue divided by that in the non-malignant specimen. Columns, mean of three separate experiments; Bars, standard deviation (SD); *, $P<0.05$. B. Immunohistochemical staining of human bladder cancer specimens with anti-IL-6 antibody. Representative slides are shown. C. The IHC data showed that IL-6 levels were significantly correlated with clinical stage. D. Urinary IL-6 levels of patients were examined by ELISA analysis. Columns, mean of three separate experiments; Bars, SD; *, $P<0.05$. (NT, patients with non-malignant diseases).

The written consents were signed by the patients for their specimen and information to be stored in the hospital and used for research. A total of 85 patients with muscle-invasive bladder TCC (39 with stage T2 and 46 with stages T3 –T4) who completed a course of definite chemoradiotherapy (CCRT) treatment were enrolled in the study. On completion of CCRT, patients underwent a repeat computed tomography scans (CT) and cystoscopy examination to determine the response to treatment. Patients were observed at 3-month intervals for the first 2 years and every 6 months thereafter. The follow-up for patients was continued until their death, and the end points were overall survival (OS), progression-free survival, failure pattern and response to definite CCRT. Disease progression was defined as documented local recurrence or distant metastases. Analyses were performed using SPSS version 17.0.

Immunohistochemical (IHC) staining

In addition to tissue specimens collected from the 85 patients with muscle-invasive bladder cancer, bladder tissue specimens were collected for immunohistochemical (IHC) staining from 17 patients suffering from bladder carcinoma with distant metastasis, 50 NMIBC patients, and 40 non-malignancy patients. Formalin-fixed, paraffin-embedded tissues obtained by transurethral resection in the diagnosis were cut into 5 μm sections, and mounted on slides for IHC staining. For histological evaluation of IL-6 staining, the staining was scored independently by two observers who were blind to the clinical outcome of patients; discordant scores were reviewed, and a consensus was reached. In the present study, a criterion of more than 10% positive staining of tumor cells was considered positive on IHC scoring, which was defined by receiver operating characteristic (ROC) curve analysis.

Cell culture and reagents

HT137 and HT1197, human bladder cancer cell lines, were obtained from the American Type Culture Collection (ATCC). The IL-6-neutralizing antibody was obtained from R&D Systems (Minneapolis, MN) and the IL-6-GFP silencing vector (human IL6 shRNA constructs in retroviral GFP vector) and GFP-control

Table 1. Baseline characteristics of patients.

	No. of	patients	
	IHC-IL-6 (−)	IHC-IL-6 (+)	p value
Patients with non-muscle invasive bladder cancer	37	13	
Age			0.52
Median	69.9	68.2	
Range	41.9–89.5	51.9–83.4	
Gender			0.94
Male	26	9	
Female	11	4	
IHC–DNMT1			0.0002*
(+)	4	8	
(−)	33	4	
Clinical stage			0.19
Ta	13	2	
Tis&T1	24	11	
Patients with muscle-invasive bladder cancer	42	43	
Age			0.554
Median	70.0	73.9	
Range	46.5–88.2	48.5–92.5	
Gender			0.19
Male	28	34	
Female	14	9	
IHC–DNMT1			0.012*
(+)	17	29	
(−)	25	14	
Clinical stage			0.0001*
T2	28	11	
T3–T4	14	32	
Histologic grade			0.097
Low-intermediate	19	12	
High	23	31	
LN involvement			0.039*
Negative	37	30	
Positive	5	13	
RT dose (cGy)			0.401
mean	5832	5736	
median	5940	5940	
Response to definite CCRT			0.056
CR (+)	35	28	
CR (−)	7	15	
Disease status			0.0001*
Control	32	13	
Failure (LR+DM)	10	30	

Abbreviations: CCRT = concurrent chemotherapy and radiotherapy; LN = lymph node; CR = complete response; LR = local recurrence; DM = distant metastasis. *, P<0.05.

vector (Non-effective scrambled shRNA cassette in retroviral GFP vector) were obtained from Origene Technologies, Inc. (Rockville, MD).

Tumor xenograft model (ectopic and orthotopic)

This study was carried out in strict accordance with the recommendations in the Guide for the Care and Use of Laboratory Animals as promulgated by the Institutes of Laboratory Animal Resources, National Research Council, U.S.A. The protocol was approved by the Committee on the Ethics of Animal Experiments of Chang Gung Memorial Hospital (Permit Number: 2010070201). Eight-week-old female athymic nude mice were used as the xenograft tumor implantation model. In the ectopic tumor implantation model, cells (5×10^6 tumor cells were injected subcutaneously per implantation, five animals per group) were implanted into the bilateral dorsal gluteal region. Tumor size was measured every three days after implantation (day 0). The tumor volume was calculated assuming an ellipsoid shape. In the orthotopic tumor implantation model, we performed intravesicular instillation of canccer cells as described previously (five animals per group). The extent of orthotopic tumor invasion was measured after implantation at the indicated times. The effect of IL-6 stimulation was also investigated in vivo. For the treated group, an intraperitoneal injection of IL-6 (60 or 100 ng per mouse, 3 times per week) was started one day before tumor implantation.

Cell migration and cell invasion assay. Capacity for cell invasion was determined by Cell Invasion Assay (Trevigen, Gaithersburg, MD). The top chambers were pre-coated with basement membrane extract (derived from EHS tumor and provided in the kit). After incubation for 24 h, the number of cells in the bottom chamber was determined by measuring the fluorescent anion calcein released from intracellular calcein acetoxymethylester. To validate experiments on cell migration, scratch assays were also done. A 2 mm wide scratch was drawn across each cell layer using a pipette tip. The plates were photographed at the times indicated.

Immunofluorescence (IF) staining

Cells were seeded onto glass coverslips at 5×10^4 cells/ml in 6-well plates for immunofluorescence (IF) staining with or without treatment. At the specified times after treatment, cells were fixed with 2% paraformaldehyde for 5 minutes, and washed in PBS with Tween-20 (PBST). Slides were incubated for 1 h at room temperature with antibodies against E-cadherin and IL-6, followed by incubation with Texas Red-conjugated secondary antibody and counterstaining with 4′,6-diamidino-2-phenylindole (DAPI).

Real-time reverse transcription-polymerase chain reaction (RT-PCR)

Real-time RT-PCR was performed on RNA extracted from cells and tissue specimens (six cancer tissue specimens and six non-malignant tissues; two specimens in each lane). The primer sequences were as follows: (forward and reverse, respectively) 5′-GTTCTTCCTCCTGGAGAATGTCA-3′ and 5′-GGGCCACGCCGTACTG-3′ for DNMT-1; 5′-TACATCCTC-GACGGCATCTC-3′ and 5′-GCTACATTTGCCGAAGA--GCC-3′ for IL-6. A β-actin primer set was used as a loading control. The optimized PCR was performed on an iCycler iQ multicolor real-time PCR detection system. Significant fluorescent PCR signals from carcinoma tissue were normalized relative to the mean value of signals obtained from non-malignant tissues.

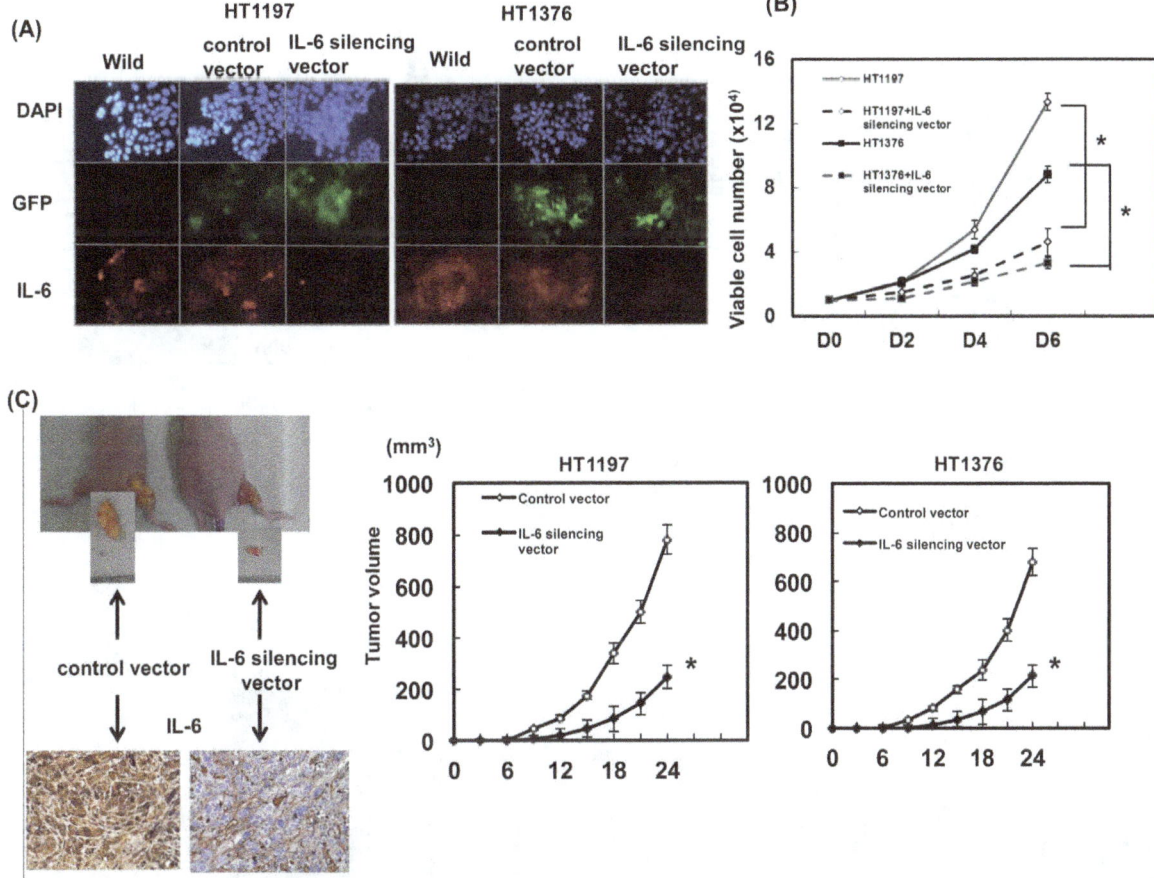

Figure 2. Role of IL-6 in tumor cell growth. A. Effects of the IL-6-GFP silencing vector on IL-6 level in HT1197 and HT1376 cells as demonstrated by immunofluorescence analysis. Representative micrographs are shown, with the respective immunofluorescent colors (DAPI, blue; GFP, green; IL-6, red). IL-6 levels were significantly decreased by the IL-6-GFP silencing vector compared with the control-GFP vector. B. Effects of the IL-6 silencing vector on he proliferation rates of HT1197 and HT1376 cancer cells. The same number of cells (10^4) was plated in each plate on day 0 and allowed to grow in their respective cultures. We counted the numbers of viable cells after incubation for 2, 4, and 6 days. The y-axis represents the viable cell number. Point, mean of three separate experiments. Bars, SD. *, $P<0.05$. C. Effects of IL-6 inhibition on xenograft tumor growth. Each point represents the mean of three separate experiments; bars, SD; *, $P<0.05$. Expression of IL-6 was also evaluated by immunochemical staining of xenografts. Representative slides are shown at ×400 magnification.

Enzyme-linked immunosorbent assay (ELISA) for IL-6 levels *in vitro* and *in vivo*

Urine specimens were obtained from 60 patients with bladder cancers (25 from patients with NMIBC, 35 from those with muscle-invasive disease), and 20 samples from patients without evidence of malignancy. Sample of 10 ml of fresh urine was collected from each subject, and subsequently centrifuged at 3000 rpm for 5 minutes. At the time of analysis urine aliquots were defrosted and urinary IL-6 were measured in the supernatants. Commercially available ELISA assay (HS human IL-6 immuno-assay kit; R&D Systems) was used to measure levels of urinary IL-6. The assays were conducted according to the manufacturer's instructions. Calibration curves were prepared using purified standards for each protein assessed. To test IL-6 level in cellular supernatant, the cells were cultured with 1 ml serum-free medium for 24 h in 6-well plate. The medium was collected and clarified by centrifugation at 3000 g. IL-6 level in the supernatant was detected by ELISA assay.

Statistical analysis

Survival probabilities were analyzed using the Kaplan–Meier method. Survival was calculated from the date of treatment started to the date of death or the most recent follow-up. The significance of differences between groups was assessed using the log-rank test. All statistical tests were two-sided, with $p<0.05$ taken to indicate significance. Significance of difference between samples was determined using Student's t-test. Data are presented as mean±''' standard error of the mean (SEM). Three repeats were carried out for evaluating each experiment, and repeat the entire set of experiments at least twice. A probability level of $p<0.05$ was adopted throughout to determine statistical significance unless otherwise stated.

Results

IL-6 expressions in patients with bladder cancers

The level of IL-6 in tissue specimens (six paired cancer and adjacent nonmalignant tissue specimens) was examined using mRNA and protein analyses. As shown in Figure 1A, bladder

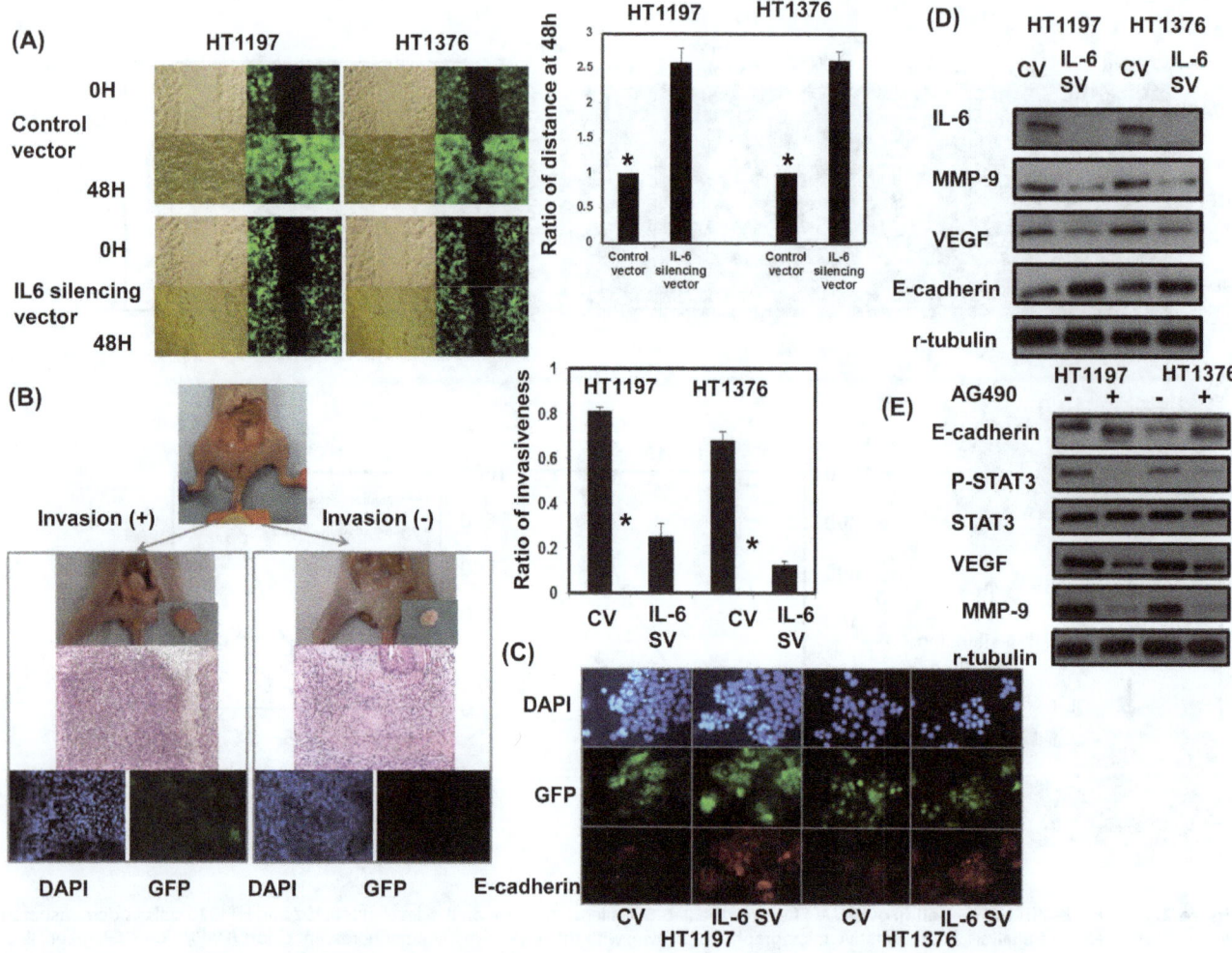

Figure 3. Effects of IL-6 inhibition on aggressive tumor behavior and EMT changes. A. The invasive capacity of bladder cancer cells with or without the IL-6 silencing vector was evaluated by migration scratch assays. The results from representative slides are shown. Column, mean of three separate experiments. Bars, SD. *, $P<0.05$. B. The invasive capacity of bladder cancer cells with or without the IL-6 silencing vector was evaluated by murine orthotopic tumor implantation. The representative slides and quantitative data are shown. The y-axis represents the ratio of mice presenting intravesicular tumors, normalized to that received orthotopic tumor implantation. The IL-6 silencing vector decreased the rate of tumor implantation in the bladder and was associated with a smaller tumor size. Column, mean of three separate experiments. Bars, SD. *, $P<0.05$. (CV, cells transfected with the control vector; IL-6 SV, cells transfected with the IL-6 silencing vector). C. Change in E-cadherin in cells was evaluated and the representative micrographs are shown, with the respective immunofluorescent colors (DAPI, blue; GFP, green; E-cadherin, red). D. Change in EMT-associated proteins in transfectants was evaluated by Western blotting analysis (CV, cells transfected with the control vector; IL-6 SV, cells transfected with the IL-6 silencing vector). E. Change in EMT-associated proteins in cells treated with JAK inhibitor- AG490.

cancer specimens expressed substantially higher level of IL-6 than non-malignant tissues. IHC analysis for bladder TCC (Fig. 1B and Table 1) indicated positive staining for IL-6 in 51% of T2 –T4 bladder cancer tissues [28% (11/39) in T2 vs. 70% (32/46) in T3 – T4; $P=0.0001$]. In addition, 65% (11/17) of the more advanced tumors (patients with distant metastases) showed positive staining for IL-6, but only 17.5% (7/40) of non-malignant bladder tissues and 26% (13/50) of early-stage tumors (CIS or T1) expressed IL-6. As shown in Figure 1C, positive staining for IL-6 was significantly correlated with clinical stage (T2 –T4 vs. T1 and CIS; $P=0.005$). Moreover, the urinary levels of IL-6 were examined by ELISA analysis. The mean IL-6 levels in urine samples from patients with NMIBC (81±30.8 pg/mL) and T2 muscle-invasive bladder cancer (98±24 pg/mL) were slightly higher than those without malignant disease (25.14±9.71 pg/mL), but the differences were not statistically significant (Fig. 1D). Urinary IL-6 levels were significantly elevated in patients with T3 –T4 local-advanced

bladder cancers (250±27 pg/mL) compared to those in patients with ≤T2 bladder cancer or non-malignant disease ($P=0.01$).

Role of IL-6 in tumor growth and invasion

To investigate whether IL-6 plays a role in the aggressive behavior of bladder cancer, HT1197 and HT1376 cells were transfected with the IL-6-GFP silencing vector. As shown in Figure 2A, the IL-6 silencing vector significantly decreased IL-6 expression in both cell lines. As determined by viable cell counts over six days (Fig.2B), the IL-6 silencing vector significantly attenuated the proliferation rate of HT1197 and HT1376 cells. Furthermore, using xenograft tumors model, inhibition of IL-6 resulted in slower tumor growth *in vivo* (Fig. 2C). The data demonstrate that the IL-6 silencing vector significantly inhibited the growth rate of bladder cancer cells. Additionally, IL-6 silencing vector significantly attenuated the invasive capacity of bladder cancer cells as demonstrated using migration scratch assays [16]

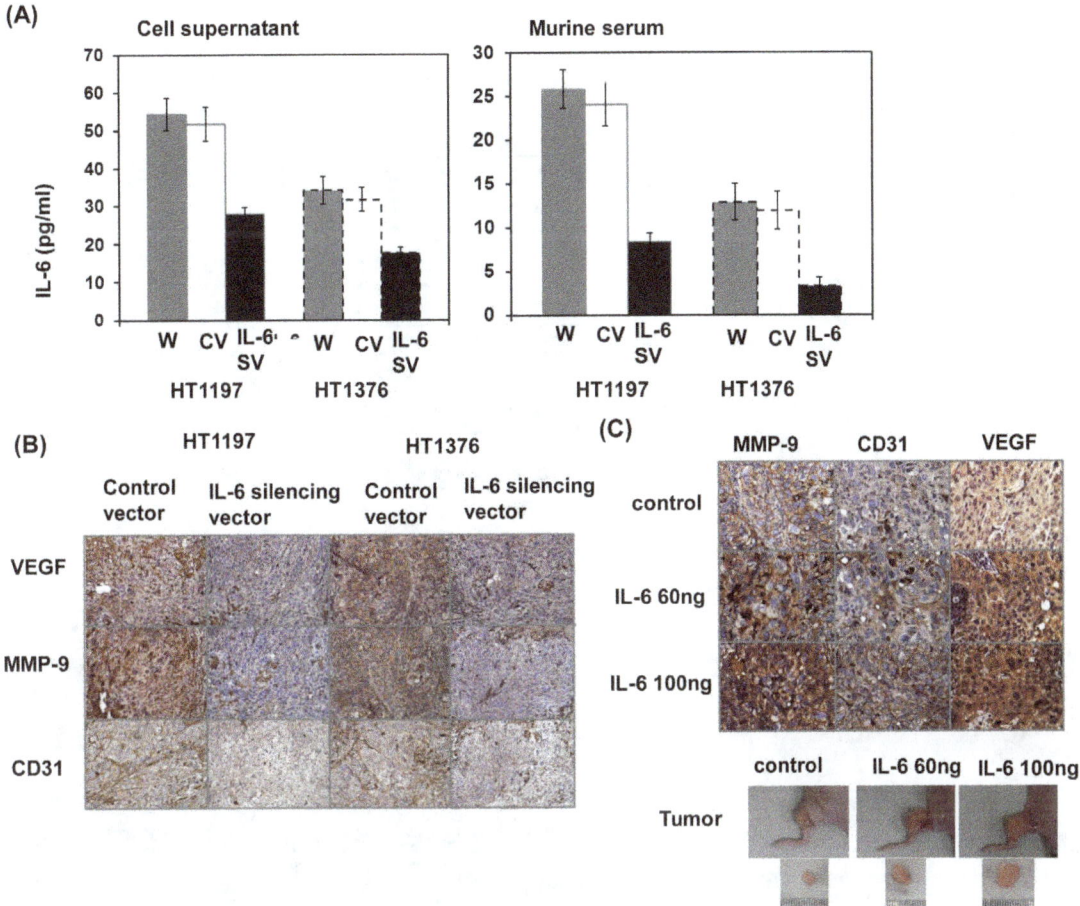

Figure 4. IL-6 is linked with the induction of angiogenesis. A. The level of IL-6 in cell culture supernatants and serum of mice bearing tumors with or without the IL-6 silencing vector was examined by ELISA *in vitro* and *in vivo*. Column, mean of three separate experiments. Bars, SD. *, *P*<0.05. B. Change in vascular endothelial growth factor (VEGF) and matrix metallopeptidase 9 (MMP-9), and CD31 in tumor xenografts was evaluated by immunohistochemical staining. The results from representative slides are shown. C. Effect of IL-6 on xenograft tumor growth and the induction of angiogenesis was evaluated in mice bearing tumors for 2 weeks. Tumor cells were injected subcutaneously into the mice with or without IL-6 injection as indicated in Materials and Methods, and tumor growth examined 2 weeks later. Immunohistochemistry using MMP-9, CD31, and VEGF stained- representative slides were demonstrated.

and invasion assay *in vitro* (Fig. 3A, Fig. S1). An orthotopic tumor implantation technique was used to examine the effects of the IL-6 silencing vector on invasive capability *in vivo* (Fig. 3B). Sixteen mice received intravesicular instillation of each bladder cancer cell line. After 28 days, 13 mice (81%) instilled with HT1197 cells, four (25%) instilled with HT1197 cells plus IL-6 silencing vector, 11 (69%) with HT1376 cells, and two (13%) with HT1376 cells plus IL-6 silencing vector developed intravesicular tumors. The data indicated that the IL-6 silencing vector decreased invasive capability *in vivo*.

Role of IL-6 in EMT changes

EMT is a key event in invasiveness [17], and we examined whether this is the mechanism underlying the aggressive behavior of IL-6-positive bladder cancer. As shown in Figure 3C-D, the IL-6 silencing vector increased expression of E-cadherin associated with decrease in vascular endothelial growth factor (VEGF) and matrix metallopeptidase 9 (MMP-9) expressions in tumor cells [18]. It has been reported that IL-6 is a major activator of STAT3 signaling, and the activation of STAT3 signaling plays a role in the induction of aggressive tumor behavior and EMT changes in cancer [19]. When we blocked STAT3 activation with JAK

inhibitor-AG490, the EMT-related proteins were decreased (Fig. 3E). These observations suggested that the increased aggressive tumor behavior and EMT changes induced by IL-6 might be mediated by STAT3 activation, a part at least.

Effects of IL-6 on angiogenesis

ELISA data revealed that IL-6 silencing vector clearly attenuated IL-6 secretion in cell culture supernatants and serum from mice after 28 days of tumor implantation (Fig. 4A). CD31-mediated endothelial cell-cell interactions are involved in angiogenesis [20]. Figure 4B showed that IL-6 silencing vector attenuated angiogenesis demonstrated by the staining of CD31 and VEGF. To further examined whether circulating IL-6 facilitating the induction of angiogenesis, an intraperitoneal injection of IL-6 (60 or 100 ng per mouse, 3 times per week) was started one day before tumor implantation. As shown in Figure 4C, IL-6 triggered angiogenesis and endothelial tube formation within the tumor by the staining of VEGF, MMP-9 and CD31 in mice bearing tumors for 2 weeks. Therefore, induction of angiogenesis may be one of the mechanisms responsible for tumor promotion by IL-6.

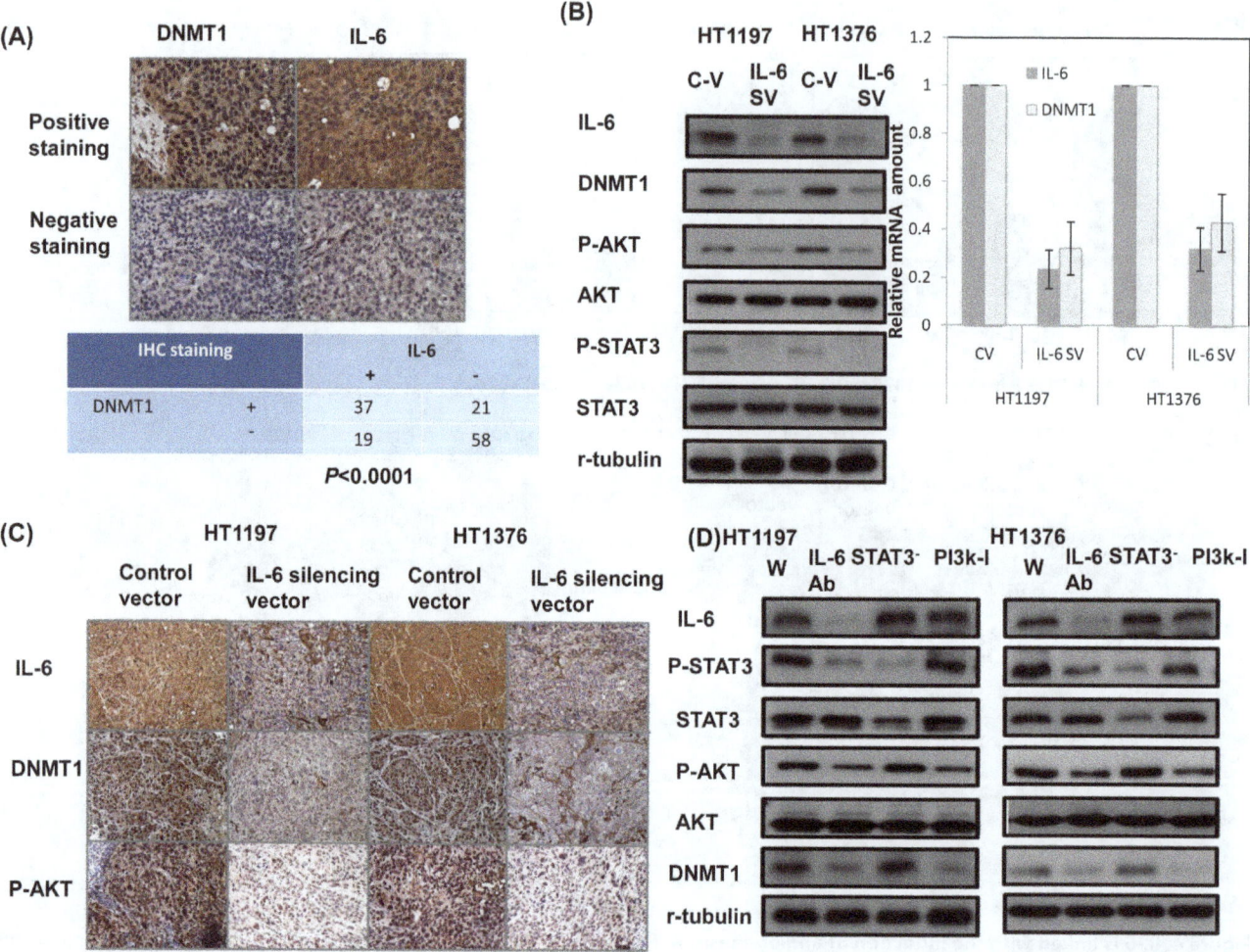

Figure 5. DNMT1 is linked to activated IL-6 signaling via Akt phosphorylation. A. IL-6 level was positively correlated with DNMT1 expression in human bladder cancer specimens ($P<0.0001$). Representative slides of a selected tumor specimen positively staining for both IL-6 and DNMT1, and another tumor specimen negative for both IL-6 and DNMT1 are shown at ×400 magnification. B. Effect of IL-6 on the level of DNMT1, p-AKT, and p-STAT3 was examined by Western blotting (CV, cells transfected with the control vector; IL-6 SV, cells transfected with the IL-6 silencing vector). C. Effect of IL-6 on the level of DNMT1 and p-AKT was evaluated by immunohistochemical staining, and the results from representative slides are shown. D. Effect of IL-6 inhibition by IL-6-neutralizing antibody, p-AKT inhibition by PI3K inhibitor, and p-STAT3 inhibition by STAT3 siRNA on the level of DNMT1 was examined by Western blotting (W, wild-type; IL-6⁻, cells treated with IL-6-neutralizing Ab; STAT3⁻, cells treated with Stat3 siRNA; PI3K-I, cells treated with PI3K inhibitor.

Relationship between expression of IL-6 and DNMT1 in bladder cancer

As we reported previously [21], higher DNMT1 levels were associated with aggressive tumor behavior and EMT changes in bladder cancers. We found there was a significant correlation between positive staining for IL-6 and DNMT1 on IHC staining of bladder cancer specimens (Fig. 5A). By mRNA and protein analysis, decreased IL-6 resulted in inhibited DNMT1 associated with attenuated STAT3 and Akt activation (Fig. 5B-C). We further examined whether the IL-6 inhibition decreased DNMT1 expression via inhibition of AKT using a PI3K inhibitor-LY294002 [22], or down regulation of STAT3 with STAT3 short interfering RNA (siRNA). As shown in Figure 5D, inhibition of Akt phosphorylation, but not decreased p-STAT3, significantly attenuated DNMT1 expression. Therefore, it is suggested that activation of AKT might be responsible to the increased DNMT1 in IL-6-positive bladder cancers.

IL-6 is related to clinical outcome of bladder TCC

The median progression-free survival time in the 85 patients completed definite CCRT treatment was 36.97 months. By univariate analysis, positive staining for IL-6 was significantly related to higher clinical stage, higher disease failure rate after definite treatment and shorter survival time (Table 1 and Figure 6). The findings strongly underscore the contribution of IL-6 to the prognosis in bladder cancer.

Discussion

We demonstrated that IL-6 was expressed at higher levels in bladder TCC than in non-malignant tissues. Moreover, positive staining for IL-6 was preferentially associated with muscle-invasive bladder TCC relative to lower stage Ta –T1 disease. Urinary levels of IL-6 were also significantly elevated in patients with locally advanced bladder TCC compared to patients with NMIBC. Therefore, IL-6 expression might be related to a more malignant phenotype.

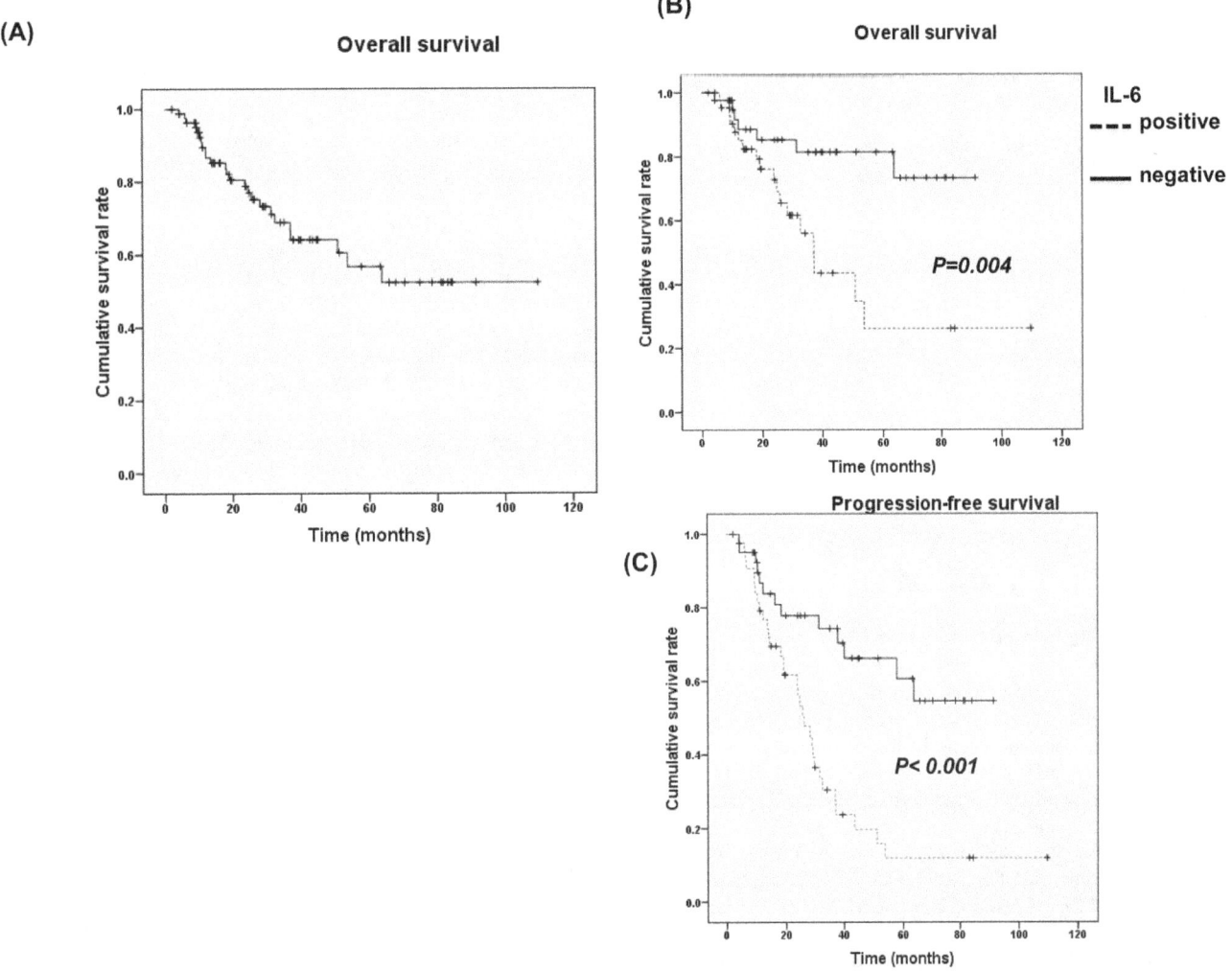

Figure 6. Effects of IL-6 on survival. A survival difference was demonstrated in accordance with positive staining of IL-6. The Kaplan–Meier overall survival curves showed that patients with higher levels of IL-6 expression had shorter survival periods.

To investigate whether IL-6 was responsible for the aggressive behavior of bladder TCC, IL-6 was suppressed in bladder cancer cells by stable transfection with a silencing vector. Data revealed that inhibiting IL-6 resulted in decreased bladder tumor growth *in vitro* and *in vivo*. Moreover, the IL-6 silencing vector significantly attenuated the invasive ability detected in cellular invasion assays and mouse orthotopic models. IL-6 is a major activator of JAK/STAT3 signaling [10,11], and activated STAT3 signaling has been reported to contribute to oncogenesis by promoting proliferation and EMT [18,23]. Moreover, STAT3 activation has been shown a role in predisposing urothelial basal cells toward the CIS progression pathway into invasive bladder cancer [24]. Our data revealed that inhibition of IL-6 attenuated STAT3 activation associated with increased E-cadherin and decreased VEGF and MMP-9 expressions. Increased expressions of VEGF and MMP-9 are reported to correlate with EMT change and poor prognosis of bladder cancer [25,26]. Therefore, it is likely that STAT3 activation plays a role in IL-6 transmitting to downstream targets that regulate EMT and invasiveness.

We showed that IL-6 levels in serum and urine were elevated in a subgroup of patients with muscle-invasive bladder cancer, consistent with other research [13,27]. Angiogenesis is one of the

mechanisms that promote tumor progression, and the expression of angiogenic factors is suggested to have predictive value for treatment response and outcome in patients with cancer [28]. Furthermore, IL-6 has been reported to play multiple functions in angiogenesis and vascular modeling [29], and increase angiogenesis by transcriptional of VEGF and MMP-9 in STAT3-dependent manner. STAT3 activation was demonstrated to modulate the expression of genes that mediate angiogenesis; *e.g.*, VEGF [30]. Accordingly, the links between IL-6, angiogenesis, and promotion of bladder cancer in tumor-bearing mice were further investigated in the present study. Using a xenograft tumor model, our data demonstrated that IL-6 level positively linked with angiogenesis and STAT3 activation. These findings suggested that the induction of angiogenesis mediated by STAT3 activation may be one of the mechanisms underlying the aggressiveness of IL-6-positive bladder cancer.

We previously reported [21] that DNMT1 could be a significant clinical predictor of bladder cancer. Studies have identified that DNMT1 expression may be directly altered by pro-inflammatory cytokines such as IL-6 in some types of malignancies [5,31,32]. A positive correlation between IL-6-positive samples and nuclear staining for DNMT1 was found by IHC analysis in the present

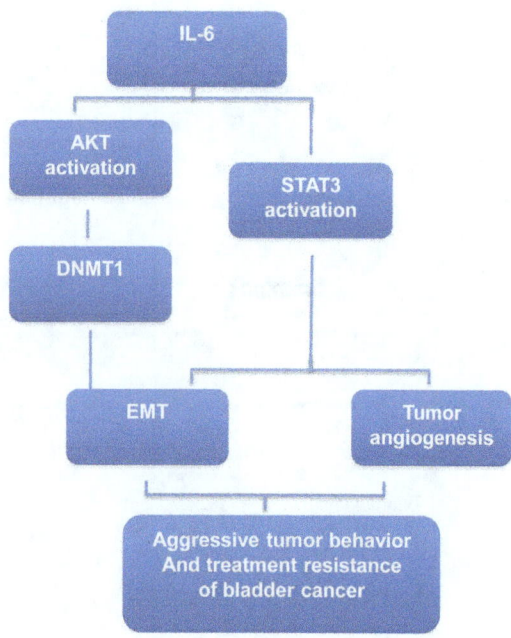

Figure 7. IL-6 signaling pathway in bladder cancer.

study. The relationship between IL-6/STAT3 signaling and DNMT1 in bladder cancer was further examined to see whether regulation of IL-6/STAT3 signaling results in changes of DNMT1 expression. The mRNA and protein analysis revealed that inhibited IL-6 signaling suppressed nuclear DNMT1 expression associated with decreased p-AKT and p-STAT3. However, directly inhibiting STAT3 by STAT3 siRNA had no obvious effect on DNMT1 expression. Phosphorylation of Akt kinase has been reported to be the mechanism responsible for enhanced expression of DNMT1 stimulated by IL-6 [33,34]. When we blocked phosphoinositide 3 kinase/Akt signaling using the specific inhibitor LY294002, the attenuation of AKT activation was associated with decreased DNMT1. We therefore suggest that activated IL-6 signaling enhanced activation of DNMT1 is mediated by activation of Akt in bladder TCC.

Identification of potential factors has important implications for the development and selection of molecular targets in cancer therapy. Our experimental data indicated that the level of IL-6 is important for the aggressive tumor behavior seen in bladder cancer. Therefore, we further examined the predictive power of IL-6 regarding the clinical outcome of bladder TCC after definite CCRT. Our data showed that enhanced expression of IL-6 was significantly associated with a lower complete response rate after treatment, a higher disease failure rate and a shorter survival period, demonstrating a role of IL-6 in predicting prognosis. The

data obtained from the present study revealed that increased IL-6 production is critical in tumor aggressiveness and prognosis of bladder cancer. We outlined the main signaling pathways that are thought to link IL-6 to bladder cancer (Fig. 7).

In addition to IL-6, several cytokines were reported to be important in studies of bladder cancer. TNF-α was shown to stimulate bladder cancer cells to produce MMP-9, which has been implicated in tumor invaαsion and metastasis [35]. Mian et. al. reported that IL-8 blockade significantly inhibited the expressions of MMP-2 and MMP-9, resulting in decreasing invasion [36]. Moreover, increased expression of IL-8 is correlated with poor prognosis of bladder cancer [37]. Inflammation can be considered as enabling for its contribution to the acquisition of core hallmark capabilities. The biological mechanisms linking tumor aggressiveness in IL-6, IL-8 and TNF- α are not clearly understood. The issue needs further investigation in future.

Our study has some limitations. First, we retrospectively examined the predictive value of IL-6 in bladder cancer patients only by the fraction of positive staining. Also, it is a retrospective analysis of a population with different clinical stages from a single institution. Therefore, further investigations of the levels of IL-6 in patients with different stages in a prospective trial are needed.

Taken together, our findings suggest that IL-6 is crucial for aggressive tumor growth, and the clinical outcome of bladder cancer after definite radiotherapy. The data support the emerging hypothesis that IL-6 is a clinically significant prognostic predictor and may represent a suitable target for bladder cancer treatment.

Supporting Information

Figure S1 IL-6 inhibition attenuated the invasion capacity. The invasive capacity in bladder cancer cells with or without IL-6 silencing vector was evaluated. The results are shown by representative slides and quantitative data. Quantification of invasion ability was counting the number of invading cells for each condition. The y-axis represents the ratio normalized by the value of the respective cell line under control condition. Column, mean of three separate experiments; Bar, SD. *, $P < 0.05$

Acknowledgments

The authors thank Dr. S. P. Huang, Department of Urology, Kaohsiung Medical University Hospital, for his advice and support in this study. The work was support by Chang Gung Memorial Hospital, Taiwan, grant CMRPG690332-3

Author Contributions

Conceived and designed the experiments: MFC CTW. Performed the experiments: MFC PYL CTW. Analyzed the data: PYL CFW WCC. Wrote the paper: MFC CTW.

References

1. Dinney CP, McConkey DJ, Millikan RE, Wu X, Bar-Eli M, et al. (2004) Focus on bladder cancer. Cancer Cell 6:111–116.
2. Stein JP, Lieskovsky G, Cote R, Groshen S, Feng AC, et al. (2001) Radical cystectomy in the treatment of invasive bladder cancer: long-term results in 1,054 patients. J Clin Oncol 19:666–675.
3. Coussens LM, Werb Z (2002) Inflammation and cancer. Nature 420:860–867.
4. Balkwill F, Mantovani A (2001) Inflammation and cancer: back to Virchow? Lancet 357:539–545.
5. Gonda TA, Tu S, Wang TC (2009) Chronic inflammation, the tumor microenvironment and carcinogenesis. Cell Cycle 8:2005–2013.
6. Smyth MJ, Cretney E, Kershaw MH, Hayakawa Y (2004) Cytokines in cancer immunity and immunotherapy. Immunol Rev 202:275–293.

7. Abdel-Latif MM, Duggan S, Reynolds JV, Kelleher D (2009) Inflammation and esophageal carcinogenesis. Curr Opin Pharmacol 9:396–404.
8. Zhu Z, Shen Z, Xu C (2012) Mediators Inflamm. 2012:528690
9. Lee H, Herrmann A, Deng JH, Kujawski M, Niu G, et al. (2009) Persistently activated Stat3 maintains constitutive NF-kappaB activity in tumors. Cancer Cell. 15: 283–93.
10. Kishimoto T (2005) Interleukin-6: from basic science to medicine--40 years in immunology. Annu Rev Immunol 23:1–21.
11. Schafer ZT, Brugge JS (2007) IL-6 involvement in epithelial cancers. J Clin Invest 117:3660–3663.
12. Chen CC, Chen WC, Lu CH, Wang WH, Lin PY, et al. (2010) Significance of interleukin-6 signaling in the resistance of pharyngeal cancer to irradiation and

the epidermal growth factor receptor inhibitor. Int J Radiat Oncol Biol Phys 76:1214–1224.

13. Andrews B, Shariat SF, Kim JH, Wheeler TM, Slawin KM, et al. (2002) Preoperative plasma levels of interleukin-6 and its soluble receptor predict disease recurrence and survival of patients with bladder cancer. J Urol 167:1475–1481.

14. George DJ, Halabi S, Shepard TF, Sanford B, Vogelzang NJ, et al. (2005) The prognostic significance of plasma interleukin-6 levels in patients with metastatic hormone-refractory prostate cancer: results from cancer and leukemia group B 9480. Clin Cancer Res 11:1815–1820.

15. Scambia G, Testa U, Benedetti Panici P, Foti E, Martucci R, et al. (1995) Prognostic significance of interleukin 6 serum levels in patients with ovarian cancer. Br J Cancer 71:354–356.

16. Liang CC, Park AY, Guan JL (2007) In vitro scratch assay: a convenient and inexpensive method for analysis of cell migration in vitro. Nat Protoc. 2(2):329–33.

17. McConkey DJ, Choi W, Marquis L, Martin F, Williams MB, et al. (2009) Role of epithelial-to-mesenchymal transition (EMT) in drug sensitivity and metastasis in bladder cancer. Cancer Metastasis Rev 28:335–344.

18. Rieger-Christ KM, Ng L, Hanley RS, Durrani O, Ma H, et al. (2005) Restoration of plakoglobin expression in bladder carcinoma cell lines suppresses cell migration and tumorigenic potential. Br J Cancer 92:2153–9

19. Bromberg J (2002) Stat proteins and oncogenesis. J Clin Invest 109:1139–1142.

20. Sharma S, Sharma MC, Sarkar C (2005) Morphology of angiogenesis in human cancer: a conceptual overview, histoprognostic perspective and significance of neoangiogenesis. Histopathology 46:481–489.

21. Wu CT, Wu CF, Lu CH, Lin CC, Chen WC, et al. (2011) Expression and function role of DNA methyltransferase 1 in human bladder cancer. Cancer 117:5221–5233.

22. Lin J, Guan Z, Wang C, Feng L, Zheng Y, et al. (2010) Inhibitor of differentiation 1 contributes to head and neck squamous cell carcinoma survival via the NF-kappaB/survivin and phosphoinositide 3-kinase/Akt signaling pathways. Clin Cancer Res 16:77–87.

23. Levy DE, Darnell JE Jr (2002) Stats: transcriptional control and biological impact. Nat Rev Mol Cell Biol 3:651–662

24. Ho PL, Lay EJ, Jian W, Parra D, Chan KS (2012) Stat3 activation in urothelial stem cells leads to direct progression to invasive bladder cancer. Cancer Res 72:3135–42

25. Reis ST, Leite KR, Piovesan LF, Pontes-Junior J, Viana NI, et al. (2012) Increased expression of MMP-9 and IL-8 are correlated with poor prognosis of Bladder Cancer. BMC Urol. 12:18

26. Nakanishi R, Oka N, Nakatsuji H, Koizumi T, Sakaki M, et al. (2009) Effect of vascular endothelial growth factor and its receptor inhibitor on proliferation and invasion in bladder cancer. Urol Int. 83:98–106

27. Seguchi T, Yokokawa K, Sugao H, Nakano E, Sonoda T, et al. (1992) Interleukin-6 activity in urine and serum in patients with bladder carcinoma. J Urol 148:791–794.

28. Kozin SV, Duda DG, Munn LL, Jain RK (2012) Neovascularization after irradiation: what is the source of newly formed vessels in recurring tumors? J Natl Cancer Inst. 104(12): 899–905.

29. Wei LH, Kuo ML, Chen CA, Chou CH, Lai KB, et al. (2003) Interleukin-6 promotes cervical tumor growth by VEGF-dependent angiogenesis via a STAT3 pathway. Oncogene. 22:1517–27.

30. Aggarwal BB, Kunnumakkara AB, Harikumar KB, Gupta SR, Tharakan ST, et al. (2009) Signal transducer and activator of transcription-3, inflammation, and cancer: how intimate is the relationship? Ann N Y Acad Sci. 1171: 59–76

31. Feinberg AP, Tycko B (2004) The history of cancer epigenetics. Nat Rev Cancer 4:143–153.

32. Wehbe H, Henson R, Meng F, Mize-Berge J, Patel T (2006) Interleukin-6 contributes to growth in cholangiocarcinoma cells by aberrant promoter methylation and gene expression. Cancer Res 66:10517–10524.

33. Chen CC, Chen WC, Wang WH, Lu CH, Lin PY, et al. (2011) Role of DNA methyltransferase 1 in pharyngeal cancer related to treatment resistance. Head Neck 33:1132–1143.

34. Hodge DR, Cho E, Copeland TD, Guszczynski T, Yang E, et al. (2007) IL-6 enhances the nuclear translocation of DNA cytosine-5-methyltransferase 1 (DNMT1) via phosphorylation of the nuclear localization sequence by the AKT kinase. Cancer Genomics Proteomics 4:387–398.

35. Lee SJ, Park SS, Cho YH, Park K, Kim EJ, et al. (2008) Activation of matrix metalloproteinase-9 by TNF-alpha in human urinary bladder cancer HT1376 cells: the role of MAP kinase signaling pathways. Oncol Rep. 19:1007–13.

36. Mian BM, Dinney CP, Bermejo CE, Sweeney P, Tellez C, et al. (2003) Fully human anti-interleukin 8 antibody inhibits tumor growth in orthotopic bladder cancer xenografts via down-regulation of matrix metalloproteases and nuclear factor-kappaB. Clin Cancer Res. 9:3167–75.

37. Reis ST, Leite KR, Piovesan LF, Pontes-Junior J, Viana NI, et al. (2012) Increased expression of MMP-9 and IL-8 are correlated with poor prognosis of Bladder Cancer. BMC Urol. 12:18

10

MicroRNA-1280 Inhibits Invasion and Metastasis by Targeting ROCK1 in Bladder Cancer

Shahana Majid[1], Altaf A. Dar[2], Sharanjot Saini[1], Varahram Shahryari[1], Sumit Arora[1], Mohd Saif Zaman[1], Inik Chang[1], Soichiro Yamamura[1], Takeshi Chiyomaru[1], Shinichiro Fukuhara[1], Yuichiro Tanaka[1], Guoren Deng[1], Z Laura Tabatabai[1], Rajvir Dahiya[1]*

1 Department of Urology, VA Medical Center and UCSF, San Francisco, California, United States of America, 2 Research Institute, California Pacific Medical Center, San Francisco, California, United States of America

Abstract

MicroRNAs (miRNAs) are non-protein-coding sequences that can function as oncogenes or tumor suppressor genes. This study documents the tumor suppressor role of miR-1280 in bladder cancer. Quantitative real-time PCR and in situ hybridization analyses showed that miR-1280 is significantly down-regulated in bladder cancer cell lines and tumors compared to a non-malignant cell line or normal tissue samples. To decipher the functional significance of miR-1280 in bladder cancer, we ectopically over-expressed miR-1280 in bladder cancer cell lines. Over-expression of miR-1280 had antiproliferative effects and impaired colony formation of bladder cancer cell lines. FACS (fluorescence activated cell sorting) analysis revealed that re-expression of miR-1280 in bladder cancer cells induced G2-M cell cycle arrest and apoptosis. Our results demonstrate that miR-1280 inhibited migration and invasion of bladder cancer cell lines. miR-1280 also attenuated ROCK1 and RhoC protein expression. Luciferase reporter assays demonstrated that oncogene ROCK1 is a direct target of miR-1280 in bladder cancer. This study also indicates that miR-1280 may be of diagnostic and prognostic importance in bladder cancer. For instance, ROC analysis showed that miR-1280 expression can distinguish between malignant and normal bladder cancer cases and Kaplan-Meier analysis revealed that patients with miR-1280 high expression had higher overall survival compared to those with low miR-1280 expression. In conclusion, this is the first study to document that miR-1280 functions as a tumor suppressor by targeting oncogene ROCK1 to invasion/migration and metastasis. Various compounds are currently being used as ROCK1 inhibitors; therefore restoration of tumor suppressor miR-1280 might be therapeutically useful either alone or in combination with these compounds in the treatment of bladder cancer.

Editor: Natasha Kyprianou, University of Kentucky College of Medicine, United States of America

Funding: This research was supported by the National Center for Research Resources of the National Institutes of Health through Grant Number RO1CA138642, RO1CA130860, RO1CA160079 and VA Merit Review and VA Program Project. The funders had no role in study design, data collection and analysis, decision to publish, or preparation of the manuscript.

* E-mail: rdahiya@urology.ucsf.edu

Introduction

MicroRNAs (miRNAs) are non-protein-coding sequences thought to regulate >90% of human genes [1]. Deregulation of miRNA expression has been identified in a number of cancers [2,3], and accumulating evidence indicates that some miRNAs can function as oncogenes or tumor suppressor genes. miRNAs are expressed in a tissue-specific manner and can play important roles in cell proliferation, apoptosis, and differentiation [4,5]. Inactivation of oncogenic miRNAs [6,7] or restoration of tumor-suppressor miRNAs [8,9,10] may have great potential for cancer treatment.

Alterations in cellular functions such as cell proliferation, adhesion and motility are based on the morphological changes that result from actin cytoskeleton reorganization. Rho family proteins interact with the actin cytoskeleton regulating formation of stress fibers and focal adhesions within cells. Rho-associated serine-threonine protein kinase, ROCK [11,12], one of the best characterized downstream effectors of Rho, is activated when it selectively binds to the active GTP-bound form of Rho. Activated

ROCK interacts with the actin cytoskeleton to promote stress-fiber formation and assembly of focal contacts [13]. Rearrangements of the actin cytoskeleton are involved in cancer cell migration which is central to the process of metastasis. Tang et al [14] examined the effects of ROCK1 inhibition on the activity of upstream RhoA and Rac1. ROCK1 indirectly diminishes the activity of upstream RhoA by stimulating Tiam1-induced Rac1 activity. ROCK1 provides a feedback mechanism, mediating upstream Rac1 and RhoA activity, thus reflecting the diverse effects of ROCK1 on the functional balance of small GTPases [14]. Rearranging the actin cytoskeletal proteins in response to Rho is important for the ability of tumor cells to metastasize [15]. The Rho/ROCK pathway plays role in cancer progression by regulating actin cytoskeleton reorganization and a specific ROCK inhibitor was found to suppress tumor growth and metastasis [16,17]. In prostate carcinoma PC-3 cells, RhoA is a critical endogenous promoter of cell invasion and migration [18]. Inhibition of RhoA or its major downstream effector, ROCK1, diminishes motility of prostate carcinoma cells [18]. In bladder cancer, the Rho/ROCK

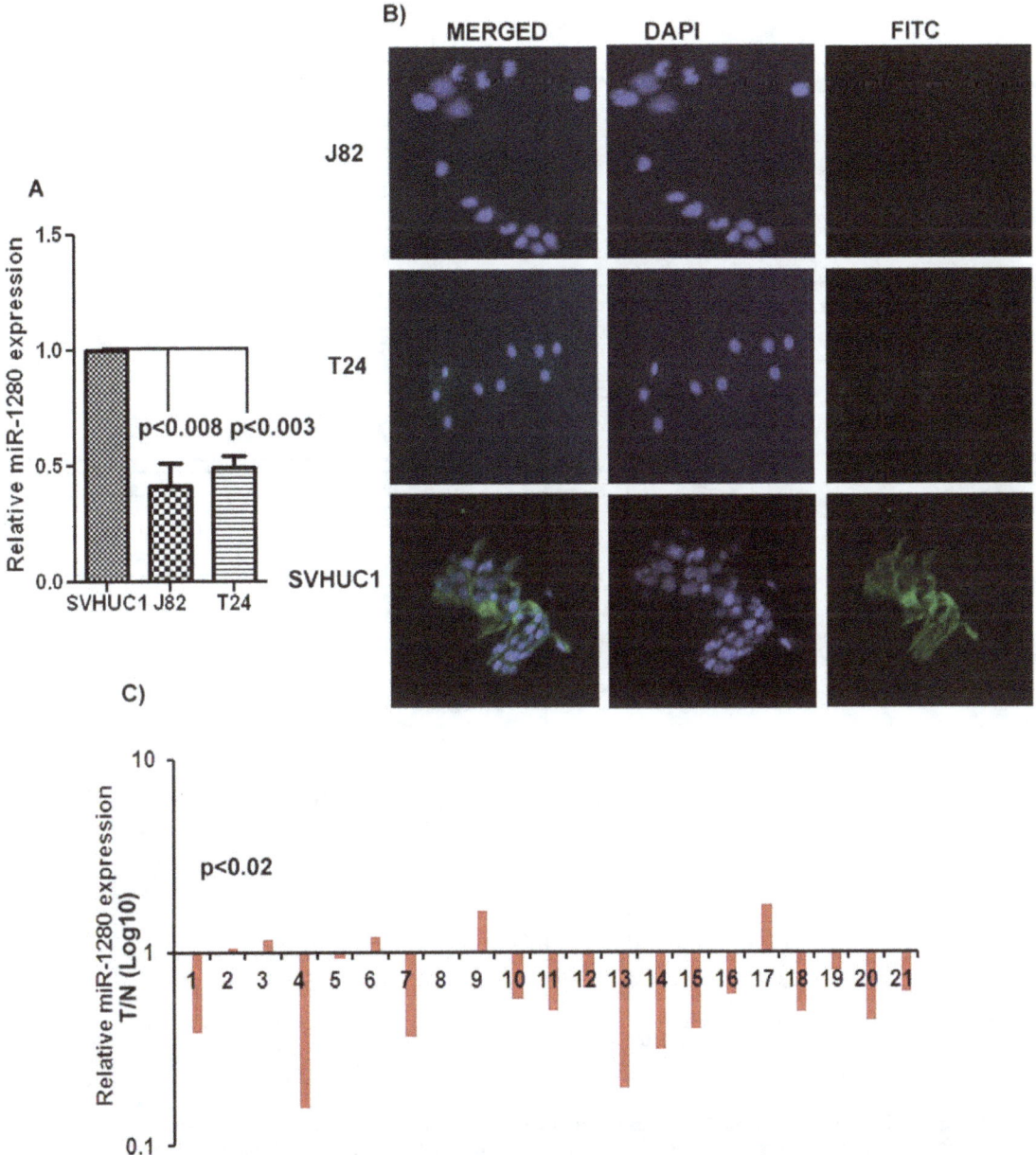

Figure 1. miR-1280 expression is downregulated in bladder cancer. A) Quantitative RT-PCR analysis of miR-1280 in cell lines. B) *Fluorescence In-situ* hybridization (FISH) in cell lines. C) Quantitative real time PCR analysis of mir-23b expression in matched Laser-Captured Microdissected tissue samples. (T/N- Tumor/Normal).

pathway was reported to be involved in occurrence and progression of bladder cancer [19]. These observations suggest that the Rho/ROCK pathway may be a molecular target for prevention of cancer invasion and metastasis. Here for the first time we report on the tumor suppressor activity of microRNA-1280 (miR-1280) in bladder cancer and show that it bladder cancer migration and invasion by directly targeting ROCK1.

Materials and Methods

Cell Lines and Cell Culture

SV-HUC-1, T24 and J82 cells were purchased from the American Type Culture Collection (ATCC) and grown according to ATCC protocols. SV-HUC-1 cells were cultured in F-12K Medium (ATCC) with 10% FBS. T24 cells were cultured in McCoy's 5A medium supplemented with 10% FBS and J82 cells were cultured in Minimum Essential Media (MEM) supplemented with 10% FBS.

Plasmids, Precursors and Transfection

TaqMan probes and precursors for hsa-miR-1280 and negative control pre-miR were purchased from Applied Biosystems (Foster City, CA). pmir-GLO Dual-Luciferase miRNA Target Expression Vector was purchased from Promega. Lipofectamine 2000 (Invitrogen) was used for all transfections.

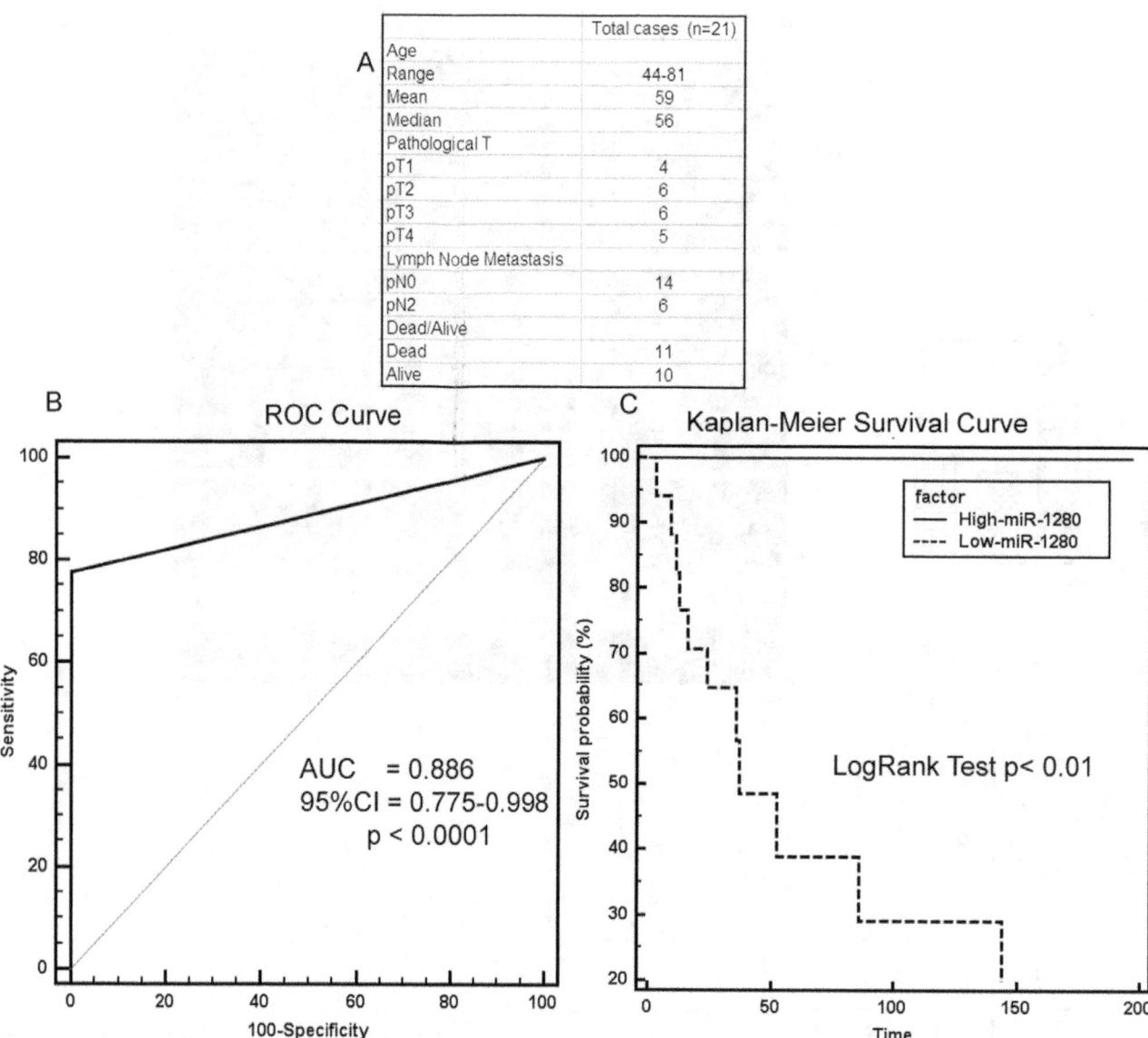

Figure 2. Diagnostic and prognostic significance of miR-1280 in bladder cancer. A) Clinicopathological characteristics of patient cohort. B) ROC curve analysis showing performance of miR-1280 expression to discriminate between malignant and non-malignant tissue samples. C) Kaplan-Meier analysis for overall survival based on miR-1280 expression.

RNA Extraction

miRNA and total RNA were extracted from cell lines using a miRNeasy Mini Kit and an RNeasy Mini Kit (Qiagen). miRNAs from clinical samples were extracted using laser capture micro-dissection techniques with a miRNeasy FFPE kit (Qiagen).

Human Clinical Samples

Clinical samples were obtained from the San Francisco Veterans Affairs (VA) Medical Center. Written informed consent was obtained from all patients and the study was approved by the UCSF Committee on Human Research (Approval number: H9058-35751-01).

Quantitative Real-time PCR

Mature miRNAs were assayed using the TaqMan MicroRNA Assays in accordance with the manufacturer's instructions (Applied Biosystems). All RT reactions, including no-template controls and RT minus controls, were run in a 7500 Fast Real Time PCR System (Applied Biosystems). RNA concentrations were determined with a NanoDrop (Thermo Scientific, Rockford, IL). Samples were normalized to RNU48 (Applied Biosystems). Gene expression levels were quantified using the 7500 Fast Real Time Sequence detection system Software (Applied Biosystems). Comparative real-time PCR was performed in triplicate, including no-template controls. Relative expression was calculated using the comparative Ct.

In Situ Hybridization

In situ hybridization was performed as described previously [20]. Briefly cell lines were stained using DIG-labeled locked nucleic acid (LNA)-based probes specific for mir-1280 following the manufacturer's protocol (Exiqon,Inc Woburn, MA) and detected using anti-DIG-Fluorescein, Fab Fragments (Roche Applied Science, Indianapolis, IN).

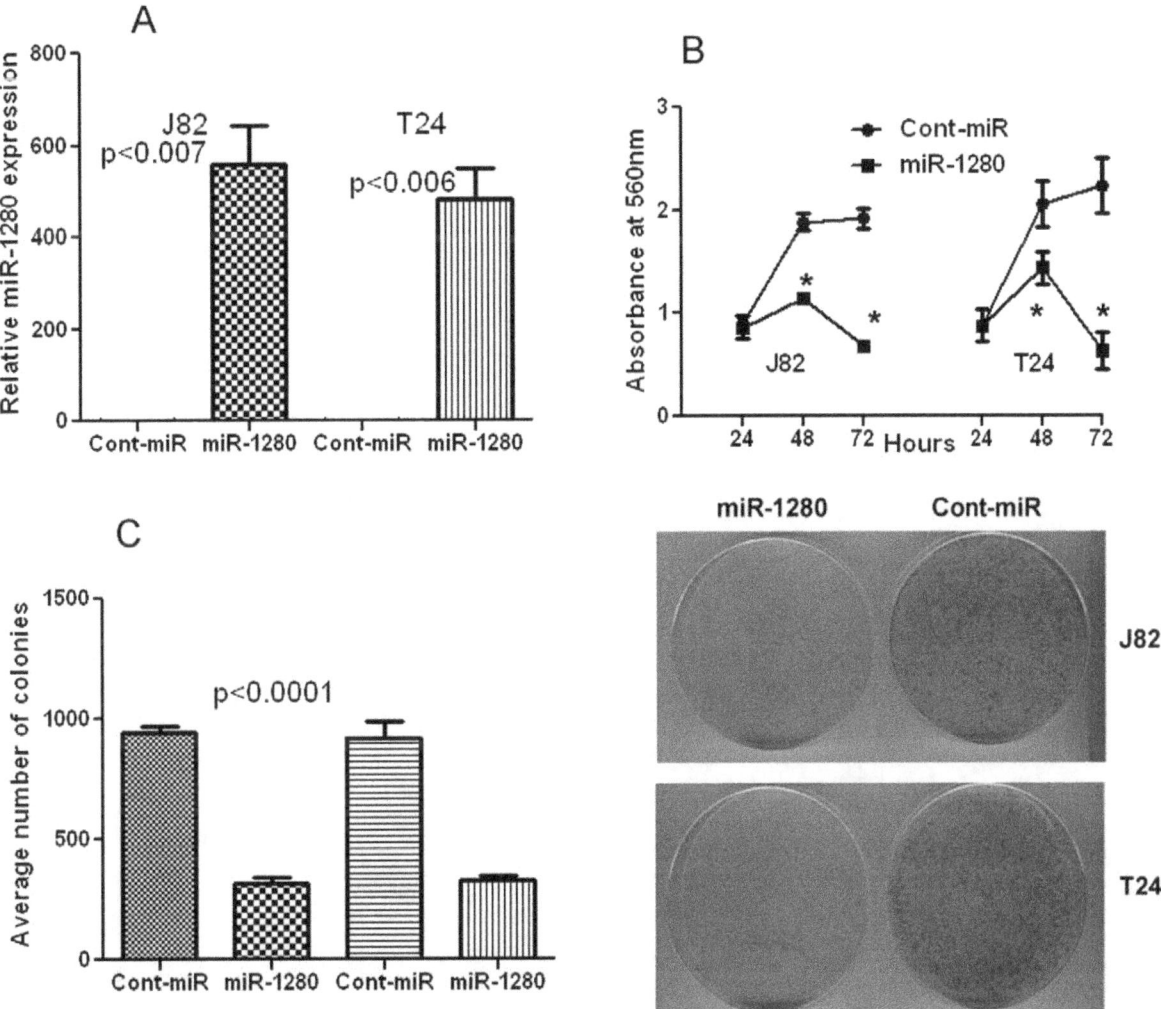

Figure 3. Transient transfection of miR-1280 inhibits bladder cancer cell proliferation and colony formation capability of bladder cancer cells. A) Transient transfection of miR-1280 precursor significantly increased expression of miR-1280 in bladder cancer cells. B) Proliferation of J82 and T24 cells after miR-1280 transfection was significantly reduced compared to cont-miR. C) miR-1280 over-expression significantly inhibits colony forming ability of bladder cancer cells.

Cell Viability and Clonability Assay

Cell viability was determined at 24, 48 and 72 h by using the CellTiter 96 AQueous One Solution Cell Proliferation Assay kit (Promega, Madison, WI) according to the manufacturer's protocol. Absorbance was measured at 490 nm using Spectra-MAX 190 (Molecular Devices). Data are presented as the mean value for triplicate experiments compared to the negative control. For colony formation assay, cells were seeded at low density (1000 cells/plate) and allowed to grow untill visible colonies appeared. Then, cells were stained with Giemsa and colonies were counted.

Migration and Invasion Assays

Cytoselect 24-well cell migration and invasion assay kits (Cell Biolabs, Inc) were used for migration and invasion assays according to the manufacturer's protocol. Briefly, T24 and J82 cells transfected with Pre-miR miRNA precursor or negative control were harvested 72 hours after transfection and resuspended in serum-free Opti-MEM. Cells (10×10^4 per 300 µl media without serum) were added to the upper chamber, and the lower

chamber was filled with 500 µl of media containing 10% FBS. Cells were incubated for 16 hours at 37°C in a 5% CO2 tissue culture incubator. After 16 hours, non-migrated/non-invading cells were removed from upper side of transwel membrane filter inserts using a cotton-tipped swab. Migrated/invaded cells on the lower side were stained and the absorbance was read at 560 nm according to the manufacturer's protocol.

Immunoblotting

Protein was isolated from 70–80% confluent plates of cultured cells using the M-PER Mammalian Protein Extraction Reagent (Pierce Biotechnology, Rockfield, IL) following the manufacturer's directions. Protein concentrations were determined by the Bradford method. Equal amounts of protein were resolved on 4–20% sodium dodecyl sulfate (SDS) polyacrylamide gels and transferred to a nitrocellulose membrane by voltage gradient transfer. The resulting blots were blocked with 5% non-fat dry milk and probed with specific antibodies. Blots were then incubated with appropriate peroxidase-conjugated secondary

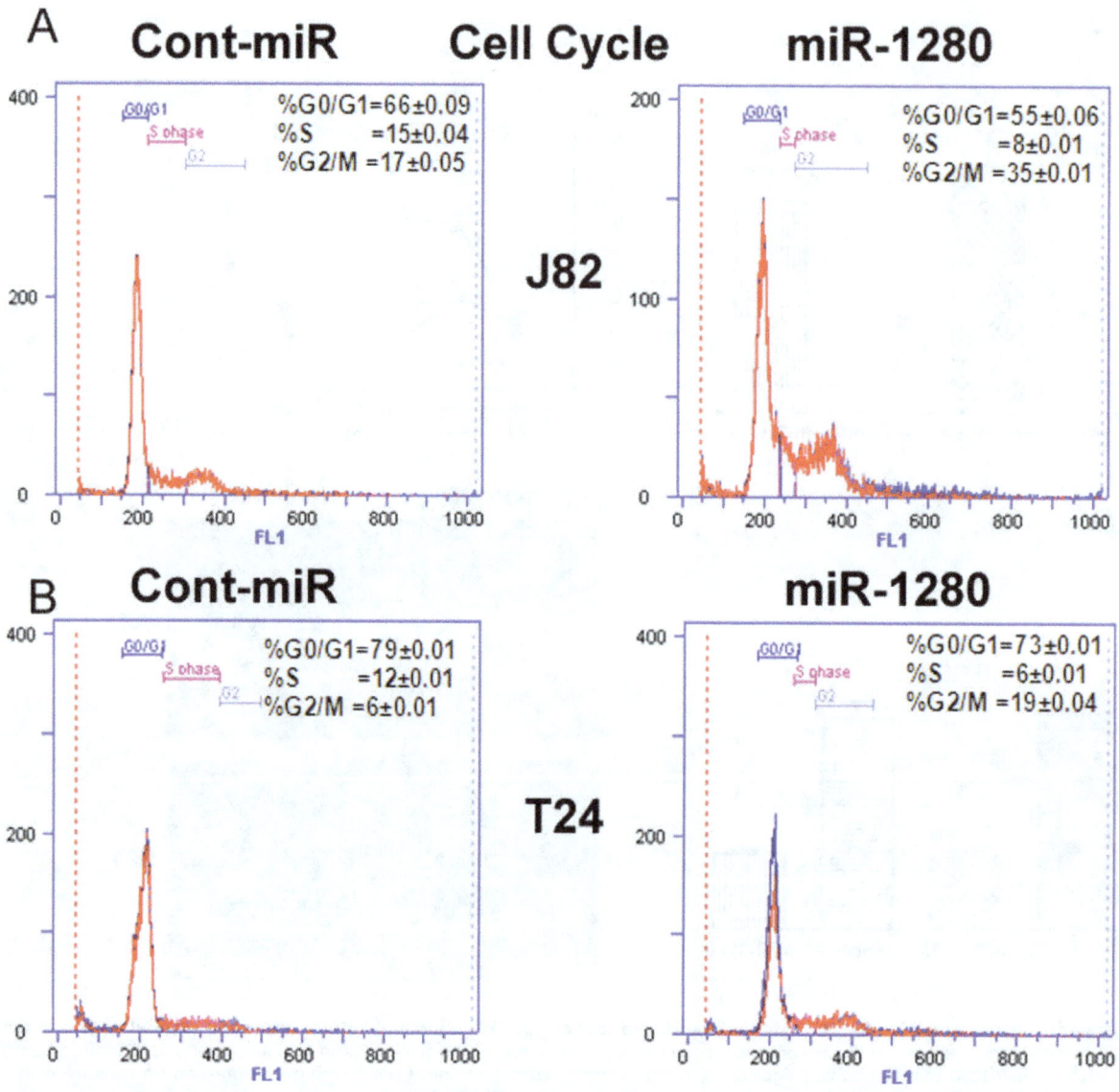

Figure 4. miR-1280 induces cell cycle arrest in bladder cancer cells. A-B) FACS analysis shows miR-1280 over-expression induces G2-M cell cycle arrest in J82 and T24 cells with a corresponding decrease in S-phase cells. Values are shown from triplicate experiments ±SD.

antibodies and visualized using enhanced chemiluminescence (Pierce Biotechnology, Rockford, IL).

Luciferase Reporter Assay

A pmirGLO Dual-Luciferase miRNA target expression vector was used for 3′-UTR luciferase assays (Promega, Madison, WI). The target oncogene of miRNA-1280 was selected on the basis of online microRNA target database http://www.microrna.org/microrna/home.do. The primer sequences for the wild type 3′UTR were: Forward 5′ CGCGGCCGCTAGTCTGTG-GAATCGTGTGGGAT 3′ and Reverse 5′ ctagatcccacacgattcca-cagactagcggccgcgagct 3′. For the mutant 3′UTR, the primer sequences were: Forward 5′ CGCGGCCGCTAGTCTGTG-GAATCGTTCATACT 3′ and reverse 5′ ctagagtatgaacgattcca-cagactagcggccgcgagct 3′. For luciease assay, T24 and J82 cells were cotransfected with hsa-miR-1280 and pmirGLO Dual-Luciferase miRNA target expression vectors with wild-type or mutant target sequence using Lipofectamine 2000. Firefly luciferase activities were measured using the Dual Luciferase Assay (Promega, Madison, WI) 18 hr after transfection and the results were normalized with Renilla luciferase. Each reporter plasmid was transfected at least three times (on different days) and each sample was assayed in triplicate.

Statistical Analysis

Statistical analyses were performed with GraphPad Prism 5 and MedCalc version 10.3.2. All quantified data represents an average of at least triplicate samples or as indicated. Error bars represent standard deviation of the mean. All tests were performed two tailed and p-values <0.05 were considered statistically significant. Receiver operating curves (ROC) were calculated to determine the potential of miR-1280 to discriminate between malignant and non-malignant samples. For disease progression, Kaplan-Meier (log-rank test) analysis was performed.

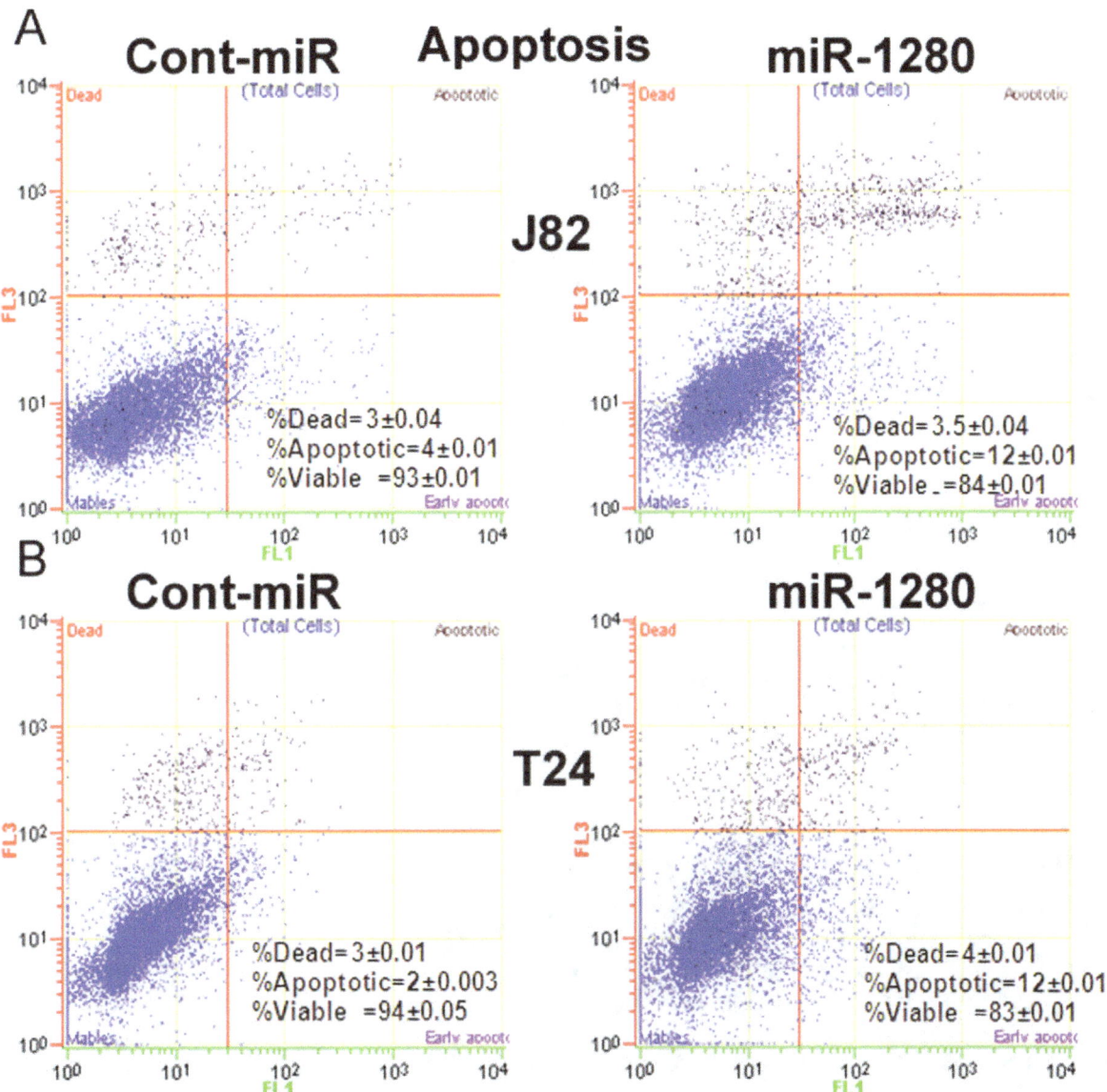

Figure 5. Reconstitution of miR-1280 induces apoptosis in bladder cancer cell lines. A–B) miR-1280 over-expression induces apoptosis in J82 and T24 cells with a concomitant decrease in the viable number of cells. Values shown are from triplicate experiments ±SD.

Results

Expression of miR-1280 in Bladder Tumors and Cancer Cell lines

Expression of miR-1280 was examined by real-time PCR in bladder cancer cell lines J82, T24 and compared to non-malignant cell line SV-HUC1. The results indicated that miR-1280 was downregulated in cancer cell lines (Figure 1A). *In-situ* hybridization also confirmed the presence of miR-1280 expression (green signal) in SV-HUC1 cells compared to cancer cell lines (Figure 1B). To examine the biological significance of miR-1280, its expression was analyzed in laser captured microdissected (LCM) human bladder tumor tissue and compared to normal matched control tissue. The expression of miR-1280 was found to be significantly downregulated in all the tumor samples compared to their matched normal samples (Figure 1C). These results indicate a putative tumor suppressor role for miR-1280 in bladder cancer.

Diagnostic and Prognostic Significance of miR-1280 in Bladder Cancer

Clinical demographics of the patient cohort are summarized in Figure 2A. Receiver operating curve (ROC) analyses were performed to evaluate the ability of miR-1280 expression to discriminate between normal and tumor cases using tissue samples. An area under the ROC curve (AUC) of 0.886 (P<0.0001; 95% CI = 0.775 to 0.998) (Figure 2B) was obtained suggesting that miR-1280 expression can discriminate between malignant and non-malignant samples and hence can be used as a diagnostic marker for bladder cancer though additional samples may strengthen these results. To determine whether miR-1280 has any prognostic significance, we divided cases into low miR-1280 (expression T/N<0.8 fold) and high miR-1280 (expression T/N>0.8 fold) groups and performed Kaplan-Meier survival analysis. In Kaplan-Meier analysis, the high miR-1280 group had significantly higher overall survival probability compared to the low miR-1280 group (Logrank Test p<0.02) (Figure 2C).

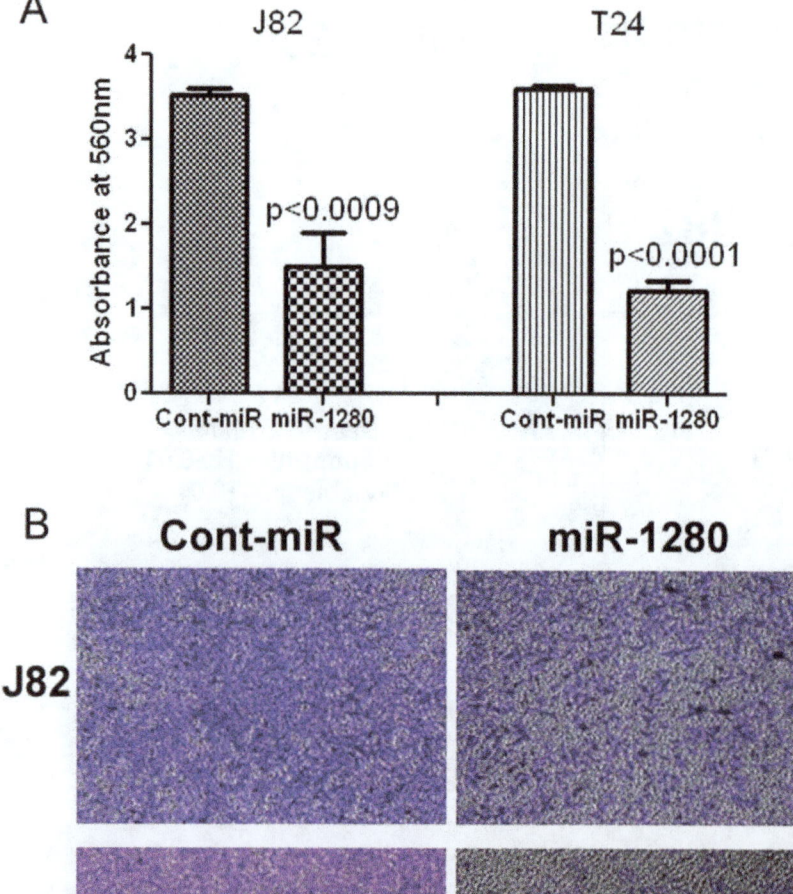

Figure 6. Ectopic expression of miR-1280 inhibits bladder cancer cell migration. A) Migration assays of J82 and T24 cells transfected with miR-1280. B) Representative pictures of migration assay.

These findings suggest that miR-1280 has the potential to be a diagnostic and prognostic marker for bladder cancer.

MicroRNA-1280 Overexpression Suppresses Bladder Cancer Cell Proliferation and Colony Formation

To determined the functional significance of miR-1280 overexpression in bladder cancer, we transfected bladder cancer cell lines J82 and T24 with miR-1280 precursors. miR-1280 was significantly overexpressed in J82 and T24 cell lines after transient transfection with miR-1280 precursor compared to the cont-miR precursor (Figure 3A). Ectopic expression of miR-1280 significantly decreased cell proliferation as compared to cells expressing cont-miR (Figure 3B). miR-1280 transfected cells also had low colony formation ability as the number of foci in miR-1280 expressing cells were decreased when compared with cont-miR transfected cells (Figure 3C). These results indicate anti-proliferative effect of miR-1280 in bladder cancer.

miR-1280 Triggers Cell Cycle Arrest and Induces Apoptosis in Bladder Cancer Cells

FACS (fluorescence activated cell sorting) analysis revealed that re-expression of miR-1280 lead to a significant increase in the number of cells in the G2-M phase of the cell cycle (17% to 35%) while the S-phase population decreased from 15% to 8% in J82 cells (Figure 4A). Similar results were observed in T24 cells with an increase in G2-M population of cells (6% to 19%) and a decrease in S-phase population (12% to 6%), suggesting that miR-1280 triggers a G2-M arrest in miR-1280 transfected cells compared to cont-miR. FACS analysis for apoptosis was performed using Annexin-V-FITC-7-AAD dye. The percentage of total apoptotic cells (early apoptotic + apoptotic) was significantly increased (4% to 12%) in response to miR-1280 overexpression compared to cont-miR with a corresponding 10% decrease in the viable cell population in J82 cells (Figure 5A). In T24 cells, an increase (2% to 12%) in apoptotic cells was observed with miR-1280 overexpres-

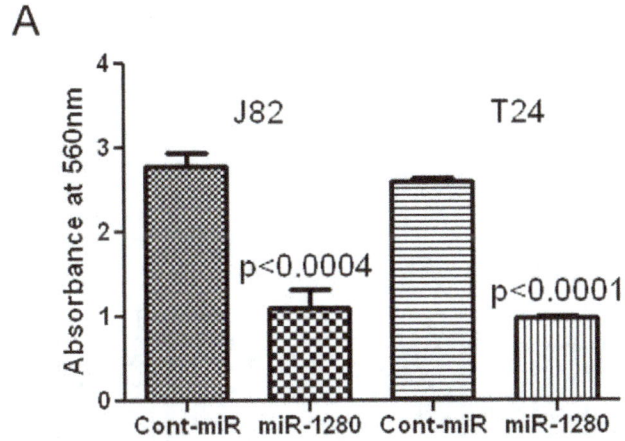

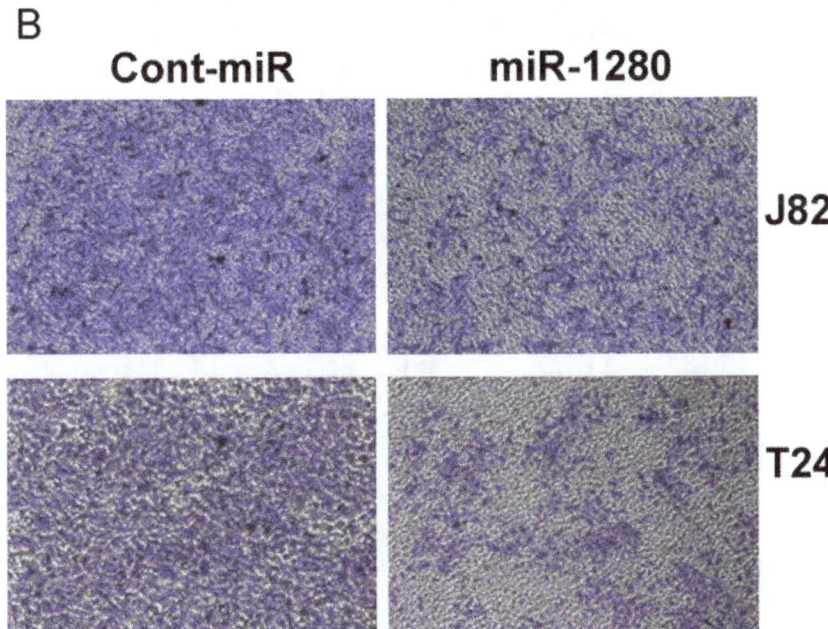

Figure 7. Overexpression of miR-1280 inhibits bladder cancer cell invasion. A) Invasion assay shows a significant decrease in the number of invading J82 and T24 cells transfected with miR-1280. B) Representative pictures of invasion assay.

sion compared to cont-miR (Figure 5B). These results indicate a tumor suppressor role for miR-1280 in bladder cancer.

Anti-migration/Invasion Effects of miR-1280 in Bladder Cancer

Overexpression of miR-1280 had anti-migratory and anti-invasive effects on bladder cancer cell lines. Less absorbance was observed at 560 nm with miR-1280 transfected cells compared to cont-miR in the migration assay (Figure 6) and miR-1280 overexpression also significantly reduced the invasiveness of bladder cancer cells (Figure 7).

miR-1280 Directly Targets Oncogene ROCK1

ROCK1 has been reported to be an important molecule that drives bladder cancer migration and invasion. Using an online microRNA target database we found oncogene ROCK1 as the putative target of miR-1280 with complementary 3′UTR sites for the seed sequence of miR-1280 (Figure 8A). We performed Western analysis for ROCK1 expression in miR-1280 transfected

cells and found that miR-1280 attenuated the protein expression of ROCK1 compared to the cont-miR (Figure 8B). We also found a decrease in the protein levels of RohC, another oncogenic protein that is upstream of ROCK1. To check whether a direct interaction is involved between miR-1280 and its target oncogene ROCK1, we performed luciferase reporter assays. We found that co-transfection of miR-1280 along with the wild type 3′UTR of oncogene ROCK1 caused a significant decrease in luciferase units compared to controls (Figure 8C). These results suggest that miR-1280 targets oncogene ROCK1 directly.

Discussion

Though little is known about microRNA-1280, one study has shown that miR-1280 is expressed in colon and pancreatic cancers based on expression analysis of 19 colorectal and 17 pancreatic human cancer samples [21]. Here we for the first time report that miR-1280 plays a tumor suppressor and has diagnostic and prognostic potential in bladder cancer. We also performed

Majid et al Figure 8

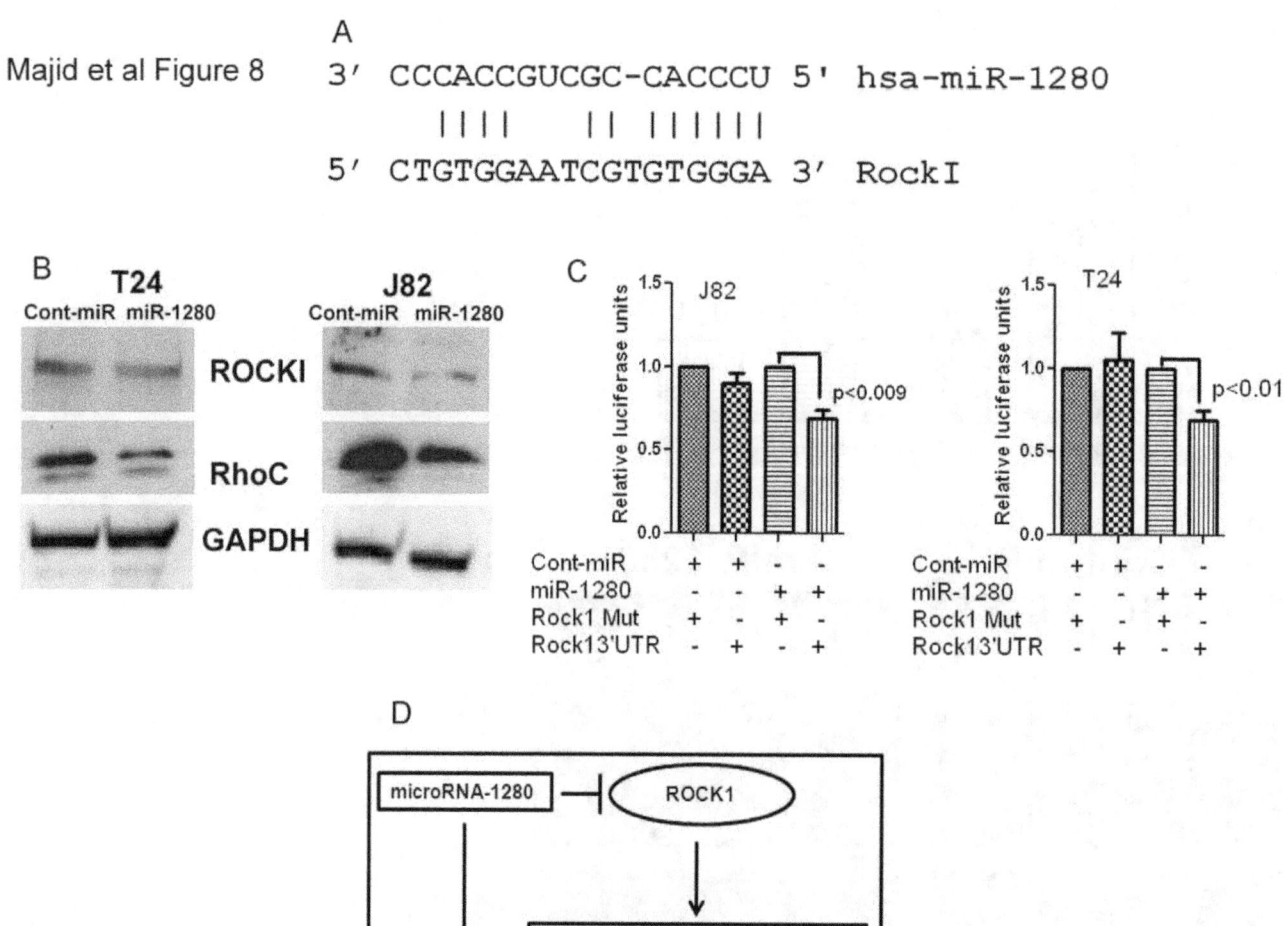

A

3' CCCACCGUCGC-CACCCU 5' hsa-miR-1280
   | | | | | | | | | | | |
5' CTGTGGAATCGTGTGGGA 3' RockI

Figure 8. miR-1280 directly targets oncogene ROCK1. A) Complimentary miR-1280 binding sequences in the ROCK1 3′UTR. B) Western blot analysis shows that miR-1280 represses translation of oncogenes ROCK1 and RhoC. C) Luciferase assays showing decreased reporter activity after co-transfection of either the wild type or mutant Src-3′UTR with miR-1280 in J82 and T24 cells. Mut- Mutated 3′UTRROCK1 sequence. D) Schematic representation of role of miR-1280 in bladder cancer.

functional analyses to confirm the anti-tumor effects of miR-1280 and show that miR-1280 directly targets oncogene ROCK1, an important molecule in bladder cancer cell migration and invasion.

We also observed that miR-1280 is significantly downregulated in bladder cancer cell lines and tumor tissues compared to non-malignant cell line or normal tissues indicating that miR-1280 might be a tumor suppressor in bladder cancer. Previous studies have shown that microRNAs are highly tissue specific and they can act as tumor suppressor or oncogenes [5,6]. MicroRNAs possess several features that make them attractive candidates as new prognostic biomarkers and powerful tools for the early diagnosis of cancer [22]. In this study, we found that miR-1280 was predictive of overall survival such that patients with higher miR-1280 expression had longer overall survival compared to patients with low miR-1280 expression. MicroRNA-1280 expression also distinguished malignant from normal tissues indicating the diagnostic significance of miR-1280 in bladder cancer although this needs to be confirmed in a larger cohort of tissue

samples. Our functional assays revealed that miR-1280 has anti-proliferative effects, inducing cell cycle arrest and apoptosis in bladder cancer. It also showed anti-migratory and anti-invasive effect on bladder cancer cells.

Since ROCK1 is an important molecule that is involved in bladder cancer migration and invasion [19], we examined whether ROCK1 is a target of miR-1280 in bladder cancer. Overexpression of ROCK1 has been reported to occur in various cancers [14,19] and the Rho/ROCK pathway has been found to be associated with progression of bladder cancer [19]. ROCK mediates responses in the pathway initiated by Rho, and regulates the reorganization of cytosleletal proteins such as formation of stress fibers and focal adhesions [23]. Rearranging cytoskeletal proteins is important for the ability of tumor cells to metastasize [15] and our study showed that miR-1280 attenuated expression of oncogene ROCK1. Luciferase assays also revealed direct interaction of miR-1280 and ROCK1. Therefore these results indicate that miR-1280 inhibits migration/invasion and thus metastasis of bladder cancer that is mediated through downregulation of oncogene ROCK1 (Figure 8D). We also found decreased expression of oncogene RhoC that is upstream of ROCK1. A previous study has reported that ROCK1 diminishes activity of its upstream RhoA family members indirectly [14]. By the same principal, inhibition of ROCK1 by miR-1280 may have an indirect inhibitory action on the RhoC oncogene.

In conclusion, our study is the first report to document the tumor suppressor role of miR-1280 in bladder cancer. miR-1280 directly targets oncogene ROCK1, inhibiting migration/invasion which are central to the process of metastasis. Various compounds such as Y-27632, have been found to inhibit ROCK1. Our findings indicate that restoration of tumor suppressor miR-1280 might be useful therapeutically either alone or in combination with these compounds in the treatment of bladder cancer.

References

1. Miranda KC, Huynh T, Tay Y, Ang YS, Tam WL, et al. (2006) A pattern-based method for the identification of MicroRNA binding sites and their corresponding heteroduplexes. Cell 126: 1203–1217.
2. Porkka KP, Pfeiffer MJ, Waltering KK, Vessella RL, Tammela TL, et al. (2007) MicroRNA expression profiling in prostate cancer. Cancer Res 67: 6130–6135.
3. Volinia S, Calin GA, Liu CG, Ambs S, Cimmino A, et al. (2006) A microRNA expression signature of human solid tumors defines cancer gene targets. Proc Natl Acad Sci U S A 103: 2257–2261.
4. Bartels CL, Tsongalis GJ (2009) MicroRNAs: novel biomarkers for human cancer. Clin Chem 55: 623–631.
5. Sempere LF, Christensen M, Silahtaroglu A, Bak M, Heath CV, et al. (2007) Altered MicroRNA expression confined to specific epithelial cell subpopulations in breast cancer. Cancer Res 67: 11612–11620.
6. Medina PP, Nolde M, Slack FJ (2010) OncomiR addiction in an in vivo model of microRNA-21-induced pre-B-cell lymphoma. Nature 467: 86–90.
7. Obad S, dos Santos CO, Petri A, Heidenblad M, Broom O, et al. (2011) Silencing of microRNA families by seed-targeting tiny LNAs. Nat Genet 43: 371–378.
8. Lujambio A, Calin GA, Villanueva A, Ropero S, Sanchez-Cespedes M, et al. (2008) A microRNA DNA methylation signature for human cancer metastasis. Proc Natl Acad Sci U S A 105: 13556–13561.
9. Lujambio A, Ropero S, Ballestar E, Fraga MF, Cerrato C, et al. (2007) Genetic unmasking of an epigenetically silenced microRNA in human cancer cells. Cancer Res 67: 1424–1429.
10. Saito Y, Liang G, Egger G, Friedman JM, Chuang JC, et al. (2006) Specific activation of microRNA-127 with downregulation of the proto-oncogene BCL6 by chromatin-modifying drugs in human cancer cells. Cancer Cell 9: 435–443.
11. Bishop AL, Hall A (2000) Rho GTPases and their effector proteins. Biochem J 348 Pt 2: 241–255.
12. Ishizaki T, Maekawa M, Fujisawa K, Okawa K, Iwamatsu A, et al. (1996) The small GTP-binding protein Rho binds to and activates a 160 kDa Ser/Thr protein kinase homologous to myotonic dystrophy kinase. EMBO J 15: 1885–1893.
13. Ishizaki T, Naito M, Fujisawa K, Maekawa M, Watanabe N, et al. (1997) p160ROCK, a Rho-associated coiled-coil forming protein kinase, works downstream of Rho and induces focal adhesions. FEBS Lett 404: 118–124.
14. Tang AT, Campbell WB, Nithipatikom K (2012) ROCK1 feedback regulation of the upstream small GTPase RhoA. Cell Signal 24: 1375–1380.
15. del Peso L, Hernandez-Alcoceba R, Embade N, Carnero A, Esteve P, et al. (1997) Rho proteins induce metastatic properties in vivo. Oncogene 15: 3047–3057.
16. Itoh K, Yoshioka K, Akedo H, Uehata M, Ishizaki T, et al. (1999) An essential part for Rho-associated kinase in the transcellular invasion of tumor cells. Nat Med 5: 221–225.
17. Imamura F, Mukai M, Ayaki M, Akedo H (2000) Y-27632, an inhibitor of rho-associated protein kinase, suppresses tumor cell invasion via regulation of focal adhesion and focal adhesion kinase. Jpn J Cancer Res 91: 811–816.
18. Sequeira L, Dubyk CW, Riesenberger TA, Cooper CR, van Golen KL (2008) Rho GTPases in PC-3 prostate cancer cell morphology, invasion and tumor cell diapedesis. Clin Exp Metastasis 25: 569–579.
19. Kamai T, Tsujii T, Arai K, Takagi K, Asami H, et al. (2003) Significant association of Rho/ROCK pathway with invasion and metastasis of bladder cancer. Clin Cancer Res 9: 2632–2641.
20. Majid S, Saini S, Dar AA, Hirata H, Shahryari V, et al. (2011) MicroRNA-205 inhibits Src-mediated oncogenic pathways in renal cancer. Cancer Res 71: 2611–2621.
21. Piepoli A, Tavano F, Copetti M, Mazza T, Palumbo O, et al. (2012) Mirna expression profiles identify drivers in colorectal and pancreatic cancers. PLoS One 7: e33663.
22. Schaefer A, Jung M, Mollenkopf HJ, Wagner I, Stephan C, et al. (2009) Diagnostic and prognostic implications of microRNA profiling in prostate carcinoma. Int J Cancer 126: 1166–1176.
23. Amano M, Fukata Y, Kaibuchi K (2000) Regulation and functions of Rho-associated kinase. Exp Cell Res 261: 44–51.

Acknowledgments

We thank Dr. Roger Erickson for his support and assistance with the preparation of the manuscript.

Author Contributions

Conceived and designed the experiments: SM AAD RD. Performed the experiments: SM AAD SS VS GD. Analyzed the data: SM AAD RD SS. Contributed reagents/materials/analysis tools: SM AAD SS VS SA MSZ IC SY TC SF YT GD. Wrote the paper: SM. Designed the research plan: SM RD. Conducted experiments: SM AAD VS. Analyzed data: SM AAD SS VS SA MSZ IC SY TC SF YT GD RD. Provided necessary reagents for research: SM AAD SS VS SA MSZ IC SY TC SF YT GD. Wrote manuscript: SM. Supervise the research and review manuscript: SM RD. Board certified pathologist to identify tumor and normal tissues: ZLT.

11

Does Occupational Exposure to Solvents and Pesticides in Association with Glutathione S-Transferase A1, M1, P1, and T1 Polymorphisms Increase the Risk of Bladder Cancer? The Belgrade Case-Control Study

Marija G. Matic[1,5⑨], **Vesna M. Coric**[1,5⑨], **Ana R. Savic-Radojevic**[1,5], **Petar V. Bulat**[2,5], **Marija S. Pljesa-Ercegovac**[1,5], **Dejan P. Dragicevic**[3,5], **Tatjana I. Djukic**[1,5], **Tatjana P. Simic**[1,5], **Tatjana D. Pekmezovic**[4,5]*

1 Institute of Medical and Clinical Biochemistry, Faculty of Medicine, University of Belgrade, Belgrade, Serbia, 2 Institute of Occupational Health, Belgrade, Serbia, 3 Clinic of Urology, Clinical Center of Serbia, Belgrade, Serbia, 4 Institute of Epidemiology, Faculty of Medicine, University of Belgrade, Belgrade, Serbia, 5 Faculty of Medicine, University of Belgrade, Belgrade, Serbia

Abstract

Objective: We investigated the role of the glutathione S-transferase A1, M1, P1 and T1 gene polymorphisms and potential effect modification by occupational exposure to different chemicals in Serbian bladder cancer male patients.

Patients and Methods: A hospital-based case-control study of bladder cancer in men comprised 143 histologically confirmed cases and 114 age-matched male controls. Deletion polymorphism of glutathione S-transferase M1 and T1 was identified by polymerase chain reaction method. Single nucleotide polymorphism of glutathione S-transferase A1 and P1 was identified by restriction fragment length polymorphism method. As a measure of effect size, odds ratio (OR) with corresponding 95% confidence interval (95%CI) was calculated.

Results: The glutathione S-transferase A1, T1 and P1 genotypes did not contribute independently toward the risk of bladder cancer, while the glutathione S-transferase M1-null genotype was overrepresented among cases (OR = 2.1, 95% CI = 1.1–4.2, p = 0.032). The most pronounced effect regarding occupational exposure to solvents and glutathione S-transferase genotype on bladder cancer risk was observed for the low activity glutathione S-transferase A1 genotype (OR = 9.2, 95% CI = 2.4–34.7, p = 0.001). The glutathione S-transferase M1-null genotype also enhanced the risk of bladder cancer among subjects exposed to solvents (OR = 6,5, 95% CI = 2.1–19.7, p = 0.001). The risk of bladder cancer development was 5.3–fold elevated among glutathione S-transferase T1-active patients exposed to solvents in comparison with glutathione S-transferase T1-active unexposed patients (95% CI = 1.9–15.1, p = 0.002). Moreover, men with glutathione S-transferase T1-active genotype exposed to pesticides exhibited 4.5 times higher risk in comparison with unexposed glutathione S-transferase T1-active subjects (95% CI = 0.9–22.5, p = 0.067).

Conclusion: Null or low-activity genotypes of the glutathione S-transferase A1, T1, and P1 did not contribute independently towards the risk of bladder cancer in males. However, in association with occupational exposure, low activity glutathione S-transferase A1 and glutathione S-transferase M1-null as well as glutathione S-transferase T1-active genotypes increase individual susceptibility to bladder cancer.

Editor: Keitaro Matsuo, Kyushu University Faculty of Medical Science, Japan

Funding: This work was supported by the Ministry of Education and Science of the Republic of Serbia (Grants number: 175052 and 175087. The funders had no role in study design, data collection and analysis, decision to publish, or preparation of the manuscript.

Competing Interests: The authors have declared that no competing interests exist.

* E-mail: pekmezovic@sezampro.rs

⑨ These authors equally contributed to this work.

Introduction

Bladder cancer is the second most common malignancy of the urinary tract and has the second highest mortality rate among urological neoplasms [1]. It affected 73,510 patients and lead to 14,880 deaths in 2012 worldwide [2]. Demographic characteristics associated with the greatest risk for bladder cancer include male gender, white race and the increasing age [3]. It is generally estimated that the male:female incidence ratio is 3.8:1.0 [3]. The most frequent pathohistological type of bladder cancer is urothelial carcinoma, also called transitional cell carcinoma (TCC), accounting for approximately 90% of all bladder cancers [3]. It has been known that uroepithelial cells are most vulnerable to metabolic end products of different compounds, including carcinogens. This malignancy is characterized by multifactorial etiology, involving both genetic and environmental factors.

The well established risk factors for bladder cancer include cigarette smoking (50% cases in men, 30% cases in women), but also exposure to occupational agents [3]. Occupational exposures account for 5 to 25% of all bladder cancer cases. [4]. Over 40 occupations have been associated with an elevated risk of bladder cancer in epidemiologic studies, but the evidence is compelling for only a few. Those established at risk industries include the manufacturing of products such as synthetic dyes and paints, cables, textiles, leather works, and aluminum and the petrochemical, coal tar, and rubber industries [5,6]. A number of specific occupations have also been identified to be associated with increased risk of bladder cancer. These include, but are not limited to, cooks and kitchen workers, electricians, hairdressers, leather workers, machinists, petroleum workers, rubber workers, coalminers, truckers, and vehicle mechanics, as summarized by Schulte et al. [7] in 1987, as well as coke oven workers, roofers, dry cleaners, chimney sweeps, and painters, as addressed by others in more recent literature [5,8–10].

Despite the fact that occupations associated with bladder cancer have been well established, the question still arises why individuals with seemingly equal exposure to occupational carcinogens develop bladder cancer in an unpredictable manner. This is probably attributed to genetic polymorphisms of the genes coding for the xenobiotic metabolizing enzymes, particularly glutathione S-transferase (GST). GSTs catalyze the conjugation of glutathione on electrophilic substrates and are an important line of defense in the protection of cellular components against reactive species. The most well characterized GST classes have been named alpha (GSTA), mu (GSTM), pi (GSTP) and theta (GSTT). Appreciable GST activities are seen in bladder epithelium [11]. GST enzymes that belong to various classes have different, but sometimes overlapping, substrate specificities. Several types of allelic variations have been identified within GST classes, with that in the GSTM1, GSTT1 and GSTP1 genes receiving the most attention in genetic epidemiological studies [12]. Individuals homozygous for the GSTM1*0 and GSTT1*0 alleles (frequently referred to as GSTM1-null and GSTT1-null genotypes), which comprise for 50% and 11–18% of white population, respectively [13,14], exhibit loss of GSTM1 and GSTT1 enzymatic activity. Single-nucleotide polymorphism (SNP) leading to amino acid substitution from isoleucine (Ile) to valine (Val) changes catalytic activity of the GSTP1 enzyme [15]. In healthy Caucasians, the frequencies of the genotype variants of GSTP Ile/Ile, -Ile/Val and -Val/Val are 51.5, 39.4, and 9.1%, respectively [15]. The role of GSTA1 polymorphism has emerged relatively recently in genetic epidemiological studies. It is represented by three, apparently linked, single nucleotide polymorphisms (SNPs): -567TOG, -69COT, -52GOA [16]. These substitutions result in differential expression with lower transcriptional activation of variant GSTA1*B (-567G, -69T, -52A) than common GSTA1*A allele (-567T, -69C,-52G) [16]. The relative frequencies of GSTA1-AA, AB and BB genotype in Caucasians are 38%, 48% and 14%, respectively [16].

Many of the well known occupational agents, such as polycyclic aromatic hydrocarbons, aromatic amines, halogenated hydrocarbons, associated with bladder cancer risk are substrates for GST. Although this reaction generally results in detoxification, in selected cases GST-mediated conjugation may lead to a more toxic or mutagenic metabolite. Still the data on association between GST gene variants and risk of occupational bladder cancer are scarce. We hypothesized that GST gene variants coding for enzymes involved in biotransformation of specific occupational agents may influence the risk of occupational bladder cancer.

Therefore, in this case-control study we investigated the role of the polymorphisms GSTA1, GSTM1, GSTP1 and GSTT1 gene and potential of effect modification by occupational exposure to different chemicals in Serbian male TCC patients.

Methods and Materials

Ethics Statement

This study was approved by the Ethical Committee of Faculty of Medicine, University of Belgrade and conducted according to the principles expressed in the Declaration of Helsinki. All the participants provided written informed consent.

Study subjects

A hospital-based case-control study of urinary bladder cancer in men was carried out between September 2007 and January 2010. A total of 143 histologically confirmed incident urinary bladder carcinoma male cases were recruited from the Clinics of Urology and Nephrology, Clinical centre of Serbia, Belgrade. This is the national reference center for urology and nephrology and the majority of bladder cancer patients from Serbia are diagnosed and treated at this clinic. The control group consisted of 114 male subjects which were recruited from individuals with nephrolithiasis admitted to the same hospital during the same period of time and had no history of any malignant disease. Urinary bladder carcinoma patients and corresponding controls did not differ with respect to mean age (Table 1).

After the informed consent was obtained, each subject was interviewed by well-trained interviewers using a standard questionnaire to collect information including demographic characteristics, history of cigarette smoking and occupational exposure. Response rate was 92% and the most frequent reason for no participation was personal.

In our study, smokers were defined as persons who reported every day smoking during a minimum of 60-day period prior to completing the questionnaire. Participants were asked about the number of cigarettes smoked per day and duration of smoking. The amount of pack-years was calculated using the following formula: pack-years = (cigarettes/day÷20)×(smoked years).

The life-time occupational history listed all jobs (including official jobs and jobs done outside normal working hours) lasting more than six months and consisted of the job title, the industry or type of business, employment dates and duration, company name and location, tasks as well as the exposure to at least one of the categories of agents under study, solvents and pesticides. In order to analyze occupational exposure occupational reports of patients were evaluated by experienced specialist in occupational medicine (author, P.B.). The exposure categories were defined as no exposure and exposure. Based on the evaluation patients were exposed to the following organic solvents: tetrachloroethylene, toluene, xylene, ethyl acetate, acetone, petrol ether and ethanol, as well as pesticides: organophosphate, carbamates, aminophosphonic analogues, chloroacetanilides, derivative of benzoic acid. All exposure data referred to a time period prior to the diagnosis of bladder cancer for the cases, and a corresponding period for the controls.

DNA extraction and genotyping

Genomic DNA was isolated from whole blood using the QIAGEN QIAmp (Qiagen, Inc., Chatsworth, CA, USA) 96-spin blood protocol according to the manufacturer's instructions. Blood was collected when patients were admitted to the clinic.

GSTM1 genotyping was performed by multiplex PCR method [17]. Primers used were GSTM1 forward: 5'-GAACTCCCT-

Table 1. Selected characteristics of male patients with bladder cancer and controls.

Characteristic	Cases n (%)	Controls n (%)	OR (95%CI)	P
Group				
Male	143	114		
Age (years)	63.6±10.7	61.1±9.9		N.S.
Smoking habits				
Never smokers	25 (18)	37 (34)	1.0 (reference group)	
Current smokers	112 (82)	72 (66)	2.3 (1.3–4.1)	0.005
No of pack-years of smoking	46.4±28.1	41.9±30.3	1.3 (0.7–2.5)	0.357
Occupational exposure				
No	77 (54)	80 (70)	1.0 (reference group)	
Yes	66 (46)	34 (30)	3.2 (1.6–6.6)[a]	0.001
Organic solvents	48 (34)	22 (19)	3.4 (1.5–7.3)[a]	0.002
Pesticides	15 (10)	9(8)	3.5 (0.9–12.9)[a]	0.058
Other chemicals	3 (2)	3 (3)	2.6 (0.4–17.7)[a]	0.323

N.S. not significant, *OR-* odds ratio, *CI*-confidence interval,
[a]*OR adjusted by age and pack-years.*

GAAAAGCTAAAGC-3′ and *GSTM1* reverse: 5′-GTTGGG-CTCAAATATACGGTGG-3′. Exon 7 of the *CYP1A1* gene was co-amplified and used as an internal control using the following primers: *CYP1A1* forward: 5′-GAACTGCCACTT CAGCTG-TCT-3; and *CYP1A1* reverse: 5′-CAGCTGCATTTG GAAGTG-CTC-3′. The presence of the *GSTM1-active* genotype was detected by the band at 215 bp, since the assay does not distinguish heterozygous or homozygous wild-type genotypes. Internal positive control (*CYP1A1*) PCR product corresponded to 312 bp.

GSTT1 genotyping was performed by multiplex PCR method [17]. Primers used were *GSTT1*-forward: 5′-TTCCTTACT-GGTCCTCACATCTC-3′ and *GSTT1*-reverse: 5′-TCACGG-GATCATGGCCAGCA-3′. Exon 7 of CYP1A1 genes were co-amplified and used as an internal control. The assay does not distinguish between heterozygous or homozygous wild-type genotypes; therefore, the presence of 480 bp bands was indicative for the *GSTT1-active* genotype. Internal positive control (*CYP1A1*) PCR product corresponded to 312 bp.

GSTP1 Ile105Val polymorphism was analyzed using the polymerase chain reaction–restriction fragment length polymorphism (PCR–RFLP) [18]. Primers used were: *GSTP1 Ile105Val* forward: 5′-ACCCCAGGGCTCTATGGGAA-3′ and *GSTP1 Ile105Val* reverse: 5′-TGAGGGCACAAGAAGCCCCT-3′. The amplification 176 bp products (20 µl) were digested by 10 U of restriction endonuclease Alw261at 37°C over night. The presence of restriction site resulting in two fragments (91 and 85 bp) indicated mutant allele (*Val/Val*), while if *Ile/Val* polymorphism incurred, it resulted in one more fragment of 176 bp.

GSTA1 C-69T polymorphism was determined by polymerase chain reaction–restriction fragment length polymorphism (PCR–RFLP) according to Coles et al [16]. The primers used were *GSTA1 C-69T* forward:5′-TGTTGATTGTTTGCCTGAAATT-3′ and *GSTA1 C-69T* reverse: 5′-GTTAAACGCTGT-CACCCGTCCT-3′. The amplification 481 bp products (20 µl) were digested by 10 U of restriction endonuclease Ear1 at 37°C over night. The presence of restriction site resulting in two fragments (385 and 96 bp) indicated mutant allele (*B/B*) and if *A/*

B polymorphism incurred, it resulted in one more fragment of 481 bp.

All genotyping was performed by laboratory personnel blinded to case-control status, and blinded quality control samples were inserted to validate genotyping identification procedures; concordance for blinded samples was 100%.

Statistical analysis

The distribution of the *GSTA1* and *GSTP1* polymorphisms for the case and control populations was tested for the Hardy–Weinberg equilibrium by χ^2 test. As a measure of effect size, odds ratio (OR) with corresponding 95% confidence interval (95%CI) was used to describe the strength of association between the genotypes and bladder cancer modified by occupational exposure. Unconditional logistic regression analysis is applied. Bearing in mind that age and smoking are well established risk factors for bladder cancer, we adjusted OR by these variables as potential confounders. Interactions between GST polymorphisms and occupational exposure were included in the logistic regression models and also adjusted by potential confounding variables. The probability level of ≤ 0.05 was considered statistically significant. For statistical analysis the SPSS 17.0 statistical software package (SPSS Inc, Chicago, IL, USA.) was used.

Results

Table 1 shows selected characteristics of male patients with bladder cancer and their controls. The smoking prevalence among cases was higher (82%) than the prevalence found in controls (66%) with the smokers being at 2.3-fold higher risk for TCC than non-smokers (95% CI = 1.3–4.1,p = 0.005). Furthermore, occupationally exposed men had 3.2 times higher risk for TCC than those unexposed (95% CI = 1.6–6.6, p = 0.001). We observed the significantly higher risk in those men occupationally exposed to organic solvents (OR = 3.4, 95% CI = 1.5–7.3, p = 0.002).

Genotyping was conducted for all recruited patients (Table 2). The *GSTA1* and *GSTP1* genotype frequencies were in Hardy-Weinberg equilibrium both for cases and controls (p>0.05). The observed genotype frequencies in controls were not significantly different from frequencies previously described among Caucasians. However, the frequency of *GSTT1-null* genotype in control group (28%) was higher than values reported among Caucasians (18.1%). As shown in Table 2, the frequencies of *GST null/low-activity* genotypes were higher in cases compared to controls with the exception of the *GSTT1-null* genotype. Although *GST A1, T1* and *P1* genotypes did not contribute independently toward the risk of TCC, the *GSTM1-null* genotype was overrepresented among cases (56%) compared to *M1-active* genotype with an adjusted OR of 2.1 reaching a statistical significance (95% CI = 1.1–4.2, p = 0.032).

Combined effects of *GSTA1, GSTM1, GSTP1* and *GSTT1* polymorphisms and occupational exposure on bladder cancer risk in male patients are shown in Table 3. When both cases and controls were dichotomized according to both genotype and occupational exposure, exposed subgroup was at TCC risk regardless of *GST* genotype. We found that occupationally exposed individuals with *GSTT1-active* genotype exhibited 4.3-fold increased risk compared to the unexposed *T1-active* subjects (95% CI = 1.7–10.6, p = 0.002). However, only for the *GSTP1* gene is there evidence of a gene–occupational exposure interaction (p = 0.017).

In order to test whether GST-occupational exposure interaction is modified by the specific type of exposure, cases and controls were further stratified into exposed to solvents and exposed to pesticides. Combined effect of occupational exposure to solvents and *GST* genotype on bladder cancer risk in male patients is shown on Table 4. The results of gene-occupational exposure to solvents interaction analyses indicated a significant effect between occupational exposure to solvents and all common *GST* polymorphisms tested. The most pronounced effect regarding occupational exposure to solvents and *GST* genotype on bladder cancer risk was observed for the *GSTA1* genotype, since men exposed to solvents with *GSTA1-low activity* genotype had 9 times higher risk of

bladder cancer than *GSTA1-active* unexposed men (95% CI = 2.4–34.7, p = 0.001). Similarly to that observed for *GSTA1-low activity*, the *GSTM1-null* genotype enhanced the risk of TCC among subjects exposed to solvents compared to the unexposed *GSTM1-active* individuals (OR = 6.5, 95% CI = 2.1–19.7, p = 0.001). These results point to the importance of antioxidant GSTA1 and GSTM1 activity protection against free radicals produced during solvent metabolism. The risk of TCC development was 5.3–fold elevated among *GSTT1-active* patients exposed to solvents in comparison with *GSTT1-active* unexposed patients (95% CI = 1.9–15.1, p = 0.002). Significant association was also found for *GSTP1 Ile/Ile* individuals who had 3.3 higher TCC risk compared to the unexposed *Ile/Ile* individuals (95% CI = 1.0–10.8, p = 0.047). However, only for GSTP1 statistically significant interaction between genotype and occupational exposure to solvents was found (p = 0.044)

Combined effect of occupational exposure to pesticides and *GST* genotype on bladder cancer risk in male patients is shown on Table 5. Men with *GSTT1-active* genotype exposed to pesticides exhibited 4.5 times higher risk in comparison with unexposed *GSTT1-active* subjects (95% CI = 0.9-22.5, p = 0.067).

Discussion

Our results showed that occupationally exposed men had 3 times higher risk for TCC. This result confirms the occupational exposure as a TCC risk factor [4]. Furthermore, the analysis of gene-occupational exposure interaction indicated a significant effect between occupationally exposed men and GSTP1 polymorphism. GSTP1 seems to play a role of particular importance in the detoxification of inhaled toxicants in occupationally exposed individuals since it is the most abundant GST isoform in the lung [19]. The mutated GSTP1 seems to be less effective in detoxification than the wild genotype [20]. Thus, Heuser et al. [18] showed that the mutated genotype (Ile/Val or Val/Val) was

Table 2. *GSTA1, GSTM1, GSTT1* and *GSTP1* genotypes in relation to bladder cancer risk in male patients.

GST genotype	Cases	Controls	OR (95%CI)	p
	n (%)	n (%)		
GSTA1				
AA	45 (31)	41 (36)	1.0 (reference group)	
AB	81 (57)	54 (47)	1.9 (0.9–4.2)	0.094
BB	17 (12)	19 (17)	1.1 (0.4–2.9)	0.875
AB+BB	98 (69)	73 (64)	1.7 (0.8–3.5)	0.171
GSTM1				
active[a]	63 (44)	58 (51)	1.0 (reference group)	
null[b]	80 (56)	56 (49)	2.1 (1.1–4.2)	0.032
GSTT1				
active[a]	101 (74)	82 (72)	1.0 (reference group)	
null[b]	36 (26)	32 (28)	1.0 (0.5–2.2)	0.999
GSTP1				
Ile/Ile	62 (43)	49 (43)	1.0 (reference group)	
Ile/Val	65 (46)	48 (42)	0.92 (0.5–1.9)	0.918
Val/Val	16 (11)	17 (15)	0.6 (0.2–1.9)	0.401
Ile/Val+Val/Val	81 (57)	65 (47)	0.9 (0.4–1.7)	0.876

[a]Active (present) if at least one active allele present.
[b]Inactive (null) if no active alleles present. *OR*- odds ratio adjusted for age and pack-years. *CI*- confidence interval.

Table 3. Combined effect of occupational exposure and *GST* genotype on bladder cancer risk in male male patients.

GST/exposure	Cases	Controls	OR (95%CI)	p
	n (%)	n (%)		
GSTA1				
AA/unexposed	21 (15%)	32 (28%)	1.0 (reference group)	
AB+BB/unexposed	56 (39%)	48 (42%)	2.4 (0.8–7.3)	0.121
AA/exposed	24 (17%)	9 (8%)	6.2 (1.4–27.1)	0.015
AB+BB/exposed	42 (29%)	25 (22%)	6.4 (2.0–20.2)	0.002
P interaction between genotype and occupational exposure =0.104				
GSTM1				
active[a]/unexposed	35 (24%)	44 (39%)	1.0 (reference group)	
null[b]/unexposed	42 (29%)	36 (32%)	3.3 (1.2–9.4)	0.023
active/exposed	28 (20%)	14 (12%)	5.4 (1.9–15.8)	0.002
null/exposed	38 (27%)	20 (17%)	6.0 (2.2–16.5)	0.001
P interaction between genotype and occupational exposure =0.601				
GSTT1				
active[a]/unexposed	54 (40%)	57 (50%)	1.0 (reference group)	
null[b]/unexposed	22 (16%)	23 (20%)	1.3 (0.5–3.9)	0.577
active/exposed	47 (34%)	25 (22%)	4.3 (1.7–10.6)	0.002
null/exposed	14 (10%)	9 (8%)	2.6 (0.8–8.9)	0.124
P interaction between genotype and occupational exposure =0.770				
GSTP1				
Ile/Ile/unexposed	31 (22%)	32 (28%)	1.0 (reference group)	
Ile/Val+Val/Val/unexposed	46 (32%)	48 (42%)	0.8 (0.3–2.1)	0.605
Ile/Ile/exposed	31 (22%)	17 (15%)	2.8 (1.0–7.9)	0.049
Ile/Val+Val/Val/exposed	35 (24%)	17 (15%)	2.8 (1.0–8.0)	0.049
P interaction between genotype and occupational exposure =0.017				

[a]Active (present) if at least one active allele present.
[b]Inactive (null) if no active alleles present. *OR*- odds ratio adjusted for age and pack-years. *CI*- confidence interval.

associated with greater DNA damage in Brazilian footwear workers than the wild (Ile/Ile) genotype [21]. These studies point to an interaction between the exposure and GSTP1 genotype. In our study, the most significant TCC risk was found for solvents. Epidemiologic evidence on the relationship between solvents and various cancers, such as gastrointestinal cancers, lung cancer and lymphohematopoietic malignancies, is well established [22]. Among compounds that have carcinogenic role halogenic aliphatic solvents have been mostly described. There are few reports about relationship between urinary bladder risk and solvents. Previous case-control studies reported significantly increased risks (between 3.1 and 8.8 times) among workers in the dyestuffs industry [23,24]. Several other investigators have reported elevated risks for spray painters [25,26], who have been reported to be exposed to many known or suspected carcinogens, including solvents. On the other hand, Lohi and others [27] found that among Finnish workers exposure to solvents was positively associated with the incidence of bladder cancer in women, but not in men.

It is important to note that risk imposed by occupational hazards was modified by GST polymorphism. We observed that individuals occupationally exposed to solvents with at least one *low activity GSTA1 allele* had the highest risk (about 9 times), while *GSTM1-null* carriers had 6.5 times higher bladder cancer risk when compared to unexposed *GSTA1 AA* and *GSTM1-active*

persons, respectively. This result was expected since in several malignant diseases, such as colorectal, prostate and hepatocellular cancer, *GSTA1*B allele* with lower transcriptional activity was associated with increased risk. GSTA1 protein belongs to the most promiscuous GSTs that acts upon a broad range of substrates which bind to its active site [28]. Our findings that *low-activity GSTA1* and *GSTM1-null* genotype increase susceptibility to bladder cancer in occupationally exposed men can be explained by the role of GST enzymes in detoxification and in antioxidant defense. Namely, GSTA1 and GSTM1 possess strong peroxidase activity and are key components in cellular defense against free radicals [29]. It may be speculated that free radicals are produced during solvent metabolism [30]. Regarding potential place of solvent detoxification, it is important to note that uroepithelial cells do not express GSTA1, while their GSTM1 protein level is also relatively low [31]. On the other hand, liver cells abundantly express GSTA1 and GSTM1 and thus participate in GSTA1 and GSTM1 mediated conjugation of different metabolites with glutathione, thereby enhancing their excretion in urine [32]. Taken together, these data suggest that liver, by its GSTs conjugating and peroxidase activity plays a key role in protection against bladder carcinogens present in halogenated solvents. On the other hand, *GSTT1-active* individuals occupationally exposed to solvents exhibited 5 times higher risk of TCC in comparison with *GSTT1-active* unexposed subjects. These results are biologically

Table 4. Combined effect of occupational exposure to solvents and *GST* genotype on bladder cancer risk in male patients.

GST/exposure	Cases	Controls	OR (95%CI)	p
	n (%)	n (%)		
GSTA1				
AA/unexposed	21 (1%)	32 (32%)	1.0 (reference group)	
AB+BB/unexposed	56 (46%)	48 (49%)	2.4 (0.8–7.3)	0.121
AA/solvents	14 (11%)	6 (6%)	5.9 (1.0–33.1)	0.046
AB+BB/solvents	31 (25%)	13 (13%)	9.2 (2.4–34.7)	0.001
P interaction between genotype and occupational exposure to solvents = 0.228				
GSTM1				
active[a]/unexposed	35 (28%)	44 (43%)	1.0 (reference group)	
null[b]/unexposed	42 (34%)	36 (35%)	3.3 (1.2–9.4)	0.023
active/solvents	21 (17%)	10 (10%)	4.7 (1.6–13.8)	0.006
null/solvents	27 (22%)	12 (12%)	6.5 (2.1–19.7)	0.001
P interaction between genotype and occupational exposure to solvents = 0.896				
GSTT1				
active[a]/unexposed	54 (46%)	57 (56%)	1.0 (reference group)	
null[b]/unexposed	22 (18%)	23 (22%)	1.3 (0.5–3.9)	0.577
active/solvents	34 (29%)	15 (15%)	5.3 (1.9–15.1)	0.002
null/solvents	8 (7%)	7 (7%)	1.7 (0.4–7.3)	0.470
P interaction between genotype and occupational exposure to solvents = 0.224				
GSTP1				
Ile/Ile/unexposed	31 (25%)	32 (31%)	1.0 (reference group)	
Ile/Val+Val/Val/unexposed	46 (37%)	48 (47%)	0.8 (0.3–2.1)	0.605
Ile/Ile/solvents	22 (18%)	9 (9%)	3.3 (1.0–10.8)	0.047
Ile/Val+Val/Val/solvents	26 (21%)	13 (13%)	2.6 (0.9–7.9)	0.089
P interaction between genotype and total occupational exposure to solvents = 0.044				

[a]Active (present) if at least one active allele present.
[b]Inactive (null) if no active alleles present. *OR*- odds ratio adjusted for age and pack years; *CI*- confidence interval.

plausible since GST-mediated conjugation with halogenated substrates may lead to a more toxic or mutagenic metabolites. Namely, substrates with ≥2 halogenes are activated because the conjugated product is instable, leading to reactions with nucleophiles, particularly DNA and proteins [33]. The human polymorphic GSTT1 catalyze conjugation of halomethanes, dihalomethanes, ethylene oxide and a number of other industrial compounds. Our results confirm the assumption of Avima M Ruder et al. [34] that humans with fully functional *GST* genes produce enzymes that metabolize some solvents to cytotoxic metabolites; while those with less functional or nonfunctioning genes have little or no enzyme and apparently do not produce cytotoxic metabolites from solvent exposure. Until now, the association between *GST* polymorphism and occupationally related cancers has been studied mostly in renal cell carcinoma. Results of these studies showed that *GSTT1-active* genotype enhanced the risk of renal cell carcinoma among subjects exposed to solvents. Our results on higher bladder carcinoma risk in *GSTT1-active* individuals occupationaly exposed to solvents are in accordance with previously published results in renal cell carcinoma [35,36]. Regarding the potential mechanism of solvent metabolism by GST, it is generally assumed that the main site is liver, followed by a mandatory transfer of conjugates to the kidney. However, the initial bioactivation step of halogenated solvents, can take place in the kidney itself [37]. Uroepithelium is also capable of

metabolizing some procarcinogens to inactive or genotoxic metabolites, and is, therefore, not exposed only to preformed reactive metabolites in the urine [38]. As the renal parenchyma and uroepithelium are exposed to the same broad range of potentially genotoxic compounds, the potential genotoxicity of carcinogens also depends on the biotransformation capacity of these tissues. As a result of GST polymorphism, great interindividual differences in GST isoenzyme profiles exist, in both renal parenchyma and uroepithelial cells [37].

Although it has been postulated that exposure to pesticides and/or fertilizers might be responsible for higher urinary bladder risk, the evidence is still conflicting. Some studies have shown that TCC risk was significantly elevated among men in the landscape and horticultural services industry, as well as in gardeners, and lawn care service employees [39,40], while others did not [41]. Some suggestions of a possible relation between GST status and early markers of genotoxic effects in humans exposed to pesticides are available. An increased frequency of micronuclei in cultured peripheral lymphocytes has been found among pesticide exposed greenhouse workers with the *GSTM1-active* genotype [42]. Significantly higher levels of sister hromatid exchanges were also found among *GSTT1-active* individuals exposed to pesticides when compared to *GSTT1-null* workers similarly exposed [43]. Until now only one study investigated association between *GST* polymorphism and occupational exposure to pesticide with respect

Table 5. Combined effect of occupational exposure to pesticides and *GST* genotype on bladder cancer risk in male patients.

GST/exposure	Cases	Controls	OR (95%CI)	p
	n (%)	n (%)		
GSTA1				
AA/unexposed	21 (22%)	32 (36%)	1.0 (reference group)	
AB+BB/unexposed	56 (60%)	48 (54%)	2.4 (0.8–7.3)	0.121
AA/pesticides	8 (9%)	3 (3%)	4.2 (0.5–36.0)	0.190
AB+BB/pesticides	8 (9%)	6 (7%)	2.0 (0.5–7.9)	0.239
P interaction between genotype and occupational exposure to pesticides = 0.957				
GSTM1				
active[a]/unexposed	35 (37%)	44 (49%)	1.0 (reference group)	
null[b]/unexposed	42 (45%)	36 (41%)	3.3 (1.2–9.4)	0.023
active/pesticides	7 (8%)	3 (3%)	2.9 (0.7–12.2)	0.138
null/pesticides	9 (10%)	6 (7%)	1.9 (0.5–6.7)	0.264
P interaction between genotype and occupational exposure to pesticides = 0.125				
GSTT1				
active[a]/unexposed	54 (59%)	57 (64%)	1.0 (reference group)	
null[b]/unexposed	22 (24%)	23 (25%)	1.3 (0.5–3.9)	0.577
active/pesticides	11 (12%)	7 (8%)	4.5 (0.9–22.5)	0.067
null/pesticides	5 (5%)	2 (3%)	2.6 (0.4–20.6)	0.264
P interaction between genotype and occupational exposure to pesticides = 0.508				
GSTP1				
Ile/Ile/unexposed	31 (33%)	32 (36%)	1.0 (reference group)	
Ile/Val+Val/Val/unexposed	46 (49%)	48 (53%)	0.8 (0.3–2.1)	0.605
Ile/Ile/pesticides	9 (10%)	6 (7%)	2.9 (0.6–13.6)	0.181
Ile/Val+Val/Val/pesticides	7 (8%)	3 (4%)	2.4 (0.5–10.1)	0.231
P interaction between genotype and occupational exposure to pesticides = 0.320				

[a]Active (present) if at least one active allele present.
[b]Inactive (null) if no active alleles present. *OR*- odds ratio adjusted for age and pack years. *CI*- confidence interval.

to risk of carcinoma of urinary tract. Namely, Karami and others reported that renal cell carcinoma risk associated with pesticide exposure was highest among individuals with *active GSTM1/T1* genotypes [44]. Although we did not observe significant effect between exposure to pesticides and GST polymorphisms we found borderline significance for *GSTT1-active* genotype. One of the reasons for non-significant association between *GSTT1-active* genotype may be the relatively small number of pesticide exposed participants in both case and control groups. Nevertheless, it is well known that pesticides produced from halogenated alkanes, alkenes undergo bioactivation in the liver and kidney after conjugation to glutathione by GSTT1 [41]. Therefore, an active GSTT1 enzyme will be required to conjugate substrates and form more reactive intermediates that directly damage tissues. Conversely, the deleted variant of *GSTT1-genotype* will form an inactive enzyme and therefore metabolism of halogenated compounds will occur through oxidation, without formation of reactive intermediates [44].

The principal limitations of this study are the relatively small sample size which limiting the precision of the odds ratios, hospital-based control group and qualitative evaluation of occupational exposure. Concerning the actual sample size (143 cases and 114 controls), the statistical power is 66%. Furthermore, it is well known that relatively small numbers of both study participants and *GST* polymorphisms studied might be sources of

potential biases which may influence the study findings. However, we tested effects of four *GST* polymorphisms and occupational exposure on bladder cancer risk and therefore significantly decreased chance for publication bias. Additionally, we cannot entirely rule out the possibility that some of our results could be caused by confounding, although we included only men and adjusted all results by age and smoking status. Further studies with larger samples and more rigorous designs are needed to investigate the gene effects and the potential effect modification by environmental factors.

Conclusions

GSTM1-null genotype increased the risk of bladder cancer in males. Null or low-activity genotypes of the *GSTA1*, *GSTT1*, and *GSTP1* did not contribute independently towards the risk of bladder cancer in males. However, in association with occupational exposure, both *low activity GSTA1* and *GSTM1-null* genotype increase individual susceptibility to bladder cancer suggesting the protective role of these detoxification and antioxidant enzymes in metabolism of occupational hazards, specifically organic solvents. On the other hand, the presence of *GSTT1-active* genotype in occupationally exposed subjects, resulting in GSTT1 protein expression and GSTT1 mediated bioactivation, increases the risk of bladder cancer.

Acknowledgments

The authors would like to thank technician Miss Sanja Zivotic for collecting data and support in manuscript preparation as well as Professor Goran Trajkovic, for final statistical consultancy.

Author Contributions

Conceived and designed the experiments: MGM VMC TPS TDP. Performed the experiments: MGM VMC TID. Analyzed the data: MGM VMC ARSR MSPE TID TPS TDP. Contributed reagents/materials/analysis tools: PVB DPD. Wrote the paper: MGM VMC ARSR MSPE TPS TDP.

References

1. Kim JJ (2012) Recent advances in treatment of advanced urothelial carcinoma. Curr Urol Rep 13:147–52.
2. Siegel R, Naishadham D, Jemal A (2012) Cancer statistics. CA Cancer J Clin 62:10–29.
3. American Cancer Society (2012) Bladder Cancer 2012. American Cancer Society, Atlanta, USA.
4. Olfert SM, Felknor SA, Delclos GL (2006) An updated review of the literature: risk factors for bladder cancer with focus on occupational exposures. South Med J 99:1256–63.
5. Clapp RW, Howe G, Lefevre MJ (2005) Environmental an Occupational Causes of Cancer, A Review of Recent Scientific Literature. Lowell Center for Sustainable Production. Lowe Mass, USA
6. International Agency for Research on Cancer (2010) Painting, fire- fighting, and shiftwork. IARC Monographs on the Evaluation of Carcinogenic Risks to Humans. pp. 43–394.
7. Schulte PA, Ringen K, Hemstreet GP, Ward E (1987) Occupational cancer of the urinary tract. Occup Med 2: 85–107.
8. International Agency for Research on Cancer (2010) Some aromatic amines, organic dyes, and related exposures. IARC Mono-graphs on the Evaluation of Carcinogenic Risks to Humans. pp. 1–692.
9. International Agency for Research on Cancer (2010) Some non-heterocyclic polycyclic aromatic hydrocarbons and some related compounds. IARC Monographs on the Evaluation of Carcinogenic Risks to Humans. pp. 754–759.
10. Pukkala E, Martinsen JI, Lynge E, Gunnarsdottir HK, Sparén P, et al. (2009) Occupation and cancer follow-up of 15 million people in five Nordic countries. Acta Oncologica 48: 646–790.
11. Simic T, Mimic-Oka J, Savic-Radojevic A, Opacic M, Pljesa M, et al. (2005) Glutathione S-transferase T1-1 activity upregulated in transitional cell carcinoma of urinary bladder. Urology 65: 1035–40.
12. Di Pietro G, Magno LA, Rios-Santos F (2010) Glutathione S-transferases: an overview in cancer research. Expert Opin Drug Metab Toxicol 6: 153–70.
13. Eaton DL, Bammler TK (1999) Concise review of the glutathione S-transferases and their significance to toxicology. Toxicol Sci 49: 156–64.
14. Landi S (2000) Mammalian class θ GST and differential susceptibility to carcinogens: a review. Mutat Res 463: 247–83.
15. Watson MA, Stewart RK, Smith GB Massey TE, Bell DA (1998) Human glutathione S-transferase P1 polymorphisms: relationship to lung tissue enzyme activity and population frequency distribution. Carcinogenesis 19: 275–80.
16. Coles FB, Kadlubar FF (2005) Human alpha class glutathione S-transferases: genetic polymorphism, expression, and susceptibility to disease. In: Helmut S, Lester P, editors. Glutathione Transferases and Gamma-Glutamyl Transpeptidases, Methods Enzymology. London: Elsevier Academic Press. pp 9–42.
17. Abdel-Rahman SZ, El-Zein RA, Anwar WA, Au WW (1996) A multiplex PCR procedure for polymorphic analysis of GSTM1 and GSTT1 genes in population studies. Cancer Lett 107: 229–33.
18. Harries LW, Stubbins MJ, Forman D, Howard GC, Wolf CR (1997) Identification of genetic polymorphisms at the glutathione S-transferase Pi locus and association with susceptibility to bladder, testicular and prostate cancer. Carcinogenesis 18: 641–44.
19. Hirvonen A (2005) Gene–environment interaction and biological monitoring of occupational exposures. Toxicol Appl Pharmacol 207: 329–335.
20. Miller DP, Asomaning K, Liu G, Wain JC, Lynch TJ, et al. (2006) An association between glutathione S-transferase P1 gene polymorphism and younger age at onset of lung carcinoma. Cancer 107: 1570–7.
21. Heuser VD, Erdtmann B, Kvitko K, Rohr P, da Silva J (2007) Evaluation of genetic damage in Brazilian footwear-workers: Biomarkers of exposure, effect, and susceptibility. Toxicology 232: 235–47.
22. Lynge E, Anttila A, Hemminki A (1997) Organic solvents and cancer. Cancer Causes Control 8: 406–19.
23. Risch HA, Burch JD, Miller AB, Hill GB, Steele R, et al. (1988) Occupational factors and the incidence of cancer of the bladder in Canada. Br Industr Med 45: 361–367.
24. Bonassi S, Merlo F, Pearce N, Puntoni R (1989) Bladder cancer an occupational exposure to polycyc aromatic hydrocarbons. Int Cancer 44: 648–651.
25. La Vecchia C, Negri E, D'Avanzo B, Franceschi S (1990) Occupation and the risk of bladder cancer. Int J Epidemiol 19: 264–8.
26. Cordier S, Clavel J, Limasset JC, Boccon-Gibod L, Le Moual N, et al. (1993) Occupational risks of bladder cancer in France: A multicentre case-control study. Int J Epidemiol 22: 402–11.
27. Lohi J, Kyyrönen P, Kauppinen T, Kujala V, Pukkala E (2008) Occupational exposure to solvents and gasoline and risk of cancers in the urinary tract among Finnish workers. Am J Ind Med 51: 668–72.
28. Honaker MT, Acchione M, Zhang W, Mannervik B, Atkins WM (2013) Enzymatic detoxication, conformational selection, and the role of molten globule active sites. J Biol Chem 288: 18599–611.
29. Hayes JD, Strange RC (2000) Glutathione S-transferase polymorphisms and their biological consequences. Pharmacology 61: 154–66.
30. Weber LW, Boll M, Stampfl A (2003) Hepatotoxicity and mechanism of action of haloalkanes: carbon tetrachloride as a toxicological model. Crit Rev Toxicol 33: 105–36.
31. Savic-Radojevic A, Mimic-Oka J, Pljesa-Ercegovac M, Opacic M, Dragicevic D, et al. (2007) Glutathione S-transferase-P1 expression correlates with increased antioxidant capacity in transitional cell carcinoma of the urinary bladder. Eur Urol 52: 470–7.
32. Rossi AM, Guarnieri C, Rovesti S, Gobba F, Ghittori S, et al. (1999) Genetic polymorphisms influence variability in benzene metabolism in humans. Pharmacogenetics 9: 445–51.
33. Guengerich P (2005) Activation of alkyl halides by glutathione transferases. In: Helmut S, Lester P, editors. Glutathione Transferases and Gamma-Glutamyl Transpeptidases, Methods Enzymology. London: Elsevier Academic Press.pp 9–42.
34. Ruder AM, Yiin JH, Waters MA, Carreón T, Hein MJ, et al. (2013) The Upper Midwest Health Study: gliomas and occupational exposure to chlorinated solvents. Occup Environ Med 70: 73–80.
35. Buzio L, De Palma G, Mozzoni P, Tondel M, Buzio C, et al. (2003) Glutathione S-transferases M1-1 and T1-1 as risk modifiers for renal cell cancer associated with occupational exposure to chemicals. Occup Environ Med 60: 789–93.
36. Moore LE, Boffetta P, Karami S, Brennan P, Stewart PS, et al. (2010) Occupational trichloroethylene exposure and renal carcinoma risk: evidence of genetic susceptibility by reductive metabolism gene variants. Cancer Res 70: 6527–36.
37. Simic T, Savic-Radojevic A, Pljesa-Ercegovac M, Matic M, Mimic-Oka J (2009) Glutathione S-transferases in kidney and urinary bladder tumors. Nat Rev Urol 6: 281–9.
38. Thier R, Golka K, Brüning T, Ko Y, Bolt HM (2002) Genetic susceptibility to environmental toxicants: the interface between human and experimental studies in the development of new toxicological concepts. Toxicol Lett 127: 321–7.
39. Band PR, Le ND, MacArthur AC, Fang R, Gallagher RP (2005) Identification of occupational cancer risks in British Columbia: a population-based case-control study of 1129 cases of bladder cancer. J Occup Environ Med 47: 854–8.
40. Zahm SH (1997) Mortality study of pesticide applicators and other employees of a lawn care service company. J Occup Environ Med 39: 1055–67.
41. Viel F-F, Challier B (1995) Bladder cancer among French farmers: does exposure to pesticides in vineyards play a part? Occup Environ Med 52: 587–92.
42. Falck GC, Hirvonen A, Scarpato R, Saarikoski ST, Migliore L, et al. (1999) Micronuclei in blood lymphocytes and genetic polymorphism for GSTM1, GSTT1 and NAT2 in pesticide-exposed greenhouse workers. Mutat Res 441: 225–37.
43. Scarpato R, Migliore L, Hirvonen A, Falck G, Norppa H (1996) Cytogenetic monitoring of occupational exposure to pesticides: characterization of GSTM1, GSTT1, and NAT2 genotypes. Environ Mol Mutagen 27: 263–9.
44. Karami S, Boffetta P, Rothman N, Hung RJ, Stewart T, et al. (2008) Renal cell carcinoma, occupational pesticide exposure and modification by glutathione S transferase polymorphisms. Carcinogenesis 29: 1567–71.

12

Reproducibility and Prognostic Value of WHO1973 and WHO2004 Grading Systems in TaT1 Urothelial Carcinoma of the Urinary Bladder

Ok Målfrid Mangrud[1,2], Rune Waalen[3], Einar Gudlaugsson[1,2], Ingvild Dalen[4], Ilker Tasdemir[5], Emiel A. M. Janssen[1], Jan P. A. Baak[1,2]*

1 Department of Pathology, Stavanger University Hospital, Stavanger, Norway, 2 Clinical Institute-1, University of Bergen, Bergen, Norway, 3 Department of Pathology, Innlandet Hospital Trust, Lillehammer, Norway, 4 Department of Research, Stavanger University Hospital, Stavanger, Norway, 5 Department of Urology, Stavanger University Hospital, Stavanger, Norway

Abstract

Background: European treatment guidelines of TaT1 urinary bladder urothelial carcinomas depend highly on stage and WHO1973-grade but grading reproducibility is wanting. The newer WHO2004 grading system is still debated and both systems are currently used.

Aims: To compare reproducibility and prognostic value (of stage progression) of the WHO1973 and WHO2004.

Methods: One hundred and ninety-three primary urothelial carcinomas were reviewed. Follow-up data were retrieved from the patient records. Kappa statistics and Harrell's C-index were used.

Results: Median follow-up was 75 months (range 1–127). 17 patients (9%) progressed, 82% of these within and 18% after 60 months. The distribution of WHO73-grades 1, 2 and 3 was 23%, 51% and 26%, interobserver agreement for each individual grade was 66% (kappa = 0.68), while for grades 1&2 versus 3 89% (kappa = 0.68). Intraobserver reproducibility was 68–63% for WHO73 and 88–89% for WHO73 as 1&2 vs.3. Progression free survival rates at 5 years were 95% (grade 1), 98% (grade 2) and 82% (grade 3) and 96% and 82% for grades 1&2 versus 3 (Hazard Ratio, HR, 5.4, p = 0.003). Using WHO2004, 62% were low grade and 38% high grade, inter-observer agreement 87% (kappa = 0.70), intraobserver reproducibility 93%, and progression free 5-year survival rates 97% and 85% (HR 6.6, p = 0.004). Positive and negative predictive values for stage progression within 5 years for the WHO73 (1&2 vs. 3) were 18% and 96%, and 15% and 97% for the WHO04. Using Harrell's C-index, none of the grading systems was prognostically superior.

Conclusion: None of the grading systems is prognostically stronger than the others. Most importantly, inter-observer reproducibility and sensitivies for stage progression of both systems are low and need improvement for optimal treatment.

Editor: Konradin Metze, University of Campinas, Brazil

Funding: The authors have no support or funding to report.

Competing Interests: The authors have declared that no competing interests exist.

* E-mail: jpabaak47@yahoo.com

Introduction

Superficial (TaT1) urothelial carcinoma (UC) is the most common urinary bladder cancer in the Western world. Approximately 70% recur and 8–30% progress to a higher T-stage [1,2]. Prognosis in TaT1 UCs depends largely on lamina propria invasion, and grade. European treatment guidelines [3] are based on the 1973 World Health Organization (WHO73) grading system. The WHO73 discerns three grades (1, 2, and 3) based on the degree of anaplasia [4] (Figure 1) but intra- and inter-observer reproducibility is wanting and efforts have been made to develop a more reliable grading system. Following a WHO/International Society of Urological Pathology (ISUP) consensus conference, a new grading system was introduced in 1998 [5] and adopted in the

WHO 2004 blue book (WHO04) [6]. The WHO04 divides the neoplasms into benign papillomas, papillary urothelial neoplasm of low malignant potential (PUNLMP), and low and high grade carcinomas. The WHO04 was thought to be more reproducible than the WHO73, but several studies have shown considerable inter-observer variability [7,8]. There have also been discussions on the incidence of PUNLMP with rates ranging from 12–39%, and stage progression rates between 2 and 8% [9–11], very similar to the low grade carcinomas.

Therefore, the aims of the current study were to compare the inter-observer reproducibility and prognostic value (on stage progression) of the WHO73 and WHO04 in patients with TaT1 urothelial urinary bladder cancer and the clinical significance of distinguishing PUNLMP and low grade cancers.

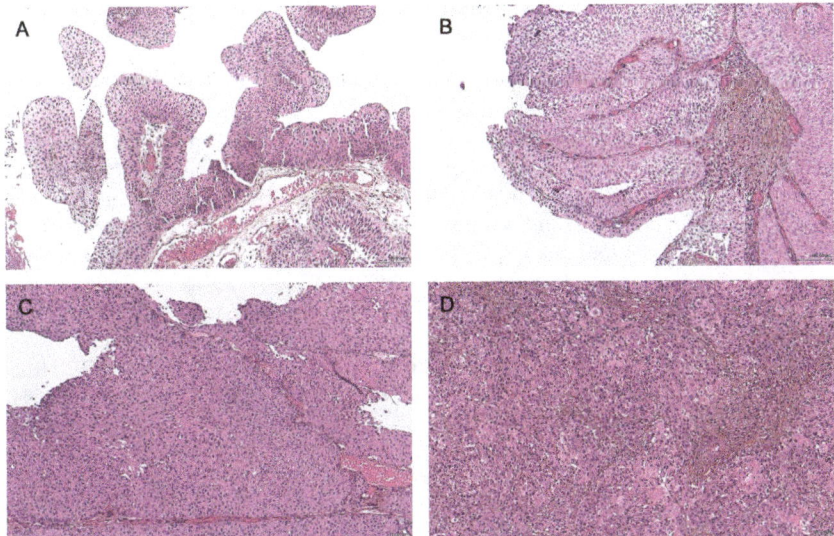

Figure 1. Grading of urothelial carcinomas. A. WHO73 Grade 1/WHO04 Low grade. **B.** WHO73 Grade 2/WHO04 Low grade. **C.** WHO73 Grade 2/WHO04 High grade. **D.** WHO73 Grade 3/WHO04 High grade.

Methods

Ethics statement

The study was approved by the Norwegian Regional Ethics Committee (REK Vest, #106/09) before the start of the study. With approval from REK Vest, informed consent was not obtained as the tissue samples had already been removed for diagnostic and treatment purposes.

Patients

Two hundred and forty nine consecutive cases of primary (first diagnosis) non-muscle invasive urothelial carcinoma of the urinary bladder were diagnosed at the Departments of Urology and Pathology, Stavanger University Hospital (SUH) January 1, 2002 through December 31, 2006.

Tumour tissue was obtained by transurethral resection or biopsy at the Department of Urology, SUH. All samples were originally routinely diagnosed as primary urothelial carcinoma WHO73 grade 1–3, pTaT1, by seven different pathologists. The tumour tissue was fixed in 4% buffered formaldehyde, dehydrated and embedded in paraffin. Four μm thick sections stained with haematoxylin-erythrosine-saffron were used for routine diagnostics. In total fifty-six cases were excluded from this study; the majority of these due to inadequate sample quality (Table 1).

The patients were uniformly treated according to the national guidelines at the time of diagnosis. All patients underwent transurethral resection (TUR) followed by a single instillation of a cytotoxic agent (normally 40 mg Mitomycin C). High risk patients were treated with BCG-instillations (alternatively chemotherapy) over 1 to 3 years. High risk patients included Ta grade 3 tumours, T1 grade 2 or 3 tumours, primary carcinoma in situ (CIS) without evidence of urothelial carcinoma, or concurrent CIS in several localisations. Patients who had 3 or more separate tumours diagnosed within 18 months of follow-up or recurrences at multiple sites at first or second follow-up following TUR also received instillation treatment.

Grading of urothelial carcinomas

All specimens were independently reviewed according to the WHO73 classification (grades 1 through 3) and WHO04 (low grade or high grade) by experienced pathologists (EG, RW, OM). Two of the pathologists (EG and OM) repeated the classification at a later stage. The pathologists did their evaluations in separate sessions, independently and without prior knowledge of the original stage, grade, each other's assessments, their own assessments, treatment or follow-up of the patients. In case of discrepancies, consensus was reached after discussion using a multihead microscope.

The WHO04 low grade tumours were also reviewed with regards to discerning low grade and PUNLMP tumours.

Patient follow-up

Follow-up data were retrieved from medical records and from any available new specimens at the Department of Pathology, SUH.

The follow up protocol depended on the grade and stage of the primary tumour. Provided that follow up cystoscopies were

Table 1. Exclusion criteria, number of excluded and included patients.

Primary pTaT1 urothelial carcinomas at SUH 2002–2006	249
Insufficient material	21
Thermal damage	11
Fragmented specimen	1
Necrotic specimen	2
Sarcomatoid differentiation	1
Previous urothelial carcinoma (on review of clinical notes)	1
cT3 or cT4 (on review of clinical notes)	3
pT2 at re-TURV	2
pT2 at review	1
Clinical metastasis at time of diagnosis	2
Lost to follow-up	11
Included in study	**193**

negative, patients with Ta grade 1 tumours would undergo cystoscopy 3 months after initial diagnosis followed by cystoscopy after 9 months and consequently annually for 5 years. All other patients would have cystoscopies every 3 months for the first 2 years, every 4 months the 3rd year, every 6 month the 4th and 5th years followed by annual cystoscopies thereafter.

Recurrence was defined as the reappearance of histopathologically confirmed urothelial carcinoma in the bladder. Progression was defined as an advance in stage, histologically proven metastasis or death of disease.

Statistical analysis

The inter- and intra-observer reproducibility was measured by unweighted or quadratically weighted kappa statistics as appropriate. Unweighted kappa statistics were used for dichotomized variables (WHO04 and WHO73 (1&2 vs. 3)). Weighted kappa statistics were applied for WHO73 as this classification system has 3 categories. Quadratic weight, rather than linear weight, was used as the difference between the second and third category (grade 2 and 3) has greater clinical implications than the difference between the first and second category (grades 1 and 2). To evaluate the consistency of the grading systems, mean grade was calculated [12].

For comparison between different groups of patients, log rank test, Kaplan-Meier survival curves and the Mann Whitney U test were used. Median ages for patients with different WHO73 or WHO04 grade tumours were compared by Mann Whitney U tests. Log rank tests were used to compare survival times between the groups of patients. The reported p-values are two-sided, i.e. the null hypothesis is that there is no difference between the groups and the alternate hypothesis that there is a difference. As a measure of predictive discrimination of those who did vs. those who did not experience progression within 5 years, we present sensitivities, specificities, and positive and negative predictive values (PPV and NPV). Continuity corrected confidence intervals were estimated. Positive predictive value was defined as patients with stage progression and high grade or grade 3 tumours (true positives) divided by the total number of true positives and patients with high grade (or grade 3 tumours) who did not experience progression (false positives). Conversely, negative predictive value was defined as patients without stage progression (true negatives) divided by the total number of true negatives and patients with low grade (or grade 1 and 2 tumours) who did experience progression (false negatives). Sensitivity was defined as true positives divided by the total number of patients with progression, and specificity was defined as true negatives divided by the total number of patients without progression.

The time of progression was considered in survival analyses, using Kaplan-Meier plots and univariable Cox proportional hazards models. The proportional hazards assumption was tested by inspection of stratified log minus log survival plots and by introducing time-dependent covariates into the models. The predictive ability with regard to time of progression was measured by Somers' D rank correlation R function rcorr.cens of the package Hmisc, which was transformed into Harrell's (concordance) C-index by the formula $C = 0.5 * (|D| + 1)$ [13]. Confidence intervals for the C-indices were bootstrapped percentile intervals, using simple nonparametric bootstrapping with 2000 samples. Finally, in order to correct for the "optimism" in a concordance measure evaluated on the same data that was used to fit the survival model, adjusted ("bootstrapped") C-indices were estimated (R function validate.cph of the package rms, with B = 150).

Statistical analyses were performed using IBM SPSS for Windows version 21.0 (IBM Corp, Armonk, NY, USA), Vassar-Stats (http://vassarstats.net) and R Project for Statistical Computing (http://www.R-project.org)

Results

The median age at diagnosis was 74 years (range 39 to 95). One hundred and forty-eight patients were male (76.7%) and 45 (23.3%) female (ratio = 3.3). Median age depended on WHO73-grade and was 65.5 years for grade 1, 74.0 years for grade 2 and 75.0 years for grade 3 tumours (Mann Whitney U tests gave p = 0.005 for grade 1 versus 2, p = 0.22 for 2 versus 3). For WHO04, the median age was 71.0 years for low grade and 75.5 years for high grade tumours (p = 0.006).

Median follow-up time was 75 months (range 1–127). Histologically proven recurrences occurred in 111 patients (57.5%). Stage progression at recurrence occurred in 17 patients (15.3% of the patients with recurrence or 8.8% of all patients), 14 of these within 36 months and 3 more than 5 years (at 61, 62 and 101 months) after the original diagnosis. We used recurrence and progression within 5 years after the initial diagnosis as the endpoint because of the obvious dichotomous progression pattern (<3years versus >5 years), and also as it seemed unlikely to us that biomarkers can predict progression after such a long interval.

The excluded patients had a median age of 75 years (range 49–90). 71% were male, 29% female. Median follow-up time was 35 months (0–137 months). There were no differences in sex, age, stage, initial diagnosis (grade), or occurrence of carcinoma in situ between the excluded and the included patients. Of the excluded patients, 36 had true non-muscle-invasive urothelial carcinomas with adequate follow-up. Of these, 28% recurred and 14% progressed to a higher T-stage.

Reproducibility

The distribution of consensus WHO73-grades 1, 2 and 3 was 44 (23%), 98 (51%) and 51 (26%). One hundred and nineteen tumours (62%) were low grade and 74 (38%) were high grade according to the WHO04. For the final consensus WHO73 grades, there was pre-discussion consensus between the reviewing pathologists on the grade of 39 of the grade 1 tumours (88.6%), 55 of the grade 2 tumours (56.1%), and on 34 of the grade 3 tumours (65.4%). Regarding the final consensus WHO04 grades, there was pre-discussion agreement on 119 of the low grade (100%) and 49 of the high grade tumours (66%). On consensus diagnosis, all WHO73 grade 1 tumours were classified as low grade. Twenty-four (24.5%) of the grade 2 and 50 (98.0%) of the grade 3 tumours were re-classified as high grade tumours, and one grade 3 downgraded to a low-grade tumour.

Tables 2 and 3 summarize inter- and intraobserver overall agreement and kappa-values with 95% confidence intervals (95% CI). The interobserver reproducibility of the WHO73, both as three-tiered and grades 1&2 versus 3, and the WHO04 were very similar with overlapping confidence intervals. For pathologist 1, intraobserver reproducibility for the WHO73 (both two-tiered and three-tiered) is very similar to the interobserver reproducibility. For pathologist 2 there is more variation as the WHO73 (three tiered) seems less reproducible and the WHO04 more reproducible for this observer than the interobserver reproducibility, however wide and overlapping confidence intervals makes a clear-cut conclusion difficult.

In our study, only one pathologist assessed both grading systems (OM). The mean grade difference for this pathologist is 0.3 grade points in both grading systems (table 4). For the other pathologist who did to reviews of a grading system (EG, WHO73), the mean grade difference was 0.4. Due to the very low number of

Table 2. Interobserver reproducibility.

	Overall agreement (95% CI)	Kappa (95% CI)
WHO73	66% (59–73%)	0.68 (0.57–0.78)*
WHO73 (1&2 vs. 3)	89% (83–93%)	0.68 (0.56–0.80)
WHO04	87% (81–91%)	0.70 (0.59–0.81)

*: Quadratic weighted kappa.
CI: Confidence interval.

Table 4. The difference in mean grade between the reviewers.

	EG 1	EG 2	RW 1	OM 1	OM 2
WHO73	1.83	1.79	NP	2.00	1.97
WHO04	NP	NP	2.33	2.31	2.31

EG: Pathologist 1, 1st review. EG2: Pathologist 1, 2nd review. RW 1: Pathologist 2 (only one review). OM: Pathologist 3, 1st review. OM2: pathologist 3, 2nd review. NP: Not performed.

PUNLMPS, direct comparison of the mean grade of the two systems is not feasible.

Prognostic comparison

The patients' age was a statistically significant factor for progression, (p = 0.004), with median time to progression 8 months for patients ≤73 years and 24 months for patients >73 years,), but not for recurrence (p = 0.14). Gender was not prognostically significant (recurrence: p = 0.88; stage progression: p = 0.96).

The recurrence rates of the three WHO73 grades were 57%, 46% and 61% after 5 years. There were no significant differences in recurrence rates of the WHO73, the WHO73 as grades 1&2 versus 3 or the WHO04 high and low grades (51% and 54%, p = 0.25), table 5. The progression-free survival rates for grades 1, 2 and 3 were 95%, 97% and 82% at five years after the index specimen. The progression rate of grade 3 cases differed (p = 0.001) from grades 1 or 2, but the progression rates between grades 1 and 2 did not (p = 0.70).

Stage progression of the WHO04 low and high grades differed greatly (3% versus 15%, p = 0.003). Sensitivity, specificity, hazard ratio (HR), p-values and Harrell's C-index for stage progression-or-not of WHO73 and WHO04 are summarized in Tables 6–7. With very similar Harrell's C-indices, none of the grading systems is prognostically stronger than the others with regard to time to stage progression. The PPV and NPV for the two classification systems are similar with overlapping confidence intervals upholding that none of the grading systems is stronger than the other for predicting stage progression, The specificity of the WHO73 (1&2 vs. 3) is somewhat better than the WHO04. The sensitivity of the WHO04 seems better than for the WHO73 (1&2 vs. 3), but 95% confidence intervals are wide and overlapping making the conclusion ambiguous.

There were 154 pTa (80%) and 39 pT1 (20%) tumours, with 79 (51%) and 22 (56%) recurrences (p = 0.22) and 6 and 8 progression cases respectively (4% and 20%, p<0.001, HR = 7.0, 95% CI = 2.4–20.3). When analysing progression in the two stages

Table 5. Recurrence free survival at 5 years.

	Threshold	Recurrence/patients n (%)
WHO73	Grade 1	25/44 (57)
	Grade 2	45/98 (46)
	Grade 3	31/51 (61)
WHO73 (1&2 vs. 3)	Grades 1&2	70/142 (49)
	Grade 3	31/51 (61)
WHO04	Low grade	61/119 (51)
	High grade	40/74 (54)

CI: Confidence interval.

separately, for pTa tumours there were significant differences between the grades of both the WHO73 (grades 1&2 versus 3) and the WHO04, but more so in the WHO73 (p<0.001 versus p = 0.015, Figure 2). There were no significant differences between the progression rates of the different grades in pT1 tumours.

The progression free survival rates (PFSR) of WHO73 grades 1&2 (n = 142) and WHO04 low grade (n = 117) overlapped (PSFR = 97% and 96% respectively), although the number of grades 1&2 was much higher than the WHO04 low grades. As expected, the WHO73 grades 3 had a worse PFSR (82%) than the WHO04 high grades (85%).

Papillary urothelial neoplasms of low malignant potential

Three cases were classified by the reviewing pathologists as PUNLMP, two by the first and another case by the other. When the cases were evaluated independently by two other pathologists, one of these three cases was classified as low grade, leaving 2 cases as undeniable PUNLMP. The recurrence rate was 50% and none showed stage progression. Comparison with the original WHO grades showed that the 2 PUNLMPs had been classified by all

Table 3. Intraobserver reproducibility.

	Pathologist 1		Pathologist 2	
	Overall agreement (95% CI)	Estimated kappa (95% CI)	Overall agreement (95% CI)	Estimated kappa (95% CI)
WHO73	68% (61–74%)	0.69 (0.59–0.79)*	63% (56–70%)	0.61 (0.48–0.74)*
WHO73 (1&2 vs. 3)	88% (82–92%)	0.66 (0.54–0.79)	89% (83–93%)	0.68 (0.55–0.80)
WHO04	Not performed	Not performed	93% (88–96%)	0.83 (0.74–0.92)

*: Quadratic weighted kappa.
CI: Confidence interval.

Table 6. Progression free survival at 5 years.

	Threshold	Progression/patients, n (%)	HR (95% CI)	Wald p	Harrell's C-index (95% CI)	Harrell's C-index Boot-strapped
WHO73	Grade 1	2/44 (5)	0.71 (0.12–4.23)	0.010	0.70 (0.53–0.84)	0.68
	Grade 2	3/98 (3)	4.34 (0.94–20.1)			
	Grade 3	9/51 (18)				
WHO73 (1&2 vs. 3)	Grades 1&2	5/142 (4)	5.42 (1.82–16.2)	0.003	0.70 (0.56–0.83)	0.69
	Grade 3	9/51 (18)				
WHO04	Low grade	3/119 (3)	6.59 (1.84–23.6)	0.004	0.72 (0.60–0.82)	0.71
	High grade	11/74 (15)				

CI: Confidence interval. HR: Hazard ratio.

Table 7. Sensitivities, specificities, positive and negative predictive values of 5 years progression of the WHO73 (1&2 vs. 3) and WHO04.

	Sensitivity (95% CI)	Specificity (95% CI)	PPV (95% CI)	NPV (95% CI)
WHO73 (1&2 vs. 3)	64% (36–86%)	77% (70–82%)	18% (9–31%)	96% (92–99%)
WHO04	79% (49–94%)	65% (57–72%)	15% (8–25%)	97% (92–99%)

CI: Confidence interval. PPV: positive predictive value. NPV: Negative predictive value.

pathologists as WHO73 grade 1 or WHO04 low grade at review. The 44 grade 1 cases recurred in 57% and 4% showed stage progression, which was not statistically different from the 2 PUNLMPs (p = 0.64 and p = 0.75). Of the low grade tumours, 58% recurred and 3% showed stage progression. Recurrence and stage progression in the PUNLMPs and the low grade tumours by univariate survival analysis were not different (p = 0.81 and 0.79).

Discussion

The clinical course of urinary bladder cancer is strongly heterogeneous. Tumour stage is the most important classical clinicopathological parameter for the prognosis of urothelial carcinoma of the urinary bladder, but the extent of invasion is hard to determine on (superficial) biopsies alone. Additional prognostic value is obtained by the histology of the tumour. Well differentiated urothelial carcinoma usually grows superficially, while poorly differentiated urothelial carcinoma more often has an infiltrating growth pattern at the time of presentation. In 2006, the European Organization for Research and Treatment of Cancer (EORTC) developed a scoring system for risk of recurrence and progression [14]. The system is based on the following factors: tumour size, number of tumours, prior recurrence rate, histological grade and stage, and the presence of concomitant carcinoma

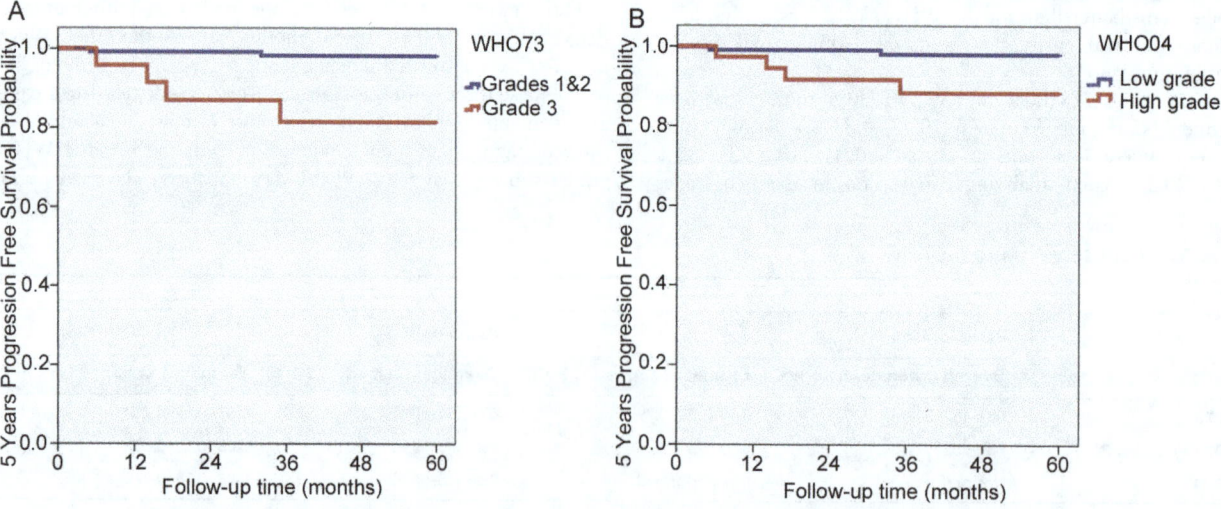

Figure 2. Five years progression free survival, pTa. A. WHO73 Grades 1&2 versus 3. **B.** WHO04 Low grade versus high grade.

Table 8. Comparison of the studies by Pan et al (2010), Chen et al (2012) and Mangrud et al (2013).

	Pan	Chen	Mangrud
Period	1991–2005	1999–2009	2002–2006
Time	15 years	10 years	5 years
Patients	2191	392	249
Included	1515	348	193
Men	1307 (86%)	287 (82.5%)	148 (76.7%)
Women (%)	208 (14%)	61 (17.5%)	45 (23.3%)
Mean age	71 (23–92)	N/A	71 (39–95)
Median age	N/A	68 (21–92)	74 (39–95)
Reviewers	1	1	3
Grading system	WHO04	WHO73/WHO04	WHO73/WHO04
Patients with complete follow-up	874	?	193
Median follow-up, months	74 (1–215)	47 (2–124)	75 (1–127)
IVI Treatment*	592 (39%)	?	35 (18%)
PUNLMP	212 (14.0%)	40 (11.5%)	2 (1.0%)
Low grade	706 (46.6%)	223 (64.1%)	117 (61%)
High grade	597 (39.4%)	85 (24.4%)	74 (38%)
Grade 1	N/A	125 (35.9%)	44 (23%)
Grade 2	N/A	176 (50.6%)	98 (51%)
Grade 3	N/A	47 (13.5%)	51 (26%)
pTa	1006 (66.4%)	220 (63.2%)	154 (80%)
pT1	509 (33.6%)	128 (46.8%)	39 (20%)
Recurrence, total	484 (31.9%)	122 (35.1%)	111 (57.5%)
Recurrence, PUNLMP	17.9%	25.0%	50%
Recurrence, low grade	35.0%	30.0%	59%
Recurrence, high grade	34.0%	52.9%	56%
Recurrence, grade 1	N/A	15.2%	57%
Recurrence, grade 2	N/A	42.0%	46%
Recurrence, grade 3	N/A	61.7%	61%
Progression, total	222 (14.7%)	41 (11.8%)	17 (8.8%)
Progression, PUNLMP	1.9%	0.0%	0%
Progression, low grade	6.5%	6.7%	3%
Progression, high grade	28.8%	30.6%	15%
Progression, grade 1	N/A	2.4%	4.5%
Progression, grade 2	N/A	27.0%	3.1%
Progression, grade 3	N/A	38.3%	18%
Progression, definition	Advanced stage, metastasis or death.	pT2 or higher	Advanced stage, metastasis or death.

*IVI Treatment: Intra-vesical instillation treatment.
N/A: Not applicable.

in situ. These variables are weighted and the combined score determines risk stratification of the patients. High risk patients are routinely treated with BCG-instillations. The EORTC risk scores have not been calculated in our study. The clinical information was extracted from patient records several years after the treatment was given. For a large proportion of the patients the tumour size or number of tumours was not recorded, hence the risk score is impossible to calculate.

The WHO73 grading system is a well-established and accepted system. There have however been discussions over the reproducibility of this system, and the WHO04 grading system was designed and hoped to be universally acceptable and better

reproducible. However, several studies have shown considerable inter-observer variability using the WHO04 as well. In our material, the WHO73 (as grades 1&2 versus 3) and WHO04 (as low grade versus high grade) have nearly the same interobserver reproducibility, which was not perfect, and slightly more variation in the intraobserver reproducibility for one of the observers as the WHO04 is possibly better reproducible than the WHO73. The WHO04 has many more high-grade tumours (n = 74) than the WHO73 (grade 3, n = 51). None of the grading systems is superior with regards to predicting recurrence or stage progression.

The current European guidelines on treatment of non-muscle-invasive bladder carcinoma recommends reporting according to both grading systems as the clinical guidelines are based on the WHO73 but the WHO04 is also used. The improvement of the 2004 classification has been disputed by several authors with the main debate being the PUNLMP [8,15–18]. A two-tier system differentiating only between low grade and high grade tumours would yield better reproducibility results. The WHO04 has not been implemented in the clinical guidelines as the predictive value of the grading system with respect to recurrence and stage progression is not yet fully investigated.

Table 8 summarizes the results from the largest study on WHO04, by Pan et al [15], a recent study comparing the WHO73 and the WHO04 grading systems by Chen et al [19] and our study. In Pan's study a very large number of cases were evaluated, but it does not compare the WHO73 with the WHO04. Moreover, the WHO04 evaluations have been done by one pathologist only. Chen et al (2012) did compare both grading systems, but again only one pathologist did the review. We used three independent reviewers. Statistically, none of the grading systems was stronger than the others with regards to predicting recurrence or progression in our study. The proportion of WHO73 grade 3 tumours was 26% whereas there were 38% WHO04 high grade tumours, both considerably higher than the overall progression rate of 9%. For patients with otherwise similar risk factors for progression (multiplicity, tumour size, progression rate, and stage), this could lead to overtreatment if the WHO04 high grade tumours were treated similarly to the WHO73 grade 3 tumours. This could point to a slight preference for the WHO73. In addition, Table 6 shows that there are considerable differences between the populations from different countries. Multicentre international studies are needed to give a better impression about the real value of the WHO73 and WHO04; however, a more reasonable conclusion would be that both systems have a very low predictive value. It therefore seems better to study new molecular quantitative biomarkers which may have stronger prognostic value and also can be better reproducible than conventional microscopic evaluations, as has been found for Ki67 in breast cancer [20]. In 2010, van Rhijn et al showed that using a molecular grade, consisting of a combination of FGFR3 mutations status and Ki67%, could predict recurrence and progression more accurately and more reproducibly [21]. Combining the molecular grade and the EORTC risk score could provide clinicians with an even more precise tool for therapy decision making with regard choice of follow-up and treatment.

The median age in our study population was somewhat higher than reported by others [6,22], but in Norway, the median age at diagnosis of new cancers (primary diagnosis) of the bladder, urethra and ureters in Norway in 2005–2009 falls within the 70–74 years bracket [23]. Although the median age might be higher than in other publications, the population of the catchment area of SUH does not differ from the Norwegian population as a whole.

The clinical impact of PUNLMP is not yet established. As reproducibility is low, recurrence and progression rates should be interpreted with caution. Recurrence rates vary from 3 to 60% [24], including several patients who have been diagnosed with muscle-invasive carcinoma at a later stage [25]. The follow-up of this group is controversial. Some authors believe they should be grouped with the low grade carcinomas, as recurrence rates and disease-specific mortality rates do not differ significantly [18,26]. However, there are also authors who argue that patients with PUNLMP need not be followed as closely as patients with low grade urothelial carcinomas as some studies show low recurrence rates for PUNLMP [17]. Others add to this by arguing that the psychological trauma may be less if the patients are not given a cancer-label. This view has not been validated in clinical trials. Avoiding the cancer-label might be of importance in areas where universal health care is not available, and a history of cancer may be negative with regards to insurance issues [16].

PUNLMPs are very rare in our material. Other studies report PUNLMP-rates of 12–39%. As specimens from all the patients treated for bladder cancer in the South Rogaland region are sent to our laboratory, ours is a population based material. Both urothelial carcinomas and papillomas from the study period were reviewed to ensure that no PUNLMPs were falsely labelled as papillomas. The very low incidence therefore seems real and representative for our region. One could hypothesise that the scarcity of PUNLMPs could be due to the tendency of a rather medically conservative attitude in the population of the catchment area of our hospital as preventative screening for bladder carcinoma is not performed, and investigation and diagnosis depend on clinical presentation.

In conclusion, there are still challenges with respect to reproducibility and specificity to predict stage progression. We propose further studies of the additional value of quantitative molecular biomarkers such as proliferation markers (Ki67, PPH3 and FGFR3) and possibly also host immune response to improve the reproducibility and prognostic value of predicting stage progression.

Author Contributions

Conceived and designed the experiments: OMM EAMJ JPAB IT. Performed the experiments: OMM RW EG IT. Analyzed the data: OMM ID EAMJ JPAB. Wrote the paper: OMM ID EAMJ JPAB. Built the database: OMM IT EAMJ.

References

1. Holmang S, Hedelin H, Anderstrom C, Johansson SL (1995) The relationship among multiple recurrences, progression and prognosis of patients with stages Ta and T1 transitional cell cancer of the bladder followed for at least 20 years. J Urol 153: 1823–1826; discussion 1826–1827.

2. Larsson P, Wijkstrom H, Thorstenson A, Adolfsson J, Norming U, et al. (2003) A population-based study of 538 patients with newly detected urinary bladder neoplasms followed during 5 years. Scand J Urol Nephrol 37: 195–201.

3. Babjuk M, Oosterlinck W, Sylvester R, Kaasinen E, Bohle A, et al. (2011) EAU guidelines on non-muscle-invasive urothelial carcinoma of the bladder, the 2011 update. Eur Urol 59: 997–1008.

4. Mostofi FK, Sobin LH, Torloni H, editors (1973) Histological typing of urinary bladder tumours. Geneva: World Health Organization.

5. Epstein JI, Amin MB, Reuter VR, Mostofi FK (1998) The World Health Organization/International Society of Urological Pathology consensus classification of urothelial (transitional cell) neoplasms of the urinary bladder. Bladder Consensus Conference Committee. Am J Surg Pathol 22: 1435–1448.

6. Eble JN, Sauter G, Epstein JI, Sesterhenn IA, editors (2004) World Health Organization Classification of Tumours. Pathology and Genetics of Tumours of the Urinary System and Male Genital Organs. Lyon: IARC Press.

7. Bol MG, Baak JP, Buhr-Wildhagen S, Kruse AJ, Kjellevold KH, et al. (2003) Reproducibility and prognostic variability of grade and lamina propria invasion in stages Ta, T1 urothelial carcinoma of the bladder. J Urol 169: 1291–1294.

8. Yorukoglu K, Tuna B, Dikicioglu E, Duzcan E, Isisag A, et al. (2003) Reproducibility of the 1998 World Health Organization/International Society of Urologic Pathology classification of papillary urothelial neoplasms of the urinary bladder. Virchows Arch 443: 734–740.

9. Samaratunga H, Makarov DV, Epstein JI, Samaratunga H, Makarov DV, et al. (2002) Comparison of WHO/ISUP and WHO classification of noninvasive papillary urothelial neoplasms for risk of progression. Urology 60: 315–319.

10. Yin H, Leong AS (2004) Histologic grading of noninvasive papillary urothelial tumors: validation of the 1998 WHO/ISUP system by immunophenotyping and follow-up. Am J Clin Pathol 121: 679–687.

11. Engers R (2007) Reproducibility and reliability of tumor grading in urological neoplasms. World J Urol 25: 595–605.

12. van Rhijn BW, van Leenders GJ, Ooms BC, Kirkels WJ, Zlotta AR, et al. (2010) The pathologist's mean grade is constant and individualizes the prognostic value of bladder cancer grading. Eur Urol 57: 1052–1057.

13. Harrell FE, Lee KL, Mark DB (1996) Multivariable prognostic models: Issues in developing models, evaluating assumption and adequacy, and measuring and reducing errors. Statistics in Medicine 15: 361–387.

14. Sylvester RJ, van der Meijden AP, Oosterlinck W, Witjes JA, Bouffioux C, et al. (2006) Predicting recurrence and progression in individual patients with stage Ta T1 bladder cancer using EORTC risk tables: a combined analysis of 2596 patients from seven EORTC trials. Eur Urol 49: 466–465; discussion 475–467.

15. Pan CC, Chang YH, Chen KK, Yu HJ, Sun CH, et al. Prognostic significance of the 2004 WHO/ISUP classification for prediction of recurrence, progression, and cancer-specific mortality of non-muscle-invasive urothelial tumors of the urinary bladder: a clinicopathologic study of 1,515 cases. Am J Clin Pathol 133: 788–795.

16. MacLennan GT, Kirkali Z, Cheng L (2007) Histologic grading of noninvasive papillary urothelial neoplasms. Eur Urol 51: 889–897; discussion 897–888.

17. Epstein JI (2003) The new World Health Organization/International Society of Urological Pathology (WHO/ISUP) classification for TA, T1 bladder tumors: is it an improvement? Crit Rev Oncol Hematol 47: 83–89.

18. Murphy WM, Takezawa K, Maruniak NA (2002) Interobserver discrepancy using the 1998 World Health Organization/International Society of Urologic Pathology classification of urothelial neoplasms: practical choices for patient care. J Urol 168: 968–972.

19. Chen Z, Ding W, Xu K, Tan J, Sun C, et al. (2012) The 1973 WHO Classification is more suitable than the 2004 WHO Classification for predicting prognosis in Non-muscle-invasive bladder cancer. PLoS One 7: e47199.

20. Gudlaugsson E, Skaland I, Janssen EA, Smaaland R, Shao Z, et al. (2012) Comparison of the effect of different techniques for measurement of Ki67 proliferation on reproducibility and prognosis prediction accuracy in breast cancer. Histopathology 61: 1134–1144.

21. van Rhijn BW, Zuiverloon TC, Vis AN, Radvanyi F, van Leenders GJ, et al. (2010) Molecular grade (FGFR3/MIB-1) and EORTC risk scores are predictive in primary non-muscle-invasive bladder cancer. Eur Urol 58: 433–441.

22. Murphy W, Grignon DJ, Perlman EJ (2004) Tumors of the Kidney, Bladder, and Related Urinary Structures. Washington, DC: Armed Forces Institute of Pathology.

23. Haldorsen T (2011) Cancer in Norway 2009. Oslo: Cancer Registry of Norway.

24. Fujii Y, Kawakami S, Koga F, Nemoto T, Kihara K (2003) Long-term outcome of bladder papillary urothelial neoplasms of low malignant potential. BJU International 92: 559–562.

25. Cheng L, Neumann RM, Bostwick DG (1999) Papillary urothelial neoplasms of low malignant potential. Clinical and biologic implications. Cancer 86: 2102–2108.

26. Cheng L, MacLennan GT, Lopez-Beltran A (2012) Histologic grading of urothelial carcinoma: a reappraisal. Hum Pathol 43: 2097–2108.

13

Use of the Comet-FISH Assay to Compare DNA Damage and Repair in p53 and hTERT Genes following Ionizing Radiation

Declan J. McKenna*, Bernadette A. Doherty, C. Stephen Downes, Stephanie R. McKeown, Valerie J. McKelvey-Martin

Biomedical Sciences Research Institute, University of Ulster, Coleraine, Northern Ireland, United Kingdom

Abstract

The alkaline single cell gel electrophoresis (comet) assay can be combined with fluorescent *in situ* hybridisation (FISH) methodology in order to investigate the localisation of specific gene domains within an individual cell. The number and position of the fluorescent signal(s) provides information about the relative damage and subsequent repair that is occurring in the targeted gene domain(s). In this study, we have optimised the comet-FISH assay to detect and compare DNA damage and repair in the p53 and hTERT gene regions of bladder cancer cell-lines RT4 and RT112, normal fibroblasts and Cockayne Syndrome (CS) fibroblasts following γ-radiation. Cells were exposed to 5Gy γ-radiation and repair followed for up to 60 minutes. At each repair time-point, the number and location of p53 and hTERT hybridisation spots was recorded in addition to standard comet measurements. In bladder cancer cell-lines and normal fibroblasts, the p53 gene region was found to be rapidly repaired relative to the hTERT gene region and the overall genome, a phenomenon that appeared to be independent of hTERT transcriptional activity. However, in the CS fibroblasts, which are defective in transcription coupled repair (TCR), this rapid repair of the p53 gene region was not observed when compared to both the hTERT gene region and the overall genome, proving the assay can detect variations in DNA repair in the same gene. In conclusion, we propose that the comet-FISH assay is a sensitive and rapid method for detecting differences in DNA damage and repair between different gene regions in individual cells in response to radiation. We suggest this increases its potential for measuring radiosensitivity in cells and may therefore have value in a clinical setting.

Editor: Anthony W.I. Lo, The Chinese University of Hong Kong, Hong Kong

Funding: Funding for this project was provided in part by a Vice-Chancellor's Research Studentship from the University of Ulster, awarded to BAD. The funders had no role in study design, data collection and analysis, decision to publish, or preparation of the manuscript. No additional external funding received for this study.

Competing Interests: The authors have declared that no competing interests exist.

* E-mail: dj.mckenna@ulster.ac.uk

Introduction

The comet-FISH assay is a method that allows DNA damage and repair to be detected in specific gene regions relative to the overall genome [1]. It has been used in several studies that have successfully localised DNA damage within comets using both chromosome and gene-specific probes (reviewed in [2]). The ability to obtain this type of information would be useful because this assay could benefit many areas of clinical investigation by providing valuable information about the intrinsic DNA characteristics of individual cells and their responses to various external factors, such as radiation, chemicals and drugs. This information would prove particularly relevant in the diagnosis, prognosis and treatment of cancer by allowing analysis of tumour cells, since the repair of important gene regions is integral in determining individual patient response to therapy [3]. Indeed, the Comet assay in its various forms is an attractive candidate for a predictive test for radiosensitivity in a clinical setting [4]. The ability to predict the radiosensitivity of individual tumours would represent a major step forward in radiation biology, since there is still no definitive way of predicting whether an individual patient will respond to radiotherapy or not.

A number of different techniques have been developed to address this problem with varying degrees of success, such as the SF2 clonogenic survival assay [5], potential doubling time (Tpot) of the tumour [6], tumour hypoxia measured by pO2 [7], the percentage of apoptotic or viable cells [8], index of thymidine and BudR labelling [9], immunohistochemical detection of specific proteins [10] and microarray technology [11]. However, the comet assay offers many advantages over these, since it is a relatively simple and inexpensive technique, which requires only a few cells and results can be obtained within a matter of hours. Encouragingly, several studies have shown that the comet assay is a reliable and comparable alternative to the time-consuming clonogenic survival assay, currently considered the gold standard method for predicting tumour sensitivity [12–15]. However, for the comet assay to gain widespread acceptance for this application, more studies are required to demonstrate what sort of unique information it can provide. If information about damage and repair in specific gene regions could also be obtained by employing the comet-FISH version of the assay, this would increase the diagnostic and prognostic potential of this technique as a routine application in the clinical laboratory.

With this in mind, we have used the comet-FISH assay to simultaneously probe two gene regions in order to compare DNA damage and repair in different gene regions within the same cell. We have targeted the p53 (17p13.1) and hTERT (5q15.33) gene loci since these genes are known to have different transcriptional activities and should therefore exhibit differences in DNA repair efficiency in our assay. The p53 gene is actively transcribed [16], is induced by γ-radiation [17] and is known to be preferentially repaired in comparison to other genes [18], whereas the hTERT gene is transcriptionally inactive in normal cells but activated in the majority of tumour cells [19,20]. hTERT codes for human telomerase reverse transcriptase, the catalytic subunit of the enzyme telomerase and transcriptional up-regulation of hTERT has been shown to occur in >85% of human neoplasms clearly identifying it as a potentially useful biomarker for tumourigenesis [20]. This makes both genes ideal candidates for testing in the comet-FISH protocol.

Previous studies in our laboratory have optimised the comet-FISH assay and shown that the p53 gene region in two bladder cancer cell lines was more rapidly repaired than the overall genome following treatment with both γ-irradiation [21] and the DNA cross-linking agent mitomycin C [22]. We hypothesised that this preferential repair might be a reflection of transcription-coupled repair (TCR) occurring within the cell and proposed that the comet-FISH assay offered considerable potential for further study of gene-region specific repair. Therefore, in this current report, we build upon these previous studies and compare γ-radiation-induced DNA damage and repair between the p53 and hTERT gene regions in bladder cancer cell lines (RT4 & RT112), normal fibroblast cells (GM38) and in two Cockayne Syndrome fibroblast cell lines (CSA & CSB), which are defective in TCR. Since we are employing alkaline conditions in the Comet-FISH assay, we will be measuring a combination of frank strand breaks and other alkaline labile sites that give rise to secondary strand breaks. Therefore, when we make reference to DNA repair, it is of these particular DNA lesions we are considering. We demonstrate that this assay can successfully detect differences in DNA repair between two separate gene regions following radiation, thereby establishing it as a technique which offers great potential for monitoring the gene-specific response to DNA damage in individual cells and populations.

Materials and Methods

Cell Lines and Cell Culture

The normal, CSA and CSB fibroblast cell lines used in this study are commercially available from the Human Genetic Mutant Repository (Coriell Institute, Camden, NJ). The normal fibroblast cells (GM38) [23] were cultured in Eagle's minimum essential medium (EMEM), supplemented with 20% foetal bovine serum (FBS), 4% essential amino acids, 2% non-essential amino acids and 1% penicillin-streptomycin. The CS fibroblast cell lines used in this study, CSA (GM01856) and CSB (GM00739), were maintained in EMEM, supplemented with 15% FBS and containing 1% penicillin-streptomycin. RT112 bladder cancer cell line [24] was obtained from the European Collection of Cell Cultures (ECACC) (Salisbury, UK) and RT4 [25] bladder cancer cell line was obtained from the American Tissue Culture Collection (ATCC) (Rockville, MD). RT112 cells were cultured in Minimum Essential Medium (MEM), supplemented with 10% FBS and containing 1% penicillin-streptomycin. RT4 cells were cultured in McCoy's 5A medium, supplemented with 10% FBS and 1% penicillin-streptomycin. Werner syndrome (WS) [26] cells obtained from the Coriell Cell Repository (Camden, NJ) were

maintained in MEM, supplemented with 15% FBS and 1% penicillin-streptomycin. This cell line has been immortalised with hTERT and was used in our PCR experiments as a positive control for this gene (Simpson, unpublished). The GM38 cell line [27], RT4 cell line [28] and both CS cell lines (Alan Lehman, personal communication) all actively express wild type p53, whereas the RT112 cell line contains a point mutation at codon 248 resulting in an Arg-Gly amino acid change and therefore expresses mutant p53 [29].

RT-PCR Analysis of hTERT Gene Expression

Total RNA was extracted from the CSA, CSB, GM38 and WS cell lines using the RNeasy midi kit (Qiagen, Crawley, UK) according to the manufacturer's instructions. The quantification and quality of RNA was determined spectrophotometrically and by 1% agarose gel electrophoresis. Complementary DNA (cDNA) was obtained for each cell line using a Superscript™II RNASE H-Reverse Transcriptase Kit (Invitrogen, UK) and PCR performed. The specific primers used for PCR amplification of hTERT were 5'-CTCACCTTCAACCGCGG-3'(sense) and 5'-TTGCTGAT-GAAATGGGAGCT-3' (antisense), generating a 200 bp amplicon (genbank accession number = NM198253). For GAPDH, used as a positive control, the primers were 5'-ACCCCTTCATT-GACCTCAACTACA-3' (sense) and 5' TACTGGTGTCAGG-TACGGTAGTGA-3' (antisense), generating a 440 bp amplicon. For hTERT expression, a sample from a WS patient immortalised with hTERT was used as a positive control. Reaction conditions were 31 cycles of denaturation at 94°C for 45 seconds, annealing at 60°C for 45 seconds and extension at 72°C for 90 seconds for hTERT and 30 cycles of denaturation at 95°C for 1 minute, annealing at 56°C for 1 minute and extension at 72°C for 5 minutes for GAPDH. The amplified PCR products were separated by electrophoresis on a 1% agarose gel and visualised by staining with ethidium bromide (Sigma). The expression of hTERT mRNA relative to GAPDH mRNA was determined using gel analysis software Scion Image (Scion, Frederick, MD, USA) to measure the density of respective DNA bands.

Comet-FISH Assay

Gel preparation and comet assay. The alkaline comet assay was performed according to a standard protocol of McKelvey-Martin et al [2]. Cells were harvested and washed twice in 10 ml phosphate buffered saline (PBS). Cell viability was assessed using the trypan blue exclusion method. In all experiments, cell viability was >99%. One millilitre aliquots of the cell suspensions in Ca^{2+} and Mg^{2+} free PBS, at a concentration of 2×10^5 cells/ml were pipetted into eppendorf tubes and centrifuged at 1500 rpm for 5 minutes at 4°C. Meanwhile, Dakin fully frosted microscope slides (Labcraft, UK) were each covered with 100 μl of 0.6% normal-melting-point agarose (prepared in Ca^{2+} and Mg^{2+} free PBS) at 37°C. A 22×22 mm cover slip was placed on top and the slide was kept on ice until the agarose had solidified. Low-melting-point agarose (1.2%) was mixed in a 1:1 ratio with repair medium (growth medium containing 20% FBS), and 80 μl of this mixture was used to resuspend each pellet of cells. After the cover slip was gently removed, the cell/agarose suspension was quickly pipetted onto the first agarose layer, the cover slip was replaced, and the slide was left on ice to solidify the agarose. Following removal of the cover slips, 5Gy γ-irradiation (at a rate of 2cGy/s, using a Cs^{137} source) was administered and the slides were either (i) immediately placed in lysis solution (2.5 M NaCl, 100 mM Na_2EDTA, 10 mM Tris, pH 10, with 1% Triton X-100 added) for 1hour at 4°C or (ii) the slides were immersed in the appropriate growth medium at 37°C for 15, 30 and 60 minutes

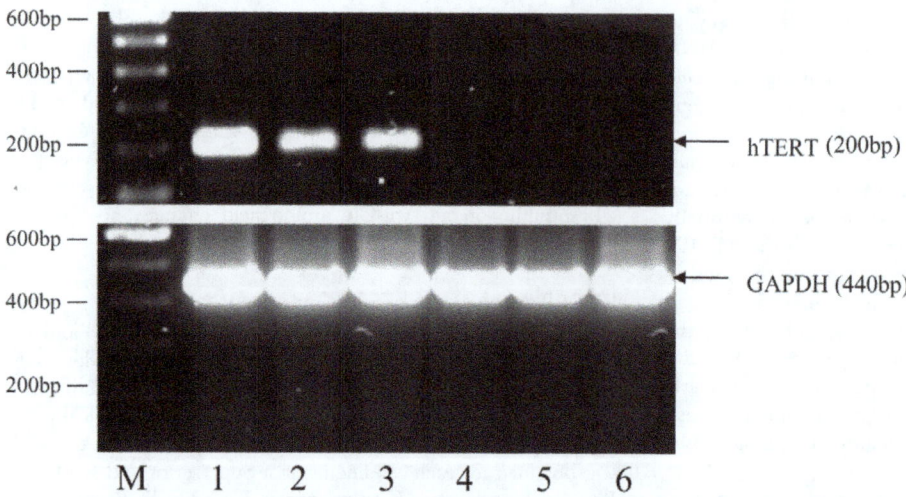

Figure 1. hTERT Expression in Cell Lines. Top image shows hTERT expression detected at 200 bp in a Werner syndrome cell line (positive control) immortalised for hTERT (Lane1). hTERT expression is also detected in the bladder cancer cell lines RT112 and RT4 (Lanes 2 and 3 respectively). No hTERT expression was found in the normal GM38 fibroblast cell line (Lane 4) or in the two Cockayne Syndrome cell lines, CSA and CSB (Lanes 5 and 6 respectively). Bottom image shows the expression of housekeeping control gene GAPDH at 440 bp in all six cell lines (Lanes 1–6). (Lane M, 100 bp size marker.).

before placing in lysis solution for 1 hour at 4°C. All slides were then placed in a horizontal gel electrophoresis tank filled with fresh chilled electrophoresis buffer (300 mM NaOH, 1 mM Na$_2$EDTA, pH >13) to a level of approximately 0.25 cm above the slides. They were left for 20 minutes to allow DNA unwinding to occur before electrophoresis at 25 V (0.66 V/cm) and 300 mA for 20 minutes. Slides were then neutralised by 3 X 5 minute washes in 0.4 M Tris, pH 7.5, followed by a 5 minute wash in 2X SSC (3 M saline sodium citrate; 0.3 M sodium citrate, pH 5.3). The slides were then drained and subsequently dehydrated in an ascending series of ethanol solutions (70%, 85%, 100% for 2 minutes each) and air-dried.

Preparation of probes and hybridization. FISH was performed on prepared comet slides using a mix of 2 probes: (i) A locus-specific identifier (LSI) Spectrum-Orange-labelled p53 DNA probe, comprised of randomly sheared 50–140 bp lengths of DNA covering approximately a 145 kb region, including the

20 kb p53 locus (17p13.1) (Vysis, Surrey, UK); (ii) A LSI Spectrum-Green-labelled hTERT DNA probe, spanning a 180 kb region including the 40 kb hTERT locus (5q15.33) (Q-Biogene, UK). For each individual slide, a hybridisation mixture containing equal concentrations of the p53 probe and the hTERT probe was added and a 22 mm × 22 mm coverslip was placed on top. Co-denaturation of both target DNA and probe DNA was performed at 80°C for 2 minutes. Hybridisation of both probes took place simultaneously at 37°C for 16 hours in a dark, humidified chamber.

Post-hybridisation and Counterstaining

Following hybridisation, the slides were placed in a solution of 50% formamide and 2X SSC for 10 minutes at 45°C. Once in the solution, the slides were gently agitated to detach the coverslips. This wash was repeated three times, followed by a 10 minute wash in 2X SSC at 45°C and a 5 minute wash in 2X SSC containing

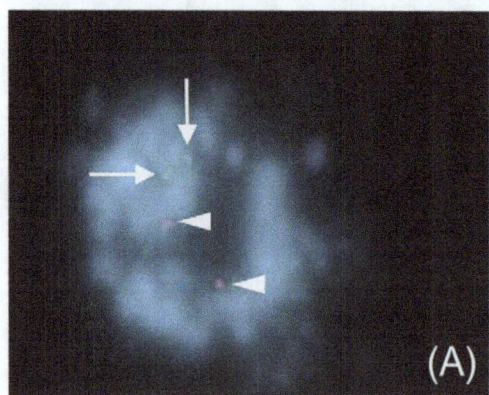
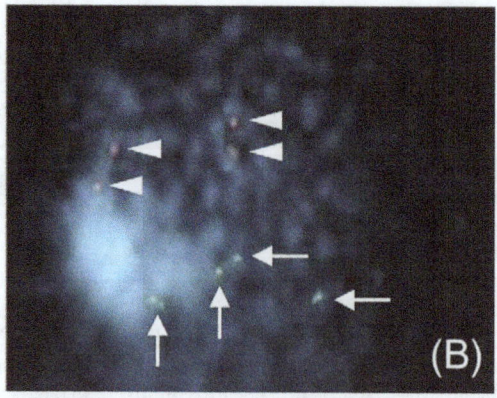

Figure 2. Representative images of comet-FISH cells. A. An untreated RT112 cell displays hardly any DNA damage evidenced by a relatively intact comet head and the absence of a comet tail. Two pink p53 (arrowheads) and two green hTERT (arrows) hybridisation spots are visible in the intact comet head. **B.** Immediately following 5Gy γ-irradiation, a large, dispersed comet tail is visible, indicating a significant amount of overall DNA damage. Cells display several p53 and hTERT hybridisation spots in both the comet head and tail, indicating that some radiation-induced strand breaks have occurred within, or close to, both gene regions.

Table 1. Table shows data generated by comet-FISH assay for all 5 cell lines at 0, 15, 30 & 60 minutes following 5Gy radiation.

		Control	0	15	30	60
RT4	% Tail DNA	6.75±0.88	47.16±1.87	34.82±2.04	30.33±4.6	24.7±4.94
	% Cells showing DNA Damage	38±4	100±0	99±1	87±7.06	80±8
	% Cells with p53 Tail Spots	29±1	100±0	69±5	67±3	55±3
	% Cells with hTERT Tail Spots	71±5	100±0	91±3	89±3	83±1
RT112	% Tail DNA	9.9±0.65	45.89±0.35	31.25±2.23	23.19±3.64	24.4±0.99
	% Cells showing DNA Damage	47±1	100±0	92±2	81±5	72±0
	% Cells with p53 Tail Spots	22±2	75±5	54±2	37±3	29±1
	% Cells with hTERT Tail Spots	65±1	91±7	86±0	76±8	71±1
GM38	% Tail DNA	6.10±0.45	30.78±1.17	28.71±0.09	21.22±1.24	17.05±0.62
	% Cells showing DNA Damage	47±5	99±1	98±0	91±5	78±4
	% Cells with p53 Tail Spots	3±2.16	90±2	54±6	46±5.5	50±2
	% Cells with hTERT Tail Spots	16±2	82±2	83±3	77±3	73±3
CSA	% Tail DNA	6.41±0.3	44.14±2.47	33.44±4.33	21.94±2.28	23.43±4.48
	% Cells showing DNA Damage	38±4	98±2	97±1	90±2	90±6
	% Cells with p53 Tail Spots	25±1	90±4	84±4	85±7	77±3
	% Cells with hTERT Tail Spots	41±1	92±2	91±1	88±4	86±6
CSB	% Tail DNA	6.28±0.55	44.90±0.36	28.99±0.9	26.63±2.11	19.08±0.59
	% Cells showing DNA Damage	39±1	99±1	91±5	81±3	89±3
	% Cells with p53 Tail Spots	12±4	97±3	87±1	88±4	82±0.02
	% Cells with hTERT Tail Spots	26±4	98±0.02	84±4	90±2	76±4

Each measurement is the mean ± SEM of two independent experiments, representing 100 cells in total.

0.1% Igepal (Sigma). Slides were left to air dry for 30 min before being counterstained with 16 µl DAPI in antifade mounting solution (Vysis, UK). Subsequently, the slides were left in the dark at 4°C for no longer than 2 hours prior to observation. All experiments were carried out under yellow light to prevent additional DNA damage by natural light. All reagents were purchased from Sigma, Poole, UK unless otherwise indicated.

Comet-FISH Analysis

Observations were made at a final magnification of x600 (Nikon x60 Fluor lens) using an epifluorescence microscope (Olympus BH2); equipped with Hitachi KP571 CCD camera interfaced through a Matrox IP8 board using Hewlett Packard Super VGA and Kromascan software (Andor Technology, UK). A triple bandpass filter set (Chroma HiQ) tuned for: DAPI (excitation 370 nm, emission 450 nm, bandwidth 20 nm), spectrum orange (excitation 560 nm, emission 590 nm, bandwidth 60 nm) and spectrum green (excitation 547 nm, emission 572 nm, bandwidth 30 nm), was utilised for comet-FISH. This enabled the simultaneous detection of: DAPI (overall genome damage), spectrum orange (p53 gene region) and spectrum green (hTERT gene region) labels. In addition to the number and position of p53 and hTERT hybridisation spots within each comet being noted, standard comet parameter measurements including tail moment and % tail DNA were also recorded for each comet. Comet analysis was performed using the Komet 5.0 digital imaging system (Andor Technology, UK), which measures a wide range of densitometric and geometric parameters for each comet. The primary measurement used in this study was % Tail DNA. One slide (50 cells) was analysed from each dose point. Two independent experiments were conducted to generate each data point (100 cells). Mean values for each measurement were

generated standard error of the mean (SEM) was calculated from the standard deviation. Student t-test was used to generate statistics.

Results

It has previously been established that the p53 gene is actively expressed in the RT4, RT112, CSA, CSB and GM38 cell lines used in our studies [27–29]. However, since we were not aware of the transcriptional activity of the hTERT gene in our cell lines, we measured the hTERT gene expression using RT-PCR. Figure 1 demonstrates that the hTERT PCR product was clearly detected in WS cells (positive control) and the RT112 and RT4 tumour cell lines, but not in the three fibroblast cell lines. These results agree with the findings of de Kok *et al* [19] and Abdul-Ghani *et al* [30] who demonstrated high levels of hTERT expression in RT112 and RT4 tumour cell lines but not in normal cells.

Representative images of cells processed in the comet-FISH assay demonstrate the typical appearance of cells when viewed through the microscope (Figure 2). By recording standard comet measurements, such as % Tail DNA, as well as the number and location of p53 and hTERT hybridisation signals for each cell, we could generate data at each time-point measured for all 5 cell lines (Table 1). The fluorescent signals were referred to as 'head spots' or 'tail spots', depending on their location within the comet.

We first focused our attention the γ-irradiation-induced DNA damage and repair in RT112 and RT4 bladder cancer cells. To measure overall DNA repair in the cells following 5Gy γ-irradiation, the mean % Tail DNA value was recorded for each time point (Table 1). A cell was considered to have radiation-induced DNA damage if its mean % tail DNA measurement had a value greater than the mean % tail DNA value for untreated cells.

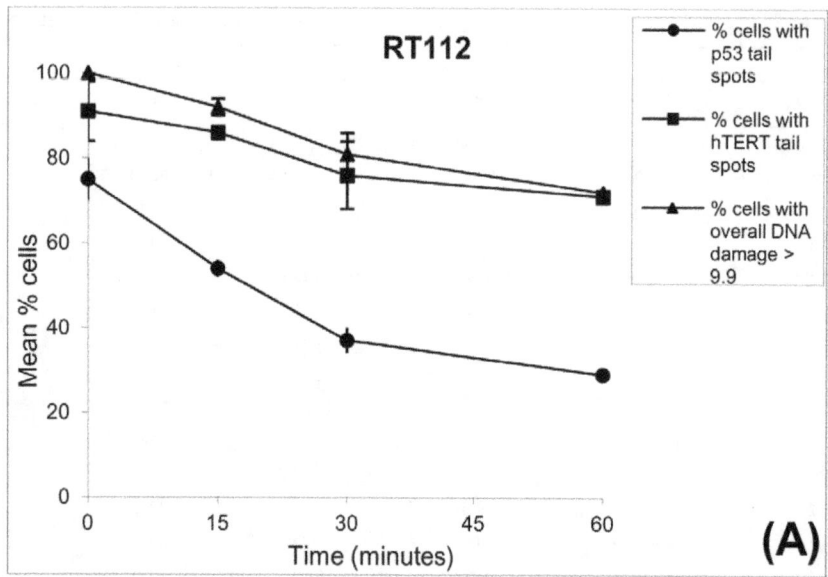

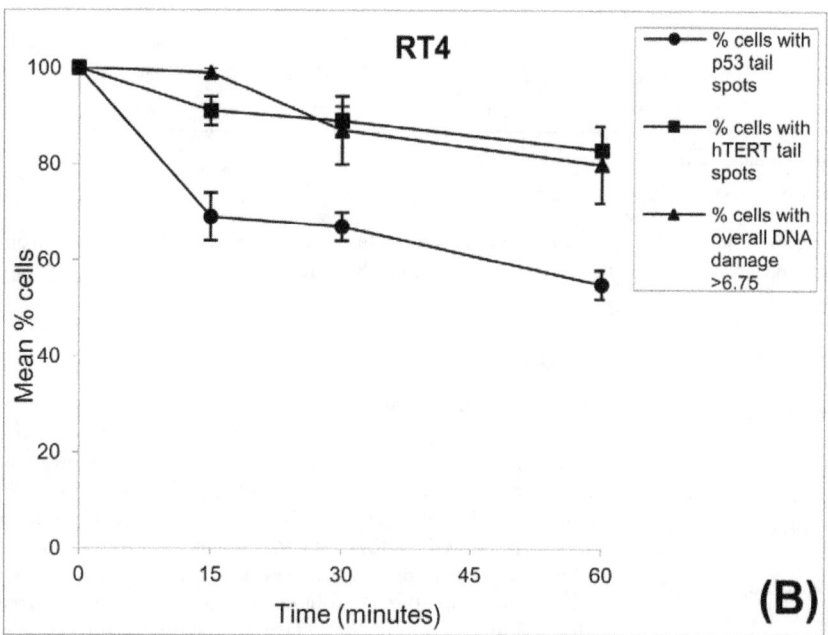

Figure 3. Comparison of repair of overall genomic DNA damage and of the p53 and hTERT gene regions in (A) RT112 cells (B) RT4 cells following 5Gy radiation. Each graph shows the mean % of cells showing γ-radiation-induced damage (▲). A cell was considered to have γ-radiation-induced DNA damage if its mean % DNA measurement had a greater value than the mean % DNA value for control cells for that cell line (control values shown in key on each graph). The mean % of cells showing p53 (●) and hTERT (■) hybridisation spots in the comet tail is also shown for each cell line. For both cell-lines the rate of repair of overall genomic DNA and hTERT is similar (as shown by slope of lines), whereas the rate of repair of p53 is significantly faster during the first 15 minutes ($P<0.05$ for both cell lines). Each data point represents the mean ± SEM of two independent experiments.

Immediately following irradiation, 100% of RT112 cells exhibited radiation-induced DNA damage as expected (Figure 3a). As the repair time increased, the number of RT112 cells showing damage decreased slowly, but steadily, to 72% by 60 minutes. hTERT tail spots were observed in 91% of RT112 cells immediately after irradiation, and this was repaired with a very similar rate to the overall genome with 71% of cells showing hTERT tail spots at 60 minutes. p53 tail spots were observed in 75% of RT112 cells

immediately following irradiation. This was significantly reduced to 54% over the first 15 minutes of repair ($p<0.05$) and was further reduced by 30 minutes to 37%. Thereafter, a similar repair rate to hTERT and the overall genome was observed from 30–60 minutes.

Similar results were demonstrated by the RT4 cells (Table 1 and Figure 3b). Immediately following irradiation, 100% of RT4 cells showed radiation-induced DNA damage, and p53 and hTERT

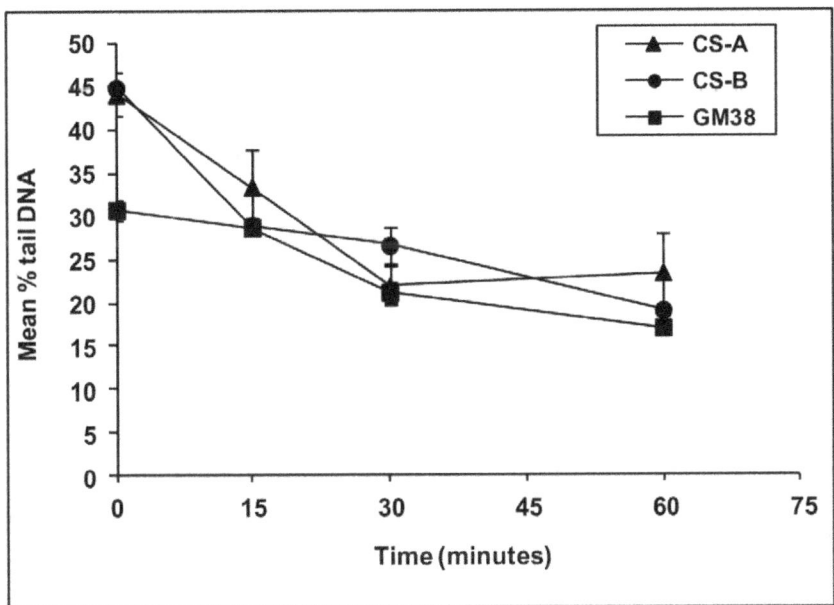

Figure 4. Repair of overall DNA damage in fibroblast cell lines measured by comet-FISH. Graph shows DNA damage and repair following the exposure to γ-radiation of normal GM38 fibroblasts and Cockayne Syndrome cell lines CSA and CSB. DNA damage is measured using mean % Tail DNA. Error bars shown are ±95% confidence limits.

tail spots. As repair time increased, the % of cells showing overall DNA damage decreased at a slow, but steady rate to 80% at 60 minutes; a similarly slow rate of reduction to 83% by 60 minutes was found for cells with hTERT tail spots. Once again, the % of cells with p53 tail spots decreased significantly within the first 15 minutes to 69% (p<0.05). From 15–60 minutes, the rate of reduction was similar to that for hTERT and the overall genome.

Having identified preferential repair of the p53 gene region in tumour cells we then investigated if this phenomenon could be replicated in normal and repair deficient fibroblasts. To establish that the comet assay could measure overall DNA repair in these cell lines following γ-irradiation, we confirmed that a decrease in the mean % tail DNA measurements over the 60 minutes for all cell lines was apparent, thereby indicating active overall DNA repair (Table 1 and Figure 4). Greater initial damage, as measured by % Tail DNA, was observed in both CS cell lines compared to the GM38 cell line, since they contain intrinsically higher levels of baseline DNA damage. Similar results were obtained using Tail Moment results (data not shown).

We then wanted to see if the defective TCR in CS lines could be detected by comet-FISH. Figure 5 shows the repair of the overall genome in each fibroblast cell line as well as repair in the p53 and hTERT gene regions. For normal GM38 fibroblasts (Figure 5a), immediately following irradiation, 99% of cells exhibited significant radiation-induced damage. The majority of cells also showed damage in the p53 gene region (90% cells show p53 tail spots) and the hTERT gene region (82% cells show hTERT tail spots). The mean % of cells showing radiation-induced damage slowly decreased to 78% by 60 minutes. The repair of the hTERT gene region followed a similarly slow decrease with 73% of cells showing hTERT tail spots after 60 minutes. However, the mean % of cells with p53 tail spots was significantly reduced within 15 minutes to 54% (p<0.001). From 15 to 60 minutes, this measurement showed little significant reduction and followed a similar repair rate to hTERT and the overall genome.

A different trend was noted in both CS cell lines. Immediately following irradiation, 98% of CSA cells exhibited radiation-induced DNA damage and this decreased only slightly to 90% over 60 minutes (Figure 5b). The most notable difference from normal fibroblasts was the lack of change in the number and location of p53 hybridisation spots over the 60 minutes. Immediately following irradiation, p53 tail spots were observed in 90% of CSA cells, reducing to 77% after 60 minutes. Likewise, 92% of CSA cells displayed hTERT tail spots immediately after irradiation, reducing to 86% at 60 minutes. The CSB cell line demonstrated similar results to CSA (Figure 5c). Immediately following irradiation, 99% of CSB cells showed induced DNA damage, and all of these also exhibited p53 and hTERT tail spots. As repair time increased, the % of cells showing overall DNA damage decreased slightly to 89% at 60 minutes. As with CSA cells, the % of cells with p53 tail spots decreased slowly with 82% of CSB cells showing p53 tail spots after 60 minutes repair. Similarly, the percentage of cells showing hTERT tail spots was only slightly reduced from 98% to 76% over 60 minutes.

Recording the number and location of hybridisation spots also gives information about the extent of DNA damage and repair, since breaks within the probed target DNA can result in an increase in spot number, whilst a reduction in spot number may indicate a rejoining of strand breaks. Figure 6 shows the frequency distribution analysis of p53 and hTERT hybridisation spot number per tail in each fibroblast cell line at each repair time-point following treatment with 5Gy γ-irradiation. As expected, the majority of untreated GM38 cells have zero p53 or hTERT tail spots (Figure 6a and 6b). Following γ-irradiation (t=0), the majority of cells display hybridisation signals for both probes in the comet tail, with some showing as many as six or eight spots. This indicates that breaks within, or near, the probed regions have occurred, and this broken DNA has migrated into the comet tail. Within 15 minutes, the number of cells displaying no p53 hybridisation spots in the comet tail is increased (see first bar in distribution profile). This indicates a rejoining of strand breaks in

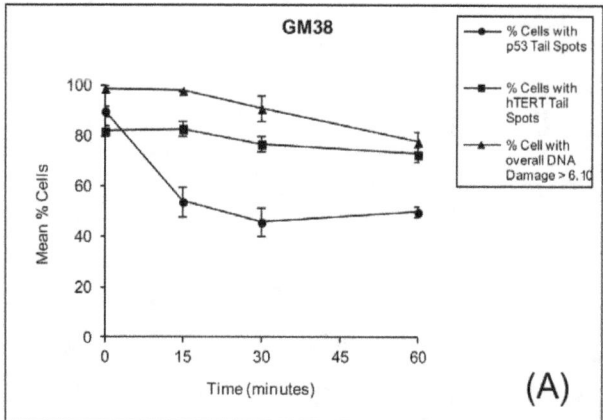

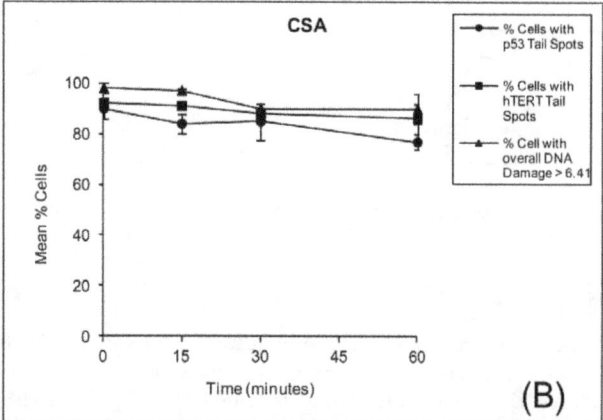

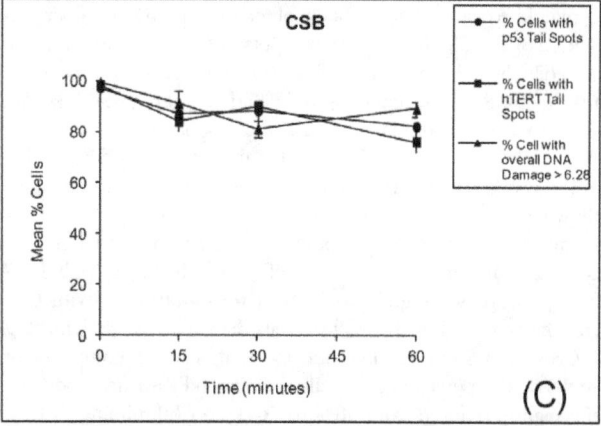

Figure 5. Comparison of repair of overall genomic DNA damage and of the p53 and hTERT gene regions in (A) GM38 cells (B) CSA cells (C) CSB cells following exposure to 5Gy γ-radiation. Each graph shows the mean % of cells showing γ-radiation-induced damage (▲). A cell was considered to have γ-radiation-induced DNA damage if its mean % DNA measurement had a greater value than the mean % DNA value for control cells for that cell line (control values shown in key on each graph). The mean % of cells showing p53 (●) and hTERT (■) hybridisation spots in the comet tail is also shown for each cell line. In GM38 fibroblasts, the rate of repair of overall genomic DNA and hTERT is similar (as shown by slope of lines), whereas the rate of repair of p53 is significantly faster during the first 15 minutes (p<0.001). However, in CSA and CSB fibroblast, the rapid repair of p53 is not apparent and all three repair rates are similar with no significant differences observed between measurements. Each data point represents the mean ± SEM of two independent experiments.

this gene region has occurred in a significant number of cells. By contrast, the distribution profile of hTERT hybridisation spots remains relatively unaffected over the repair time, indicating that repair of strand breaks is not as efficient in this region.

In CSA (Figure 6c and 6d) and CSB (Figure 6e and 6f) fibroblasts, no significant difference in the distribution profile is observed for either p53 or hTERT hybridisation signals. As with GM38 fibroblasts, irradiation increases the number of hybridisation signals for each probe, with the majority of cells in each population displaying several hybridisation spots in the comet tail (t = 0). Over the repair time, however, no clear differences are exhibited in either cell line between the distribution profiles of hybridisation signals. This demonstrates that the repair of stand breaks in the p53 gene region evidenced in GM38 fibroblasts is lost in these cells.

Discussion

The comet-FISH assay enables us to assess both overall genomic repair (by measurement of the standard comet parameters) and gene region specific repair (by analysis of hybridisation spot location and number) in individual cells. In the current study, our results demonstrate that the p53 gene region is more rapidly repaired than the hTERT gene region in the bladder cancer cell lines RT4 and RT112 (Figure 3a & 3b), which expands on our previous observations that the p53 gene region is repaired more rapidly than the overall genome following DNA damage [21,22]. This preferential repair of the p53 gene region compared to both the overall genome and the hTERT gene region was also observed in normal fibroblast cells (Figure 5a and 6a), indicating that repair of strand breaks within, or in the vicinity of, the p53 probe region is carried out quickly (ie within 15 minutes) in a significant number of analysed cells, whereas breaks in or near the hTERT gene region were not. As we have previously explained [22], these changes in hybridisation spot number and location within cells are consistent with our calculations of the likelihood of breaks occurring within (or near) the probed regions during radiation, as well as our understanding of how DNA migrates during the Comet assay. This interpretation is reviewed and supported by Spivak et al. [31] and the findings of Horvathova et al. [32], which suggest that the patterns of migration of domain-specific signals may depend on the localisation of breaks within or around the probed region.

These results mean it is clear that we are able to measure differences in repair of gene regions using the comet-FISH assay, which is not particularly surprising since it is known that DNA repair is not uniform across the genome. For example, it is well established that transcriptionally active regions of the genome are preferentially repaired in contrast to the inactive regions [33–35], whilst other studies have used other methods to demonstrate variations in repair rates between different actively transcribed genes [18] and even within the exons of a single active gene [36,37]. Our study allows us to compare the results from the bladder cancer cell lines (which have active hTERT) with those from normal fibroblasts (which have inactive hTERT). The results show that the preferential repair observed in the cancer cells is not simply a function of transcriptional activity, otherwise we would expect both the p53 and the hTERT gene regions to be preferentially repaired in comparison to overall genome in the cancer cells. Since this is not the case, other contributory factors must be involved in these cells.

Another consideration is that the efficiency of DNA repair may be dependent on the chromatin configuration and nuclear architecture of different regions of the genome [37,38], a view

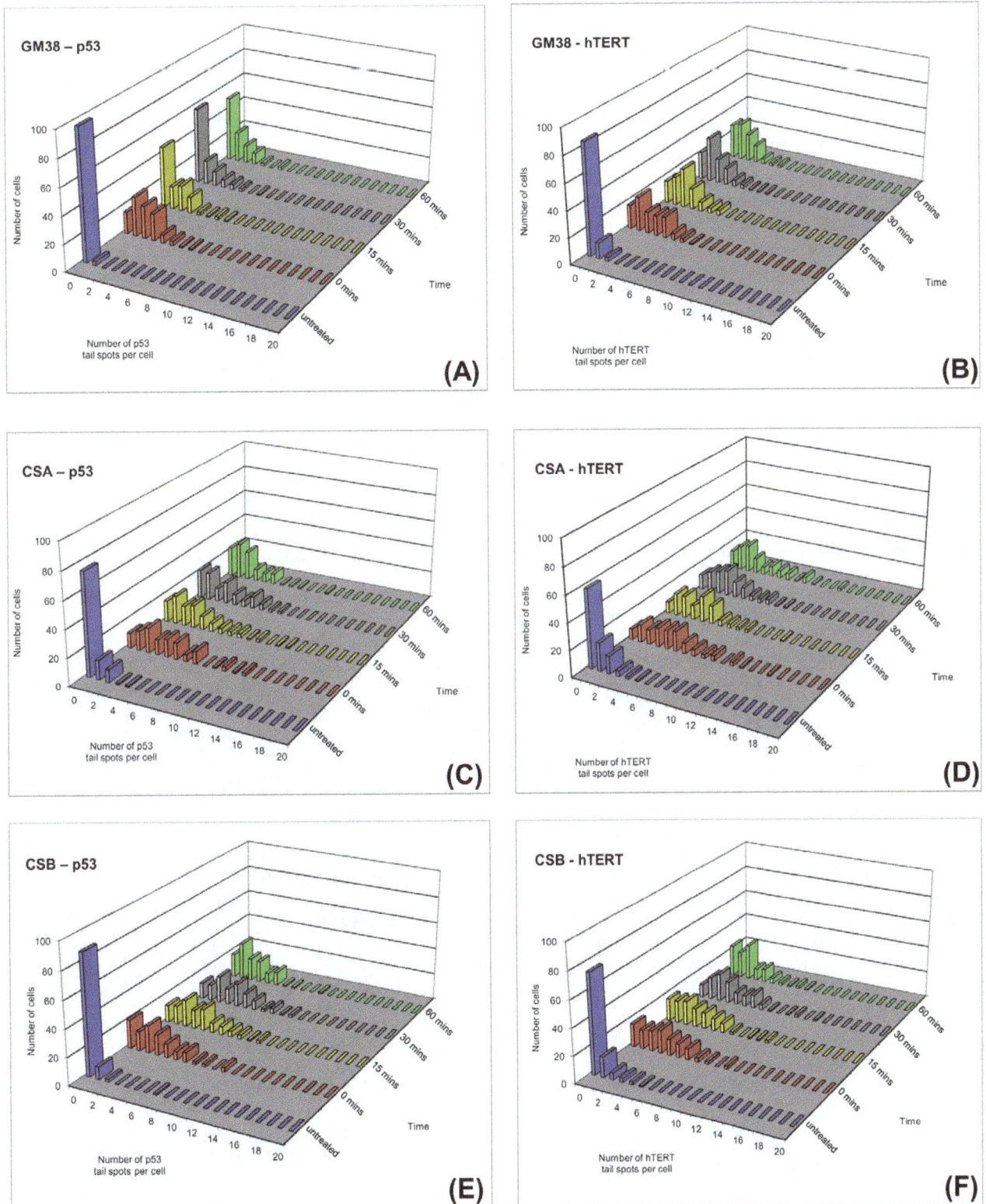

Figure 6. Frequency distribution analysis of p53 and hTERT hybridisation spot number at each repair time point following 5Gy γ-irradiation of fibroblasts. Each plot shows the number of p53 or hTERT tail spots per fibroblast in untreated cells and 0, 15, 30 and 60 minutes following irradiation. GM38 cells: (A) p53 (B) hTERT; CSA cells: (C) p53 (D) hTERT; CSB cells: (E) p53 (F) hTERT. For each cell line, the number of hybridisation signals detected in the tail is increased immediately after irradiation (t = 0). As repair occurs in GM38 fibroblasts, the number of cells displaying no p53 hybridisation spots in the comet tail is increased (see first bar in distribution profile). By contrast, the distribution profile of hTERT hybridisation spots remains relatively unaffected over the repair time. In CSA and CSB fibroblasts, no significant difference in the distribution profile is observed for either p53 or hTERT over the repair time-points.

supported by previous comet-FISH studies from our laboratory [22] and others [39]. Although active genes are normally found in a more open chromatin configuration than inactive regions, thereby enabling easier access for DNA repair proteins, the hTERT gene is known to be embedded in a condensed chromosomal region in various normal, immortal and cancer cell lines regardless of the status of hTERT expression [40]. It has also been suggested that hTERT transcription does not require global chromatin de-condensation but the loss of repressors of hTERT expression [40,41]. This repressive environment may limit the access to, and the binding of repair proteins to, the sites of damage. Indeed, this would explain why the hTERT gene region exhibits higher levels of damage than the p53 gene region during repair in our experiments and may also go some way to explaining why a number of untreated cells in our experiments showed significant damage in the hTERT gene region. It is possible that even the low amount of background DNA damage in these control cells was sufficient to affect particularly susceptible regions of the genome, such as the hTERT gene region. A final consideration for the high level of damage in the hTERT gene region is its very close location to telomeres at the extreme terminus of chromosome 5p [42]. Using the comet-FISH technique, telomeres were found to be more fragile compared to total DNA to particular cytostatics in both treated and non-treated cells [43]. It has been suggested that the location of most telomeres near the nuclear membrane may offer them a greater chance of migration following DNA damage [44].

Comparison of results from normal fibroblasts with CS fibroblasts presents some intriguing data and invites some speculation on TCR activity in these cells. Normal fibroblasts carry out rapid preferential repair of the active p53 gene region in comparison to the inactive hTERT gene region following γ-radiation exposure (Figure 5a). However, in CS cell lines the active p53 gene region is not preferentially repaired following γ-radiation and repairs at a rate similar to the inactive hTERT gene region and the overall genome (Figures 5b & 5c). Although the comet-FISH assay is not an established method for measuring TCR, it is tempting to propose that these observations reflect the TCR-defective status of CS cells, whereby overall genome repair can be carried out but the rapid preferential repair of actively transcribed genes cannot occur (e.g. in the p53 gene). If this is true, this raises some interesting questions since TCR is not normally associated with the repair of DNA damage induced by ionising radiation. However, it is worth noting that recent evidence has demonstrated that CSA and CSB proteins may have a role to play in DNA repair distinct from NER, since fibroblasts deficient in CSA or CSB have been shown to exhibit sensitivity to ionising radiation [45–49].

The results presented here would suggest that fibroblasts defective in CSA or CSB proteins do have reduced ability to repair strand breaks and DNA damage induced by ionising radiation. Whether this is due to defective TCR or not cannot be determined conclusively using the comet-FISH assay, but it would be interesting to see if this method could detect a similar lack of preferential repair in these fibroblasts following UV-radiation, which is more traditionally accepted to be linked to TCR.

It should be noted that, due to the size of the probes and the nature of the comet assay, we are precluded from stating categorically that damage and repair are occurring within a given gene. Rather, the assay enables us to conclude whether or not the damage and repair are occurring in the region including, and surrounding, the gene of interest. However, chromatin structure and rearrangement in the locality of the gene are likely to be important for efficient DNA repair, therefore investigation of DNA regions which include the gene of interest, as well as the individuals genes, is warranted. We also accept that the results probably reflect a number of cells in late S, G2 or mitosis, in which the relevant sequences have been replicated, accounting for those normal cells that show hybridisation spots. However, given the relatively short time-frame employed, this is evidently a small population of cells and would be presumably similar in each sampling. Therefore, we can still make comparison between samples.

In conclusion, we present evidence that the comet-FISH assay can detect differences in DNA repair between two separate gene regions in a variety of cell lines. It may be possible that this approach can be used to evaluate TCR and therefore will merit further investigation. From the results presented in this paper, however, it is clear that this assay is a promising technique that offers great potential for gaining further insight into the process of preferential repair in gene regions within cells. The ability to obtain such information increases the potential value of the Comet-FISH assay as the basis for a predictive test for radiosensitivity in a clinical setting.

Acknowledgments

The authors wish to thank Dr Dennis Simpson for the use of the hTERT-immortalised Werner Syndrome cell line.

Author Contributions

Conceived and designed the experiments: DJM CSD SRM VJM. Performed the experiments: BAD. Analyzed the data: DJM BAD SRM VJM. Contributed reagents/materials/analysis tools: DJM SRM VJM. Wrote the paper: DJM SRM VJM.

References

1. McKelvey-Martin VJ, Ho ETS, McKeown SR, Johnston SR, McCarthy PJ, et al. (1998) Emerging applications of the single cell gel electrophoresis (Comet) assay. IManagement of invasive transitional cell human bladder carcinoma II. Fluorescent in situ hybridization comets for the identification of damaged and repaired DNA sequences in individual cells. Mutagenesis 13: 1–8.

2. McKelvey-Martin VJ, McKenna DJ (2009) Development and Applications of the Comet-FISH Assay for the Study of DNA Damage and Repair. In: Dhawan A, Anderson D, editors. The Comet Assay in Toxicology. 129–150.

3. Filippi AR, Franco P, Ricardi U (2006) Is clinical radiosensitivity a complex genetically controlled event? Tumori 92: 87–91.

4. McKenna DJ, McKeown SR, McKelvey-Martin VJ (2008) Potential use of the Comet assay in the clinical management of cancer. Mutagenesis 23: 183–190.

5. Bjork-Eriksson T, West C, Karlsson E, Mercke C (2000) Tumor radiosensitivity (SF2) is a prognostic factor for local control in head and neck cancers. Int J Radiat Oncol Biol Phys 46: 13–19.

6. Alsner J, Hoyer M, Sorensen SB, Overgaard J (2001) Interaction between potential doubling time and TP53 mutation: predicting radiotherapy outcome in squamous cell carcinoma of the head and neck. Int J Radiat Oncol Biol Phys 49: 519–525.

7. Nordsmark M, Eriksen JG, Gebski V, Alsner J, Horsman MR, et al. (2007) Differential risk assessments from five hypoxia specific assays: the basis for biologically adapted individualized radiotherapy in advanced head and neck cancer patients. Radiother Oncol 83: 389–397.

8. Burcombe R, Wilson GD, Dowsett M, Khan I, Richman PI, et al. (2006) Evaluation of Ki-67 proliferation and apoptotic index before, during and after neoadjuvant chemotherapy for primary breast cancer. Breast Cancer Res 8: R31.

9. Tachibana M, Miyakawa A, Nakamura K, Baba S, Murai M, et al. (1996) Role of proliferative activity estimated by bromodeoxyuridine labeling index in determining predictive factors of recurrence in superficial intermediately malignant bladder tumors. J Urol 156: 63–69.

10. Komuro Y, Watanabe T, Tsurita G, Muto T, Nagawa H (2005) Evaluating the combination of molecular prognostic factors in tumor radiosensitivity in rectal cancer. Hepatogastroenterology 52: 666–671.

11. Kruse JJ, Stewart FA (2007) Gene expression arrays as a tool to unravel mechanisms of normal tissue radiation injury and prediction of response. World J Gastroenterol 13: 2669–2674.

12. McKeown SR, Robson T, Price ME, Ho ET, Hirst DG, et al. (2003) Potential use of the alkaline comet assay as a predictor of bladder tumour response to radiation. Br J Cancer 89: 2264–2270.

13. Dunne AL, Price ME, Mothersill C, McKeown SR, Robson T, et al. (2003) Relationship between clonogenic radiosensitivity, radiation-induced apoptosis and DNA damage/repair in human colon cancer cells. Br J Cancer 89: 2277–2283.

14. Moneef MA, Sherwood BT, Bowman KJ, Kockelbergh RC, Symonds RP, et al. (2003) Measurements using the alkaline comet assay predict bladder cancer cell radiosensitivity. Br J Cancer 89: 2271–2276.

15. Eastham AM, Marples B, Kiltie AE, Orton CJ, West CM (1999) Fibroblast radiosensitivity measured using the comet DNA-damage assay correlates with clonogenic survival parameters. Br J Cancer 79: 1366–1371.

16. Calabretta B, Kaczmarek L, Selleri L, Torelli G, Ming PM, et al. (1986) Growth-dependent expression of human Mr 53,000 tumor antigen messenger RNA in normal and neoplastic cells. Cancer Res 46: 5738–5742.

17. McKay BC, Ljungman M, Rainbow AJ (1999) Potential roles for p53 in nucleotide excision repair. Carcinogenesis 20: 1389–1396.

18. Evans MK, Taffe BG, Curtis CH, Bohr VA (1993) DNA strand bias in the repair of the p53 gene in normal human and xeroderma pigmentosum group C fibroblasts. Cancer Res 53: 5377–5381.

19. de Kok JB, Ruers TJ, van Muijen GN, van Bokhoven A, Willems HL, et al. (2000) Real-time quantification of human telomerase reverse transcriptase mRNA in tumors and healthy tissues. Clin Chem 46: 313–318.

20. Hiyama E, Hiyama K (2003) Telomerase as tumor marker. Cancer Lett 194: 221–33.

21. McKenna DJ, Rajab NF, McKeown SR, McKerr G, McKelvey-Martin VJ (2003) Use of the comet-FISH assay to demonstrate repair of the p53 gene region in two human bladder carcinoma cell lines. Radiat Res 159: 49–56.

22. McKenna DJ, Gallus M, McKeown SR, Downes CS, McKelvey-Martin VJ (2003) Modification of the alkaline comet assay to allow simultaneous evaluation of mitomycin C-induced DNA cross-link damage and repair of specific DNA sequences in RT4 cells. DNA Repair 2: 879–890.

23. Tan YH, Chou EL, Lundh N (1975) Regulation of chromosome 21-directed anti-viral gene(s) as a consequence of age. Nature. 257: 310–312.

24. Marshall CJ, Franks LM, Carbonell AW (1977) Markers of neoplastic transformation in epithelial cell lines derived from human carcinomas. J Natl Cancer Inst. 58: 1743–51.

25. Rigby CC, Franks LM (1970) A human tissue culture cell line from a transitional cell tumour of the urinary bladder: growth, chromosone pattern and ultrastructure. Br J Cancer 24: 746–754.

26. Ouellette MM, McDaniel LD, Wright WE, Shay JW, Schultz RA (2000) The establishment of telomerase-immortalized cell lines representing human chromosome instability syndromes. Hum Mol Genet 9: 403–411.

27. Tong Z, Singh G, Rainbow AJ (2000) The role of the p53 tumor suppressor in the response of human cells to photofrin-mediated photodynamic therapy. Photochem Photobiol 71: 201–10.

28. Hinata N, Shirakawa T, Zhang Z, Matsumoto A, Fujisawa M, et al. (2003) Radiation induces p53-dependent cell apoptosis in bladder cancer cells with wild-type- p53 but not in p53-mutated bladder cancer cells. Urol Res 31: 387–396.

29. Warenius HM, Jones M, Gorman T, McLeish R, Seabra L, et al. (2000) Combined RAF1 protein expression and p53 mutational status provides a strong predictor of cellular radiosensitivity. Br J Cancer 83: 1084–1095.

30. Abdul-Ghani R, Ohana P, Matouk I, Ayesh S, Ayesh B, et al. (2000) Use of transcriptional regulatory sequences of telomerase (hTER and hTERT) for selective killing of cancer cells. Mol Therapy 2: 539–544.

31. Spivak G, Cox RA, Hanawalt PC (2009) New applications of the Comet assay: Comet-FISH and transcription-coupled DNA repair. Mutat Res 681: 44–50.

32. Horvathova E, Dusinska M, Shaposhnikov S, Collins AR (2004) DNA damage and repair measured in different genomic regions using the comet assay with fluorescent in situ hybridization. Mutagenesis 19: 269–276.

33. Bohr VA, Smith CA, Okumotao DS, Hanawalt PC (1985) DNA repair in an active gene: removal of pyrimidine dimmers from the DHFR gene of CHO cells is much more efficient than in the genome overall. Cell 40: 359–369.

34. Boulikas T (1996) The non-uniform repair of active and inactive chromatin domains. Int J Oncol 8: 65–75.

35. Tornaletti S, Pfeifer GP (1994) Slow repair of pyrimidine dimmers at p53 mutation hotspots in skin cancer. Science 263: 1436–1438.

36. Hu W, Feng Z, Chasin LA, Tang M (2002) Transcription-coupled and transcription-independent repair of cyclobutane pyrimidine dimers in the dihydrofolate reductase gene. J Biol Chem 277: 38305–38310.

37. Feng Z, Hu W, Chasin LA, Tang MS (2003) Effects of genomic context and chromatin structure on transcription-coupled and global genomic repair in mammalian cells. Nucleic Acids Res 31: 5897–5906.

38. Lukas J, Lukas C, Bartek J (2011) More than just a focus: The chromatin response to DNA damage and its role in genome integrity maintenance. Nat Cell Biol 13: 1161–9.

39. Rapp A, Bock C, Dittmar H, Greulich KO (2000) UV-A breakage sensitivity of human chromosomes as measured by COMET-FISH depends on gene density and not on the chromosome size. J Photochem Photobiol B 56: 109–117.

40. Wang S, Zhu J (2004) The hTERT gene is embedded in a nuclease-resistant chromatin domain. J Biol Chem 279: 55401–55410.

41. Szutorisz H, Lingner J, Cuthbert AP, Trott DA, Newbold RF, et al. (2003) A chromosome 3-encoded repressor of the human telomerase reverse transcriptase (hTERT) gene controls the state of hTERT chromatin. Cancer Res 63: 689–695.

42. Bryce LA, Morrison N, Hoare SF, Muir S, Keith WN (2000) Mapping of the gene for the human reverse transcriptase, htert, to chromosome 5p15.3 by fluorescence in situ hybridization. Neoplasia 2: 197–201.

43. Arutyunyan R, Rapp A, Greulich KO, Hovhannisyan G, Haroutiunian S, et al. (2005) Fragility of telomeres after bleomycin and cisplatin combined treatment measured in human leukocytes with the Comet-FISH technique. Exp Oncol 27: 38–42.

44. Glei M, Hovhannisyan G, Pool-Zobel BL (2009) Use of Comet-FISH in the study of DNA damage and repair: Review. Mutat Res 681: 33–43.

45. de Waard H, de Wit J, Andressoo JO, van Oostrom CT, Riis B, et al. (2004) Different effects of CSA and CSB deficiency on sensitivity to oxidative DNA damage. Mol Cell Biol 24: 7941–7948.

46. de Waard H, de Wit J, Gorgels TG, van den Aardweg G, Andressoo JO, et al. (2003) Cell type-specific hypersensitivity to oxidative damage in CSB and XPA mice. DNA Repair (Amst) 2: 13–25.

47. Tuo J, Jaruga P, Rodriguez H, Bohr VA, Dizdaroglu M (2003) Primary fibroblasts of Cockayne syndrome patients are defective in cellular repair of 8-hydroxyguanine and 8-hydroxyadenine resulting from oxidative stress. FASEB J 17: 668–674.

48. Gorgels TG, van der Pluijm I, Brandt RM, Garinis GA, van Steeg H, et al. (2007) Retinal degeneration and ionizing radiation hypersensitivity in a mouse model for Cockayne syndrome. Mol Cell Biol 27: 1433–1441.

49. Cramers P, Verhoeven EE, Filon AR, Rockx DA, Santos SJ, et al. (2011) Impaired repair of ionizing radiation-induced DNA damage in Cockayne Syndrome cells. Radiat Res 175: 432–443.

14

Cell-Free Urinary MicroRNA-99a and MicroRNA-125b are Diagnostic Markers for the Non-Invasive Screening of Bladder Cancer

Ding-Zuan Zhang[1], Kin-Mang Lau[2], Eddie S. Y. Chan[1], Gang Wang[3], Cheuk-Chun Szeto[3], Kenneth Wong[4], Richard K. W. Choy[4], Chi-Fai Ng[1]*

1 Division of Urology, Department of Surgery, The Chinese University of Hong Kong, Hong Kong SAR, China, 2 Department of Anatomical and Cellular Pathology, The Chinese University of Hong Kong, Hong Kong SAR, China, 3 Division of Nephrology, Department of Medicine and Therapeutic, The Chinese University of Hong Kong, Hong Kong SAR, China, 4 Department of Obstetrics & Gynaecology, The Chinese University of Hong Kong, Hong Kong SAR, China

Abstract

Background: Evidence implicated the diagnostic significance of microRNAs in whole urine/urine sediments in urothelial carcinoma of the bladder (UCB). However, the contaminated blood cells in patients with haematouria significantly altered the expression profiles of urinary microRNA, influencing the test accuracy.

Methods: MicroRNA profiles of the urine supernatants of UCB patients and controls without any malignancy and profiles of malignant and corresponding normal mucosa tissues from the patients were determined by microRNA microarray and compared to identify differentially expressed microRNAs. The differential expression was verified in the tissues of an independent patient cohort by RT-qPCR. The diagnostic significance of selected microRNAs as biomarkers in the urine supernatant was investigated in the expanded cohorts.

Results: MicroRNA-99a and microRNA-125b were down-regulated in the urine supernatants of UCB patients. The degree of down-regulation was associated with the tumor grade. A diagnostic model was developed using a combined index of the levels of microRNA-99a and microRNA-125b in the urine supernatant with a sensitivity of 86.7%, a specificity of 81.1% and a positive predicted value (PPV) of 91.8%. Discriminating between high- and low-grade UCB, the model using the level of microRNA-125b alone exhibited a sensitivity of 81.4%, a specificity of 87.0% and a PPV of 93.4%.

Conclusions: The results revealed a unique microRNA expression signature in the urine supernatants of UCB patients for the development of molecular diagnostic tests. An effective cell-free urinary microRNA-based model was developed using a combined index of the levels of microRNA-99a and microRNA-125b to detect UCB with good discriminating power, high sensitivity and high specificity.

Editor: Rajvir Dahiya, UCSF / VA Medical Center, United States of America

Funding: This study was supported by the Direct Grant for Research (2009.1.096), The Chinese University of Hong Kong. The funders had no role in study design, data collection and analysis, decision to publish, or preparation of the manuscript.

Competing Interests: The authors have declared that no competing interests exist.

* Email: ngcf@surgery.cuhk.edu.hk

Introduction

Urothelial carcinoma of the bladder (UCB) is the second most common malignancy in the urinary system [1]. Due to its high incidence and frequent recurrence, effective diagnostic and disease monitoring tools are essential for the clinical management of patients. Cystoscopy is currently the standard clinical test for diagnosis and cancer surveillance. However, the procedure is invasive and unpleasant, and has several practical limitations. For example, it may not be able to detect small and/or flat tumors like carcinoma *in situ*. Therefore, an alternative non-invasive approach exhibiting high specificity and sensitivity is required. Although many blood- and urine-based biomarkers have been identified and evaluated in the literature, none have been ideal and powerful enough to replace cystoscopy [2].

MicroRNAs, which are small non-coding RNAs, have recently demonstrated significant diagnostic and prognostic value in various types of cancer [3–5]. MicroRNAs exhibit high stability and easy detectability even at low levels in various types of clinical samples [6–8]. It is considered an excellent disease biomarker for detection and monitoring. One study demonstrated that a number of microRNAs were aberrantly expressed in UCB tumor tissues and that these aberrations could be engaged in diagnosis and the staging of bladder cancer biopsies [9]. In addition, the assessment of the levels of these aberrantly expressed microRNAs that show unique signatures in whole urine or urine exfoliated cells is even more promising for the diagnosis and disease surveillance of UCB [10–11]. However, the results are sometimes unreliable when studying patients with haematuria, in whom contaminated blood cells significantly alter the urinary microRNA profiles and thus mask the signatures. In fact, 85% of patients exhibit varying degrees of haematuria [12–13]. As a result, an alternative approach to measuring microRNAs is required. Evidence has suggested that free nucleic acids, such as DNA biomarkers in urine supernatants, provide a higher detection rate and higher sensitivity than those in sediment for UCB diagnosis [14–16]. Therefore, assessment of the levels of microRNAs in urine supernatant could improve the use of microRNAs as diagnostic biomarkers for detecting UCB, especially in patients with haematuria. In this study, the feasibility of using cell-free urinary microRNAs for diagnosing UCB was determined and models for diagnosing UCB and discriminating tumor grades were developed.

Methods

Patients and samples

An overview of this study is shown in Figure S1. With the written consent of the donors and the approval of the Joint Chinese University of Hong Kong - New Territories East Cluster Clinical Research Ethics Committee, tissue and urine samples were collected in the Urology Unit, Department of Surgery, Prince of Wales Hospital, Hong Kong. Mid-stream urine was collected from bladder cancer patients before surgery. Both tumor tissue and normal bladder mucosa located >3 cm away from the tumor edge were obtained by cystoscopy. The 1973 WHO diagnosis and grading system for bladder cancer [17] was used for diagnosis. For the normal controls, urine samples were collected from patients who had normal cystoscopic findings, absence of malignancies with a >6 months follow-up and haematuria. All of the urine samples were centrifuged at 2,500 r.c.f. for 20 minutes and the urine supernatants were collected.

MicroRNA microarray

The total RNA of the urine supernatants and frozen tissue was extracted using the MirVanaPARIS Kit (Ambion) in accordance with the manufacturer's recommended protocols. The Agilent Human miRNA Microarray Chip (Release 13.0, Agilent Technologies, Santa Clara, CA, U.S.A.), which encompasses 866 human microRNAs and 89 viral microRNAs, was used to profile the expression of these microRNAs in the urine supernatants and cancer and control tissues. The dataset was deposited to ArrayExpress (https://www.ebi.ac.uk/arrayexpress/) and the accession number is E-MTAB-2573. The signal intensity of each spot was median-normalized and further normalized by linear regression.

Reverse transcription-quantitative polymerase chain reaction (RT-qPCR)

First strand cDNA was synthesized from the total RNA of the urine supernatants and tissue samples using a universal cDNA synthesis kit (Exiqon, Vedbaek, Denmark) in accordance with the manufacturer's recommended protocol. The resultant cDNA was subjected to quantitative polymerase chain reaction (qPCR) with SYBR Green master mix and microRNA LNA PCR primer (Exiqon) that specifically recognized the targeted microRNA in an ABI 7900HT fast RT-qPCR machine (Applied Biosystem/Life Technologies, Grand Island, NY, U.S.A.). RNU6B was used as the reference control. All of the samples were tested in duplicate. The relative level of microRNA was determined using the $\Delta\Delta C_q$ method.

Statistical methods

The microarray data were analyzed using the Gene Spring 11.0 software (Agilent) to normalize and identify the differentially expressed microRNAs. ABI SDS 2.3 software (ABI/Life Technologies) was used to analyze the RT-qPCR data. The quantitative data were subjected to a Mann-Whitney U test and a Wilcoxon signed-rank test using the SPSS 16.0 software (IBM Co, Armonk, NY, U.S.A.). In subsequent post-hoc analysis, a bivariate logistic regression analysis was performed to determine the Combined Index (CI) for the combination of two microRNAs expression levels. A receiver operating characteristic (ROC) curve analysis was carried out using the SPSS 16.0 software. The sensitivity, specificity, positive and negative predictive values, and positive and negative likelihood ratios were calculated.

Results

Identification of differentially expressed microRNAs between the urine supernatants of UCB patients and controls and between cancer and normal tissues by microRNA microarray

Urine supernatants from six UCB patients and three normal controls together with four pairs of UCB tissues and their corresponding normal bladder mucosal tissues were subjected to microRNA microarray analysis. The patient characteristics are shown in Table 1. To determine the presence and absence of microRNAs in the samples, a threshold signal was defined as the average background plus three standard deviations. Signals above this threshold were considered a "presence" and signals below the threshold were considered an "absence." After global normalization, 117 ± 63.8 out of 866 human microRNAs were detected in the urine supernatants and 314 ± 83.4 microRNAs were detected in the bladder tissues. There was no significant difference in the total number of microRNAs detected between the urine supernatants from cancer patients and controls and between the cancer and control tissues. Comparing the profiles in the urine supernatants of the UCB patients with those of the normal controls, 39 microRNAs showed differential expression (Mann-Whitney test, $p<0.05$; fold differences >1.60). There were 78 differentially expressed microRNAs between the cancer and normal tissues (paired Mann-Whitney test, $p<0.05$; fold differences >2.0). Ten microRNAs were commonly dysregulated in both the urine supernatants and tissue samples (Figure 1 and Figure S1). Of these, the levels of microRNA-1, microRNA-99a, microRNA-125b, microRNA-133a, microRNA-133b, microRNA-143 and microRNA-1207-5p significantly decreased and those of microRNA-16, microRNA-96 and microRNA-183 increased in the UCB samples (Figure 1).

Validation of the 10 selected microRNAs in independent cohorts of tissue and urine supernatant samples

To validate the microarray results, the levels of the 10 selected microRNAs were quantified by RT-qPCR in another 18 pairs of bladder cancer and corresponding normal mucosa tissues (Table 1). Of these, the differential expression of six microRNAs between cancer and normal tissues was validated (Wilcoxon signed-rank two-related-samples test, $p<0.05$) (Figure 2). MicroRNA-1 was down-regulated in all 18 pairs of cancer tissues ($p<0.01$) and 17 out of 18 pairs showed down-regulation ($p<0.01$) in the remaining five microRNAs (microRNA-99a, microRNA-125b, microRNA-133a, microRNA-133b and microRNA-143). MicroRNA-1, microRNA-99a, microRNA-125b, microRNA-133a, microRNA-133b and microRNA-143 were down-regulated 266.87 ± 2.06, 130.69 ± 2.30, 49.52 ± 3.39, 263.20 ± 1.99, 261.38 ± 2.11 and 67.18 ± 1.83 times over in the cancer tissues, respectively.

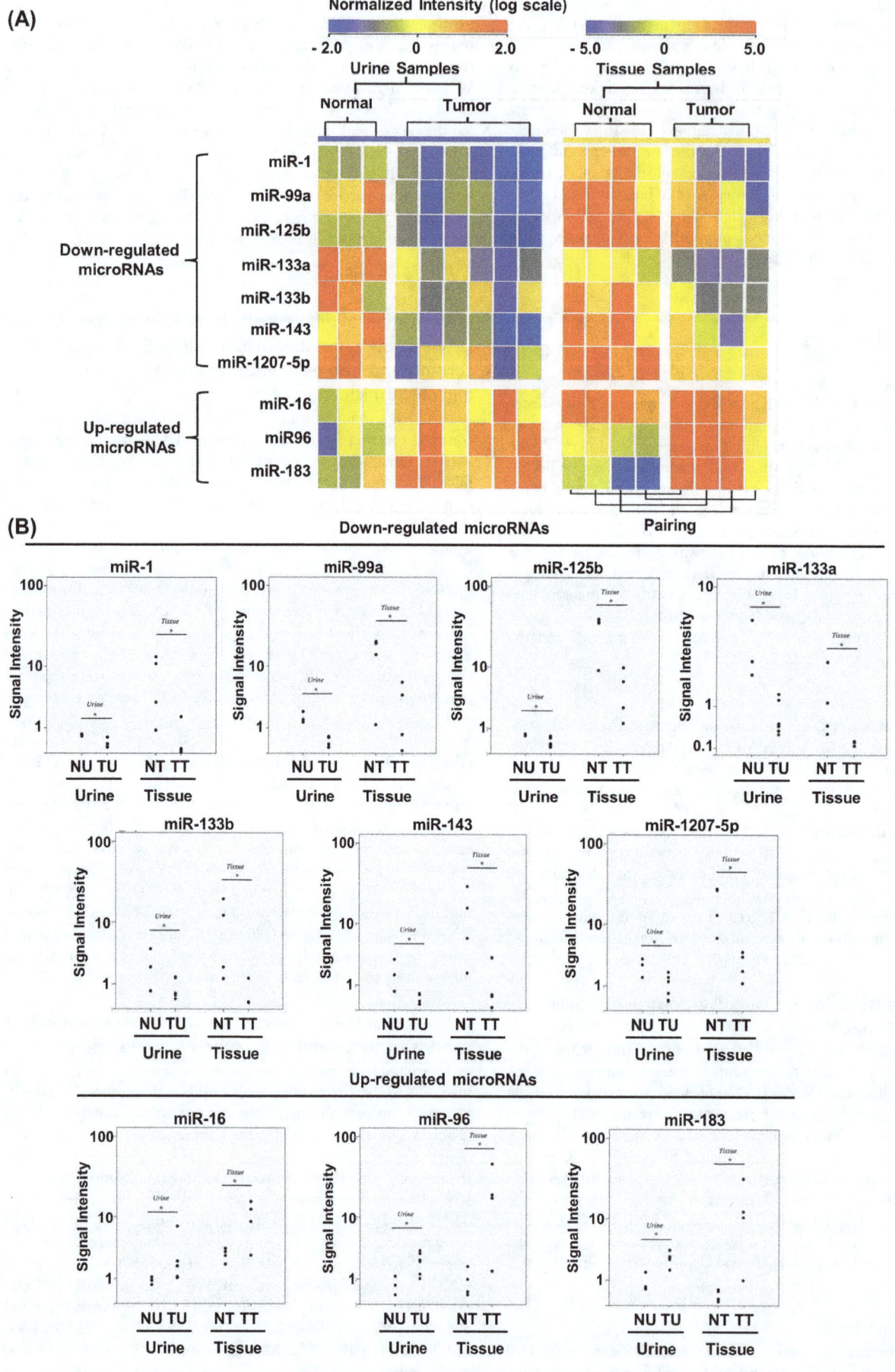

Figure 1. Results of microRNA microarray analysis. (A) Heat map of the levels of 10 selected microRNAs in nine urine supernatant samples and four pairs of tissue samples. The total RNA was extracted and subjected to microRNA microarray analysis using an Agilent Human microRNA Microarray Chip. The signal intensity of each spot was median-normalized and further normalized by linear regression. The normalized signal intensities for each microRNA in the urine supernatant and tissue samples of UCB patients and controls are presented. (D) Scatter plots of the normalized signal sensitivities of the 10 selected microRNAs. A Mann-Whitney U test was conducted to compare the levels of microRNAs in the urine supernatant of UCB patients (TU) (n = 6) and controls (NU) (n = 3), and a paired Mann-Whitney U test was conducted to compare the tumors (TT) (n = 4) and their corresponding normal mucosa tissues (NT) (n = 4) in the UCB patients. A significance level of 0.01 was used for all of the comparisons. Asterisks (*) indicate a statistically significant difference (p<0.01).

The discrimination power of the six validated microRNAs in the urine supernatants was then assessed using 71 urine supernatant samples, including 50 samples from bladder cancer patients (15 cases of low-grade cancer and 35 cases of high-grade cancer) and 21 samples from controls (Table 1). In this expanded set of samples, the urine supernatants of the UCB patients possessed lower levels of microRNA-99a (p<0.01), microRNA-125b (p< 0.01), microRNA-133b (p<0.05) and microRNA-143 (p<0.01) than that of the controls (Figure 3A), but not of microRNA-133a and microRNA-1.

Development of cell-free urinary microRNA models for the detection of UCB and the discrimination of tumor grades

The ROC curve was determined to evaluate the diagnostic strength of these microRNAs in detecting UCB. High area under the curve (AUC) values were found for microRNA-99a (0.800, ranging from 0.715 to 0.886) and microRNA-125b (0.813, ranging from 0.729 to 0.897) (Figure 3B), whereas microRNA-133b and microRNA-143 exhibited low diagnostic strength with AUC values around 0.6. To further determine the diagnostic significance of microRNA-99a and microRNA-125b, related cut-off points were determined from the ROC curves based on Youden's Index rule. The cut-off points for the normalized expression levels of microRNA-99a and microRNA-125b were $2^{2.18}$ and $2^{4.1}$, respectively. A patient with a urine supernatant whose microRNA level was lower than or equal to the cut-off point was considered a cancer case, and considered normal if the level was higher than the cut-off point. According to this system, the sensitivity, specificity, positive prediction value (PPV), negative prediction value (NPV), positive likelihood (LR+) and negative likelihood (LR-) for microRNA-99a were 78.0%, 85.7%, 92.7%, 61.0%, 5.46 and 0.26, respectively, and for microRNA-125b were 84.8%, 76.2%, 89.3%, 68.1%, 3.57 and 0.20, respectively (Table 2). To achieve better diagnostic performance, a combination of the expressions of microRNA-99a and microRNA-125b was subjected to a bivariate logistic regression. The CI performed better than the use of each microRNA alone. The AUC value increased to 0.876. The CI formula was CI = $1/\{1+\exp[-(2.332+0.425 \ x\Delta Cq_{microRNA-125b}+ 0.069 \ x\Delta Cq_{microRNA-99a})]\}$. When the cut-off point was set at 0.6244 based on Youden's Index rule, the prediction system improved with an increased sensitivity (86.7%) and NPV (71.4%) and a decreased LR- (0.16), with comparable values for the specificity, PPV and LR+ (Table 2).

The clinical relevance of the four microRNAs selected to discriminate low-grade from high-grade cancers was also assessed. The levels of urinary microRNA-99a and microRNA-125b were significant lower in patients with high-grade cancers (G2 and G3) than in those with low-grade cancers (G1) (Mann-Whitney U test, p<0.01). The levels of microRNA-133b and microRNA-143 showed no tumor grade discrimination value (Figure 3A). The AUC values differentiating between high- and low-grade cancers for microRNA-99a and microRNA-125b were 0.819 and 0.791, respectively (Figure 3B). The cut-off points of the normalized levels

of microRNA-99a and microRNA-125b for tumor grading were $2^{1.71}$ and $2^{0.91}$, respectively. Based on these cut-off points, the system using the level of microRNA-99a exhibited a sensitivity of 74.2%, a specificity of 83.3%, a PPV of 91.5%, an NPV of 58.1%, an LR+ of 4.46 and an LR- of 0.31. In the case of microRNA-125b, these values were 81.4%, 87.0%, 93.4%, 67.0%, 6.11 and 0.21, respectively, for discriminating tumor grades (Table 2). When combining the levels of microRNA-99a and microRNA-125b in the system, the CI formula became CI = $1/\{1+\exp[-(1.742 +0.0295 x\Delta Cq_{microRNA-125b} +0.496 x\Delta Cq_{microRNA-99a})]\}$, with 0.7398 as the cut-off point. The sensitivity, specificity, PPV, NPV, LR+ and LR- were 79.4%, 88.0%, 94.7%, 61.1%, 6.61 and 0.23, respectively (Table 2). All of these values were either comparable with or lower than those for the systems using either microRNA-99a or microRNA-125b alone. Taken altogether, the system using microRNA-125b alone performed better at differentiating between high- and low-grade UCB.

Correlation between expressions of microRNA-99a and microRNA-125b in urine supernatants and bladder cancer and control tissues

Via a Pearson correlation analysis, the microRNA-99a and microRNA-125b levels in both the tissues and urine supernatants of the patients and controls were highly correlated (R = 0.896, p< 0.001 for the tissue samples; R = 0.982, p<0.001 for the urine supernatant samples) (Figure 3C), suggesting that their expression may have been co-regulated. In fact, these genes were clustered at the q21.1 region of chromosome 21 (Figure 3D).

Restoration of microRNA-99a and microRNA-125b expressions in post-operative patients

To demonstrate the crucial link between bladder cancer status and decreased microRNA-99a and microRNA-125b levels in the urine supernatants, these two microRNAs were quantified in the urine supernatants of pre-operative and post-operative patients. Twenty patients were recruited (Table 1). Post-operative urine was collected 4 weeks after a transurethral resection. After the resection, the patients were able to restore the microRNA-99a and microRNA-125b levels in the urine supernatant (Wilcoxon signed-rank two-related-samples test, p<0.01) (Figure 4) to levels comparable with those of the normal control samples (Figure S2).

Discussion

This study developed an effective cell-free urinary microRNA-based model for detecting UCB with good discriminating power (AUC = 0.876) and high sensitivity (86.7%) and specificity (81.1%). The feasibility of using urinary microRNAs as bladder cancer diagnostic biomarkers was previously investigated. The ratio of microRNA-126 to microRNA-152 in urine was studied to detect UCB at a sensitivity of 82% and a specificity of 72%, with an AUC value of 0.768 [7]. By studying the expression levels of microRNA-96 and microRNA-183 in urine sediment, tests using these two microRNA biomarkers independently showed sensitiv-

Table 1. Patient characteristics.

Characteristics	microRNA microarray			qRT-PCR			qRT-PCR
	Tissues (TT and NT)	Urine supernatant		Tissues (TT and NT)	Urine supernatant		Urine supernatant - pre- and post-operative
		TU	CU		TU	CU	
Total number	4 pairs	6	3	18 Pairs	50	21	20 pairs
Median age	74	71	62	71	75	65	75
(years old)	(58–81)	(58–81)	(61–70)	(45–88)	(43–85)	(32–87)	(43–85)
Gender							
Male	3	5	2	17	10	13	14
Female	1	1	1	1	40	8	6
Stage							
Superficial	2	2	-	8	41	-	17
Invasive	2	4	-	10	9	-	3
Grade							
Low grade (G1)	1	1	-	2	15	-	5
High grade (≥G2)	3	5	-	16	35	-	15
Tumor status							
New case	3	3	-	12	27	-	9
Recurrent case	1	5	-	6	23	-	11

TT: cancer tissue; NT: normal mucosa tissue; TU: urine supernatant from tumor patient; CU: urine supernatant from control.

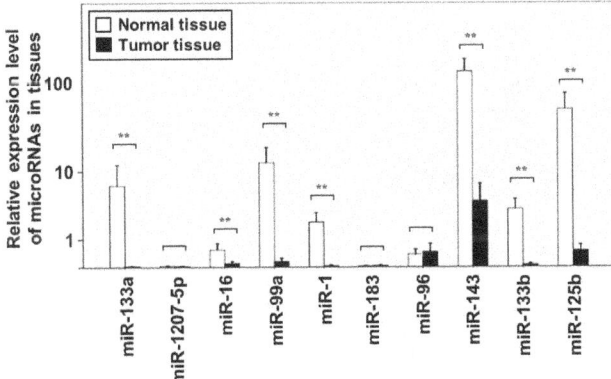

Figure 2. Validation study of the down-regulated expression of 10 selected microRNAs in bladder cancer tissues by RT-qPCR. The total RNA was extracted from 18 pairs of bladder cancer tissues and their corresponding normal adjacent mucosa tissues. The levels of these microRNAs were quantified by RT-qPCR in duplicate. The relative expression levels (2-ΔCq) are presented. A paired Mann-Whitney U test was conducted to compare the tumors and their corresponding normal mucosa tissues in UCB patients. Columns, Means; Bars, S.D.; n = 18. ** denotes p<0.001.

ities of 71% and 74%, specificities of 89% and 77% and AUC values of 0.8331 and 0.817, respectively [18]. Using the CI of the microRNA-99a and microRNA-125b levels in urine supernatant here significantly improved the effectiveness of the diagnostic test for UCB detection. Moreover, the diagnostic performance was better than that of commercially available urine-based biomarkers (Table S1).

Unlike mRNA, which is vulnerable to environmental RNase, microRNAs are relatively stable in clinical samples. MicroRNAs remain intact even under unfavorable conditions such as high temperatures, extreme pH levels and 10 freeze-thaw cycles [6]. Moreover, they are readily detected in human plasma or serum by RT-qPCR, even at very low levels [7–8]. Tumor-associated changes to microRNA expression profiles in the circulation system have provided a new approach for cancer diagnosis and prognosis. In 2008, Lawrie et al. [19] reported that an elevated microRNA-21 serum level was associated with the relapse-free survival of patients with diffuse large B-cell lymphoma. Ng et al. [20] demonstrated the diagnostic significance of plasma microRNAs in colorectal cancer screening. These studies indicated the potential of circulating microRNAs in serum/plasma as biomarkers for cancer detection. In addition to serum/plasma, microRNAs are very stable in urine [17–18] and thus the detection of intact microRNAs in urine is promising. Wang et al. [21] identified cell-free urinary microRNA-146a and microRNA-155 as effective diagnostic biomarkers for systemic lupus erythematosus, implicating the clinical significance of cell-free urinary microRNAs in disease diagnosis and possibly prognosis. Although the yield of microRNAs from urine supernatant is relatively low compared with those from whole urine or urine sediment, urine supernatant is considered the best choice as a biomarker for disease diagnosis and prognosis [21]. Comparing the usefulness of urinary DNA in supernatant and sediment for UCB detection, Szarvas et al. [11] simultaneously analyzed urinary DNA in supernatants and sediment in patients and compared them to controls. Their results indicated that the urine supernatants yielded higher sensitivity than the sediment [11]. This was probably related to the contamination of blood cells in the urine samples of haematuria patients. The contaminated blood cells may have altered the urinary microRNA/DNA profiles in the samples and thus interfered with the cancer detection classification. In contrast, even the urine supernatants from patients with gross haematuria were relatively more homogeneous without interference due to the contaminated blood cells in the microRNA profiles. Therefore, urine supernatants may provide more convenient, reliable specimens for cancer diagnosis and disease monitoring.

Urinary microRNA profiles are subjected to various modifications such as the direct release of microRNAs from cancer tissues, immune responses to cancer and blood cells from haematuria patients. A feasibility study involving a candidate microRNA approach by qPCR was conducted to examine a small panel of microRNAs in the urine supernatants of bladder cancer patients [22]. Here, comprehensive microRNA profiles were obtained with microRNA microarrays of cell-free urine supernatants from UCB patients and controls who were confirmed to have no cystological abnormalities or other concurrent malignancies, and were compared to identify differentially expressed cell-free urinary microRNAs for UCB. The microRNAs were made a focus due to their direct release from cancer tissue and the levels of these candidates in cancer tissues and their normal counterparts were compared to validate the tissues. The microRNAs identified are probably functionally involved in UCB development and/or disease progression. They can be used as biomarkers for detection and disease monitoring. The microRNA microarray analysis results indicated the presence of more than 100 microRNAs in the urine supernatants. Among these, there were more down-regulated microRNAs than up-regulated microRNAs in the cancer patients' urine supernatants. This finding was similar to a previous finding that the majority of differentially expressed microRNAs in bladder cancer tissues were down-regulated [23]. These down-regulated microRNAs may play tumor suppressive roles in carcinogenesis [24]. The altered expression of six microRNA candidates identified by comparisons of the urinary cell-free microRNA profiles of UCB patients and controls were also observed in bladder tumor tissue in. Using an independent set of urine samples, the down-regulated expressions of four microRNAs were confirmed. As tumor tissue can directly secrete microRNAs into a patient's plasma [25], it is likely that urinary microRNAs are originally secreted by bladder cancer tissues and/or released from the necrotic/apoptotic malignant and even non-malignant epithelial cells, molding the microRNA profiles of urine supernatants. Thus, the expression patterns of various microRNAs in bladder cancer cells could be reflected by their urine supernatant profiles. However, not all of the differentially expressed microRNAs in cancer tissues can be used as urinary diagnostic biomarkers for UCB. The expressions of microRNA-1 and microRNA-133a were previously reported to be down-regulated in bladder cancer tissues and showed functional significance in carcinogenesis via targeting TAGLN2 in the cancer cells [26]. In the present study, their levels in the urine supernatant were examined, but no statistically significant difference was shown between the cancer patients and controls. This may imply other confounding factors such as the release of microRNAs from normal urinary epithelial cells and immune cells molding the microRNA profile in the urine supernatants to mask the differential expression of some cancer-related microRNAs.

Of the four microRNAs, microRNA-99a and microRNA-125b had the largest AUC values in the ROC curves for detection and could function as diagnostic biomarkers for bladder cancer. They were also found to be more significantly down-regulated in high-grade UCB than in low-grade UCB. After a complete transurethral resection of the tumors, the levels of previously down-regulated microRNA-99a and microRNA-125b in the urine

(A)

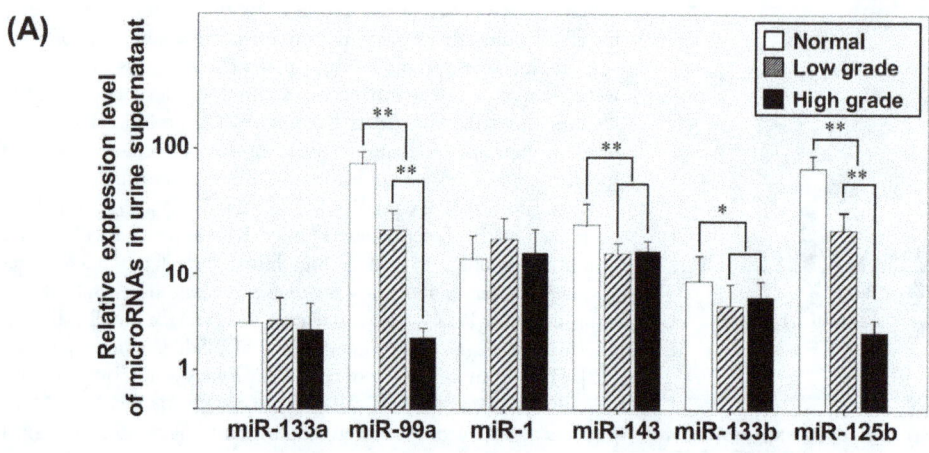

(B)

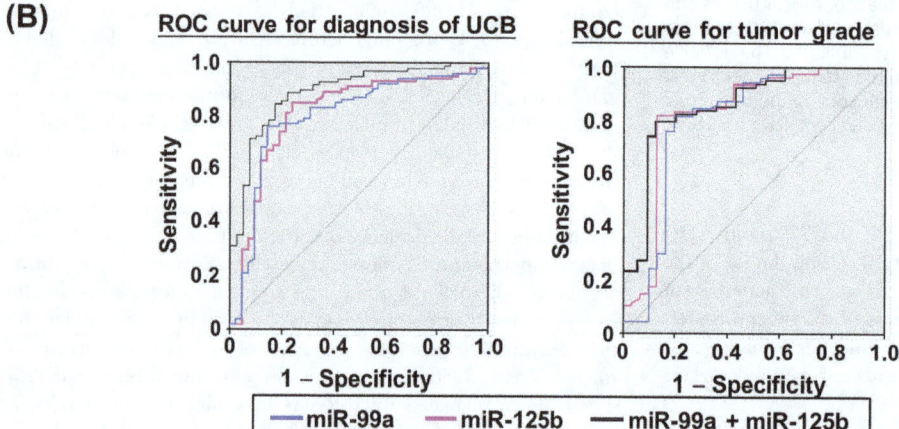

(C)

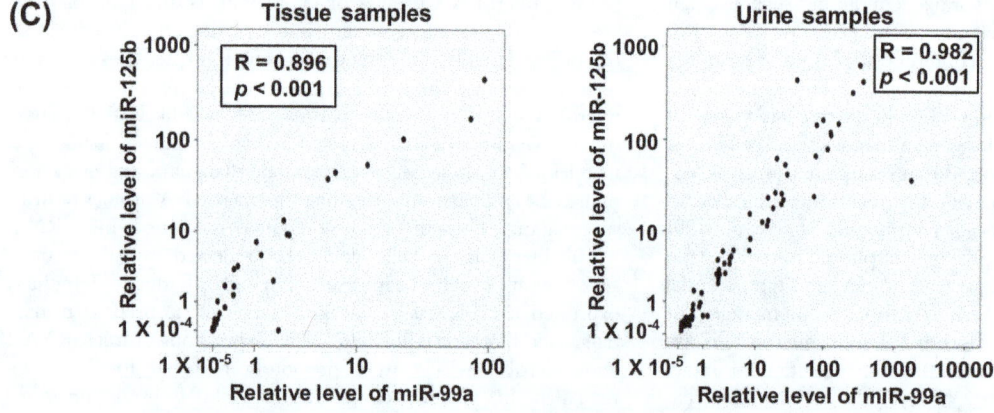

(D)

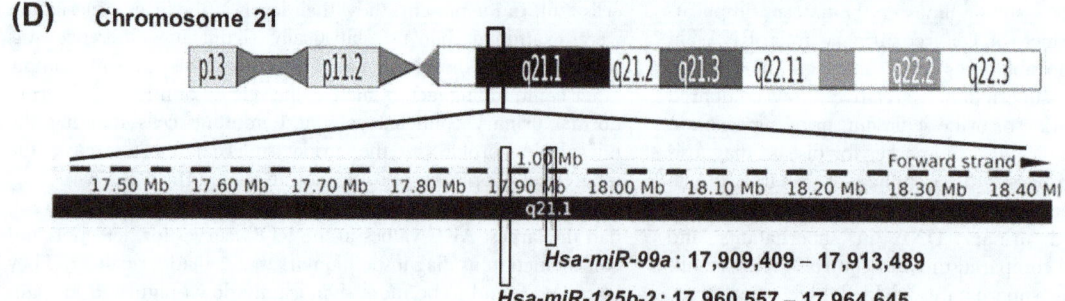

Figure 3. Expression of microRNAs in the urine supernatant of UCB patients and normal controls. The total RNA was extracted from the urine supernatants of UCB patients with low-grade (n = 15) (shaded bar) or high-grade cancers (n = 35) (black bar) and normal controls (n = 21) (white bar). The levels of six microRNAs in the samples were quantified by RT-qPCR in duplicate. (A) The relative levels (2-ΔCq) of microRNA-133a, microRNA99a, microRNA-1, microRNA-143, microRNA-133b and microRNA-125b in the urine supernatant samples are presented. A Mann-Whitney U test was conducted to compare the UCB patients and normal controls. Columns, Means; Bars, S.D.; ** denotes p<0.01; * denotes p<0.05. (B) ROC curves of microRNA-99a alone (blue line), microRNA-125b alone (red line) and microRNA-99a and microRNA-125b in combination (black line) for the diagnosis of UCB (left) and discrimination between low- and high-grade tumors (right). The cut-off points were set and the AUC values determined based on Youden's Index. (C) Results of a Pearson correlation analysis of the levels of microRNA-99a and microRNA-125b in the tissues and urine supernatant samples. Scatter plots of the relative levels of these two microRNAs in the samples are presented. The Pearson correlation coefficient R was calculated via a Pearson correlation analysis and the p-value was determined. (D) Chromosomal regions of the genes (*hsa-miR-99a* and *hsa-miR-125b-2*). Human Genome Reference Consortium GRCh37 Patch Release 12 assembly was used. *Hsa-miR-99a* is located at chromosome 21:17,909,409–17,913,489, and *hsa-miR-125b-2* is located at chromosome 21:17,960,557–17,964,645.

supernatants increased, implicating a strong association between their levels and the patients' tumor statuses. This further supports their potential roles as diagnostic biomarkers for UCB and surveillance biomarkers for monitoring tumor recurrence. Based on these models, when a patient has a positive urine supernatant test result with a CI larger than the cut-off (0.6244), he or she probably has bladder cancer, with an accuracy rate of 91.8%. If the normalized expression level of microRNA-125b is lower than $2^{1.71}$, there is a 93.4% chance that the patient has high-grade cancer. However, because the negative predicting value was 71.4% in this study, negative results cannot be used to rule out the possibility of bladder cancer in patients.

The present study showed that the levels of microRNA-99a and microRNA-125b in the urine supernatant of UCB patients and controls were highly correlated with those in the tissues. In fact, the two genes (*hsa-miR-99a* and *hsa-miR-125b-2*) are located in intron 6 of the long intergenic non-protein coding RNA 478 (*LINC00478*) in chromosome 21. Their expressions are probably co-regulated by the promoter that controls the transcription of the *LINC00478* gene. The underlying mechanism for the down-regulation of these two microRNAs in UCB may be related to the frequently observed loss of genomic 21q in UCB. Tzai et al. [27] reported a frequent allelic loss of 36.6% in the long arm of chromosome 21, where the two genes are located, in UCB. In addition, patients with Down syndrome exhibited a decreased risk of dying from urological neoplasms, suggesting the presence of genes in chromosome 21 suppressing urological cancer tumors [28].

MicroRNA-99a and microRNA-125b have been demonstrated to have tumor-suppressive roles in various human cancers [29-34].

In prostate cancer, microRNA-99a suppresses the expression of prostate-specific antigens and prostate cancer cell proliferation by interfering with the expression of two chromatin remodeling factors, SMARCA5 (SWI/SNF-related matrix-associated actin-dependent regulator of chromatin subfamily A member 5) and SMARCD1 (SWI/SNF-related matrix-associated actin-dependent regulator of chromatin subfamily D member 1), and the growth regulatory kinase mTOR (mammalian target of rapamycin) [29]. In fact, a high expression of phosphorylated mTOR was found in 74% of muscle-invasive urothelical carcinomas, in association with increased pathological stages and decreased disease-related survival [30]. The inhibition of mTOR was found to decrease *in vitro* and *in vivo* bladder cancer cell growth [30]. As microRNA-99a targets mTOR in prostate cancer cells [29], the down-regulation of this microRNA in UCB demonstrated in the present study may abolish the tumor-promoting effects of mTOR in the cells, resulting in cancer development. However, further demonstration of the regulation of mTOR by microRNA-99a in bladder cancer cells is required. Although the data of the present study indicated a down-regulation of microRNA-99a expression in both the urine supernatants and tumor tissues of UCB patients, one report showed elevated microRNA-99a in noninvasive but not invasive lesions [31]. A down-regulation of microRNA-125b expression has been frequently observed in various tumors such as hepatocellular carcinoma HCC [32], osteosarcoma [33] and bladder cancer [34]. The ectopic expression of microRNA-125b in low-expressing cancer cells has been found to significantly decrease proliferation and promote apoptosis by targeting Bcl-2 in HCC cells [35], and to affect the proliferation and migration in osteosarcoma cell lines via the suppression of STAT3 expression in the cells [33]. In

Table 2. Diagnostic strength of microRNA-99a alone, microRNA-125b alone and microRNA-99a and microRNA-125b in combination for the detection of bladder cancer and their significance in discriminating tumor grades.

	Diagnosis of UCB			Discrimination of tumor grades		
	microRNA-99a alone	microRNA-125b alone	microRNA-99a * and microRNA-125b	microRNA-99a alone	microRNA-125b alone	microRNA-99a[#] and microRNA-125b
AUC	0.800 (0.715~0.886)	0.813 (0.729~0.897)	0.876 (0.809~0.942)	0.791 (0.673~0.908)	0.819 (0.712~0.926)	0.831 (0.770~0.951)
Cut-off point	REL: $2^{2.18}$	REL: $2^{4.1}$	CI: 0.6244	REL: $2^{0.91}$	REL: $2^{1.71}$	CI: 0.7398
Sensitivity	78.0%	84.8%	86.7%	74.2%	81.4%	79.4%
Specificity	85.7%	76.2%	81.1%	83.3%	87.0%	88.0%
PPV	92.7%	89.3%	91.8%	91.5%	93.4%	94.7%
NPV	61.0%	68.1%	71.4%	58.1%	67.0%	61.1%
+LR	5.46	3.57	4.58	4.46	6.11	6.61
-LR	0.26	0.20	0.16	0.31	0.21	0.23

*Formula of CI for bladder cancer diagnosis: CI = 1/{1+exp[−(2.332+0.425 x$\Delta Ct_{microRNA-125b}$+0.069 x$\Delta Ct_{microRNA-99a}$)]}.

[#]Formula of CI for tumor grading: CI = 1/ {1+exp [−(1.742 +0.0295 x$\Delta Ct_{microRNA-125b}$ +0.496 x$\Delta Ct_{microRNA-99a}$)]}.

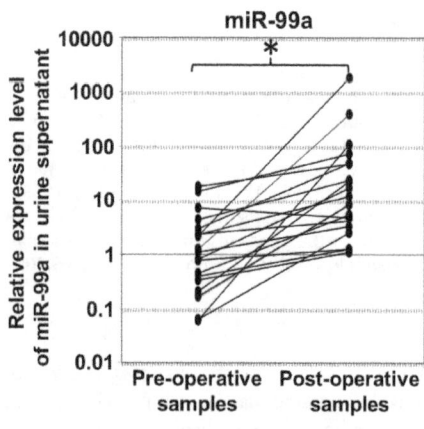 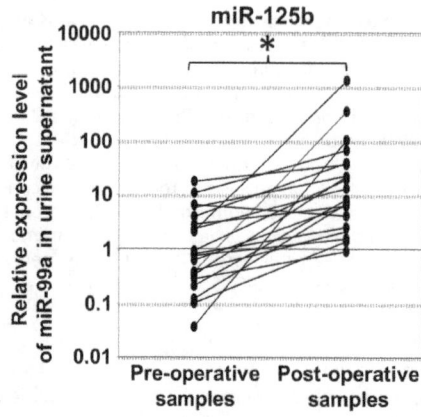

Figure 4. Restored expression of microRNA-99a and microRNA-125b in the urine supernatant of UCB patients after transurethial resection. Urine samples were collected from 20 UCB patients before (pre-operative) and after (post-operative) transurethial resection. The total RNA was extracted from the urine supernatants and subjected to RT-qPCR to quantify the levels of microRNA-99a (left) and microRNA-125b (right). A Wilcoxon signed-rank two-related-samples test was conducted to compare the levels of microRNA-99a and microRNA-125b between the pre- and post-operative samples. * denotes p<0.01.

bladder cancer, microRNA-125b inhibited colony formation in an *in vitro* cell model and *in vivo* tumor development in nude mice by targeting E2F3, which frequently showed overexpression in bladder cancer and had an expression inversely correlated with that of microRNA-125b [34]. Taken together, aberrant expressions of microRNA-99a and microRNA-125b may be involved in bladder carcinogenesis and even disease progression. Further investigations that elucidate the mechanism underlying how these two microRNAs participate in bladder cancer development and progression are required. The present study found that microRNA-99a and microRNA-125b can be used as effective biomarkers for UCB detection and disease monitoring. They can also function as therapeutic agents for UCB treatment in patients.

Conclusions

The results of this study revealed the unique microRNA expression signature in urine supernatants and tumor tissues of bladder cancer patients for the development of molecular diagnostic tests by microRNA microarray and RT-qPCR. The differential expression of microRNA-99a and microRNA-125b in an expanded patient cohort was verified. An effective cell-free urinary model using a combined index of the microRNA-99a and microRNA-125b levels for bladder cancer detection with good discriminating power, high sensitivity and high specificity was developed. The diagnostic significance of these two microRNAs was further confirmed by the reversals of the altered expression in patients after tumor resection. It was found that microRNA-99a and microRNA-125b can be used as effective biomarkers for UCB detection and disease monitoring. They can also function as therapeutic agents for UCB treatment in patients.

Supporting Information

Figure S1 Workflow of the study of microRNA profiles in urine supernatant and cancer and normal tissues of bladder cancer patients and controls. microRNA profiles were determined by microRNA microarray for identification of differentially expressed microRNAs. By RT-qPCR, the differential expression of the selected microRNAs was validated in the tissue samples of the patients and also in the urine supernatant samples of the expanded patient cohort for development of models for detection of bladder cancer. To determine the link between tumor status and the differential expression, the relative levels of the selected microRNAs in urine supernatant of pre-operative and post-operative patients was determined by RT-qPCR and compared.

Figure S2 Expression of microRNA-99a and microRNA-125b in urine supernatant of UCB patients and normal controls. Urine samples were collected from 20 UCB patients before (pre-operative) and after (post-operative) transurethial resection. Total RNA was extracted from supernatant of pre- and post-operative urine samples of UCB patients (n = 20) and also that of normal controls (n = 21). The levels of these two microRNAs in the samples were quantified by RT-qPCR in duplicate. Relative levels (2-ΔCq) of microRNA-99a and microRNA-125b in the urine supernatant samples were presented. Wilcoxon signed-rank 2 related samples test was used for the comparisons of the levels of microRNA-99a and microRNA-125b between pre-operative and post-operative samples. For the comparisons between the post-operative urine samples of UCB patients and normal controls, Mann-Whitney U test was used. Columns, Means; Bars, S.D.; * denotes $p<0.01$ for Wilcoxon signed-rank 2 related samples test; # denotes $p>0.05$ for Mann-Whitney U test.

Table S1 Median sensitivity and specificity of cytology and other urine-based markers for the detection of bladder cancer.

Author Contributions

Conceived and designed the experiments: DZZ CFN GW KW RKWC. Performed the experiments: DZZ KW. Analyzed the data: DZZ KML. Contributed reagents/materials/analysis tools: CFN. Wrote the paper: DZZ KML CFN CCS ESYC.

References

1. Timberg G, Rahu M, Gornoi K, Aareleid T, Baburin A. (1997) Bladder cancer in Estonia, 1968–1992: incidence, mortality, prevalence and survival. Scand J Urol Nephrol 31: 337–342.
2. Parker J, Spiess PE. (2011) Current and emerging bladder cancer urinary biomarkers. Sci World J 11: 1103–1112.
3. Fabbri M, Garzon R, Cimmino A, Liu Z, Zanesi N, et al. (2006) MicroRNA expression and function in cancer. Trends Mol Med 12: 580–587.
4. Iorio MV, Ferracin M, Liu CG, Veronese A, Spizzo R, et al. (2005) MicroRNA gene expression deregulation in human breast cancer. Cancer Res 65: 7065–7070.
5. Yanaihara N, Caplen N, Bowman E, Seike M, Kumamoto K, et al. (2006) Unique microRNA molecular profiles in lung cancer diagnosis and prognosis. Cancer Cell 9: 189–198.
6. Chen X, Ba Y, Ma L, Cai X, Yin Y, et al. (2008) Characterization of microRNAs in serum: a novel class of biomarkers for diagnosis of cancer and other diseases. Cell Res 18: 997–1006.
7. Weber JA, Baxter DH, Zhang S, Huang DY, Huang KH, et al. (2010) The microRNA spectrum in 12 body fluids. Clin Chem 56: 1733–1741.
8. Mraz M, Malinova K, Mayer J, Pospisilova S. (2009) MicroRNA isolation and stability in stored RNA samples. Biochem Biophys Res Commun 390: 1–4.
9. Yang H, Dinney CP, Ye Y, Zhu Y, Grossman HB, Wu X. (2008) Evaluation of genetic variants in microRNA-related genes and risk of bladder cancer. Cancer Res 68: 2530–2537.
10. Hanke M, Hoefig K, Merz H, Feller AC, Kausch I, et al. (2010) A robust methodology to study urine microRNA as tumor marker: microRNA-126 and microRNA-182 are related to urinary bladder cancer. Urol Oncol 28: 655–661.
11. Snowdon J, Boag S, Feilotter H, Izard J, Siemens DR. (2012) A pilot study of urinary microRNA as a biomarker for urothelial cancer. Can Urol Assoc J May 15: 1–5.
12. Schroeder GL, Lorenzo-Gomez MF, Hautmann SH, Friedrich MG, Ekici S, et al. (2004) A side by side comparison of cytology and biomarkers for bladder cancer detection. J Urol 172(3): 1123–1126.
13. Friedman GD, Carroll PR, Cattolica EV, Hiatt RA. (1996) Can hematuria be a predictor as well as a symptom or sign of bladder cancer? Cancer Epidemiol Biomarkers Prev 5(12): 993–996.
14. Szarvas T, Kovalszky I, Bedi K, Szendroi A, Majoros A, et al. (2007) Deletion analysis of tumor and urinary DNA to detect bladder cancer: urine supernatant versus urine sediment. Oncol Rep 18: 405–409.
15. Chang HW, Tsui KH, Shen LC, Huang HW, Wang SN, et al. (2007) Urinary cell-free DNA as a potential tumor marker for bladder cancer. Int J Biol Markers 22: 287–294.
16. Zancan M, Franceschini R, Mimmo C, Vianello M, Di Tonno F, et al. (2005) Free DNA in urine: a new marker for bladder cancer? Preliminary data. Int J Biol Markers 20: 134–136.
17. Mostofi FK, Davis CJ, Sesterhenn I. (1999) Histological typing of urinary bladder tumours. 2nd edition. Berlin, New York: Springer.
18. Yamada Y, Enokida H, Kojima S, Kawakami K, Chiyomaru T, et al. (2011) MiR-96 and miR-183 detection in urine serve as potential tumor markers of urothelial carcinoma: correlation with stage and grade, and comparison with urinary cytology. Cancer Sci 102(3): 522–529.
19. Lawrie CH, Gal S, Dunlop HM, Pushkaran B, Liggins AP, et al. (2008) Detection of elevated levels of tumor-associated microRNAs in serum of patients with diffuse large B-cell lymphoma. Br J Haematol 141: 672–675.
20. Ng EK, Chong WW, Jin H, Lam EK, Shin VY, et al. (2009) Differential expression of microRNAs in plasma of patients with colorectal cancer: a potential marker for colorectal cancer screening. Gut 58: 1375–1381.
21. Wang G, Tam LS, Li EK, Kwan BC, Chow KM, et al. (2010) Serum and urinary cell-free miR-146a and miR-155 in patients with systemic lupus erythematosus. J Rheumatol 37: 516–522.
22. Wang G, Chan ES, Kwan BC, Li PK, Yip SK, et al. (2012) Expression of microRNAs in the urine of patients with bladder cancer. Clin Genitourin Cancer 10(2): 106–113.
23. Wang G, Zhang H, He H, Tong W, Wang B, et al. (2010) Up-regulation of microRNA in bladder tumor tissue is not common. Int Urol Nephrol 42: 95–102.
24. Esquela-Kerscher A, Slack FJ. (2006) Oncomirs - microRNAs with a role in cancer. Nat Rev Cancer 6(4): 259–269.
25. Mitchell PS, Parkin RK, Kroh EM, Fritz BR, Wyman SK, et al. (2008) Circulating microRNAs as stable blood-based markers for cancer detection. Proc Natl Acad Sci USA 105: 10513–10518.
26. Yoshino H, Enokida H, Chiyomaru T, Tatarano S, Hidaka H, et al. (2011) The tumor-suppressive function of miR-1 and miR-133a targeting TAGLN2 in bladder cancer. Br J Cancer 104: 808–818.
27. Tzai TS, Chen HH, Chan SH, Ho CL, Tsai YS, et al. (2003) Clinical significance of allelotype profiling for urothelial carcinoma. Urology 62(2): 378–384.
28. Satgé D, Sasco AJ, Day S, Culine S. (2009) A lower risk of dying from urological cancer in Down syndrome: clue for cancer protecting genes on chromosome 21. Urol Int 82: 296–300.
29. Sun D, Lee YS, Malhotra A, Kim HK, Matecic M, et al. (2011) MiR-99 family of microRNAs suppresses the expression of prostate-specific antigen and prostate cancer cell proliferation. Cancer Res 71: 1313–1324.
30. Hansel DE, Platt E, Orloff M, Harwalker J, Sethu S, et al. (2010) Mammalian target of rapamycin (mTOR) regulates cellular proliferation and tumor growth in urothelial carcinoma. Am J Pathol 176: 3062–3672.
31. Wszolek MF, Rieger-Christ KM, Kenney PA, Gould JJ, Silva Neto B, et al. (2011) A microRNA expression profile defining the invasive bladder tumor phenotype. Urol Oncol 29(6): 794–801.
32. Alpini G, Glaser SS, Zhang JP, Francis H, Han Y, et al. (2011) Regulation of placenta growth factor by microRNA-125b in hepatocellular cancer. J Hepatol 55(6): 1339–1345.
33. Liu LH, Li H, Li JP, Zhong H, Zhang HC, et al. (2011) MiR-125b suppresses the proliferation and migration of osteosarcoma cells through down-regulation of STAT3. Biochem Biophys Res Commun 416(1–2): 31–38.
34. Huang L, Luo J, Cai Q, Pan Q, Zeng H, et al. (2011) MicroRNA-125b suppresses the development of bladder cancer by targeting E2F3. Int J Cancer 128(8): 1758–1769.
35. Zhao A, Zeng Q, Xie X, Zhou J, Yue W, et al. (2012) MicroRNA-125b induces cancer cell apoptosis through suppression of Bcl-2 expression. J Genet Genomics 39(1): 29–35.

15

Elevated Phospholipase A_2 Activities in Plasma Samples from Multiple Cancers

Hui Cai[1,2], Elena G. Chiorean[3], Michael V. Chiorean[3], Douglas K. Rex[3], Bruce W. Robb[3], Noah M. Hahn[3,4], Ziyue Liu[5], Patrick J. Loehrer[3], Marietta L. Harrison[6], Yan Xu[1]*

1 Department of Obstetrics and Gynecology, Indiana University School of Medicine, Indianapolis, Indiana, United States of America, 2 Department of Thoracic Oncosurgery, First Affiliated Hospital of Xi'an Jiaotong University, Xi'an, People's Republic of China, 3 Department of Medicine, Indiana University Melvin and Bren Simon Cancer Center, Indiana University School of Medicine, Indianapolis, Indiana, United States of America, 4 Hoosier Oncology Group, Indianapolis, Indiana, United States of America, 5 Department of Biostatistics, Indiana University School of Medicine, Indianapolis, Indiana, United States of America, 6 Medicinal Chemistry and Molecular Pharmacology, Oncological Sciences Center, Purdue University Center for Cancer Research, West Lafayette, Indiana, United States of America

Abstract

Only in recent years have phospholipase A_2 enzymes (PLA_2s) emerged as cancer targets. In this work, we report the first detection of elevated PLA_2 activities in plasma from patients with colorectal, lung, pancreatic, and bladder cancers as compared to healthy controls. Independent sets of clinical plasma samples were obtained from two different sites. The first set was from patients with colorectal cancer (CRC; n = 38) and healthy controls (n = 77). The second set was from patients with lung (n = 95), bladder (n = 31), or pancreatic cancers (n = 38), and healthy controls (n = 79). PLA_2 activities were analyzed by a validated quantitative fluorescent assay method and subtype PLA_2 activities were defined in the presence of selective inhibitors. The natural PLA_2 activity, as well as each subtype of PLA_2 activity was elevated in each cancer group as compared to healthy controls. PLA_2 activities were increased in late stage vs. early stage cases in CRC. PLA_2 activities were not influenced by sex, smoking, alcohol consumption, or body-mass index (BMI). Samples from the two independent sites confirmed the results. Plasma PLA_2 activities had approximately 70% specificity and sensitivity to detect cancer. The marker and targeting values of PLA_2 activity have been suggested.

Editor: Mohammad O. Hoque, Johns Hopkins University, United States of America

Funding: This work is supported in part by the Cancer Care Engineering Project, Department of Defense, USAMRMC, W81XWH-08-1-0065 and W81XWH-10-1-0540 (http://www.grants.gov/search/search.do?mode=AGENCYSEARCH&agency=DOD), as well as National Institutes of Health R21 CA133744 (http://www.cancer.gov/researchandfunding) and the Mary Fendrich Hulman Charitable Trust to YX. Funding for the Hoosier Oncology Group Study was provided by the Walther Cancer Institute Foundation, Indianapolis, IN. The funders had no role in study design, data collection and analysis, decision to publish, or preparation of the manuscript.

Competing Interests: The authors have declared that no competing interests exist. The authors have filled a PCT Patent Application "PLA2 Activity as a Marker for Ovarian and Other Gynecologic Cancers" in 2011.

* E-mail: xu2@iupui.edu

Introduction

Cancer is one of the major health burdens worldwide. More than 1.6 million new cancer cases and over 577,000 deaths from cancer are projected to occur in the United States in 2012 [1]. Lung cancer (LC) and colorectal cancer (CRC) are among the most frequent types of cancers. Pancreatic and bladder cancers count for (3–7% of all cancers), but pancreatic cancer (PC) is one of the deadest cancers, with a dismal 5-year survival rate of 6% [1]. The success of current cancer treatments depends strongly on the time of diagnosis, with early detection and identification of high risk patient populations resulting in the most favorable overall survivals in these diseases [1,2]. It is expected that early detection and screening of high risk patient populations may have the most significant impact on altering overall survival in these diseases. Thus, there is an urgent need for efficient and sensitive early detection methods [3]. While imaging-based detection methods, including spiral computerized axial tomography (CT) and colonoscopy are effective early detection methods for LC and CRC, respectively [4], they are rather expensive and inconvenient. In addition, modern imaging techniques have a high incidence of discovery of lung nodules, many of which are falsely positive, but still calling for additional and sometimes painful examinations [5]. Molecular approaches to cancer diagnosis through biomarkers measured by non-invasive means could significantly improve the specificity and sensitivity of cancer detection [5]. In particular, serologic biomarkers may be the most useful in early detection due to the minimal invasiveness, cost-effectiveness, and convenience. Moreover, serological biomarkers identifying novel cancer-related genes and/or molecules may provide new insight into the biology of cancers and may also become attractive targets for treatment [3].

Phospholipase A_2 enzymes (PLA_2s) are the major enzymes producing the cyclooxygenase-2 (COX-2) substrate, arachidonic acid (AA), as well as lysophospholipids. Both of these classes of products are signaling molecules involved in cancers. However, only in recent years have PLA_2s emerged as cancer targets [6]. More than 30 enzymes that possess PLA_2 or related activity have been identified in mammals [7]. They are divided into four groups based on their cellular localization, substrate specificity, and calcium-dependence [8], including cytosolic ($cPLA_2$), calcium-independent ($iPLA_2$), secreted ($sPLA_2$), and lipoprotein-associated

Table 1. Demographic data for participants from IUSM and HOG study.

| | No. | Age (years) | | | Sex (%) | | | Race (%) | | | |
		Mean	SD	P value	Male	Female	P value	White	African American	Others	P value
Participants from IUSM											
Healthy	77	51.6	13.5		40.3	59.7		89.6	9.1	1.3	
CRC	38	56.0	13.4	0.1075	44.7	55.3	0.6470	86.8	5.3	7.9	0.4501
Participants from HOG											
Healthy	79	42.7	12.0		77.2	22.8		89.3	2.7	8.0	
LC	95	63.2	9.5	<0.0001	64.2	35.8	0.0621	89.5	8.4	2.1	0.0654
BC	31	70.5	10.0	<0.0001	87.1	12.9	0.2438	93.6	6.5	0.0	0.1868
PC	38	68.7	8.7	<0.0001	63.2	36.8	0.1102	92.1	5.3	2.6	0.4327

CRC: colorectal cancer; LC: Lung cancer; BC: Bladder cancer; PC: Pancreatic cancer; SD, standard deviation; HOG: Hoosier Oncology Group.
In the HOG set: • For gender, the overall P value is 0.0339. • For Age, the overall P value is <0.0001. • For race, the overall P value is 0.2352. Since it was not significant, it was not recommended to perform pair-wise comparisons. Nonetheless, P values for pair-wise comparisons are given to be consistent with the other two variables. All pair-wise comparisons are against healthy controls.

PLA_2 (Lp-PLA_2). In cancer, most of the attention has been focused on $sPLA_2$ and $cPLA_2$ [8]. We and others have shown that $iPLA_2$ is functionally involved in promoting the development of ovarian cancer (OC) and other cancers, *in vitro* and *in vivo* [9–13]. $sPLA_2$ and Lp-PLA_2 are secreted enzymes. In contrast, both $cPLA_2$ and $iPLA_2$ are cytosolic enzymes and their extracellular existence has only been shown to be related to exosomes from RBL-2H3 cells (a mast and basophil cell line) [14]. Exosomes are 40–100 nm diameter membrane vesicles released from multivesicular bodies by intact cells and are known to participate in intercellular signaling [15]. We have recently detected extracellular- and exosome-free $iPLA_2$ and $cPLA_2$ activities in ascites and tissues from OC patients [16].

In the current work we have focused on PLA_2 activities rather than expression of individual PLA_2 enzymes and examined PLA_2 activities in blood plasma samples from patients with different cancers, in comparison with those from healthy controls. We used our recently validated quantitative, convenient, highly reproducible PLA_2 assay method [16] and showed for the first time that plasma PLA_2 activities from patients with CRC, LC, PC, and bladder cancer (BC) were significantly higher than those of healthy controls. In addition, PLA_2 activities were correlated with tumor stages in CRC. Other potential influential factors, including sex, age, smoking and alcohol consumption were also examined in this study.

Materials and Methods

Human sample collection and processing

Two sets of independently collected clinical plasma samples were obtained for this study. The first set from the Indiana University School of Medicine (IUSM) focused on CRC patients and healthy controls screened by colonoscopy and found negative for adenomatous polyps and CRC. Blood samples collected in the presence of EDTA were centrifuged at 1,750 g for 15 min at 15–24°C, aliquoted in siliconized Eppendorf tubes and stored at −80°C. The second set of samples was from patients with lung, bladder, or pancreatic cancers, as well as healthy controls. These samples were collected by the Hoosier Oncology Group (HOG) in Indianapolis, IN as part of the study entitled, "A Biological Sample Collection Protocol of Patients with and without Metastatic Solid Organ Malignancies: Hoosier Oncology Group Study BANK09-

138". Blood samples were centrifuged at 3,500 rpm for 30 min. The aliquoted samples were stored at −70°C. HOG is a nonprofit medical research organization. Although it is a separate entity, IUSM is a supporting organization for board appointments and IRB approvals for HOG. Three separate IRB protocols for collecting and/or use the blood samples related to this work have been approved by the same IUSM Institutional Review Board (Protocol numbers: 0670-81, 0808-24, 0905-20). Written informed consent forms were obtained from all subjects and all clinical investigation had been conducted according to the principles expressed in the Declaration of Helsinki.

Reagents and inhibitors

The PLA_2 substrate 1-O-(6-Dabcyl-Aminohexanoyl)-2-O-(6-(12-BODIPY-Dodecanoyl) Aminohexanoyl)-sn-3-Glyceryl Phosphatidylcholine (DBPC) was from Echelon Bioscience (Salt Lake City, UT, USA). Bromoenol lactone (BEL) and methyl arachidonylfluorophosphonate (MAFP) were from Santa Cruz Biotechnology (Santa Cruz, CA, USA).

PLA_2 enzymatic activity analyses

PLA_2 activities were analyzed using the fluorescent substrate DBPC, a fluorogenic phosphatidylcholine substrate [17]. Plasma samples (0.1 μL) were mixed with DBPC (0.2 μg in PBS) to final volume 200 μL. The fluorescence was read at intervals over several hours on a Victor³V plate reader (Perkin Elmer, Waltham, MA, USA). PLA_2 activities were expressed as change in fluorescence intensity/min/μL of plasma. As previously described [16], we selected conditions to distinguish PLA_2 activity derived from different subtypes: a) the "natural" PLA_2 activity without any exogenous additives, b) the $iPLA_2$ activity in the presence of 5 mM EDTA (a divalent cation chelator to block all PLA_2s requiring calcium, including $sPLA_2$ and $cPLA_2$), c) the $sPLA_2$ activity in the presence of 1.2 mM calcium chloride (the natural ionized calcium concentration in blood [18]) and MAFP (10 μM, a dual inhibitor of $cPLA_2$ and $iPLA_2$), and d) the $cPLA_2$ activity in the presence of 100 μM calcium chloride and bromoenol lactone (BEL, 10 μM, a selective inhibitor for $iPLA_2$).

A

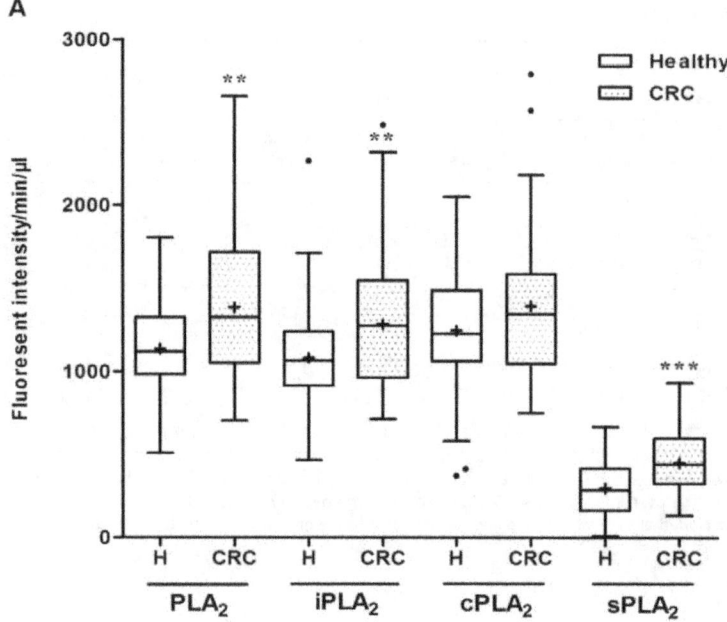

B

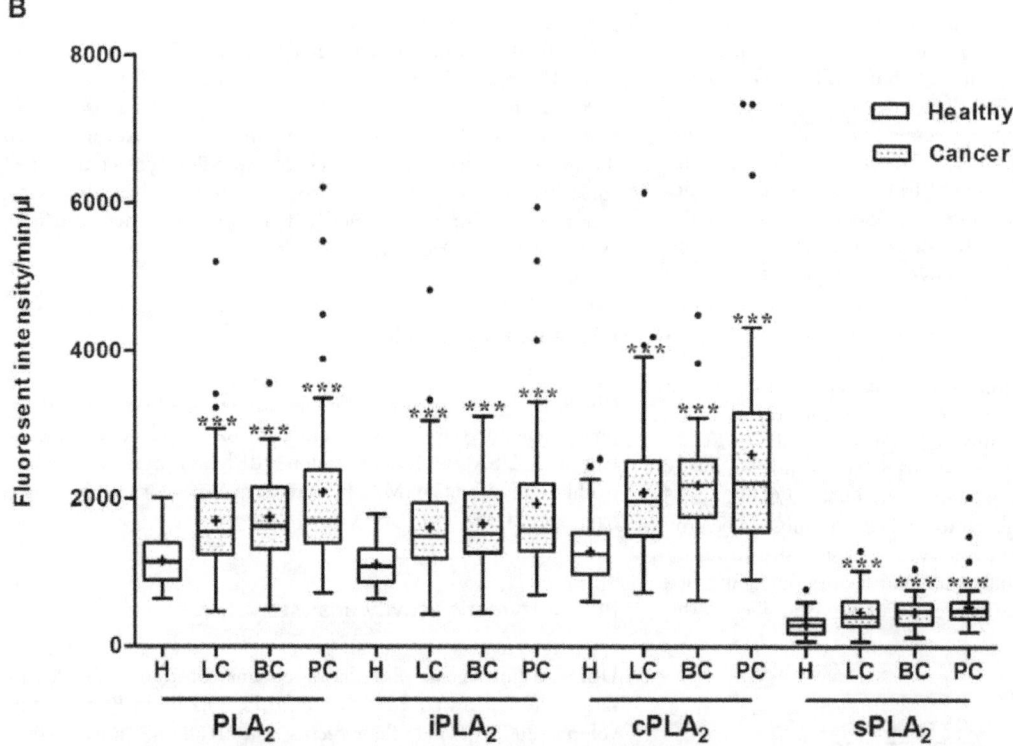

Figure 1. Plasma PLA$_2$ activities were elevated in cancer groups vs. healthy controls. Comparison of PLA$_2$ activities in the healthy control (normal colonoscopy; n = 77) and CRC (n = 38) groups. A. Comparison of PLA$_2$ activities in the healthy (n = 79) and other cancer groups. Lung cancer (LC, n = 95), bladder cancer (BC, n = 31) and pancreatic cancer (PC, n = 38). The distribution of the natural and individual groups of PLA$_2$ activities were analyzed as described in Materials and Methods. The mean values of PLA$_2$ activities were presented by the "+" in the figure. *$P<0.05$; **$P<0.01$; ***$P<0.001$.

Statistical Analysis

Categorical variables were summarized as counts with percentages and continuous variables were summarized as means with standard deviations (SD) across the healthy control, and cancer groups. The Chi-square test was used to test the associations between disease statuses and categorical covariates such as sex, race, smoking, and alcohol drinking. For continuous covariates such as age and BMI, one-way ANOVA was used to test the overall difference and Student t-test was used to test the pair-wise difference across disease statuses. Linear regression was used to assess the univariate association between PLA$_2$ measurements and

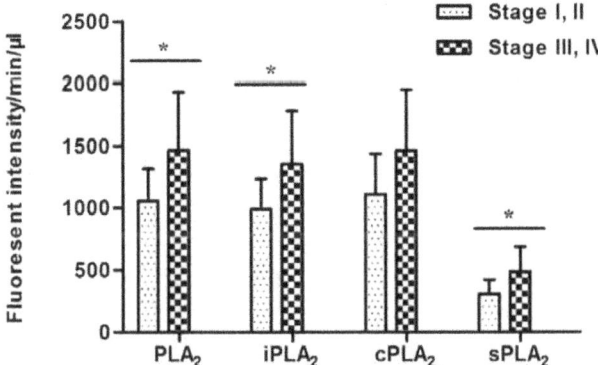

Figure 2. PLA$_2$ activities were higher in late stage CRC samples. The natural and individual groups of PLA$_2$ activities were progressively increased by tumor stage. Stage I and II (n = 7), Stage III and IV (n = 31). *Student t-test, $P < 0.05$.

covariates. Logistic regression was used to evaluate the classification performance of PLA$_2$ measurements. Bootstrap was used to internally validate the classification performance using 1000 samples [19]. Each sample had the same size as the original data set and was used to develop the model. The results were then tested in the original data. Areas under the curve (AUCs) were calculated for each repeat. All tests were two-sided. Given the exploratory nature of this study, no adjustments for multiple comparisons were adopted. P values < 0.05 were considered to be statistically significant. All analyses were performed using SAS software Version 9.3 (SAS Institute Inc., Cary, NC, USA).

Results

Subject demographic data

The demographic data for the study participants are summarized in **Table 1**. For the IUSM CRC set samples, 41.7% of the overall participants were male, 88.7% were white, and the mean age was 53.1 years. The age, sex, and race composition were not significantly different in control vs. CRC groups (P values > 0.05; **Table 1**). For the second set of samples, the age in the healthy control group was significantly younger than each of the three

cancer groups (**Table 1**). Although males were dominant in each group, they were not significantly different from the second set of healthy controls. 71.2% of the overall participants were male, 90.4% were white, and the mean age was 58.3 years (**Table 1**).

Reproducibility and stability of the PLA$_2$ assays

We have recently validated the quantitative nature of the DBPC-based PLA$_2$ assays and optimized the conditions for biological fluids and tissues samples [16]. When each of 8 representative plasma samples were analyzed three times, the PLA$_2$ activity values reproducible, with an average standard deviation (SD) 13.5 (1.3%). We also tested the PLA$_2$ activity stability by comparing them in samples before storage to those in the same samples stored at $-80°$C for one month, as well as the effect of freeze-and-thaw on the PLA$_2$ activities in 8 representative samples. As previously reported [16], PLA$_2$ activities were stable with SDs < 35.8 (5.8%). In addition, we showed that in the presence of all other assay components including inhibitor(s) used in this study, but in the absence of blood or other biological samples, the non-specific hydrolysis of the DBPC substrate was negative and negligible (data not shown).

The natural PLA$_2$, cPLA$_2$, iPLA$_2$, and sPLA$_2$ activities were elevated in cancer samples vs. healthy controls

Blood iPLA$_2$ and cPLA$_2$ activities have not been previously reported in human samples. We analyzed the natural PLA$_2$ (defined as the PLA$_2$ activities measured under the conditions without any modifiers, which may be lower than the sum of the subgroup PLA$_2$ activities measured under modified conditions), as well as cPLA$_2$, iPLA$_2$, and sPLA$_2$ activities in plasma samples.

Except for the healthy vs. CRC cPLA$_2$ activity, all other comparisons showed that PLA$_2$ activities were significantly elevated in the cancer groups (**Fig. 1A** and **1B**). PLA$_2$ activity values across plasma samples from LC, BC, and PC patients were not significantly different (P values > 0.05).

Since sPLA$_2$ is secreted, it was expected that sPLA$_2$ activity would account for the major portion of the PLA$_2$ activity detected in the blood. However, in our results, high levels of iPLA$_2$ and cPLA$_2$ and low levels of sPLA$_2$ activities were observed in all plasma samples. Blood exosomes may be the carriers of these activities [15]. We used differential centrifugation steps as we described recently [16] to determine whether these activities could

Table 2. Clinical characteristics and PLA$_2$ activities in the CRC cases.

	No.	PLA$_2$			iPLA$_2$			cPLA$_2$			sPLA$_2$		
		Mean	SD	P value	Mean	SD	P value	Mean	SD	P value	Mean	SD	P value
Primary site				0.6856*			0.7407*			0.6419*			0.3410*
Colon	24	1412.3	473.75		1302.8	428.78		1424.0	480.16		476.3	199.33	
Rectum	14	1348.0	460.33		1254.7	428.33		1347.7	489.95		408.3	195.50	
Previous treatment				0.6543**			0.3081**			0.3348**			0.6212**
Surgery only	7	1340.3	382.29		1193.1	286.55		1303.4	424.30		435.5	92.75	
CT and RT	3	1614.8	542.80		1599.5	626.64		1755.4	707.50		495.9	219.34	
Surgery and CT	10	1496.8	596.54		1399.5	543.97		1521.1	633.55		519.8	264.44	
Surgery, CT and RT	5	1459.0	437.46		1402.9	322.07		1511.8	322.27		472.8	200.95	
Untreated	13	1252.2	404.71		1128.6	341.99		1221.8	327.50		388.5	183.68	

*Student *t*-test.
**One-way ANOVA.
CT: chemotherapy; RT: radiotherapy.

Table 3. Clinical characteristics and PLA$_2$ activities in the LC, BC, and PC cases.

	No.	PLA$_2$ Mean	SD	P value	iPLA$_2$ Mean	SD	P value	cPLA$_2$ Mean	SD	P value	sPLA$_2$ Mean	SD	P value
Lung cancer													
T stage				0.4760**			0.5001**			0.4960**			0.6129**
T1	19	1714.2	548.5		1626.6	514.2		2190.2	752.6		457.1	280.7	
T2	21	1569.3	671.8		1490.6	640.6		1924.1	754.0		478.7	261.4	
T3	9	1437.9	479.0		1347.4	460.7		1721.3	480.5		356.2	166.6	
T4	35	1803.5	878.2		1691.8	823.9		2141.7	1105.9		471.5	228.4	
N stage				0.9973**			0.9685**			0.9758**			0.8009**
N0	14	1626.7	566.2		1559.5	522.6		2061.3	584.4		386.3	143.2	
N1	11	1574.8	508.1		1442.7	479.8		1960.3	671.2		404.1	200.4	
N2	21	1613.9	643.7		1524.1	631.4		1961.6	883.6		434.1	222.9	
N3	29	1604.2	671.7		1510.2	620.6		1944.3	888.0		454.8	270.0	
Bladder cancer													
T stage				0.7482**			0.7320**			0.5790**			0.1793**
Tis	2	1736.6	429.9		1568.4	406.3		2046.9	355.0		395.2	119.1	
T1	4	1326.0	525.4		1306.3	517.3		1717.4	525.6		299.2	222.9	
T2	10	1833.5	832.3		1710.5	759.0		2207.7	1074.9		451.0	160.6	
T3	7	1812.3	522.3		1833.4	506.3		2541.3	630.6		444.4	141.7	
T4	8	1800.7	582.9		1630.9	544.2		2098.4	638.9		596.2	263.3	
N stage				0.8224**			0.7579**			0.7786**			0.1010**
N0	10	1665.1	479.6		1535.2	446.2		2158.4	619.1		436.1	168.2	
N1	5	1602.0	482.3		1549.8	507.6		1872.4	726.4		411.2	173.2	
N2	8	1813.4	964.3		1806.0	881.1		2333.5	1107.6		400.4	180.1	
N3	5	1937.5	428.0		1761.7	394.4		2135.4	234.1		671.9	287.7	
Pancreatic cancer													
T stage				0.7748**			0.8479**			0.8488**			0.8453**
T1	1	1398.3			1294.2			1400.7			419.7		
T2	12	1823.2	708.6		1730.9	647.8		2413.7	897.1		476.3	139.5	
T3	8	2031.6	1477.7		1891.1	1421.5		2693.9	2009.0		556.0	286.2	
T4	15	2279.0	1509.8		2077.8	1423.9		2741.7	1919.3		595.7	506.3	
N stage				0.1928*			0.1448*			0.1243*			0.0671*
N0	9	2663.9	1855.8		2564.3	1749.6		3475.3	2290.2		699.2	377.1	
N1	19	1756.4	837.8		1598.2	738.6		2133.6	964.7		428.6	152.1	

*Student t-test.
**One-way ANOVA.

be associated with platelets, exosomes, or other microvesicles. Two blood samples were first centrifuged at 1,750 g for 15 min to remove most blood cells and the supernatant was termed S1. S1 was centrifuged at 20,000 g for 20 min, which resulted in S2 and the pellet 2 (P2; cell fragments and large vesicles). S2 was ultracentrifuged at 110,000 g for 2 hr, which resulted in S3 and P3 (exosomes). A final centrifugation of S3 at 200,000 g for 2 hr resulted in S4 and P4 (other microvesicles). We found that all PLA$_2$ activities were retained in the S1 through S4 fractions, suggesting they were "free" and not associated with microvesicles (detailed data not shown). This is similar to what we have recently reported in human ovarian cancer ascites and novel secretion mechanisms for iPLA$_2$s and cPLA$_2$s may be involved [16].

Clinical parameters and PLA$_2$ activities in cancer plasma samples

Interestingly, the natural, iPLA$_2$, and sPLA$_2$ activities in plasma of CRC patients were increased in subjects with late stages (III and IV) as compared to earlier stage (I and II) disease ($P = 0.0335$, 0.0367, 0.0778, and 0.0345 for PLA$_2$, iPLA$_2$, cPLA$_2$, and sPLA$_2$, respectively; **Fig. 2**), suggesting that these enzymatic activities may be involved in CRC progression. We compared the PLA$_2$ activities in colon (n = 24) vs. rectal (n = 14) samples. Even though the nature, as well the sub-group PLA$_2$ activities in colon cancer patients were higher than those from rectal cancer patients, the differences were not statistically significant ($P > 0.05$ in all cases; **Table 2**). In addition, no difference was found in PLA$_2$ activities

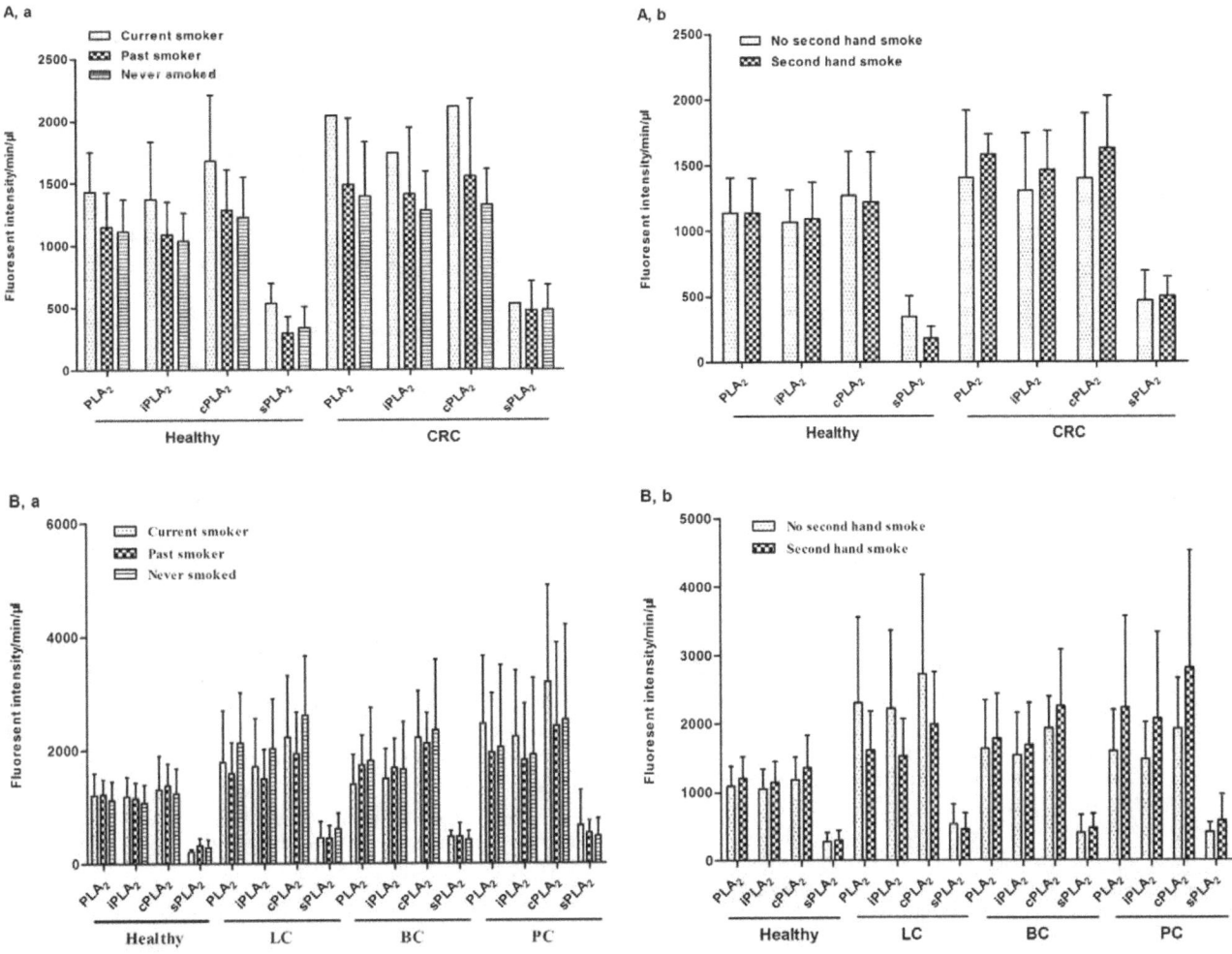

Figure 3. The influence of smoking on plasma PLA₂ activities. PLA2 activities in healthy and CRC samples with different smoking statuses(a)and second hand smoking statuses(b). A. Comparison of PLA2 activities between different smoking statuses(a) and second hand smoking statuses(b) in participants with LC, BC, and PC.

Table 4. Smoking, alcohol consumption, and the BMI status of participants from IUSM*.

	Healthy		CRC		
	No.	**%**	**No.**	**%**	**P value**
Smoking status					
Current smoker	2	3.8	1	3.7	0.4609
Past smoker	18	34.0	13	48.2	
Never smoked	33	62.3	13	48.2	
Second hand smoke					0.2185
No	48	90.6	21	80.8	
Yes	5	9.4	5	19.2	
Alcohol					0.2542
No	6	11.3	1	3.7	
Yes	47	88.4	26	96.3	
BMI (Mean ± SD)	28.2±6.96		25.4±4.01		0.0272

*These data are available from a subset of the participants.

among different subgroups of CRC patients with previous treatments (surgery, chemotherapy, radiotherapy, or untreated; **Table 2**). In contrast, we found that PLA₂ activities were not correlated to either T or N stages of LC, BC, or PC (**Table 3**).

Impact of other factors on PLA₂ activity

We have collected other factors, which might influence PLA₂ activities, including smoking, alcohol consumption, and body-mass index (BMI). For the CRC study, from the 80 subjects with available smoking information (27 CRC and 53 healthy cases), the majority (96%) of people did not smoke when the samples were collected, with an average 50.5% people never smoked and 45.7% of past smoker, and only 9.4% and 19.2% people had second hand smoking exposure in each group. The smoking statuses were similarly distributed in the two groups (P values >0.05; detailed data in **Table 4**) and there were no statistical differences in PLA₂ activities among different smoking statuses (**Fig. 3A**). In the second set of study, the smoking statuses were significantly different between healthy controls and each of the cancer groups with higher percentages of people who were current, past, or second-hand smokers in cancer groups (P values <0.05, except in one comparison, **Table 5**). Nevertheless, no statistical differences were observed in the PLA₂ activities among different smoking statuses,

Table 5. Smoking and alcohol consumption status of participants from HOG study.

	Healthy		LC			BC			PC		
	No.	%	No.	%	P value	No.	%	P value	No.	%	P value
Smoking status					<0.0001			0.0017			0.016
Current smoker	4	5.1	29	30.5		4	12.9		7	18.4	
Past smoker	25	31.6	58	61.1		19	61.3		16	42.1	
Never smoked	50	63.3	8	8.4		8	25.8		15	39.5	
Second hand smoke					<0.0001			0.0091			0.0741
No	32	40.5	10	10.5		4	13.8		9	23.7	
Yes	47	59.5	85	89.5		25	86.2		29	76.3	
Alcohol					<0.0001			0.0018			<0.0001
No	23	29.6	67	70.5		19	61.3		31	81.6	
Yes	56	70.4	28	29.5		12	38.7		7	18.4	
BMI (Mean ± SD)	28.3±5.55		26.5±6.76		0.0707	28.3±5.01		0.9625	25.9±6.17		0.0374

LC: Lung cancer; BC: Bladder cancer; PC: Pancreatic cancer.
All *P* values are comparisons between the cancer group and the healthy group.

supporting the concept obtained from the first set of study that plasma PLA_2 activities are not affected by smoking (**Fig. 3B**).

Alcohol consumption in the control and CRC groups were not significantly different (**Table 4**). The alcohol consumers in the CRC groups tend to have higher levels of plasma PLA_2 activities, but the differences were not statistically significant (**Fig. 4**). However, due to the low numbers in non-alcohol consumption group ($n = 7$), we should interpret these data with caution. For other cancers, similar results were obtained. Although there were significant higher percentages of alcohol consumption subjects in other cancer groups (**Table 5**), the PLA_2 activities were not significantly related to alcohol (**Fig. 5**).

The differences in PLA_2 activities between sexes did not reach a statistical significance in the control or any cancer groups in either set of studies (**Figs. 5A and 5B**). Similarly, there was no difference or correlation in PLA_2 activities in subjects with BMI <25 vs. BMI ≥25 groups in the CRC study (**Figs. 6A and 6B**), although the mean BMI in the CRC and PC groups were significantly less than those in control groups (**Tables 4 and 5**).

Age is one of the most clearly identified risk factors for developing CRC and other cancers. The American Cancer Society and the U.S. Preventive Services Task Force recommend that people receive colonoscopy screenings every 10 years beginning at age 50. We thus analyzed the age effects on PLA_2 activities by dividing the subjects into two groups (age <50 years, $n = 37$ and ≥50 years, $n = 78$). Although there was a trend of increased PLA_2 activities in the ≥50 years-old group in the CRC group, the differences were not statistically significant (**Fig. 7A**). Similarly, no difference was detected between the two age groups in the LC, BC, and PC set, although when all the subjects (including healthy controls) were combined, there were significant increases in PLA_2 activates in the older subjects (**Fig. 7B**).

A direct comparison of the two sets of healthy controls showed that although their sex, age, second-hand smoking, and alcohol consumption were different, there were no differences in any PLA_2 activity measured (**Table 6**). This further supports that plasma PLA_2 activities are not significantly affected by age, sex, alcohol consumption, and/or smoking.

The classification performance of plasma PLA_2 activities

Logistic regression was used to evaluate the classification performance of PLA_2 activities in cancers. All four PLA_2 measurements were kept as predictors regardless of their significance. The classification performances were summarized by receiver operating characteristic (ROC) curves (**Fig. 8**). Prediction formulas were generated using the parameter estimates.

The prediction formula to separate CRC cases from healthy subjects is:

$$\ln\left(\frac{P_{CRC}}{1 - P_{CRC}}\right) = -2.7372 + 0.00329 \times PLA_2 - 0.00286 \times$$
$$cPLA_2 + 0.000362 \times iPLA_2 + 0.00344 \times sPLA_2$$

where "P_{CRC}" stands for the probability of having CRC. The ROC curve shown in **Fig. 8A** has an area under the curve (AUC) = 0.7502.

Since external validations would require an independent study, we instead adopted internal methods to validate the classification performances. Among different internal validation methods, it has been shown that bootstrap outperforms jackknife, cross-validation and data-splitting methods [19]. Therefore, bootstrap was adopted for validation. In particular, the prediction formula was obtained by fitting the same model for each bootstrapped sample. The formula was applied to the original data to calculate the prediction probabilities. The performance for this particular bootstrap sample was summarized by AUC of the ROC curve. The overall performance was evaluated by summarizing AUCs across 1,000 bootstrapped samples. In 95% of the 1000 bootstrapped samples, AUCs are higher than 0.7143 for CRC vs. healthy. Therefore, these results internally confirm the classification performances of the models developed above.

The prediction formula and the ROC curve to separate all cancer cases from healthy subjects in the second set of study are as follows and shown in **Fig. 8B**, with an AUC = 0.8337.

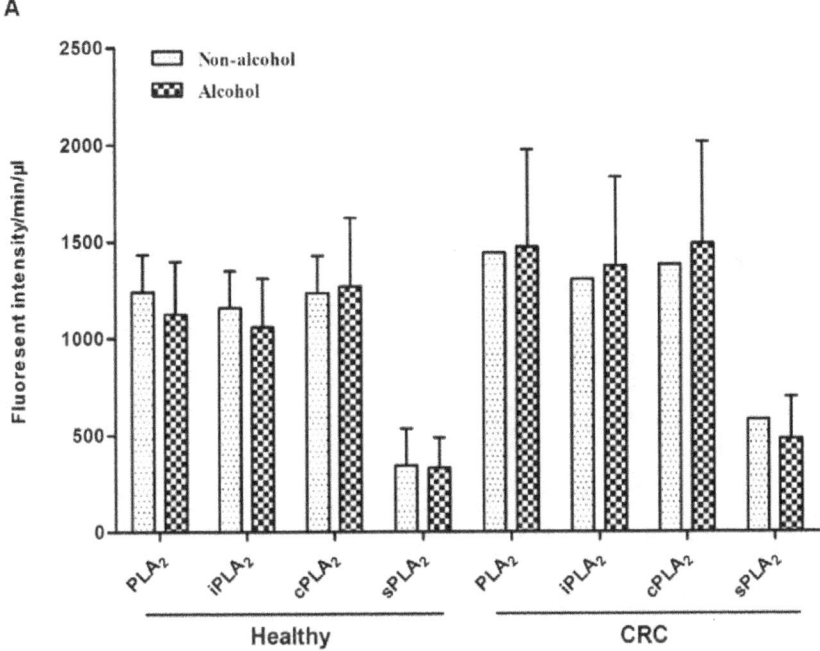

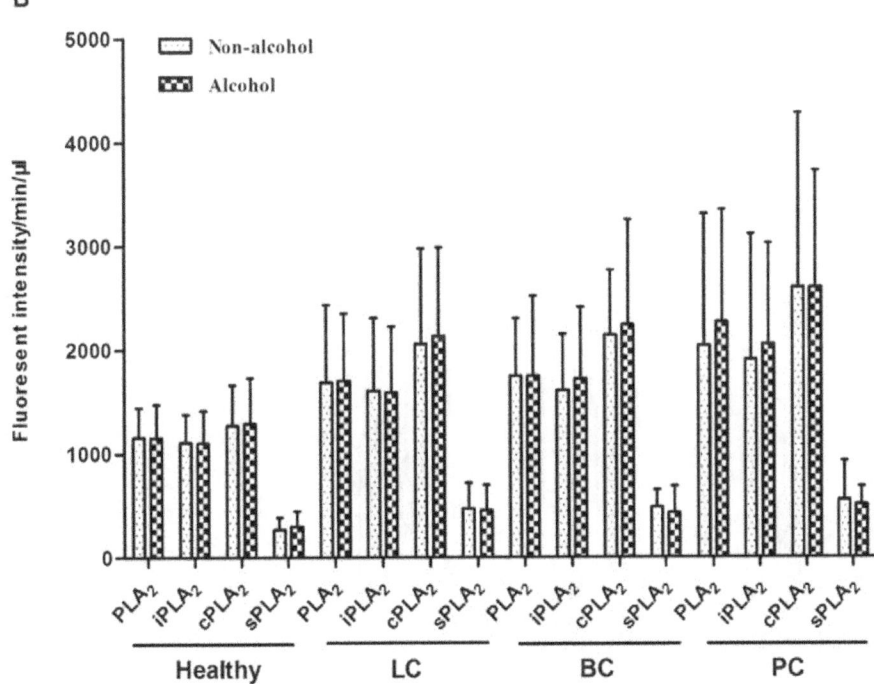

Figure 4. The influence alcohol consumption on plasma PLA$_2$ activities. Comparison of PLA2 activities between "non-alcohol" and "alcohol" groups with the healthy and CRC participants. A. Comparison of PLA2 activities between "non-alcohol" and "alcohol" groupsin the second set of studies with healthy, LC, BC, and PC participants.

$$\ln\left(\frac{P}{1-P}\right) = -2.6398 - 0.00035 \times PLA_2 - 0.00169 \times iPLA_2 +$$

$$0.00311 \times cPLA_2 + 0.00276 \times sPLA_2$$

This performance was validated in 1000 bootstrapped samples. In 95% of the 1000 bootstrapped samples, AUCs are higher than

0.8205 for LC, PC, BC combined vs. the second set of healthy controls.

The prediction formulas and the ROC curves for the separate LC, BC, and PC cases from healthy subjects in the second set of study are listed below and **Figs. 8C** to **8E**, with AUCs >0.811, indicating good classification performances of the tests. For LC versus healthy control, the AUC = 0.8119 (**Fig. 8C**). In 95% of the 1000 bootstrapped sample, AUCs are higher than 0.7923.

A

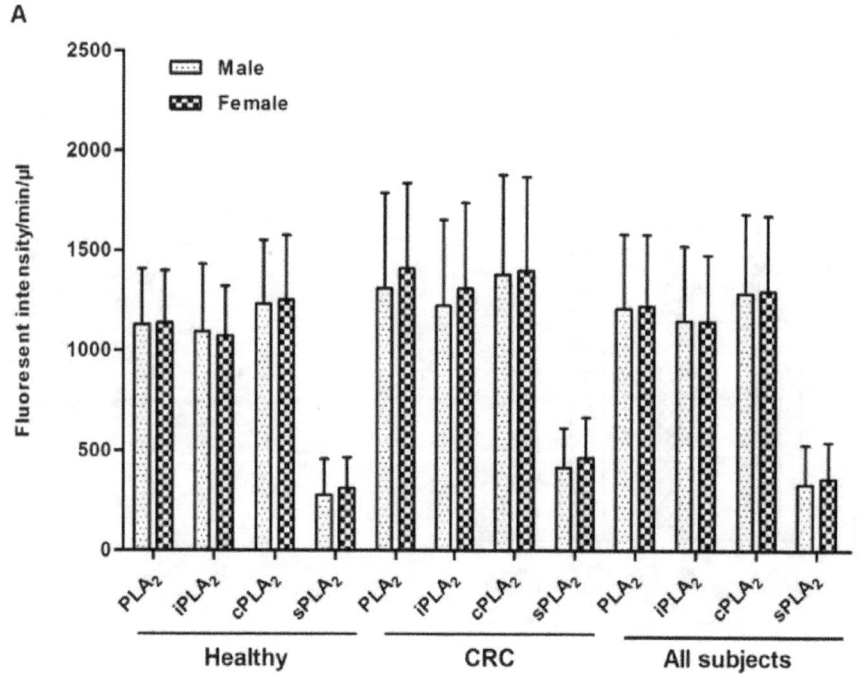

B

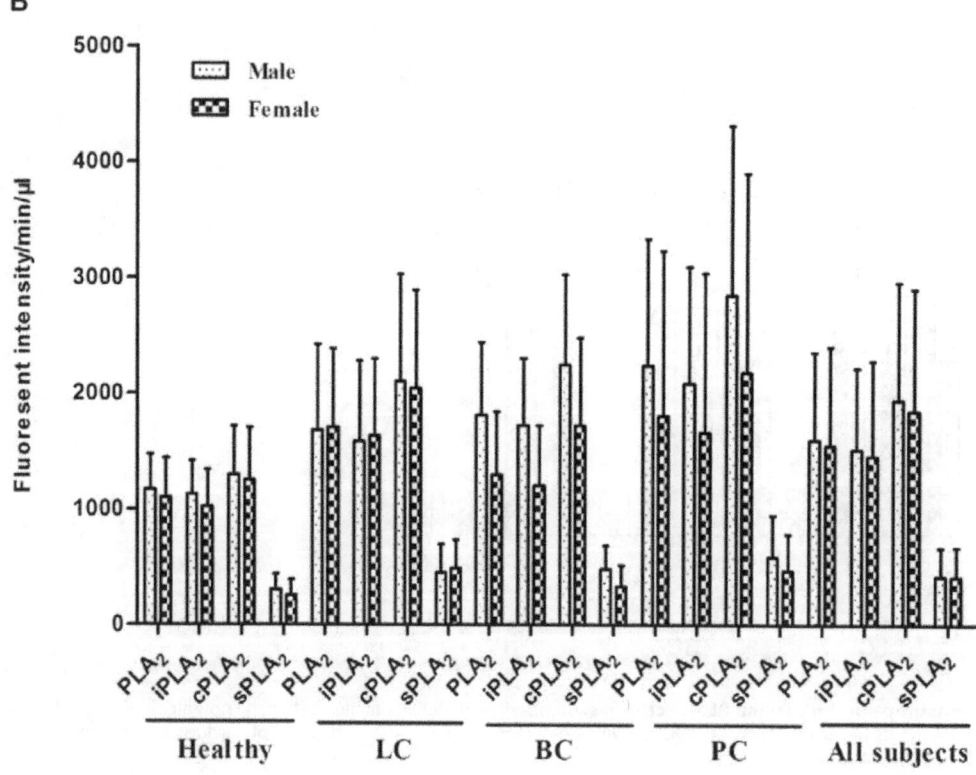

Figure 5. PLA₂activities were not significantly different between male and female. PLA2 activity comparison in males and females in the healthy and the CRC groups. A. PLA2 activity comparison in males and females in the healthy and other cancer groups. Data from all subjects in each set of studies are also presented.

A

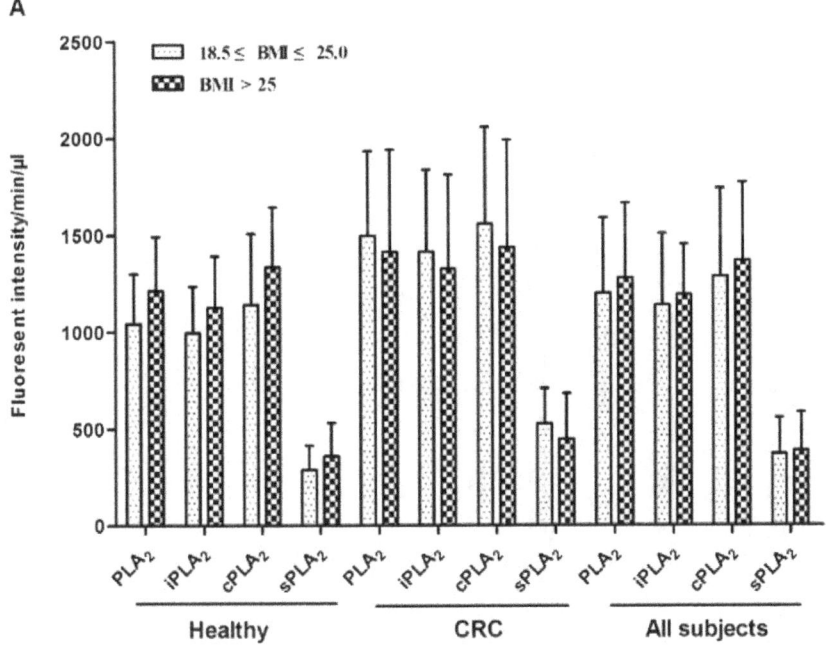

B

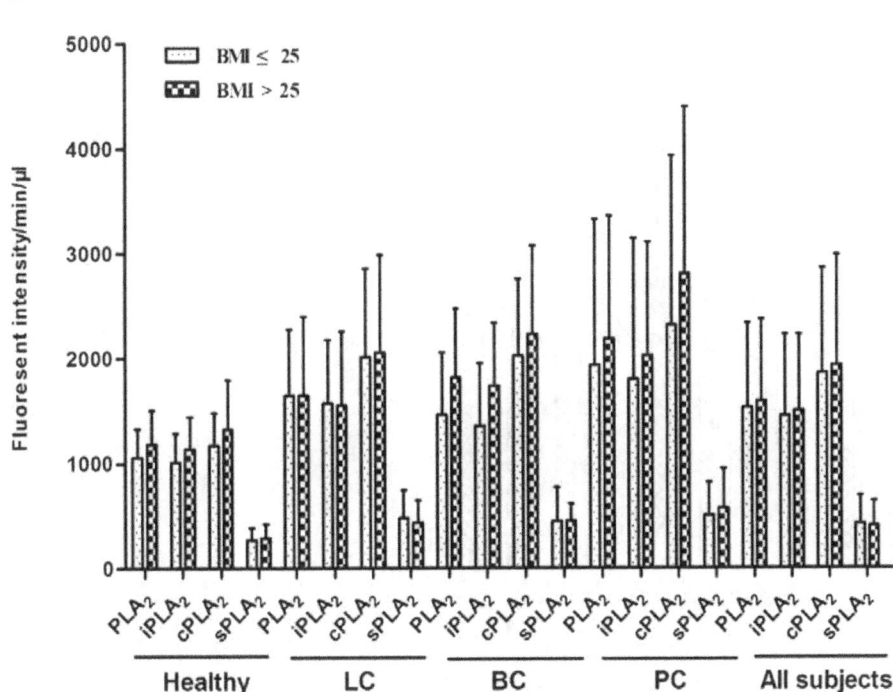

Figure 6. Comparison of PLA$_2$ activities among different BMI groups. The subjected in healthy and CRC groups were divided into two groups: BMI 18.5 to <25 (For all subjects, n=43) and BMI>25 (For all subjects, n=80). A. The subjected in healthy and other cancer groups were divided into two groups: BMI≤25 (For all subjects, n=80) and BMI>25 (For all subjects, n=148).

$$\ln\left(\frac{P}{1-P}\right) = -2.9998 - 0.00024 \times PLA_2 - 0.00136 \times iPLA_2 +$$
$$0.00278 \times cPLA_2 + 0.00230 \times sPLA_2$$

For BC versus healthy control, the AUC = 0.8624 (**Fig. 8D**). In 95% of the 1000 bootstrapped sample, AUCs are higher than 0.8161.

$$\ln\left(\frac{P}{1-P}\right) = -5.3597 - 0.002 \times PLA_2 + 0.00086 \times iPLA_2 +$$
$$0.00313 \times cPLA_2 + 0.00236 \times sPLA_2$$

For PC versus healthy control, the AUC = 0.8671. In 95% of the 1000 bootstrapped sample, AUCs are higher than 0.8426.

A

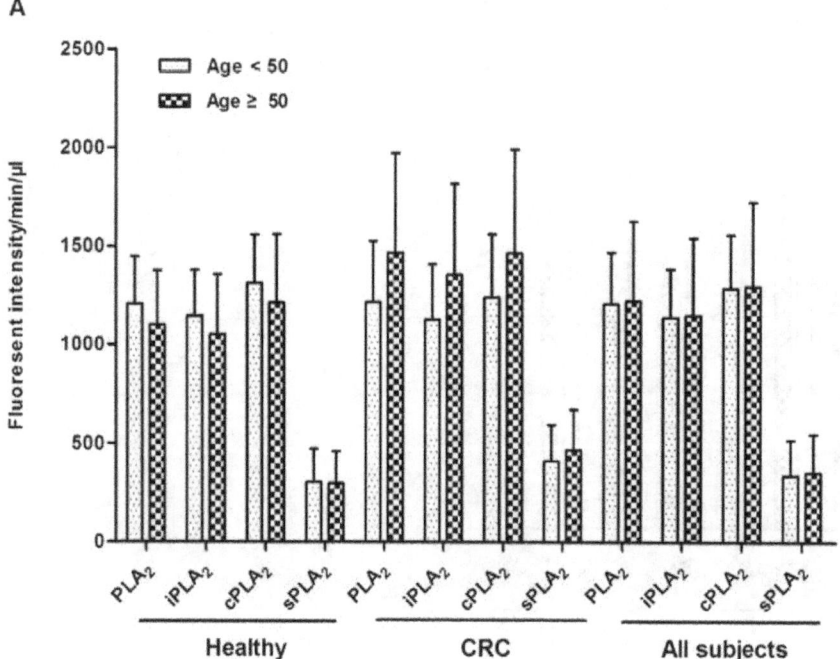

B

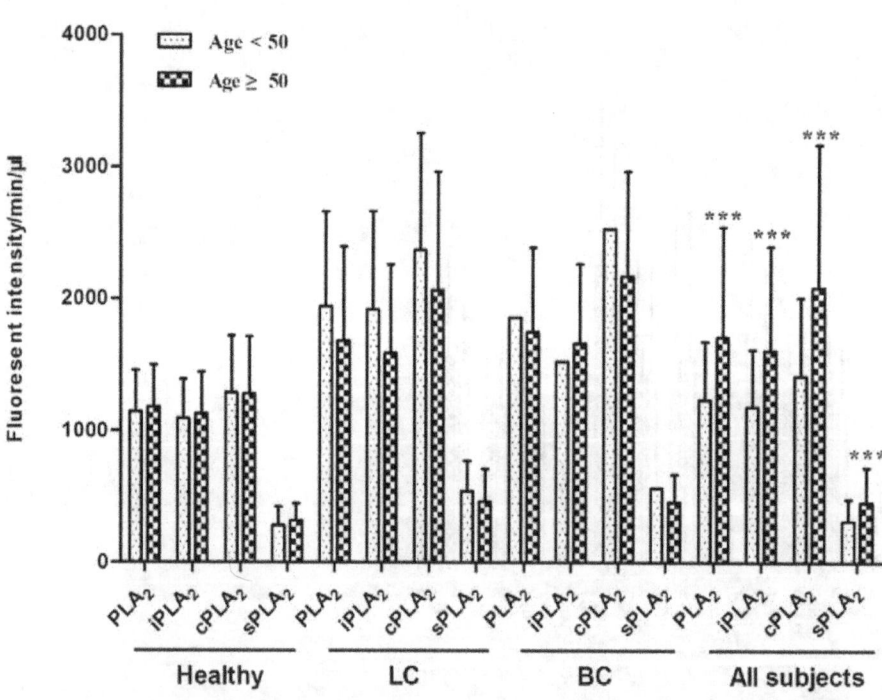

Figure 7. PLA₂activities were not significantly correlated to ages. The participants in healthy and CRC groups were divided into two groups: age<50 (For all subjects, n = 42) and age ≥50 (For all subjects, n = 153). Student t-test was performed to analyze the differences between these two groups. A. The participants in healthy and other cancer groups were divided into two groups: age<50 (For all subjects, n = 61) and age ≥50 (For all subjects, n = 144). Student t-test was performed to analyze the differences between these two groups. ***P<0.001.

$$\ln\left(\frac{P}{1-P}\right) = -4.6897 + 0.00263 \times PLA_2 - 0.00411 \times iPLA_2 +$$

$$0.00263 \times cPLA_2 + 0.00342 \times sPLA_2$$

Finally, since we have found that the PLA₂ activities were essentially no difference in the two sets of healthy controls, we combined all healthy controls and all cancer cases in both sets of studies and generated a combined formula, with an AUC = 0.8011 (**Fig. 8F**). In 95% of the 1000 bootstrapped samples, AUCs are higher than 0.7907.

Table 6. Comparison of two independent sets of healthy controls.

	1st set		2nd set		
	No.	%	No.	%	P value
Gender					<0.0001
Male	31	40.3	61	77.2	
Female	46	59.7	18	22.8	
Smoking status					
Current smoker	2	3.8	4	5.1	0.889
Past smoker	19	35.8	25	31.6	
Never smoked	32	60.4	50	63.3	
Second hand smoke					<0.0001
No	48	90.6	32	40.5	
Yes	5	9.4	47	59.5	
Alcohol					<0.0001
No	6	11.3	23	29.6	
Yes	47	88.4	56	70.4	
Age (Mean ± SD)	51.6±13.5		42.7±12.03		<0.0001
PLA$_2$ activities(Mean ± SD)					
PLA$_2$	1135.9±266.2		1156.3±311.8		0.660
iPLA$_2$	1082.0±286.1		1105.4±301.6		0.620
cPLA$_2$	1246.1±318.7		1287.8±425.9		0.488
sPLA$_2$	299.1±164.7		293.9±137.3		0.828

$$\ln\left(\frac{P}{1-P}\right) = -3.0732 + 0.000461 \times PLA_2 - 0.00131 \times iPLA_2 + $$
$$0.00222 \times cPLA_2 + 0.00254 \times sPLA_2$$

The sensitivities and specificities can be obtained from the ROC curves shown in **Fig. 8**. For the CRC set of study, 60.5% sensitivity and 77.9% of specificity were obtained (**Table 7**). For the 2nd set of study and the data combined for both sets, sensitivities >80% and the specificities >66% were obtained for all cases (**Table 7**).

The potential contributions of other factors

Although most other demographic and/or environmental factors tested were not significantly different in cancer and control groups (**Figs 3–7**), we tested their potential contributions to the performance when they are evaluated at individual levels. We kept all four PLA$_2$ measurements in the models, but let other predictors subject to model selections at the significant level 0.05.

The prediction formula and the ROC curve to separate CRC from healthy subjects in the first set of study are as follows and shown in **Fig. 9A**, with an AUC = 0.8162. In 95% of the 1000 bootstrapped sample, AUCs are higher than 0.7589.

$$\ln\left(\frac{P_L}{1-P_L}\right) = -7.1140 - 0.0006 \times PLA_2 + 0.00909 \times iPLA_2 -$$
$$0.00612 \times cPLA_2 + 0.00327 \times sPLA_2 + 3.5428 \times$$
$$Alcohol$$

The prediction formula and the ROC curve to separate all cancer cases from healthy subjects in the second set of study are as follows and shown in **Fig. 9B**, with an AUC = 0.9728.

$$\ln\left(\frac{P_{2nd,all}}{1-P_{2nd,all}}\right) = -6.7670 - 0.00034 + PLA_2 - 0.00193 \times$$
$$iPLA_2 + 0.00415 \times cPLA_2 + 0.00173 \times$$
$$sPLA_2 + 5.3434 \times (Age \geq 50) - 3.4392 \times$$
$$Alcohol + 2.8792 \times (Currently\ Smoke) +$$
$$1.4151 \times (Currently\ not\ but\ used\ to\ smoke)$$

This performance was validated in 1000 bootstrapped samples. In 95% of the 1000 bootstrapped samples, AUCs are higher than 0.9625 for LC, PC, and BC combined vs. the second set of healthy controls.

The prediction formulas and the ROC curves for the separate LC, BC, and PC cases from healthy subjects in the second set of study are listed below and **Figs. 9C** to **9E**, with AUCs >0.968, indicating high sensitivities and specifies of the tests. For LC versus healthy control, the AUC = 0.9742. In 95% of the 1000 bootstrapped sample, AUCs are higher than 0.9598.

$$\ln\left(\frac{P_L}{1-P_L}\right) = -7.5757 + 0.00136 \times PLA_2 - 0.00373 \times iPLA_2 +$$
$$0.00423 \times cPLA_2 + 0.00207 \times sPLA_2 + 4.3789 \times$$
$$(Age \geq 50) - 3.4043 \times Alcohol + 4.0312 \times$$
$$(Currently\ Smoke) + 2.3753 \times$$
$$(Currently\ not\ but\ used\ to\ smoke)$$

For BC versus healthy control, the AUC = 0.9682. In 95% of the 1000 bootstrapped sample, AUCs are higher than 0.9398.

$$\ln\left(\frac{P_B}{1-P_B}\right) = -7.6200 - 0.00424 \times PLA_2 - 0.00010 \times iPLA_2 +$$
$$0.00538 \times cPLA_2 + 0.00292 \times sPLA_2 + 5.9791 \times$$
$$(Age \geq 50) - 2.9782 \times Alcohol$$

For PC versus healthy control, the AUC = 0.9907. In 95% of the 1000 bootstrapped sample, AUCs are higher than 0.9740.

$$\ln\left(\frac{P_P}{1-P_P}\right) = -3.1927 + 0.00229 \times PLA_2 - 0.00384 \times iPLA_2 +$$
$$0.00179 \times cPLA_2 + 0.00105 \times sPLA_2 + 2.9716 \times$$
$$(Age \geq 50) - 2.1084 \times Alcohol$$

Finally, since we found that the PLA$_2$ activities were essentially no difference in the two sets of healthy controls, we combined all healthy controls and all cancer cases in both sets of studies and generated a combined formula, with an AUC = 0.9140 (**Fig. 9F**). In 95% of the 1000 bootstrapped samples, AUCs are higher than 0.9018.

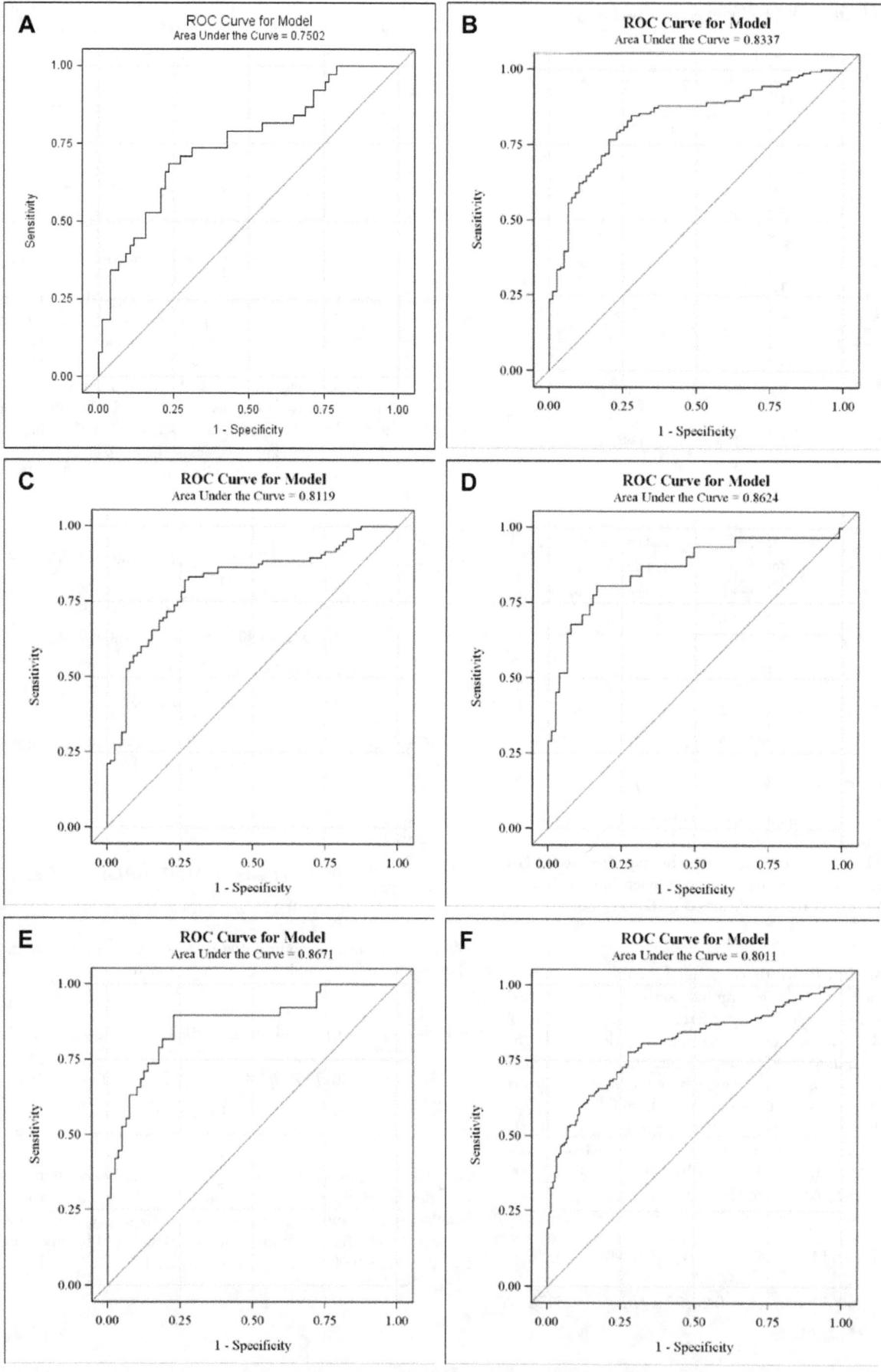

Figure 8. ROC curves of plasma PLA$_2$ activities in different groups. CRC cases vs. healthy subjects. A. All cancers vs. healthy subjects in the 2nd set. B. Lung cancer vs. healthy subjects. C. Bladder cancer vs. healthy subjects. D. Pancreatic cancer vs. healthy subjects. E. All cancers vs. all healthy subjects with combined two sets.

$$\ln\left(\frac{P_{both,all}}{1-P_{both,all}}\right) = -3.5290 + 0.000371 \times PLA_2 - 0.00066 \times$$

$$iPLA_2 + 0.0015 \times cPLA_2 + 0.00219 \times sPLA_2$$

$$+1.9213 \times (Age \geq 50) - 1.7107 \times Alcohol$$

$$+1.4619 \times (Currently\ Smoke) + 1.0802 \times$$

$$(Currently\ not\ but\ used\ to\ smoke)$$

The sensitivities and specificities obtained with these ROC curves with additional parameters are increased to >85% (except CRC vs. healthy cases; **Table 7**).

Discussion

In this work, we have presented the first measurements of plasma natural and subtype PLA$_2$ activities and their performances as potential markers for four different cancers, CRC, LC, BC, and PC. We have measured the PLA$_2$ activities in more than 20 blood samples with or without adding 1.2 mM calcium (the natural ionized calcium concentration in blood) to the final assay mixtures and did not detect any significant differences. Hence, we define the PLA$_2$ activities obtained without any additives as the "natural" PLA$_2$ activity. We have selected optimal conditions to measure each sub-family of PLA$_2$ activities. These modified conditions do not co-exist in the blood. Therefore, it is not surprising that the sum of the subfamily PLA$_2$ activities is greater than the "natural" PLA$_2$ activity. However, it is important to note that although modified conditions were used to obtain the activities for subfamilies of PLA$_2$s, the final results are from the natural PLA$_2$s present in the blood samples.

While the advantages of using convenient serologic markers are obvious, no reliable blood markers for any of these cancers are currently available. For CRC, developing/validating non-invasive or minimally invasive detection methods is a major focus in the field. Current methods include stool and blood tests, such as fecal immunochemical tests (FITs) and guaiac-based fecal occult blood testing (got). Although the specificity is high (>85%), these tests

have a low sensitivity (<23%) for colorectal adenomas and are thus unlikely to be able to increase the early detection of CRC [20,21]. Genetic stool tests detect mutations in stool that can be found in CRC. A 21 genetic change test was found to be superior to guaiac fecal occult blood test (gFOBT) for the detection of CRC [20]. However, the sensitivity only reached 51.6% [20]. The plasma PLA$_2$ activities tests presented show promising initial results in separating healthy controls from cancer patients with sensitivities and specificities approximately 70%. The majority solid cancers are highly heterogeneous, which is one of the major reasons that any single or small set of markers can hardly detect any specific cancer with very high sensitivity and specificity. Testing the potential complementary values of other identified markers in CRC and other cancers will be of high significance. Interestingly, our results suggest that PLA$_2$ activities are independent of several common demographic and environmental factors. In addition, we have compared 11 CRC blood samples collected before and after surgeries and found that 7 of 11 had reduced PLA$_2$ activities (26.1±10.9% reduction) and 4 of 11 had increased PLA$_2$ activities (37.7%±11.7%). Among them, disease progression data was available for only 6 subjects (3 from each group). Interestingly, all 3 subjects from the reduced PLA$_2$ activity group had chemotherapy and complete response and all 3 subjects from the increased PLA$_2$ activity group had chemotherapy and disease progression. These data were from a very limited number of subjects, but suggest that the prognostic value of PLA$_2$ activities warrants further testing. We are fully aware that our studies are limited to the cohort size and external validation in independent and larger scale studies will be critical and hope that our report will promote such studies.

Is a marker which may detect multiple types of cancers useful? The answer is likely to be yes. Even after decades of efforts, the success rate in finding highly specific markers for specific cancers has been low. Prostate-specific antigen is an exception, but even the value of this marker as a screening tool in prostate cancer has been recently questioned [22]. Many tumor markers are known to affect multiple cancers. Sensitive, minimally invasive, reproducible, and cost-effective blood biomarkers to detect multiple malignancies are likely to be clinically significant and highly valuable as routine first line detection. In addition, the PLA$_2$

Table 7. Sensitivities and specificities of PLA$_2$ to distinguish different cancers from healthy cases.

	Without other parameters		With other parameters	
	Sensitivity	Specificity	Sensitivity	Specificity
First set				
CRC vs. Healthy	60.5%	77.9%	63.0%	75.5%
Second set				
All cancer vs. healthy	81.1%	72.2%	87.2%	88.6%
LC vs. healthy	82.1%	67.1%	85.3%	91.1%
BC vs. healthy	80.6%	75.9%	87.1%	87.3%
PC vs. healthy	81.6%	77.2%	86.8%	96.2%
Combined two sets				
Cancer vs. healthy	80.2%	66.7%	83.2%	81.1%

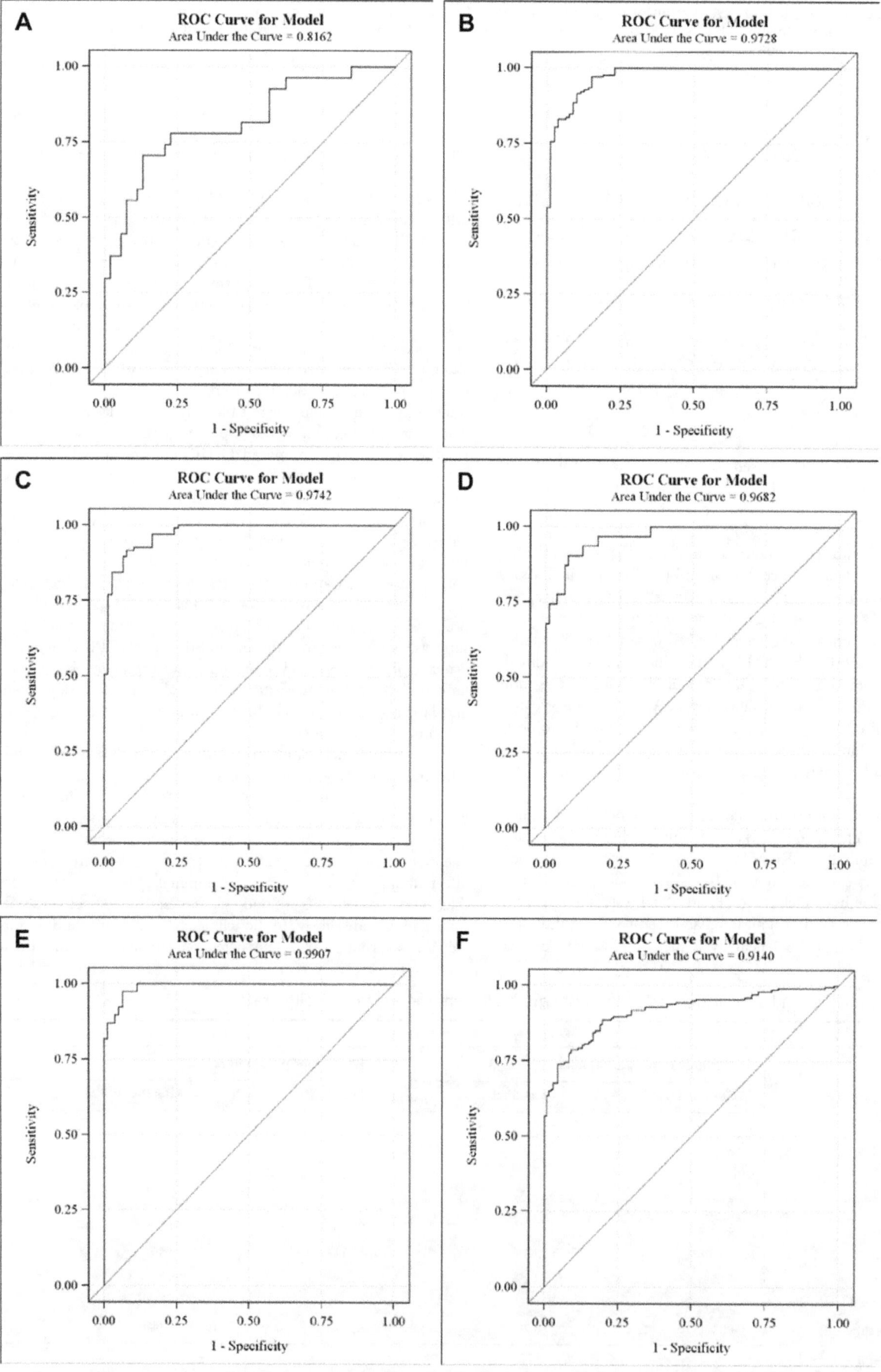

Figure 9. ROC curves of plasma PLA$_2$ activities with additional parameters. CRC cases vs. healthy subjects. A. All cancer cases vs. healthy subjects in the second set. B. Lung cancer vs. healthy subjects. C. Bladder cancer vs. healthy subjects. D. Pancreatic cancer vs. healthy subjects. E. All cancers vs. all healthy subjects with combined two sets.

activity test is very easy to perform in any laboratory with a fluorescent plate reader, and would be feasible to develop into an automated test. Moreover, very small amounts samples (1–10 μL of plasma) are needed to perform the test and the results can be obtained in 1–2 hrs. Additional markers or more specific modalities, such as colonoscopy or imaging are likely to be needed to detect specific cancers.

Another major advantage of the test is that it is reproducible, robotic, and stable. It is well-recognized that many blood markers are sensitive to how blood samples are handled, processed, and stored. It is almost impossible to unify these procedures in the USA or anywhere in the world. Freeze-and-thaw is another well-known factor affecting marker stability. These reasons account, at least in part, for the fact that although thousands of markers have been reported in the past decades, seldom have any of them been cross-validated in different centers and moved to the clinic. We have used two completely independent sets of human plasma samples, which were processed somewhat differently (see Method for details) and show that the PLA$_2$ activities are highly compatible, consistent in healthy controls, and are independent of several demographic and environmental factors, making them more likely to be useful markers. More independent studies with large samples sizes need to be conducted to further evaluate the clinical significance of our finding reported here.

A potential caveat of the clinical usage of PLA$_2$ activity is that these enzymes are known to be involved in inflammation and may be elevated in patients with benign inflammatory diseases. This needs to be experimentally tested in clinical samples. However, there are mounting lines of evidence supporting the strong causal connections between inflammation and cancers [23]. In particular, chronic inflammation plays a pivotal role in the development of CRC in patients with inflammatory bowel disease [24]. The connection between inflammation and lung cancer has been

shown not coincidental but may indeed be causal [23]. In addition, non-steroidal anti-inflammatory drugs has been associated with reduced risk to developing many types of cancers [25]. Thus, future studies on the significance of elevated PLA$_2$ activity in disease detection and progression prediction will be highly interesting.

Our results also strongly imply that the PLA$_2$ activities (which may or may not correlate to their RNA or protein expression levels) are potential targets for cancer treatment tested here. Most, if not all previous PLA$_2$ assays conducted in tissues or cell lines mainly focus on their expression levels using PCR and IHC, which are gene/protein specific, time-consuming, costly, and require relatively large amount of samples to cover different isoforms of PLA$_2$s. Since there are more than 30 PLA$_2$s, none of the previous studies provide an overall picture of PLA$_2$s in any cancer. More importantly, their enzymatic activities, but not necessarily their RNA and/or protein expression levels, are directly related to the biological effects, since PLA$_2$ activities are well-known to be regulated post-transcriptionally [26,27]. This concept has been supported in our recent pre-clinical (mouse models) and human sample studies in ovarian cancer [16] and remain to be tested further in other cancers.

Acknowledgments

We highly appreciate the proof-reading and editing of Dr. Caryl Antalis.

Author Contributions

Conceived and designed the experiments: YX. Performed the experiments: HC. Analyzed the data: HC ZL. Contributed reagents/materials/analysis tools: EGC MVC DKR BWR NMH PJL MLH. Wrote the paper: YX HC.

References

1. Siegel R, Naishadham D, Jemal A (2012) Cancer statistics, 2012. CA Cancer J Clin 62: 10–29.

2. Khochikar MV (2011) Rationale for an early detection program for bladder cancer. Indian J Urol 27: 218–225.

3. Risch A, Plass C (2008) Lung cancer epigenetics and genetics. Int J Cancer 123: 1–7.

4. Pastorino U (2010) Lung cancer screening. Br J Cancer 102: 1681–1686.

5. Mutti A (2008) Molecular diagnosis of lung cancer: an overview of recent developments. Acta Biomed 79 Suppl 1: 11–23.

6. Cummings BS (2007) Phospholipase A2 as targets for anti-cancer drugs. Biochem Pharmacol 74: 949–959.

7. Murakami M, Taketomi Y, Sato H, Yamamoto K (2011) Secreted phospholipase A2 revisited. J Biochem 150: 233–255.

8. Kudo I, Murakami M (2002) Phospholipase A2 enzymes. Prostaglandins Other Lipid Mediat 68–69: 3–58.

9. Xu Y, Xiao YJ, Zhu K, Baudhuin LM, Lu J, et al. (2003) Unfolding the pathophysiological role of bioactive lysophospholipids. Curr Drug Targets Immune Endocr Metabol Disord 3: 23–32.

10. Sengupta S, Kim KS, Berk MP, Oates R, Escobar P, et al. (2007) Lysophosphatidic acid downregulates tissue inhibitor of metalloproteinases, which are negatively involved in lysophosphatidic acid-induced cell invasion. Oncogene 26: 2894–2901.

11. Xu Y, Wang D, Wang Z (2009) Lipid generation and signaling in ovarian cacner. In: Stack MS, Fishman DA, editors. Cancer Treatment and Research-Ovarian cancer. 2 ed. New York, Dordrecht, Heidelberg, London: Springer. pp. 241–268.

12. Song Y, Wilkins P, Hu W, Murthy KS, Chen J, et al. (2007) Inhibition of calcium-independent phospholipase A2 suppresses proliferation and tumorigenicity of ovarian carcinoma cells. Biochem J 406: 427–436.

13. Li H, Zhao Z, Wei G, Yan L, Wang D, et al. (2010) Group VIA phospholipase A2 in both host and tumor cells is involved in ovarian cancer development. FASEB J 24: 4103–4116.

14. Subra C, Grand D, Laulagnier K, Stella A, Lambeau G, et al. (2010) Exosomes account for vesicle-mediated transcellular transport of activatable phospholipases and prostaglandins. J Lipid Res 51: 2105–2120.

15. Iguchi H, Kosaka N, Ochiya T (2010) Secretory microRNAs as a versatile communication tool. Commun Integr Biol 3: 478–481.

16. Cai Q, Zhao Z, Antalis C, Yan L, Del Priore G, et al. (2012) Elevated and secreted phospholipase A2 activities as new potential therapeutic targets in human epithelial ovarian cancer. FASEB J.

17. Zhao X, Wang D, Zhao Z, Xiao Y, Sengupta S, et al. (2006) Caspase-3-dependent activation of calcium-independent phospholipase A2 enhances cell migration in non-apoptotic ovarian cancer cells. J Biol Chem 281: 29357–29368.

18. Murakami M, Kudo I (2001) Diversity and regulatory functions of mammalian secretory phospholipase A2s. Adv Immunol 77: 163–194.

19. Steyerberg EW, Harrell FE, Jr., Borsboom GJ, Eijkemans MJ, Vergouwe Y, et al. (2001) Internal validation of predictive models: efficiency of some procedures for logistic regression analysis. J Clin Epidemiol 54: 774–781.

20. Pox C (2011) Colon Cancer Screening: Which Non-Invasive Filter Tests? Digestive Diseases 29: 56–59.

21. Wong MC, John GK, Hirai HW, Lam TY, Luk AK, et al. (2012) Changes in the choice of colorectal cancer screening tests in primary care settings from 7,845 prospectively collected surveys. Cancer Causes Control 23: 1541–1548.

22. Chou R, Croswell JM, Dana T, Bougatsos C, Blazina I, et al. (2011) Screening for prostate cancer: a review of the evidence for the U.S. Preventive Services Task Force. Ann Intern Med 155: 762–771.

23. Cho WC, Kwan CK, Yau S, So PP, Poon PC, et al. (2011) The role of inflammation in the pathogenesis of lung cancer. Expert Opin Ther Targets 15: 1127–1137.

24. Moossavi S, Bishehsari F (2012) Inflammation in sporadic colorectal cancer. Arch Iran Med 15: 166–170.

25. Vendramini-Costa DB, Carvalho JE (2012) Molecular Link Mechanisms between Inflammation and Cancer. Curr Pharm Des 18: 3831–3852.

26. Burke JE, Dennis EA (2009) Phospholipase A2 biochemistry. Cardiovasc Drugs Ther 23: 49–59.

27. Burke JE, Dennis EA (2009) Phospholipase A2 structure/function, mechanism, and signaling. J Lipid Res 50 Suppl: S237–242.

16

Bladder Cancer Diagnosis and Identification of Clinically Significant Disease by Combined Urinary Detection of Mcm5 and Nuclear Matrix Protein 22

John D. Kelly[1,9], Tim J. Dudderidge[1,2,9], Alex Wollenschlaeger[3]*, Odu Okoturo[4], Keith Burling[5], Fiona Tulloch[5], Ian Halsall[5], Teresa Prevost[6], Andrew Toby Prevost[7], Joana C. Vasconcelos[6], Wendy Robson[8], Hing Y. Leung[9], Nikhil Vasdev[8], Robert S. Pickard[8], Gareth H. Williams[1,3]*, Kai Stoeber[1,3]

1 Department of Pathology and Cancer Institute, University College London, London, United Kingdom, 2 The Royal Marsden National Health Service (NHS) Foundation Trust, London, United Kingdom, 3 Wolfson Institute for Biomedical Research, University College London, London, United Kingdom, 4 Department of Medicine, Imperial College London, London, United Kingdom, 5 Department of Clinical Biochemistry, Addenbrooke's Hospital, University of Cambridge, Cambridge, United Kingdom, 6 Department of Public Health and Primary Care, Centre for Applied Medical Statistics, University of Cambridge, Institute of Public Health, Cambridge, United Kingdom, 7 Department of Primary Care and Public Health Sciences, King's College London, London, United Kingdom, 8 Department of Urology, Freeman Hospital, Newcastle upon Tyne, United Kingdom, 9 Beatson Institute for Cancer Research, University of Glasgow, Bearsden, Glasgow, United Kingdom

Abstract

Background: Urinary biomarkers for bladder cancer detection are constrained by inadequate sensitivity or specificity. Here we evaluate the diagnostic accuracy of Mcm5, a novel cell cycle biomarker of aberrant growth, alone and in combination with NMP22.

Methods: 1677 consecutive patients under investigation for urinary tract malignancy were recruited to a prospective blinded observational study. All patients underwent ultrasound, intravenous urography, cystoscopy, urine culture and cytologic analysis. An immunofluorometric assay was used to measure Mcm5 levels in urine cell sediments. NMP22 urinary levels were determined with the FDA-approved NMP22® Test Kit.

Results: Genito-urinary tract cancers were identified in 210/1564 (13%) patients with an Mcm5 result and in 195/1396 (14%) patients with an NMP22 result. At the assay cut-point where sensitivity and specificity were equal, the Mcm5 test detected primary and recurrent bladder cancers with 69% sensitivity (95% confidence interval = 62–75%) and 93% negative predictive value (95% CI = 92–95%). The area under the receiver operating characteristic curve for Mcm5 was 0.75 (95% CI = 0.71–0.79) and 0.72 (95% CI = 0.67–0.77) for NMP22. Importantly, Mcm5 combined with NMP22 identified 95% (79/83; 95% CI = 88–99%) of potentially life threatening diagnoses (i.e. grade 3 or carcinoma in situ or stage ≥pT1) with high specificity (72%, 95% CI = 69–74%).

Conclusions: The Mcm5 immunoassay is a non-invasive test for identifying patients with urothelial cancers with similar accuracy to the FDA-approved NMP22 ELISA Test Kit. The combination of Mcm5 plus NMP22 improves the detection of UCC and identifies 95% of clinically significant disease. Trials of a commercially developed Mcm5 assay suitable for an end-user laboratory alongside NMP22 are required to assess their potential clinical utility in improving diagnostic and surveillance care pathways.

Editor: Clive Shiff, Johns Hopkins University, United States of America

Funding: This work was supported by Cancer Research UK (grant number C428/A3441 to KS and GHW). The funders had no role in study design, data collection and analysis, decision to publish, or preparation of the manuscript.

Competing Interests: The authors have declared that no competing interests exist.

* E-mail: gareth.williams@ucl.ac.uk

9 These authors contributed equally to this work.

Introduction

Urothelial cell carcinoma (UCC) of the urinary bladder is the 4th most common cancer in the US, with an estimated 73510 new cases and 14880 deaths from bladder cancer in 2012 [1]. Cystoscopy is the standard method of bladder tumour detection, however it is an invasive, uncomfortable and costly procedure which results in urinary infection in up to 5% of cases [2]. Detection of bladder cancer with a non-invasive tumour marker test could potentially improve the management of the disease by increasing the accuracy and decreasing the morbidity associated with current diagnostic and surveillance pathways. Through reduced frequency of cystoscopies, improvements in patient's quality of life and cost efficiency could be seen.

Urinary biomarkers for the detection of bladder cancer hold great promise and while numerous markers have regulatory approval none have been accepted as a standard diagnostic procedure [3]. Urinary cytology remains the most widely utilized because of high specificity although poor sensitivity. Novel technologies and biomarkers, however, have the potential to improve diagnostic accuracy, with the most effective diagnostic and surveillance strategies to date utilizing photodynamic cystoscopy and biomarkers [4]. Nuclear matrix protein 22 (NMP22), for example, is a nuclear mitotic apparatus protein that regulates chromatid and daughter cell separation [5,6] and has emerged as one of the promising urinary biomarkers for UCC [3]. The FDA-approved, laboratory-based quantitative NMP22® Test Kit immunoassay (Matritech, Freiburg, Germany) and a qualitative point-of-care test, NMP22® BladderChek® (Matritech; ® symbol omitted hereafter), are now available for clinical use. However, although urinary NMP22 levels are elevated in bladder cancer, dead and dying urothelial cells in many non-malignant and inflammatory conditions can also release NMP22, thus reducing specificity. Moreover, a wide marked range in test performance has been reported among different studies using NMP22, with sensitivity ranging from 33% to 100% and specificity from 40% to 93% [4].

The constrained accuracy of available biomarkers, along with their expense, has therefore limited introduction of urinary biomarkers into routine clinical practice. Hence there remains an urgent need to identify new biomarkers that might improve diagnostic accuracy, either when used in isolation or in combination with existing biomarker tests [7].

The DNA replication initiation machinery represents a final and critical step in growth control downstream of complex redundant oncogenic signalling pathways and is therefore a potentially attractive diagnostic and therapeutic target [8]. Proteins of the minichromosome maintenance (Mcm) family (Mcm2-7, collectively referred to as MCM), assemble into hexameric complexes that have DNA helicase activity, which is essential for initiation of DNA synthesis [9,10]. In epithelial-lined organ systems MCM proteins become dysregulated and overexpressed in hyperproliferative dysplastic (preinvasive) and malignant states, [8,11–13]. Indeed the degree of expression of Mcm2 and Mcm5 has been shown to predict recurrence and death in patients with bladder cancer [14–16]. Mcm2-7 protein expression in normal epithelium is restricted to the basal stem/transit compartments and is absent from surface layers as cells adopt a fully differentiated phenotype. In premalignant/dysplastic epithelial lesions there is an expansion of the proliferative compartment coupled to arrested differentiation, resulting in the appearance of cycling MCM-positive cells in superficial layers. The detection of exfoliated MCM-positive cells in clinical samples therefore provides a potentially sensitive method for detecting preinvasive and invasive cancers [8,17,18]. In a proof-of-principle study we previously showed that elevated Mcm5 levels in cells in urine sediments is predictive of the presence of bladder cancer [19].

The aim of this study was to evaluate Mcm5 as a biomarker for detection of bladder cancer alone, in comparison and in combination with NMP22. The prospective blinded observational trial utilized an immunofluorometric assay to measure Mcm5 and the FDA-approved NMP22 Test Kit.

Methods

Study Subjects

Single voided urine specimens were obtained from 1677 patients attending a one stop diagnostic clinic for investigation of

haematuria. The diagnosis was established following assessment by cystoscopy, upper urinary tract imaging, urine cytology and culture. Histological confirmation of bladder cancer at subsequent trans-urethral resection was the reference standard and all patients were followed for a period of six months from the time of initial investigations. Patients with a history of recent genito-urinary instrumentation or surgery within the previous two weeks were excluded. Patients with a history of concomitant malignancy or other malignancy within five years prior to study were also excluded. With these exceptions all consecutive patients attending for investigation during the study period were approached for recruitment into the trial.

Urine samples were split equally for: (i) urinalysis and microbiological culture, (ii) cytological analysis, (iii) Mcm5 measurement and (iv) NMP22 measurement. Patients underwent upper urinary tract imaging including ultrasound and intravenous urography. Male patients were examined by digital rectal examination for the presence of clinically detectable prostatic disease. Prostate-specific antigen (PSA) testing was not mandated and PSA levels were checked in a proportion of cases in whom cancer was suspected or who requested the test. If PSA levels were elevated patients were offered trans-rectal ultrasound guided core biopsies of the prostate. Typically all haematuria tests were completed within 24 hours and within two weeks for all patients. Clinical data were entered into a database prospectively prior to Mcm5 and NMP22 analysis. The reference standard for detection of bladder cancer was pathological confirmation following trans-urethral resection.

Urine samples were analyzed in a blinded fashion for Mcm5 detection, NMP22 testing, and cytologic analyses. On completion of the study, we decoded the patient data and compared immunofluorometric Mcm5 signals and NMP22 results with clinical diagnoses based on cystoscopy, biopsy histology, imaging and urine cytology. Staging and grading of malignant tumours was performed by a specialist uro-pathologist using the TNM (tumour-node-metastasis) classification system [20] and the 1973 World Health Organization (WHO) grading system respectively [21].

Ethics Statement

Ethical approval was obtained from the Joint UCL/UCLH Committees on the Ethics of Human Research (04/Q0502/1), Addenbrooke's Hospital Ethics Committee (00/236) and the Newcastle and North Tyneside Research Ethics Committee (2002/161). Written informed consent was received from all participants.

Urine Cytology

Urine samples (50 mL) were centrifuged at 1500 g for 5 min. Cytospin preparations were prepared on poly-L-lysine coated slides using Shandon cytospin tubes and a cytocentrifuge according to the manufacturer's instructions (Thermo Shandon, Runcorn, UK). Samples were fixed in industrial methylated spirits and stained using the Papanicolaou technique for smears [20]. Specimens were evaluated by a consultant cytologist experienced in uro-pathology. Cytology was scored as positive if atypical or malignant cells were identified.

NMP22 Assay

NMP22 was measured by enzyme-linked immunosorbent assay (ELISA) using the FDA-approved NMP22 Test Kit produced by Matritech (Freiburg, Germany). The assay run on a Dade Behring BEP 2000 automated ELISA processor (now Siemens Healthcare). All reagents, calibrators and controls were prepared as recommended by the manufacturer. All standards, quality controls and samples were analyzed in duplicate. Results were calculated using the data processing software supplied with the BEP 2000. The lower limit of detection of the assay was found to be 2 U/mL. Samples with concentrations greater than the top standard were repeated after dilution in assay buffer. The between-batch coefficient of variation was 13.3% at a concentration of 11.3 U/mL, 8.8% at 34 U/mL and 9.5% at 65 U/mL. A result for the NMP22 test was available in 1396 patients, including 195 patients (14%) with a urothelial tumour.

Immunofluorometric Assay to Measure Mcm5 Levels in Urine Sediments

Mcm5 was measured by two-site time-resolved fluorescence immunoassay on the AutoDELFIA analyzer (Perkin Elmer). All standards, quality controls and urine samples were prepared and processed as described [19]. Nunc Maxisorp microtiter plates (Perkin Elmer) were coated with 12A7 mouse anti-human Mcm5 monoclonal antibody [19] at a concentration of 8 mg/L by Dako UK Ltd (Ely, UK). A large batch (approximately 200) of plates were prepared by Dako and used throughout the study. Plates were received pre-blocked and ready for use. A second mouse anti-human Mcm5 monoclonal antibody (4B4) [19] was conjugated with europium by Dako. The europium-labelled antibody was at a concentration of 1.75 mg/mL. HeLa S3 cells were purchased commercially (Health Protection Agency Culture Collections, Porton Down, UK) and the assay was calibrated with processed HeLa cell standards at a concentration of 150000 cells/well. A series of standards spanning the concentration range 150000 to 1500 cells/well were prepared by diluting the stock standard in phosphate buffered saline containing 0.04% SDS and 0.02% sodium azide. Quality control samples containing four different concentrations of HeLa cells were analyzed at the beginning and end of each batch. The protocol for the AutoDELFIA assay was as follows. 50 μL standard, sample or quality control was added (in duplicate) to the antibody-coated microtiter plate along with 100 μL DELFIA multibuffer (Perkin Elmer product code 1380–3614). The plate was incubated for 2.5 h with continuous shaking. The plate was then washed four times with DELFIA wash buffer (Perkin Elmer product code B117-100). Europium-labelled detection antibody 4B4 was diluted 1:1,800 in DELFIA multibuffer. 100 μL of diluted antibody was added to each well and the plate incubated for a further 4 h with continuous shaking. The plate was then washed six times with DELFIA wash buffer and 200 μL DELFIA enhancement solution (Perkin Elmer product code B118-100) was added to each well. The plate was incubated on a shaker for a further 10 min. The amount of europium in each well was measured on the AutoDELFIA plate reader. Data were automatically transferred to a MultiCalc software package (Perkin Elmer), which was used to generate a calibration curve and calculate the concentration of the unknowns. The lower limit of detection of the assay was found to be 1000 cells/well. Samples with concentrations greater than the top standard were repeated after dilution in the standard dilution buffer. The between-batch coefficient of variation was 11.5% at a concentration of 2648 cells/well and 11.0% at 26382 cells/well. A result for the immunofluorometric Mcm5 test was available in 1564 patients including 210 patients (13%) with a urothelial tumour.

Statistical Analysis

Sensitivity and specificity characteristics of Mcm5 and NMP22 for the detection of UCC of the bladder are presented as receiver operating characteristic (ROC) curves. The area under the nonparametric ROC curve was used to assess the overall diagnostic performance of each test. Three cut-points were used to demonstrate test performance under different circumstances for Mcm5 as follows: (i) the lower detection limit of the assay where sensitivity of the test was maximal (1000 cells/well) (ii) sensitivity equal to specificity (2150 cells/well) and (iii) 95% specificity (8500 cells/well). Negative predictive value (NPV) and positive predictive value (PPV) were also estimated. An exact 95% confidence interval (CI) for each proportion, including sensitivity, specificity and predictive values for Mcm5 and NMP22, was derived assuming a binomial distribution. The manufacturer's recommended cut-point for NMP22, 10 U/ml was utilized for all analyses unless otherwise specified.

False positive rates (FPR) for the Mcm5 and NMP22 tests in patients with benign diagnosis were compared with clear normal patients using a Chi-squared test. The Mcm5 and NMP22 values were summarized using medians and interquartile ranges (IQR) and compared with the clear normal patients using the Mann-Whitney U-test. For each biomarker, the ROC analysis was repeated for males and females separately and the areas under the ROC curves were compared using a Chi-squared test with one degree of freedom. ROC analysis was also undertaken to examine the sensitivity of the main results to the exclusion of those with benign disease. The values of the urinary biomarkers for patients with different tumour grades and stages and normal patients were compared using Mann-Whitney U-tests between neighbouring categories, and using the Jonckheere-Terpstra test for trend across grades and stages. The Chi-squared test for linear by linear association was used to assess the evidence for a trend in the false positive rates by increasing tumour grade and stage. The sensitivity determined for urinary cytology was compared with that of the immunofluorometric Mcm5 test using McNemar's test for paired proportions. The accuracy of a biomarker was defined as the value of sensitivity and specificity where the cut-point provided these to be equal. The accuracy of the two biomarker tests was compared using McNemar's test. McNemar's test was also used to compare the sensitivity of cytology with that of each biomarker at cut-points providing the same specificity as observed for cytology. Spearman correlation was used to assess the degree to which the biomarkers were distinctive in UCC case and in normal control groups. All statistical tests were two-tailed, and a 5% level was used to indicate statistical significance.

A multi-ROC analysis [22] was performed to determine the additional performance resulting from using both biomarkers together. In this analysis, NMP22 was kept fixed at the recommended cut-point of 10 U/mL and Mcm5 was included with a varying cut-point. Raised values of either marker could predict positive for UCC. The additional performance of Mcm5 over that obtained from NMP22 (10 U/mL cut-point) was assessed using the nonparametric area under the multi-ROC curve, and assessed for statistical significance using a Chi-squared test with one degree of freedom. In order to demonstrate test performance, Mcm5 was then fixed at the cut-point that provided equal sensitivity and specificity on the multi-ROC curve from using the combined markers. This combination test accuracy was compared with the test accuracy provided by use of NMP22 alone using McNemar's test.

Results

Demographics and Clinical Investigation

The demographic characteristics, mode of presentation, final diagnosis, and tumour grade and stage for the 1677 patients included in this study are summarized in Table 1. The study population was predominantly male (62%) and had a mean age of 60.7 years (standard deviation, 16.3 years). Of those with a recorded presentation, 54% had visible haematuria and 46% had non-visible haematuria. These patients were newly presenting cases, although four patients recruited, later revealed a previous history of UCC. Investigations were omitted in a proportion of cases as follows: cystoscopy was not performed in 20 patients, ultrasound scan in 186 patients and intravenous urography in 223 patients. Urine cytology was unavailable for 109 patients due to insufficient sample collection or, alternatively, because the test was not undertaken. Neither ultrasound scan nor intravenous urography was performed in 77 patients. All patients had a clinical diagnosis attributed to them by their clinician. Data were not formally collected on the adverse effects of standard clinical testing and no adverse effects of urinary testing for Mcm5 or NMP22 were recorded.

Following clinical investigation, urinary tract tumours were identified in 222/1677 patients (13%). Nearly all tumours were UCCs, but, investigation also identified one case of adenocarcinoma and two cases of squamous cell carcinoma of the bladder. The UCCs were predominantly bladder tumours, with only seven patients with upper tract tumours. The upper tract UCCs are included alongside the bladder tumours for the analysis reported below. The diagnoses in the remaining patients included other malignancies, benign lesions or cysts of the kidney, benign inflammatory and congenital conditions, urolithiasis, benign prostatic hyperplasia and nephrological diseases. The diagnoses are listed in Table S1. As a component of the diagnostic pathway, urinary cytology had a sensitivity of 9% (95% CI, 5–14%; including atypical cytology as positive), specificity of 88% (95% CI, 86–89%) and PPV of 10% (95% CI, 7–15%).

Mcm5 and NMP22 Test Performance

The Mcm5 test discriminated, with high specificity and sensitivity, between patients with and without bladder cancer, as demonstrated by the large area under the ROC curve (AUC) (0.75 [95% CI = 0.71–0.79]) (Figure 1), statistically significantly larger than the area assumed by the null hypothesis (0.5; P<0.001) and based on 210 and 1354 patients respectively with and without UCC.

The sensitivity, specificity, and positive and negative predictive values (PPV and NPV) for Mcm5 are shown in Table 2. The cut-point analysis (cut-points correspond to (i) lower detection limit of the assay; (ii) where sensitivity is equal to specificity, and (iii) specificity of 95% for all patients tested), demonstrated a wide range of test performance levels (Table 2). At the lower detection limit of the assay, the test had 80% (167/210) (95% CI = 73–85%) sensitivity and 20% (167/846) (95% CI = 17–23%) PPV. When sensitivity is equal to specificity, the test had 69% (145/210) (95% CI = 62–75%) sensitivity and 26% (145/565) (95% CI = 22–30%) PPV. At 95% specificity (1286/1354), the test had 42% (89/210) (95% CI = 36–49%) sensitivity and 57% (89/157) (95% CI = 49–65%) PPV.

The NMP22 test discriminated with high specificity and sensitivity as demonstrated by the large AUC (0.72 [95% CI = 0.67–0.77]; null hypothesis [0.5; P<0.001] (Figure 1)) and based on 195 and 1201 patients respectively with and without UCC. The sensitivity, specificity, and positive and negative predictive values for NMP22 at the recommended 10 U/ml cut-point are shown in Table 2. Sensitivity was 53% (104/195) (95% CI = 46–60%) and PPV 36% (104/291) (95% CI = 30–42%).

In order to assess the performance of the test in patients with different stages and grades of disease the True Positive Rate (TPR) was calculated for Mcm5 (at the different cut-points), NMP22 and

Table 1. Patient demographics and clinicopathological data.

		n	%	mean	SD	median	IQR
Patients recruited		1677					
Age, years				60.7	16.3	63	49–73
Gender	Male	1040	62				
	Female	637	38				
Bladder/upper tract tumor	Positive	222	13				
	Negative	1455	87				
Grade [a]	1	26	12				
	2	129	58				
	3 (including CIS)	66	30				
Stage	T0	1455					
	Tx	1					
	Tis	8	4[b]				
	Ta	122	55				
	T1	50	23				
	≥T2	41	18				
Initial referral	Non-visible haematuria	711	46[c]				
	Visible haematuria	851	54				
	Unrecorded	115					

Abbreviations: CIS, carcinoma in situ; IQR, interquartile range; SD, standard deviation.
[a]n = 221.
[b]Percentage of patients excluding those with stage T0 and Tx.
[c]Percentage of recorded cases only.

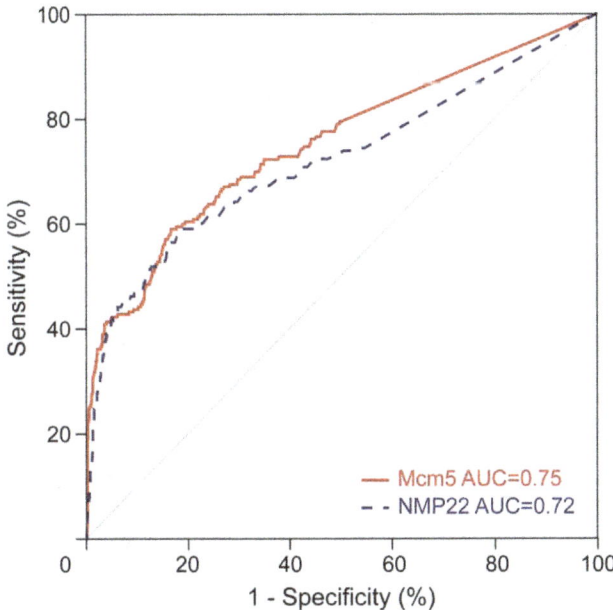

Figure 1. Receiver operating characteristics curves for Mcm5 and NMP22 tests for the detection of bladder cancer in all studied patients with valid test results.

cytology for muscle invasive vs non-muscle invasive (Table S2) and across grades (Table S3). Test performance improved for all tests in higher stage and grade categories.

Where the specificity of NMP22 (cut-point 12.1) was the same as that of positive cytology (88%; 989/1128), the sensitivity of NMP22 was significantly higher (P<0.001) (51%; 91/177 versus 8%; 14/177). Where the specificity of Mcm5 (5150-cell cut-point) was the same as that of cytology (87%; 1109/1271) the sensitivity of Mcm5 was significantly higher (P<0.001; 52%; 100/193 versus 9%; 17/193).

Biomarker False Positive Analysis

False positives were found in 400/1301 (31%) of clear normal and benign diagnosis patients with the Mcm5 test at the 2150-cell cut-point. There was a significantly higher rate of false positive results in female patients, 38% (200/520) compared to males 26% (200/781) (P<0.001). Urinary Mcm5 levels were also significantly higher in normal/benign females compared to males (median 1560 cells/well [IQR = <1000–3675 cells/well] vs median <1000 cells/well [IQR = <1000–2180 cells/well], P<0.001). Furthermore, compared to normal patients, those with, urinary calculi had a significantly higher false positive rate (44% [47/106] vs 30% [201/661], P = 0.004) and higher urinary levels of Mcm5 protein (median 1840 cells/well [<1000–3963 cells/well] vs 1040 cells/well [<1000–2645 cells/well], P<0.001; Table 3). There was no evidence of an association between the false positive rate and any of the other benign groups including inflammatory conditions and benign prostatic hyperplasia. In the clear normal and benign patient groups there were no significant differences (P = 0.99) in NMP22 levels between males and females. A raised NMP22 signal and increased false positive rate was observed for those patients with urinary tract infections (FPR: 22% vs 11%, P = 0.001; median NMP22 result: 3.35 U/mL vs 2.2 U/mL, P<0.001) and urinary calculi (FPR: 23% vs 11%, P = 0.001; NMP22:2.55 U/mL vs 2.2 U/mL, P = 0.047) (Table 3).

Table 2. Performance of Mcm5 and NMP22 tests for bladder carcinoma detection for all patients with test results available.

Test	Cut-point	n	Sens, % (CI)	Spec, % (CI)	PPV, % (CI)	NPV, % (CI)
Mcm5	1000-cell	1564	80 (73–85)	50 (47–52)	20 (17–23)	94 (92–96)
	2150-cell	1564	69 (62–75)	69 (66–71)	26 (22–30)	93 (92–95)
	8500-cell	1564	42 (36–49)	95 (94–96)	57 (49–65)	91 (90–93)
NMP22	10 U/ml	1396	53 (46–60)	84 (82–86)	36 (30–42)	92 (90–93)
Cytology		1568	9 (5–14)	88 (86–89)	10 (7–15)	87 (85–88)

Abbreviations: CI, 95% confidence interval; NPV, negative predictive value; PPV, positive predictive value; Sens, sensitivity; Spec, specificity.

The ROC analysis for Mcm5 and NMP22 was repeated observing the results in all males and females (Table S4 and Figure S1). There were no significant differences in AUC values for Mcm5 between males and females (P = 0.76), but there was a significant difference in the NMP22 AUC value between males and females (AUC 0.69 for males vs 0.80 for females, P = 0.025), apparently related to the greater NMP22 sensitivity in females.

Biomarker False Negative Analysis

Table 4 and Table S5 show the false negative rates of urinary Mcm5 and NMP22 grouped by tumour grade and stage. There was evidence of a decreasing trend in the false-negative rate with increasing tumour grade and stage for both urinary biomarkers. For grades 1, 2 and 3 respectively, the false negative rates for urinary Mcm5 at the 2150-cell cut-point were 52% (95% CI = 31–73%), 37% (95% CI = 28–46%) and 11% (95% CI = 4–22%; trend P<0.001). For NMP22 at the 10 U/mL cut-point, the corresponding false negative rates were 80% (95% CI = 59–93%), 49% (95% CI = 40–59%) and 25% (95% CI = 14–40%; trend P<0.001). Similar trends were observed for tumour stage. A significant decrease in the amplitude of the Mcm5 and NMP22 signal with lower tumour grade and stage was observed, in keeping with the increasing false negative rates observed for these groups (Table 4 and Table S5).

Combined Biomarker Multi-ROC Analysis

There were 183 bladder UCCs and 1100 normal patients with assay data available for both urinary markers. For these patients, an Mcm5 cut-point of 2180 cells/well provided equal sensitivity and specificity of 71% (130/183 and 777/1100), and for NMP22 a cut-point of 4.6 U/mL provided equal sensitivity and specificity of 67% (123/183 and 742/1100). Although there was modestly greater performance of Mcm5 compared with NMP22 in terms of accuracy (71% versus 67%, difference of 3.3%, 95% CI = −0.2–6.7%), this difference was not statistically significant (McNemar's test: P = 0.067).

The Spearman correlation coefficients between Mcm5 and NMP22 were moderately high (rho = 0.54) for UCC cases and negligible (rho = 0.08) for the normal group, indicating potential for the biomarkers to provide distinct roles within a combination. On the basis of multi-ROC analysis, the immunofluorometric Mcm5 test, in combination with NMP22 at the recommended 10 U/mL cut-point, offers a statistically significant increase in performance (P<0.001) compared with NMP22 alone at the recommended cut-point (area under multi-ROC curve = 0.65, 95% CI = 0.58–0.71). As a demonstration, if either NMP22 exceeds 10 U/mL or Mcm5 exceeds the 4200-cell cut-point, this combination provides sensitivity (131/183) and specificity (789/

Table 3. False positive rates for the Mcm5 and NMP22 tests across benign conditions.

Test	Benign condition	n	Test value, med (IQR)	P[a]	FPR, %[b]	P[c]
Mcm5[d]	Clear normal	661	1040 (<1000–2645)		30	
	BPH	132	<1000 (<1000–2438)	0.056	27	0.37
	Calculi	106	1840 (<1000–3963)	<0.001	44	0.004
	Nephrological	40	<1000 (<1000–2448)	0.25	25	0.47
	Prostatitis	14	<1000 (<1000–3433)	0.37	29	0.88
	Urethral stricture	21	1100 (<1000–2620)	0.94	29	0.86
	UTI	246	<1000 (<1000–2823)	0.84	30	0.92
	Other	81	1110 (<1000–2855)	0.68	28	0.71
NMP22[e]	Clear normal	589	2.20 (<2.00–5.30)		11	
	BPH	110	<2.00 (<2.00–5.60)	0.96	13	0.65
	Calculi	96	2.55 (<2.00–9.48)	0.047	23	0.001
	Nephrological	38	2.05 (<2.00–6.43)	0.93	11	0.9
	Prostatitis	13	<2.00 (<2.00–3.50)	0.14	0	0.2
	Urethral stricture	18	2.85 (<2.00–6.83)	0.36	17	0.47
	UTI	222	3.35 (<2.00–8.63)	<0.001	22	<0.001
	Other	68	2.80 (<2.00–8.03)	0.018	24	0.004

For each subgroup, only those patients with a test results were considered.
Abbreviations: BPH, benign prostatic hyperplasia; FPR, false positive rate; IQR, interquartile range; med, median; UTI, urinary tract infection.
[a]Mann-Whitney test, comparison of test value with normal.
[b]False positive rate determined using 2150-cell cut-point for Mcm5 test and 10 U/mL cut-point for NMP22 test.
[c]Chi-squared test, comparison of false positive rate with Normal group.
[d]Excludes 53 "other cancers" of the 1354 patients without UCC having an Mcm5 test value.
[e]Excludes 47 "other cancers" of the 1201 patients without UCC having an NMP22 test value.

1100) both equal to 72%, which indicates the improvement over use of NMP22 alone where sensitivity (123/183) and specificity (742/1100) both equal 67% (72% versus 67%, difference = 4.3% [95% CI = 1.5–7.0%], McNemar's test P = 0.002). In combination with NMP22 at 10 U/mL the MCM5 test removes false negatives from the NMP22 test, offering an improvement from the 54% sensitivity of NMP22 alone to 75% sensitivity with 65% specificity (2800-cell cut-point), or to 80% sensitivity with 58% specificity (1900-cell cut-point), or to maximal sensitivity of 85% with 45% specificity (1000-cell cut-point).

In the combination analysis, with NMP22 (10 U/mL cut-point) and Mcm5 (4200-cell cut-point, where sensitivity and specificity are equal), 100% (31/31) of muscle invasive cancers (i.e. stage ≥ T2), 93% (40/43) of pT1 tumours and 53% (54/102) of pTa tumours were detected. The total number of patients with carcinoma in situ was low and 86% (6/7) were detected. Grade 1 disease was identified in 46% (10/22), grade 2 disease in 64% (68/106) and grade 3 disease in 96% (53/55) of cases (including 6/7 cases of carcinoma in situ). Importantly, Mcm5 combined with NMP22 identified 95% (79/83, 95% CI = 88–99%) of potentially life threatening diagnoses (i.e. grade 3 or CIS or stage ≥pT1) with high specificity (72%, 95% CI = 69–74%).

Discussion

In an earlier proof-of-concept study we showed that elevated Mcm5 levels in urine cell sediments are highly predictive of bladder cancer [19]. The prospective blinded observational trial reported here, involving a large patient cohort, confirms our initial observations that Mcm5 is a sensitive and specific biomarker for detection of UCC. Importantly, through multi-ROC analysis, we show here that the Mcm5 test, in combination with NMP22 at the

established cut-point 10 U/mL, enhances diagnostic accuracy over NMP22 in isolation and identifies nearly all potentially life threatening disease.

Despite numerous studies over the last decade, the reported accuracy of the NMP22 test is highly variable. Many of the earlier studies recruited small to moderate numbers of subjects and reported high sensitivities and specificities, above 80% [23–26]. However, a wide range in test performance has been observed in more recent studies with sensitivity ranging from 33% to 100% and specificity from 40% to 93% [4]. A pooled analysis including more recent trials suggests a sensitivity of around 68% and a specificity of 79% [4]. A recent large multi-institutional international trial revealed a marked variability in the performance of the NMP22 test across participating institutions with sensitivity and specificity ranging from 36% to 86% and 50% to 94% respectively [27]. Variability has been attributed to many confounding factors including biological, analytical and epidemiological variables and methodological bias.

Our study represents the largest prospective observational trial ever undertaken using the NMP22 urinary biomarker. Notably, the performance at the 10 U/mL cut-point, with a sensitivity of 53% and specificity of 84%, is somewhat below that reported in the pooled analysis, but almost identical to the diagnostic performance reported in the Matritech supported large patient cohort trials using the NMP22 point-of-care proteomic assay [4,28]. Interestingly we observed significantly greater diagnostic accuracy of NMP22 in females compared to males. Gender differences in NMP22 test performance have been previously noted [29,30] however our data represent the largest study of this question and clearly establishes a clinically meaningful difference in test performance.

Table 4. Comparison of Mcm5 and NMP22 test performance across grade and stage.

Test			n	Test value, med (IQR)	P[a]	P[b]	P[c]	FNR, % (CI)	P[a]	P[b]	P[c]
Mcm5[d]	Normal		1354	1015 (<1000–2790)				69 (66–71)			
	Grade[e]	1	23	1300 (<1000–5310)	0.14			52 (31–73)	0.085		
		2	123	4070 (1170–12900)	<0.001	0.041		37 (28–46)	<0.001	0.16	
		3	55	40900 (5800–122000)	<0.001	<0.001	<0.001	11 (4–22)	<0.001	<0.001	<0.001
	Stage[e]	pTa	115	2590 (<1000–5710)	<0.001			46 (37–56)	<0.001		
		pT1	48	39000 (5818–136250)	<0.001	<0.001		10 (3–23)	<0.001	<0.001	
		≥pT2	38	19850 (7150–65800)	<0.001	0.28	<0.001	13 (4–28)	<0.001	0.69	<0.001
NMP22[f]	Normal		1201	2.40 (<2.00–6.30)				84 (82–86)			
	Grade[g]	1	25	<2.00 (<2.00–8.45)	0.31			80 (59–93)	0.55		
		2	112	10.20 (2.68–39.83)	<0.001	<0.001		49 (40–59)	<0.001	0.005	
		3	51	62.50 (9.90–145.50)	<0.001	<0.001	<0.001	25 (14–40)	<0.001	0.005	<0.001
	Stage[g]	pTa	109	6.00 (<2.00–24.50)	<0.001			62 (53–71)	<0.001		
		pT1	45	31.30 (5.70–125.90)	<0.001	<0.001		29 (16–44)	<0.001	<0.001	
		≥pT2	34	70.65 (22.68–258.50)	<0.001	0.099	<0.001	21 (9–38)	<0.001	0.40	<0.001

Abbreviations: CI, 95% confidence interval; IQR, interquartile range; med, median; FNR, false negative rate.
[a]Mann-Whitney test (for Test value) or Chi-squared test (for FNR), comparison with Normal group.
[b]Mann-Whitney test (for Test value) or Chi-squared test (for FNR), comparison with previous, i.e. Grade 2 vs Grade 1, Grade 3 vs Grade 2.
[c]Jonckheere-Terpstra test for trend (for Test value) or Chi-squared test for linear by linear association, across Grade or Stage, excluding Normal group.
[d]Data analysis using 2150-cell cut-point for Mcm5 test.
[e]Excludes 8 CIS and 1 adenocarcinoma from 210 UCC cases having an MCM5 test value.
[f]Data analysis using 10 U/mL cut-point for NMP22 test.
[g]Excludes 7 CIS from the 195 UCC cases having an NMP22 test value.

The analysis of false positive Mcm5 results in this study also revealed an unexpected difference between the male and female groups. The overall false positive rate in females was 38% compared to 26% in males. Rather than being related to benign pathology, the difference was most marked in the clear normal group. These findings require further investigation. Possible causes could be fungal contamination by vaginal flora (e.g. *Candida* species) or mixing of menstrual endometrial contaminants in samples, both sources of extraneous MCM expressing cells. Patients with urinary calculi had the highest incidence of false positive Mcm5 results (44%). As previously reported, higher false positive rates are expected in patients with urinary calculi due to the associated mucosal injury, which exposes the underlying MCM expressing transit amplifying compartment of the transitional epithelium to the urinary tract [8,19,31]. However, exclusion of patients with calculi from the ROC analysis did not make a significant improvement to the overall performance, presumably because they were a relatively small group (data not shown). Notably, other benign conditions such as urinary tract infection or benign prostatic hyperplasia were not associated with false positive Mcm5 results, in keeping with our proof-of-concept study [19]. In contrast to the Mcm5 test, false positive NMP22 results were linked to urinary tract infection. The different aetiologies for false positives with Mcm5 and NMP22 may account for the improved performance observed when combining the two urinary biomarkers.

Decreasing urinary Mcm5 and NMP22 signals were observed with lower stage and grade of UCC, and this was associated with an increasing false negative rate for both tests. Expression of MCM proteins in bladder cancer is closely linked to grade [15,16] and thus this trend is expected. The trend is also explained by the less spontaneous shedding of tumour cells seen in lower grade lesions due to stronger cell-cell and cell-matrix attachments. Commercial development of the Mcm5 test is currently underway

and improvements in the assay design to enhance sensitivity are planned and thus reduced false negative rates in early stage, well-differentiated tumours are anticipated. The trend for higher grade and stage tumours to exhibit higher Mcm5 levels could provide a useful predictive clinical role e.g. to target imaging and rigid cystoscopic diagnostic procedures for high risk patients identified by urinary Mcm5. This potential role requires further study.

Current routine initial investigations for haematuria or other symptoms suggestive of bladder cancer include flexible cystoscopy and rigid white light cystoscopy. However an estimated 10–40% of tumours can be missed due to poor visualization as a result of inflammatory conditions or bleeding and flat urothelial lesions such as severe dysplasia and carcinoma in situ [32–34]. Photodynamic diagnosis is a technique that can enhance tumour detection but its increased sensitivity is associated with higher false positive rates leading to additional unnecessary investigations, biopsies and thus increased cost [35]. Urinary biomarkers also have potential to enhance tumour detection and identify tumours not visualized during initial endoscopy. A systematic review of the clinical effectiveness and cost-effectiveness of photodynamic diagnosis, cytology and urine biomarkers, including FISH, ImmunoCyt and NMP22, for detection and surveillance of bladder cancer has recently been undertaken [4]. Urinary cytology had the lowest pooled sensitivity of the markers studied at 44% although specificity was highest at 96%. The range of reported sensitivity for cytology was 7–100%. Thus while our study reports low sensitivity for cytology this is not a unique finding. Pooled analyses performed by Mowatt et al showed similar diagnostic performance with NMP22 (sensitivity 84%, specificity 75%) and FISH (sensitivity 76%, specificity 85%) with ImmunoCyt slightly outperforming them (sensitivity 84% specificity 75%) [4]. Notably, of eight diagnosis and follow-up strategies included in a probabilistic sensitivity analysis using combinations of photodynamic diagnosis, flexible cystoscopy, white light cystoscopy, cytology and urinary biomarkers, four were associated with around a 20% chance of being considered cost-effective. Three of these four strategies involved the use of either a biomarker or photodynamic diagnosis. Other urinary markers of bladder cancer such as Survivin [36], various urinary micro RNAs [37,38] and epigenetic markers [38] have also been shown to have great potential as diagnostic markers with sensitivity/specificity reported >90%. As yet these markers have not been evaluated in large-scale blinded observational studies thus the initial findings from these carefully controlled trials should be interpreted with caution.

In this study, the performance of Mcm5 is similar to that of NMP22 and both markers are significantly more accurate than urinary cytology. It also outperforms the performance of cytology from studies combined in a recent systematic review [4]. The performance of Mcm5 falls below the reported accuracy of ImmunoCyt and some other novel approaches detailed above. It is worth noting that Mcm5 initially demonstrated an AUC of 0.93 in our earlier smaller study and it remains to be seen if the performance of Survivin and other novel markers is reproducible in large studies. Our current data suggest that an Mcm5 assay commercially developed for an end-user laboratory in combination with NMP22 could be used to modify diagnostic and surveillance care pathways to enhance the diagnostic accuracy in those at high risk (e.g. newly presenting visible haematuria patient) and reduce morbidity and cost of testing in low risk patients (e.g. newly presenting non-visible haematuria patient without a known risk factor or a patient with prior low grade non-muscle invasive tumour). Trials to evaluate modified against standard diagnostic pathways using a commercialised assay are currently in preparation.

In conclusion, we have demonstrated that immunofluorometric detection of Mcm5 in urine sediments is a sensitive and specific diagnostic test for bladder cancer. The test detects bladder cancers of all stages and grades. Through evaluation of different assay cut-points there could be a role for predicting high grade and stage disease. Importantly, urinary Mcm5 in combination with the urinary NMP22 measured with the FDA-approved Matritech NMP22® Test Kit, identifies nearly all life threatening disease.

Supporting Information

Figure S1   Receiver operating characteristics curves for the (A) Mcm5 and (B) NMP22 tests for detection of bladder cancer in male and female patients.

Table S1   Patient diagnoses.

Table S2   True positive rate of Mcm5 and NMP22 tests and cytology, across stage, for bladder carcinoma detection.

Table S3   True positive rate of Mcm5 and NMP22 tests and cytology, across grade, for bladder carcinoma detection.

Table S4   Comparison of Mcm5 and NMP22 test performance in male and female patients.

Table S5   True and false negative rates of the Mcm5 and NMP22 tests, by tumour grade and stage.

Acknowledgments

The authors thank Diane Walia for data entry and spreadsheet management. Mcm5 and NMP22 assays were performed by the National Institute for Health Research Cambridge Biomedical Research Centre, Core Biochemical Assay Laboratory.

Author Contributions

Conceived and designed the experiments: JDK HYL TJD GHW KS. Performed the experiments: AW OO KB FT IH WR. Analyzed the data: JDK TJD HYL AW TP ATP JCV NV RSP GHW KS. Contributed reagents/materials/analysis tools: JCV ATP. Wrote the paper: JDK TJD AW ATP GHW KS.

References

1. American Cancer Society (2012) Cancer Facts & Figures 2012. Available: http://www.cancer.org/acs/groups/content/@epidemiologysurveilance/documents/document/acspc-031941.pdf. Accessed 2012 May 22.
2. Almallah YZ, Rennie CD, Stone J, Lancashire MJ (2000) Urinary tract infection and patient satisfaction after flexible cystoscopy and urodynamic evaluation. Urology 56: 37–39.
3. Babjuk M, Oosterlinck W, Sylvester R, Kaasinen E, Bohle A, et al. (2012) Guidelines on Non-muscle-invasive Bladder Cancer (TaT1 and CIS). Uroweb 2012. Available: http://www.uroweb.org/gls/pdf/05_TaT1_Bladder_Cancer_LR%20March%2013th%202012.pdf. Accessed 2012 May 1.
4. Mowatt G, Zhu S, Kilonzo M, Boachie C, Fraser C, et al. (2010) Systematic review of the clinical effectiveness and cost-effectiveness of photodynamic diagnosis and urine biomarkers (FISH, ImmunoCyt, NMP22) and cytology for the detection and follow-up of bladder cancer. Health Technol Assess 14: 1–356.
5. Compton DA, Cleveland DW (1993) NuMA is required for the proper completion of mitosis. J Cell Biol 120: 947–957.
6. Shelfo SW, Soloway MS (1997) The role of nuclear matrix protein 22 in the detection of persistent or recurrent transitional-cell cancer of the bladder. World J Urol 15: 107–111.
7. Gaston KE, Grossman HB (2010) Proteomic assays for the detection of urothelial cancer. Methods Mol Biol 641: 303–323.
8. Williams GH, Stoeber K (2007) Cell cycle markers in clinical oncology. Curr Opin Cell Biol 19: 672–679.
9. Machida YJ, Hamlin JL, Dutta A (2005) Right place, right time, and only once: replication initiation in metazoans. Cell 123: 13–24.
10. Remus D, Diffley JF (2009) Eukaryotic DNA replication control: lock and load, then fire. Curr Opin Cell Biol 21: 771–777.
11. Williams GH, Romanowski P, Morris L, Madine M, Mills AD, et al. (1998) Improved cervical smear assessment using antibodies against proteins that regulate DNA replication. Proc Natl Acad Sci U S A 95: 14932–14937.
12. Going JJ, Keith WN, Neilson L, Stoeber K, Stuart RC, et al. (2002) Aberrant expression of minichromosome maintenance proteins 2 and 5, and Ki-67 in dysplastic squamous oesophageal epithelium and Barrett's mucosa. Gut 50: 373–377.
13. Blow JJ, Gillespie PJ (2008) Replication licensing and cancer–a fatal entanglement? Nat Rev Cancer 8: 799–806.
14. Burger M, Denzinger S, Hartmann A, Wieland WF, Stoehr R, et al. (2007) Mcm2 predicts recurrence hazard in stage Ta/T1 bladder cancer more accurately than CK20, Ki67 and histological grade. Br J Cancer 96: 1711–1715.
15. Korkolopoulou P, Givalos N, Saetta A, Goudopoulou A, Gakiopoulou H, et al. (2005) Minichromosome maintenance proteins 2 and 5 expression in muscle-invasive urothelial cancer: a multivariate survival study including proliferation markers and cell cycle regulators. Hum Pathol 36: 899–907.
16. Kruger S, Thorns C, Stocker W, Muller-Kunert E, Bohle A, et al. (2003) Prognostic value of MCM2 immunoreactivity in stage T1 transitional cell carcinoma of the bladder. Eur Urol 43: 138–145.
17. Eward KL, Obermann EC, Shreeram S, Loddo M, Fanshawe T, et al. (2004) DNA replication licensing in somatic and germ cells. J Cell Sci 117: 5875–5886.
18. Barkley LR, Hong HK, Kingsbury SR, James M, Stoeber K, et al. (2007) Cdc6 is a rate-limiting factor for proliferative capacity during HL60 cell differentiation. Exp Cell Res 313: 3789–3799.
19. Stoeber K, Swinn R, Prevost AT, De Clive-Lowe P, Halsall I, et al. (2002) Diagnosis of genito-urinary tract cancer by detection of minichromosome maintenance 5 protein in urine sediments. J Natl Cancer Inst 94: 1071–1079.
20. UICC International Union Against Cancer (2009) TNM Classification of Malignant Tumours Seventh Edition. Indianapolis: Wiley-Blackwell.
21. Mostofi FK, Sobin LH, Torloni H (1973) Histological typing of urinary bladder tumours. Geneva: World Health Organization.
22. Shultz EK (1995) Multivariate receiver-operating characteristic curve analysis: prostate cancer screening as an example. Clin Chem 41: 1248–1255.

23. Saad A, Hanbury DC, McNicholas TA, Boustead GB, Morgan S, et al. (2002) A study comparing various noninvasive methods of detecting bladder cancer in urine. BJU Int 89: 369–373.

24. Sanchez-Carbayo M, Herrero E, Megias J, Mira A, Soria F (1999) Evaluation of nuclear matrix protein 22 as a tumour marker in the detection of transitional cell carcinoma of the bladder. BJU Int 84: 706–713.

25. Zippe C, Pandrangi L, Agarwal A (1999) NMP22 is a sensitive, cost-effective test in patients at risk for bladder cancer. J Urol 161: 62–65.

26. Ponsky LE, Sharma S, Pandrangi L, Kedia S, Nelson D, et al. (2001) Screening and monitoring for bladder cancer: refining the use of NMP22. J Urol 166: 75–78.

27. Shariat SF, Marberger MJ, Lotan Y, Sanchez-Carbayo M, Zippe C, et al. (2006) Variability in the performance of nuclear matrix protein 22 for the detection of bladder cancer. J Urol 176: 919–926.

28. Grossman HB, Soloway M, Messing E, Katz G, Stein B, et al. (2006) Surveillance for recurrent bladder cancer using a point-of-care proteomic assay. JAMA 295: 299–305.

29. Redorta JP, Pascual M, Cosentino M, Caicedo JI, Rodriguez O, et al. (2011) Effect of retention time on NMP22 bladder check assay results in voided urine. Nephro-Urol Mon 3: 182–185.

30. Lotan Y, Shariat SF (2008) Impact of risk factors on the performance of the nuclear matrix protein 22 point-of-care test for bladder cancer detection. BJU Int 101: 1362–1367.

31. Ayaru L, Stoeber K, Webster GJ, Hatfield AR, Wollenschlaeger A, et al. (2008) Diagnosis of pancreaticobiliary malignancy by detection of minichromosome maintenance protein 5 in bile aspirates. Br J Cancer 98: 1548–1554.

32. Zaak D, Kriegmair M, Stepp H, Stepp H, Baumgartner R, et al. (2001) Endoscopic detection of transitional cell carcinoma with 5 aminolevulinic acid: results of 1012 fluorescence endoscopies. Urology 57: 690–694.

33. Schneeweiss S, Kriegmair M, Stepp H (1999) Is everything all right if nothing seems wrong? A simple method of assessing the diagnostic value of endoscopic procedures when a gold standard is absent. J Urol 161: 1116–1119.

34. Kriegmair M, Baumgartner R, Knuchel R, Stepp H, Hofstadter F, et al. (1996) Detection of early bladder cancer by 5-aminolevulinic acid induced porphyrin fluorescence. J Urol 155: 105–109.

35. Gakis G, Kruck S, Stenzl A (2010) Can the burden of follow-up in low-grade noninvasive bladder cancer be reduced by photodynamic diagnosis, perioperative instillations, imaging, and urine markers? Curr Opin Urol 20: 388–392.

36. Ku JH, Godoy G, Amiel GE, Lerner SP (2012) Urine survivin as a diagnostic biomarker for bladder cancer: a systematic review. BJU Int doi: 10.1111/j.1464–410X.2011.10884.x.

37. Hanke M, Hoefig K, Merz H, Feller AC, Kausch I, et al. (2010) A robust methodology to study urine microRNA as tumor marker: microRNA-126 and microRNA-182 are related to urinary bladder cancer. Urol Oncol 28: 655–661.

38. Wang G, Chan ES, Kwan BC, Li PK, Yip SK, et al. (2012) Expression of microRNAs in the Urine of Patients With Bladder Cancer. Clin Genitourin Cancer 10: 106–113.

17

Robust Prognostic Gene Expression Signatures in Bladder Cancer and Lung Adenocarcinoma Depend on Cell Cycle Related Genes

Garrett M. Dancik[1], Dan Theodorescu[2,3,4]*

1 Mathematics and Computer Science Department, Eastern Connecticut State University, Willimantic, Connecticut, United States of America, 2 Department of Surgery, University of Colorado, Aurora, Colorado, United States of America, 3 Department of Pharmacology, University of Colorado, Aurora, Colorado, United States of America, 4 University of Colorado Comprehensive Cancer Center, Aurora, Colorado, United States of America

Abstract

Few prognostic biomarkers are approved for clinical use primarily because their initial performance cannot be repeated in independent datasets. We posited that robust biomarkers could be obtained by identifying deregulated biological processes shared among tumor types having a common etiology. We performed a gene set enrichment analysis in 20 publicly available gene expression datasets comprising 1968 patients having one of the three most common tobacco-related cancers (lung, bladder, head and neck) and identified cell cycle related genes as the most consistently prognostic class of biomarkers in bladder (BL) and lung adenocarcinoma (LUAD). We also found the prognostic value of 13 of 14 published BL and LUAD signatures were dependent on cell cycle related genes, supporting the importance of cell cycle related biomarkers for prognosis. Interestingly, no prognostic gene classes were identified in squamous cell lung carcinoma or head and neck squamous cell carcinoma. Next, a specific 31 gene cell cycle proliferation (CCP) signature, previously derived in prostate tumors was evaluated and found predictive of outcome in BL and LUAD cohorts in univariate and multivariate analyses. Specifically, CCP score significantly enhanced the predictive ability of multivariate models based on standard clinical variables for progression in BL patients and survival in LUAD patients in multiple cohorts. We then generated random CCP signatures of various sizes and found sets of 10–15 genes had robust performance in these BL and LUAD cohorts, a finding that was confirmed in an independent cohort. Our work characterizes the importance of cell cycle related genes in prognostic signatures for BL and LUAD patients and identifies a specific signature likely to survive additional validation.

Editor: John D. Minna, Univesity of Texas Southwestern Medical Center at Dallas, United States of America

Funding: This work is supported in part by National Institutes of Health grants CA075115 and CA104106. The funders had no role in study design, data collection and analysis, decision to publish, or preparation of the manuscript. No additional external funding was received for this study.

Competing Interests: The authors have declared that no competing interests exist.

* E-mail: dan.theodorescu@ucdenver.edu

Introduction

Gene expression profiling of human cancers has revolutionized our understanding of the disease and expedited the discovery of prognostic and predictive biomarkers [1–3]. However, few multi-gene biomarkers have been approved for clinical use [4] in part because they lack robustness across multiple datasets. This is especially striking for bladder cancer where Lauss and associates [5] evaluated 28 published gene signatures designed for diagnostic and prognostic purposes for bladder cancer and found that none of the 6 survival signatures performed better than chance when applied to independent datasets.

Here we address this lack of robust prognostic biomarkers by postulating the existence of common cellular processes (modules) across multiple tumor types of common etiology, whose abnormal activity could be captured by a transcriptional signature. As our goal was to develop robust bladder cancer biomarkers, we selected additional cancer types with smoking as a well-defined major etiological factor. The identification of such a process would presumably allow for development of robust biomarkers that are prognostic across multiple patient cohorts and tumor types.

An overview of our analysis is provided in **Figure 1**. First, a gene set enrichment analysis of gene expression profiles from 1968 patients with tobacco-related cancers (bladder urothelial cell carcinoma, lung adenocarcinoma, lung squamous cell carcinoma, and head and neck squamous cell carcinoma) was performed and identified cycle related modules as consistently prognostic in bladder and lung adenocarcinoma. We found that a specific cell cycle gene signature was predictive of outcome in bladder and lung adenocarcinoma and that the performance of published bladder and lung adenocarcinoma signatures depended on cell cycle-correlated genes. Next we developed and evaluated a 12 gene panel of cell cycle related genes and found them effective in stratifying clinical outcome in an independent cohort. Our results characterize the core importance of cell cycle related biomarkers in prognostic gene signatures in patients with common cancer types and implicate cell proliferation as the primary driver of disease outcome. More broadly, this approach defines functionally dominant biological modules driving human cancer prognosis and identifies robust prognostic biomarkers.

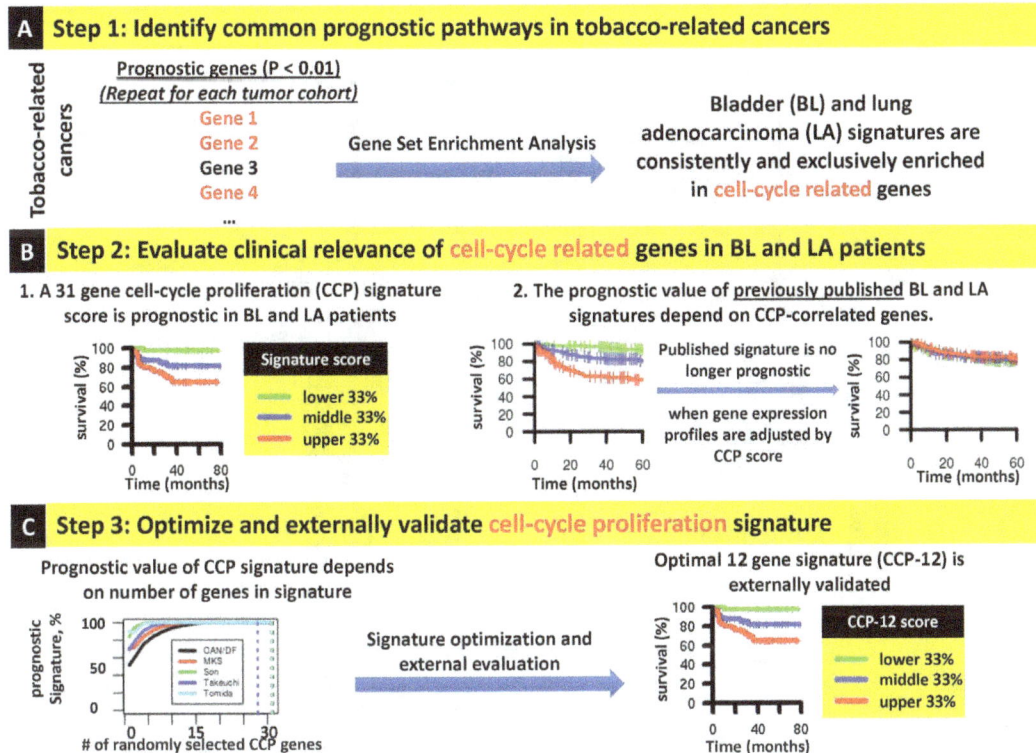

Figure 1. Study overview and summary of major findings. A, Biological processes associated with survival in tobacco-related tumors were identified through a gene set enrichment analysis. This analysis identified cell cycle as the only biological process consistently associated with outcome, in bladder and lung adenocarcinoma while no processes were identified that were predictive of outcome in lung adenocarcinoma, squamous cell lung carcinoma, or head and neck squamous cell carcinoma. **B,** Given the findings in **A,** the clinical relevance of cell cycle related genes was assessed in two ways. First, we evaluated the prognostic value of a specific 31 gene cell cycle proliferation (CCP) signature in bladder and lung adenocarcinoma in univariate and multivariate analysis. Second, we found that the prognostic value of previously published gene signatures predicting survival in bladder progression and lung adenocarcinoma was dependent on cell-cycle correlated genes. **C,** Because additional analysis revealed that the prognostic value of the CCP score was dependent on signature size, we optimized the CCP signature and found that a smaller 12 gene signature (CCP-12) was prognostic in an external dataset.

Materials and Methods

Gene expression datasets and clinical endpoints

We analyzed 20 gene expression datasets comprising 1968 patients with bladder urothelial cell carcinoma (BL, five cohorts, 42%), lung adenocarcinoma (LUAD, eight cohorts, 39%), lung squamous cell carcinoma (LUSC, three cohorts, 8%), and head and neck squamous cell carcinoma (HNSCC, four cohorts, 10%). All gene expression datasets used in this analysis are publicly available and can be downloaded from the Gene Expression Omnibus (GEO) [6] or as supplemental material to publication, as indicated in **Tables S1–S4 in File S2**. References to the original study for each cohort are also provided in **Tables S1–S4 in File S2**. For more details see **Supporting Materials and Methods in File S1**.

Endpoints included progression in BL patients. Three BL cohorts had progression information, which was defined by the original authors as increase from NMI to MI disease (Lindgren and Dyrskjot cohorts, Ref # [7,8]), or any increase in stage (CNUH, Ref # [9]). For two cohorts (Lindgren and CNUH) time to progression was not available and the ability of a gene or signature score to predict progression (progressor vs. non-progressor) was evaluated by area under the receiver operating characteristic curve (AUC). In Dyrskjot, clinical follow-up time was available allowing for progression-free survival (PFS) analysis.

The survival endpoint was selected as follows. Disease-specific survival (DSS) was always used if available (three BL cohorts). Overall survival (OS) was used if DSS was unavailable (two BL, seven LUAD, and two LUSC cohorts). Recurrence-free survival (RFS) was used if neither DSS nor OS were available (one LUAD and two HNSCC cohorts). The events for these endpoints are death from disease, death from any cause, and disease recurrence, for DSS, OS, and RFS, respectively. In one additional HNSCC cohort (Colo, Ref # [10]) recurrence status was provided but clinical follow-up times were not, and the ability of a gene to predict recurrence was evaluated by AUC. In addition, nodal involvement strongly correlates with outcome in HNSCC [11] and was used as a surrogate for survival in two cohorts allowing for a more comprehensive analysis. The clinical endpoints for each cohort are summarized in **Tables S1–S4 in File S2**.

Cell cycle proliferation (CCP) score

In microarray datasets, probes were converted to gene symbols based on Affymetrix annotation, GenBank accession number, or Unigene cluster ID. For genes with multiple probes, the probe with the highest mean expression value was used [12]. The expression of each gene was z-normalized across samples to have a mean of zero and a standard deviation of one. CCP score is the average expression of all normalized CCP signature genes on the array. In the prostate cancer dataset, CCP score is the average

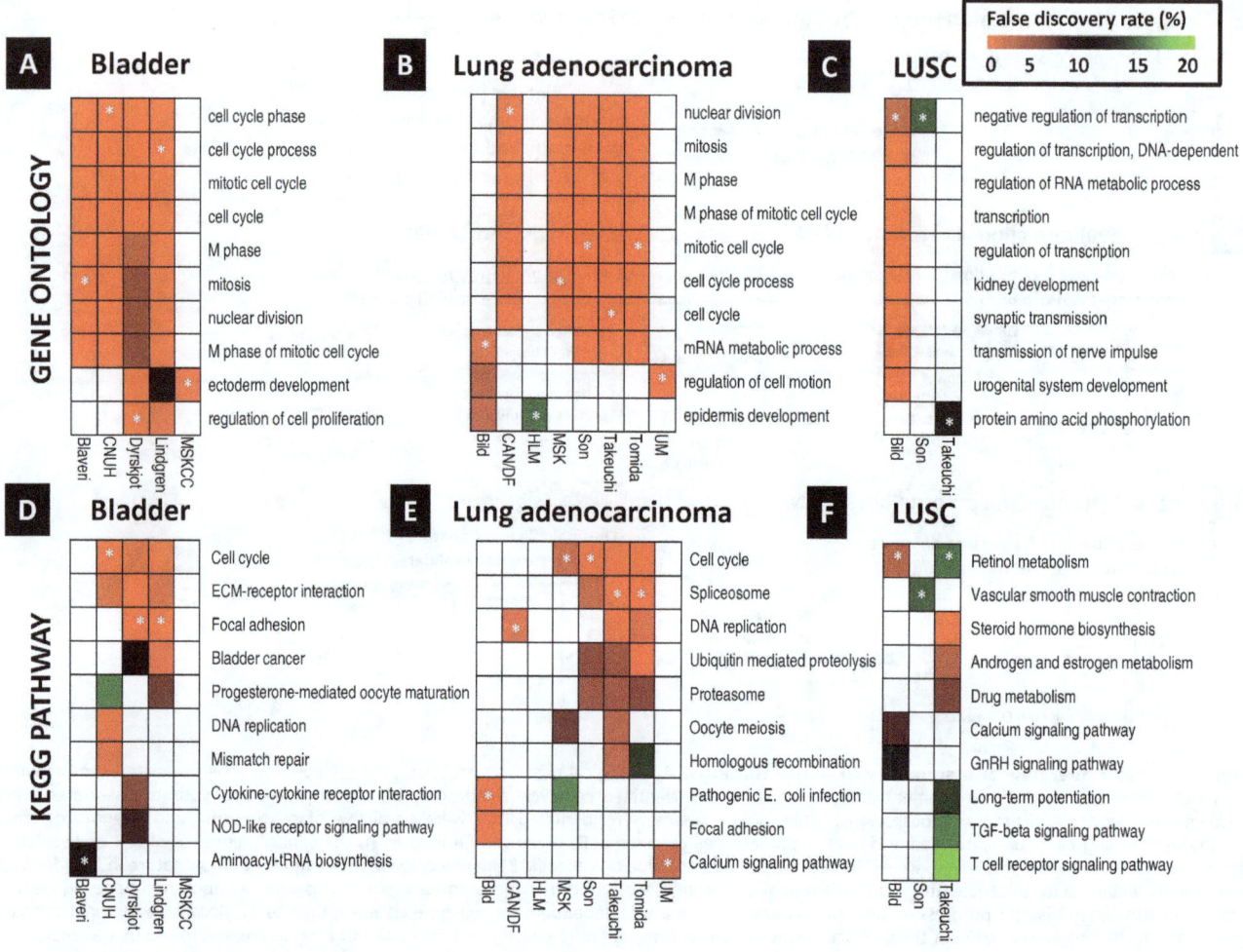

Figure 2. Prognostic modules associated with survival in tobacco-related cancers. In each cohort, over-represented Gene Ontology (GO) terms and KEGG pathways were identified from lists of genes significantly predictive of disease outcome (P<0.01) using the DAVID gene annotation enrichment analysis toolkit. Consistently prognostic modules were identified by ranking all modules first by the number of cohorts with significant results (FDR<20%) and then by average p-value. Each subfigure includes ten modules: the most consistently prognostic modules and the 'top hit' for each cohort, marked by an asterisk (*), which is defined as the module with the lowest FDR in that cohort that has an FDR<20% in multiple cohorts. **A,** over-represented GO terms associated with survival in bladder cancer. **B,** over-represented GO terms associated with survival in lung adenocarcinoma. **C,** over-represented GO terms associated with survival in squamous cell lung carcinoma. **D–F,** same as A–C except over-represented KEGG pathways are identified. There were no significantly over-represented prognostic modules in the head and neck squamous cell carcinoma cohorts at FDR<20%. LUSC: Squamous cell lung carcinoma, FDR: false discovery rate.

expression of 31 CCP genes measured by quantitative RT-PCR. For details see **Supporting Materials and Methods in File S1**.

Gene set enrichment and general statistical analyses

The Database for Visualization and Annotated Discovery (DAVID, Ref # [13]) was used for gene set enrichment analysis to identify overrepresented Gene Ontology (GO) [14] terms and KEGG pathways [15] in lists of genes. Additional details for this and general statistical analyses are provided in **Supporting Materials and Methods in File S1**. All analyses except for the gene set enrichment analysis was carried out using R (http://cran.r-project.org). Sample R code and output are provided in the form of a Sweave document that includes output from our analysis interweaved with corresponding R code (**File S3**). Additional R code is available upon request.

Results

Gene set enrichment analysis identifies cell cycle related genes as the most consistently prognostic class of biomarkers in bladder and lung adenocarcinoma

Data from 1968 patients were examined for the outcomes of tumor progression (where available) and survival (defined in **Materials and Methods**). In each cohort we identified lists of genes predictive of outcome (P<0.01) and performed an enrichment analysis that identifies overrepresented modules (GO terms [14] and KEGG pathways [15], **Figure 2, Figure S1,** and **Table S5 in File S6**) in these gene lists. Cell cycle related modules were the most consistently enriched modules across BL and LUAD patient cohorts (for details see **Supporting Results and Discussion in File S1**). In contrast, LUSC and HNSCC patient cohorts did not have a common overrepresented pathway (for details see **Supporting Results and Discussion in File S1**).

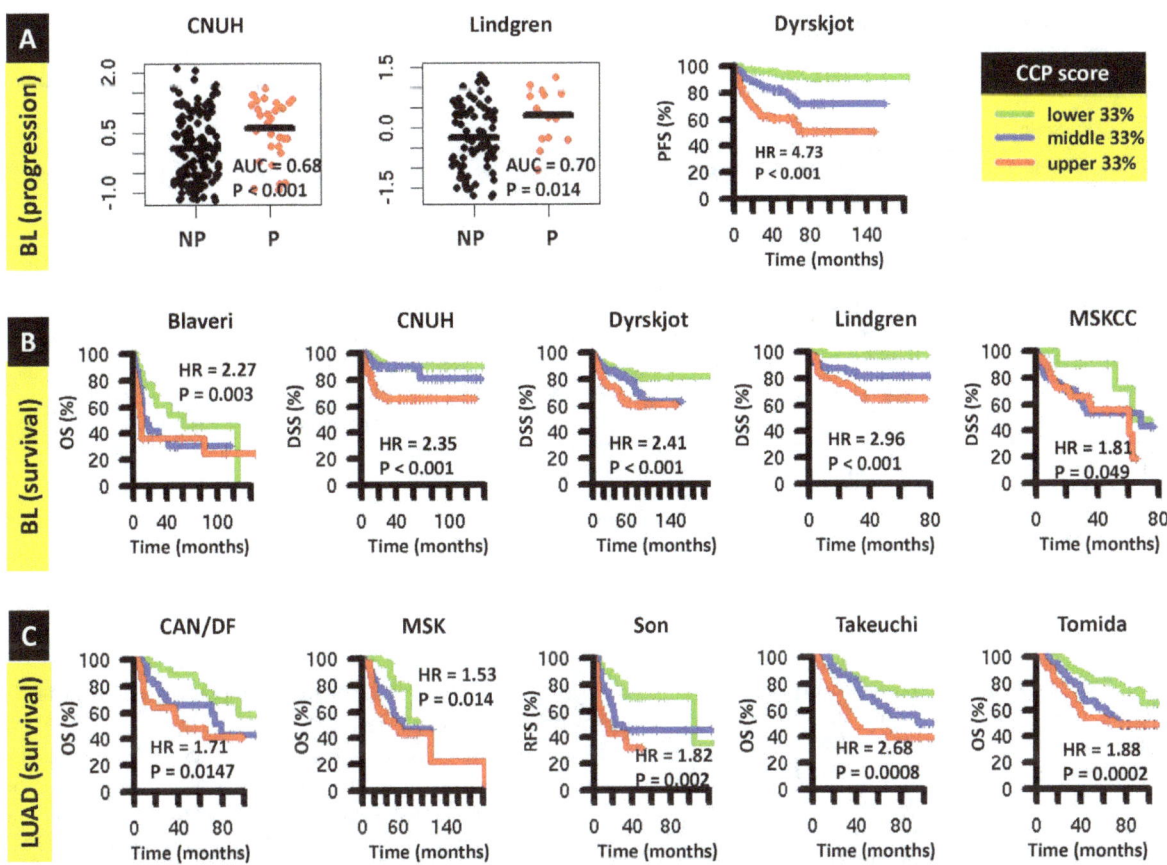

Figure 3. Prognostic value of cell cycle proliferation (CCP) gene score in bladder cancer and lung adenocarcinoma. A, prognostic value of CCP score for progression in bladder cancer in the CNUH (N = 165), Lindgren (N = 97), and Dyrskjot (N = 353) cohorts. In the CNUH and Lindgren cohorts, follow-up time was not available so we evaluated the ability of CCP score to discriminate between non-progressors (NP) and progressors (P) as described in **Materials and Methods**. In the Dyrskjot cohort, Kaplan-Meier (KM) curves for progression-free survival (PFS) were generated for patients with CCP scores at the lower (green), middle (blue), and upper (red) 33% and the log rank P-value of the continuous CCP score is reported. **B,** prognostic value of CCP score for survival in bladder cancer. KM curves were generated as in (A) for overall survival (OS) in the Blaveri (N = 74) cohort and for disease-specific survival (DSS) in the CNUH (N = 165), Dyrskjot (N = 366), Lindgren (N = 142), and MSKCC (N = 87) cohorts. **C,** prognostic value of CCP score for survival in lung adenocarcinoma. KM curves were generated for OS or recurrence-free survival (RFS) in the CAN/DF (N = 82), MSK (N = 104), Son (N = 62), Takeuchi (N = 90), and Tomida (N = 117) cohorts. Abbreviations: HR, hazard ratio, corresponding to 1-unit increase in CCP score.

Univariate and multivariate analysis of a cell cycle proliferation score in bladder and lung adenocarcinoma

To determine the clinical relevance of these findings we evaluated a previously published cell cycle proliferation (CCP) score (average expression of 31 cell cycle genes) that predicted time to recurrence or death in prostate cancer [16,17]. If the overrepresented cell cycle modules were determinant of clinical outcome, then one would also expect CCP score to be.

Overall, CCP score was significantly predictive (P<0.05) of progression and survival in all BL cohorts with these endpoints, and of survival in 5/8 LUAD cohorts, with high CCP scores associated with poor prognosis in all cases. Specifically, CCP score was predictive of progression in CNUH (AUC = 0.68, P<0.05), Lindgren (AUC = 0.70, P<0.05), and Dyrskjot (HR = 4.73, P< 0.001, **Figure 3A**) cohorts. CCP score was predictive of survival (P<0.05) in all five BL cohorts (HR 1.81–4.73, **Figure 3B**) CCP score was also predictive of outcome (P<0.05) in 5/8 LUAD cohorts (HR 1.53–2.68, **Figure 3C**).

We next evaluated whether CCP score contributes independent prognostic information. We performed a multivariate analysis and included clinically relevant variables such as age, gender, and grade in the BL and LUAD cohorts where CCP score was prognostic in the univariate analyses. For each cohort we also developed a best multivariate model (i.e., *final model*) through forward stepwise selection of informative variables (P<0.05). Such a model selects a concise, 'optimal' set of variables and may select CCP score over standard clinical variables. Because clinical variables are readily available this *final model* may not be cost-effective currently but may be so in settings where cancers are staged and graded according to their molecular pathology. Finally, we evaluated if CCP score increased the prognostic value of a *best available* model that included clinical variables that are readily available in current settings. Such an increase suggests that CCP score has clinical utility. For more details of the methodology see **Supporting Materials and Methods in File S1.**

CCP score was selected for the *final model* in all BL cohorts when progression was the endpoint (**Table 1**, **Table S6 in File S4**), and was the only significant variable in the multivariate analysis. When survival was the endpoint, CCP score was the most consistently significant variable in the multivariate analysis (P< 0.05), along with stage, which were each significant in three cohorts. CCP score was selected for the *final model* in two of these

Table 1. Multivariate progression and survival analysis in patients with bladder cancer.

Dataset	Endpoint	Clinical variables*	Multivariate analysis (P<0.05)	Final model†
CNUH (N = 165)	Progression	CCP score, stage, grade, BCG therapy, chemotherapy, age, gender	-	**CCP score**, stage
Lindgren (N = 97)	Progression	CCP score, grade	-	**CCP score**
Dyrskjot (N = 162)	PFS	CCP score, stage, grade, CIS diagnosis, BCG/MMC treatment, age, gender	**CCP score**	**CCP score**
Blaveri (N = 78)	OS	CCP score, grade, stage, surgery, age, gender	**CCP score**	**CCP score**
CNUH (N = 165)	DSS	CCP score, stage, grade, BCG therapy, chemotherapy. age gender	Stage, age	Stage, age
Dyrskjot (N = 155)	DSS	CCP score, stage, grade, CIS diagnosis, cystectomy following TURBT, BCG/MMC treatment, age, gender	**CCP score**, CIS diagnosis	**CCP score**, CIS, age
Lindgren (N = 156)	DSS	CCP score, stage, grade, cystectomy following TURBT, age, gender	Stage	Stage
MSKCC (N = 87)	OS	CCP score, stage, grade, age, gender	**CCP score**, stage, grade	Stage, grade

*Variables include the following (see **Tables S6–S7 in File S4** for complete multivariate analysis):
Stage: Ta-T1 vs. T2–T4 (CNUH, Dyrksjot - DSS, Lindgren, and MSKCC) and T1 vs. Ta (Dyrskjot -PFS);
Grade: high vs. low (CNUH, Lindgren, Blaveri, MSKCC); high vs. low vs. PUNLMP (Dyrskjot).
Surgery: cystectomy vs. transurethral resection of the bladder.
Abbreviations: PFS, progression-free survival; OS, overall survival; DSS, disease-specific survival.
†Final model is constructed from forward step-wise regression of significant variables (P<0.05).

cohorts (**Table 1**, **Table S7 in File S4**). In patients with LUAD, CCP score was the most consistently significant variable in the multivariate analysis and also the most frequently selected variable in the *final model* (**Table 2**, **Table S8 in File S4**). In the *best available* models, addition of CCP score led to an increase in prognostic ability (P<0.05) in two BL, one BL, and three LUAD cohorts when progression, survival, and survival were the endpoints, respectively (**Tables S9–S10 in File S5**). These results suggest that CCP score may be superior than standard clinical variables in both BL and LUAD cancers and that CCP score may have immediate clinical utility for predicting progression in BL patients and survival in LUAD patients. For more details see **Supporting Result and Discussion in File S1**. Consistent with the gene set enrichment analysis above, CCP score was not prognostic in patients with squamous tumors (LUSC and HNSCC) (**Figure S2**).

Prognostic signatures in bladder and lung carcinoma depend on cell cycle related genes

Because modules most consistently associated with progression in BL patients and survival in LUAD patients were cell cycle related (**Figure 2 and Figure S1**), we hypothesized that the performance of previously defined BL progression and LUAD survival signatures would be dependent on cell cycle related genes. BL survival signatures were not examined because a previous study found that their performance was poor in independent datasets [18]. We tested our hypothesis on published gene signatures using an adjustment approach (for details see **Supporting Materials and Methods in File S1**) that attenuates the predictive capability of signature genes that are correlated with CCP score [19].

In each dataset, expression levels of signature genes were adjusted for CCP score or by a constant term comprising a "negative control" (see **Supporting Materials and Methods**

Table 2. Multivariate survival analysis in patients with lung adenocarcinoma.

Dataset	Clinical variables*	Multivariate analysis (P<0.05)	Final model†
CANDF (N = 73)	CCP score, stage, grade, chemotherapy, smoking history, age, gender	**CCP score**, chemotherapy, age	**CCP score**, chemotherapy, age
MKS (N = 98)	CCP score, stage, grade, radiotherapy treatment, chemotherapy, smoking history, age, gender	Grade	Grade, chemotherapy
Takeuchi (N = 90)	CCP score, stage, grade, EGFR status, KRAS status, p53 status, smoking history, age, gender	**CCP score**	**CCP score**, stage
Tomida (N = 116)	CCP score, stage, EGFR status, KRAS status, p53 status, smoking history, age, gender	**CCP score**	**CCP score**, stage

*Variables include the following (see **Table S8 in File S4** for complete multivariate analysis):
Stage: I vs. II (CANDF), I vs. II vs. III (MKS, Takeuchi, Tomida).
Grade: Well vs. moderately vs. poorly differentiated.
Smoking history: current/former vs. never-smoker.
EGFR, KRAS, and p53 status: mutant vs. wild-type.
†Final model is constructed from forward step-wise regression of significant variables (P<0.05).

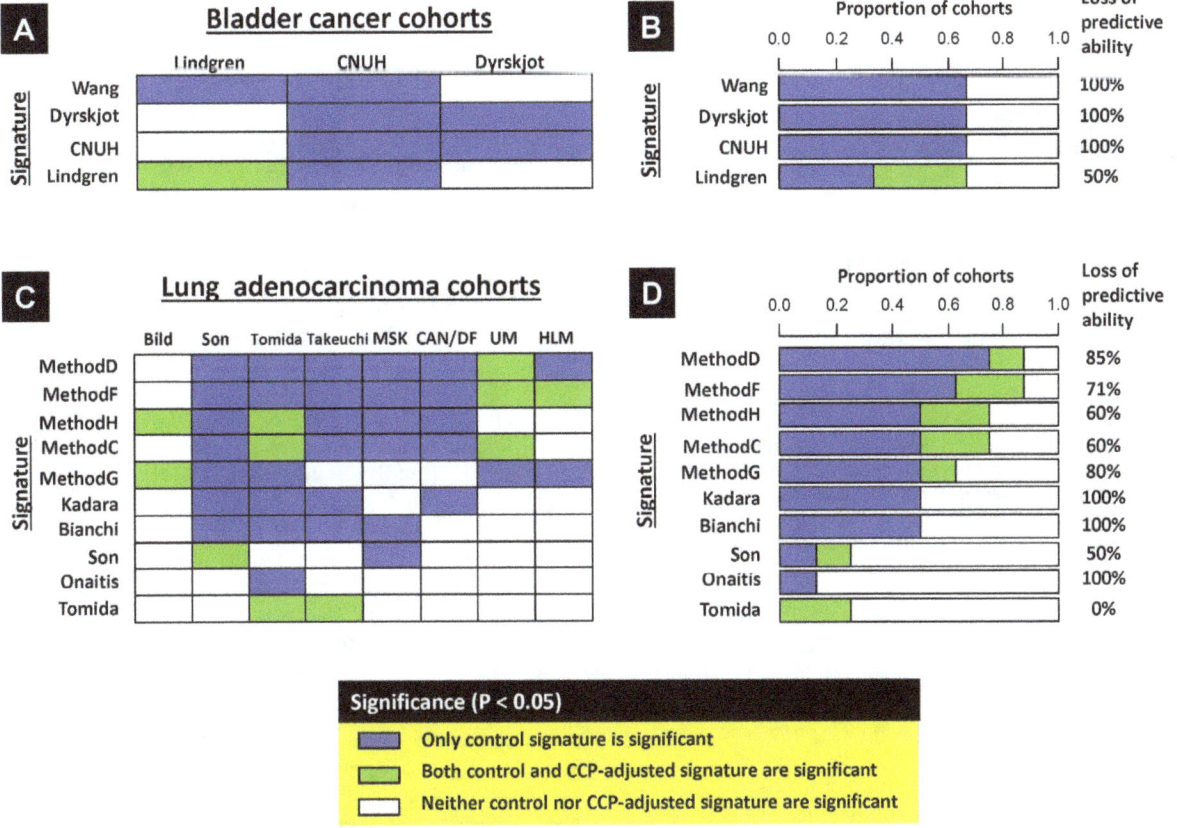

Figure 4. The prognostic value of published prognostic signatures in bladder cancer and lung adenocarcinoma. The expression values of prognostic signature genes were adjusted for CCP score or by a constant (negative control) as described in **Supporting Materials and Methods in File S1**. **A,** heatmap showing the impact of CCP score adjustment on the predictive ability of each signature (rows) on each cohort (columns). Signatures either lose their predictive ability following adjustment (P<0.05 in the control but P>0.05 in the CCP-adjusted cohort ; blue box); remain prognostic following the adjustment (P<0.05 in both the control and CCP-adjusted cohorts; green box); or were not prognostic in either case (P>0.05 in both groups, white box). **B,** stacked bar chart summarizing the prognostic value of each signature by categories described in (A). Loss of predictive ability is calculated as the percentage of signatures that lose their predictive ability following adjustment (blue boxes) with respect to the total number of control cohorts a signature is prognostic in (blue + green boxes). **C–D,** adjustment results in lung adenocarcinoma cohorts, in the same format as A–B.

in File S1 for details) and evaluated for progression in the BL cohorts and survival in the LUAD cohorts. A heatmap indicates each signature's prognostic value and whether its predictive ability is lost when adjusted for CCP score (**Figure 4**). In general, the signatures lost their predictive ability following CCP score adjustment. Specifically, bladder signatures lost their predictive ability in all independent cohorts, while lung signatures that were predictive in >2 cohorts lost their predictive ability in 83% of the

cohorts they were predictive in, on average. For details see **Supporting Results and Discussion in File S1**.

External validation of refined cell cycle expression signatures in human prostate cancer

Because CCP signature genes are highly correlated [16] and measure the same biological process, we hypothesized that a smaller gene signature would perform comparably to the full 31

Table 3. Analysis of refined CCP signatures in prostate cancer.

CCP score	Univariate HR (95% CI)	Univariate P-value	P-value adjusted by CAPRA-S	P-value for CCP- 31 adjusted by refined CCP score and CAPRA-S
CCP-31	1.99 (1.61, 2.45)	2.00E-09	7.60E-07	-
CCP-12	1.96 (1.59, 2.41)	1.70E-09	7.20E-07	0.61
CCP-10	1.87 (1.52, 2.30)	3.10E-08	5.10E-06	0.032
CCP-7	1.87 (1.50, 2.32)	1.00E-07	5.60E-06	0.033
CCP-4	1.69 (1.37, 2.08)	2.30E-06	3.90E-05	0.0037

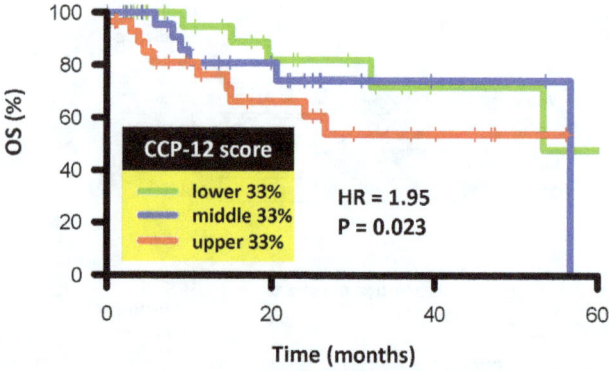

Figure 5. Prognostic value of a refined 12-gene cell cycle proliferation (CCP-12) score. Prognostic value of a refined 12-gene cell cycle proliferation (CCP-12) score in lung adenocarcinoma patients with gene expression profiling by RNASeq is shown. Kaplan-Meier (KM) curves for overall survival (OS) were generated for patients (N = 88) with CCP-12 scores at the lower (green), middle (blue), and upper (red) 33% and the log rank P-value of the continuous CCP-12 score is reported. Abbreviations: HR, hazard ratio, corresponding to 1-unit increase in CCP-12 score.

gene signature. First, we characterized the importance of signature size through repeated random sampling of CCP genes to generate gene signatures of various sizes and assessed their prognostic value in the BL and LUAD cohorts. We found that the predictive power of CCP score depends on signature size and not necessarily gene composition, and that 10–15 genes are sufficient to maintain the prognostic power of the full signature (**Figures S3, S4**) (see **Supporting Results and Discussion in File S1** for details). To independently confirm this finding and to evaluate smaller refined signatures we analyzed 4 "robust" signatures (CCP-4, -7, -10, and -12) (**Table S12 in File S8**) which include genes predictive of outcome in multiple cohorts (see **Supporting Materials and Methods in File S1** for details).

The CCP-4, -7, -10, and -12 signatures were provided to Myriad Genetics (Salt Lake City, UT) for "blinded" evaluation, i.e., without indication of our hypothesis regarding the relationship between signature size and prognostic value. The predictive ability of the signature scores for biochemical recurrence in prostate cancer was evaluated in 353 patients receiving radical prostatectomy [17], with gene expression measured by quantitative RT-PCR (see **Supporting Materials and Methods in File S1**). All scores were predictive (P<0.05) in univariate and multivariate analyses which included CAPRA-S [20], a measure of clinical risk accounting for pre-operative PSA, pathologic Gleason score, surgical margins, extra-capsular extension, seminal vesicle invasion, and lymph node invasion. In general, hazard ratios increased and p-values decreased with increasing gene number (**Table 3**). The refined signature scores were then analyzed in a multivariate analysis testing whether the full signature added predictive value to a model that also included CAPRA-S. The full signature added significant predictive value (P<0.05) to the CCP-4, CCP-7, and CCP-10 models, but not to the CCP-12 model, defining this signature (BIRC5, BUB1B, CDC20, CDCA8, CENPF, FOXM1, KIF11, NUSAP1, PTTG1, TK1, TOP2A) as sufficient.

Finally, we evaluated the CCP-12 signature in an additional cohort consisting of 88 patients with lung adenocarcinoma of mixed subtypes. Gene expression profiles for these patients were obtained through RNA sequencing (RNASeq) and downloaded from The Cancer Genome Atlas (TCGA) (http://cancergenome.nih.gov). CCP score was calculated as before (the average row-

normalized expression of the 12 CCP genes) using the normalized RNA counts (RNAseq by Expectation-Maximization, [21]) available from TCGA. **Fig. 5** shows that CCP-12 significantly predicts OS in these patients (HR = 1.95, P = 0.023), confirming the predictive ability of CCP-12 in an external cohort and indicating that CCP score is robust across multiple gene expression profiling technologies (microarray and RNAseq).

Discussion

We performed a gene set enrichment analysis of gene expression profiles in patients with four tobacco-related cancers and identified cell cycle as the functional process most consistently associated with patient outcome in tumors with non-squamous histologies. Aberrant cell proliferation is a hallmark of cancer [22] and increased expression of cell cycle genes is found in multiple tumor types [23], including those not causally associated with smoking such as breast [19] and prostate cancer [16,17]. However, it is interesting to note that smokers with prostate cancer have an increased risk of recurrence and mortality [24]. Surprisingly, cell cycle associated genes were not prognostic in tobacco-related tumors with squamous histology. However, we note these cohorts had relatively few patients (<85) which may have precluded the identification of functional processes associated with outcome in these tumor types

Our data provides important insights beyond the identification of a specific prognostic signature (CCP-12). First, it suggests that in BL and LUAD cancers, prognostic biomarkers will not validate across multiple cohorts unless they are (directly or indirectly) associated with cell cycle (**Figure 4**). Second, our finding that gene expression signatures could predict survival in multiple bladder cancer cohorts was unexpected because a recent validation study found that multiple signatures [25,26] derived from datasets examined here (Blaveri, MSKCC) had poor predictive ability [18]. Third, our data demonstrates for the first time that robust survival gene expression signatures exist in bladder cancer but only when defined based on functional gene modules. If used on other tumor types, this concept may lead to the development of robust signatures that are more likely to reach clinical practice.

Our work also tackles an important but seldom addressed issue in biomarker development, the impact of signature size on predictive ability. Cost effectiveness and feasibility of assessing multiple genes in a small quantity of biopsy tissue weigh against the need for large enough signatures that overcome technical variability from the assay and biological variability from tumor sample heterogeneity. Our results indicate the prognostic performance of cell cycle genes plateaus at 10–15. In contrast, Haibe-Kains et. al. found that in breast cancer the prognostic value of AURKA expression was comparable to multi-gene models. AURKA is one of the cell cycle genes we examined but was not as robust as CCP score, being predictive (P<0.05) in only 5/13 BL and LUAD cohorts (**Figure S5**). In general, redundancy obtained from multiple genes may overcome the variable quality of RNA derived from fixed tissue, which can cause individual gene assays to fail, thus ensuring robust analytical results. While we found that CCP-12 predicted outcome in an independent cohort additional steps such as defining thresholds that would separate patients into high and low risk groups and prospective evaluation in independent cohorts using predefined endpoints are required before this panel is ready for clinical use.

Supporting Information

File S1 Supporting Materials, Results and Discussion.

File S2   Summary of bladder cancer (Table S1), lung adenocarcinoma (Table S2), lung squamous cell carcinoma (Table S3), and head and neck squamous cell carcinoma (Table S4) patient cohorts.

File S3   Sweave document containing sample _R_ code and output.

File S4   Multivariate analyses of progression in bladder cancer (Table S6), survival in bladder cancer (Table S7), and survival in lung adenocarcinoma (Table S8).

File S5   Comparison of prognostic power of CCP score and best available clinical variables in bladder (Table S9) and lung adenocarcinoma (Table S10).

File S6   Prognostic modules associated with outcome in tobacco-related cancers (Table S5) (Excel XLSX file). In each cohort, over-represented Gene Ontology (GO) terms and KEGG pathways were identified from lists of genes significantly predictive of disease outcome (progression in BL patients and survival in BL, LUAD, LUSC, and HNSCC patients, $P<0.01$) using the DAVID gene annotation enrichment analysis toolkit. Consistently prognostic modules were identified by ranking all modules first by the number of cohorts with significant results (FDR<20%) and then by average p-value. There were no significantly over-represented prognostic modules in HNSCC patient cohorts at FDR<20%.

File S7   Prognostic bladder progression and lung adenocarcinoma survival gene signatures used in the adjustment analysis (Table S11) (Excel XLSX file).

File S8   CCP genes in five refined signatures (Table S12). Signatures are denoted by the number of CCP genes.

File S9   Prognostic modules associated with bladder progression and lung adenocarcinoma survival signatures (Table S13) (Excel XLSX file). Over-represented Gene Ontology (GO) terms and KEGG pathways were identified for each signature using the DAVID gene annotation enrichment analysis toolkit. Modules are ranked first by the number of signatures with significant results (FDR<20%) and then by average p-value.

Figure S1   Prognostic modules associated with progression in bladder cancer. In each cohort, over-represented Gene Ontology (GO) terms and KEGG pathways were identified from lists of genes significantly predictive of progression ($P<0.01$) using the DAVID gene annotation enrichment analysis toolkit. Consistently prognostic modules were identified by ranking all modules first by the number of cohorts with significant results (FDR<20%) and then by average p-value. Each subfigure includes ten modules: the most consistently prognostic modules and the 'top hit' for each cohort, marked by an asterisk (*), which is defined as the module with the lowest false discovery rate (FDR) in that cohort that has an FDR<20% in multiple cohorts. **A,** over-represented GO terms associated with progression in bladder cancer. **B,** over-represented KEGG pathways associated with progression in bladder cancer.

Figure S2   Prognostic value of CCP score in squamous cell lung cancers and head and neck squamous cell carcinomas. A, prognostic value of CCP score in squamous cell lung carcinomas (SCLC). Kaplan-Meier (KM) curves were generated for overall survival (OS) in the Bild (N = 53) and Takeuchi (N = 35) cohorts and for recurrence-free survival (RFS) in the Son (N = 76) cohort. KM curves were generated for patients with CCP scores at the lower (green), middle (blue), and upper (red) 33% and the log rank P-value of the continuous CCP score is reported. **B,** prognostic value of CCP score in head and neck squamous cell carcinomas (HNSCC). The Colo (N = 81) cohort did not include clinical follow-up time and so we evaluated the ability of CCP score to discriminate between node negative (N0) and node positive (N+) patients or between patients with non-recurrent (NR) and recurrent (R) tumors. The Pavon cohort (N = 63) did not include any clinical endpoints and so we evaluated the ability of CCP score to discriminate between N0 and N+ patients. In the Cohen cohort (N = 44), KM curves were generated for RFS. Abbreviations: HR, hazard ratio, corresponding to 1-unit increase in CCP score.

Figure S3   Relationship between prognostic value of CCP score and signature size based on proportion of significant signatures. Up to 10,000 gene signatures of sizes 1, 2, 4, …30, 31 were generated as described in **Supporting Materials and Methods in File S1**. Solid lines indicate proportion of signatures at each size that predicted survival ($P<0.05$) and are colored according to **A,** bladder patient cohort and **B,** lung adenocarcinoma cohort. Vertical dotted lines correspond to number of CCP genes (of 31) profiled in each cohort and are colored according to cohort.

Figure S4   Relationship between prognostic value of CCP score and signature size based on p-values. Up to 10,000 gene signatures of sizes 1, 2, 4, …30, 31 were generated as described in **Supporting Materials and Methods in File S1**. Boxplots of log10 p-values of signature scores for each signature size are plotted in **A,** bladder patient cohorts and **B,** lung adenocarcinoma cohorts. The blue horizontal line corresponds to a p-value of 0.05.

Figure S5   Prognostic value of CCP signature genes in **A,** bladder cancer and **B,** lung adenocarcinoma cohorts. In each cohort a gene is either significantly predictive of outcome (red box, $P<0.05$), not significantly predictive of outcome (gray box, $P\geq 0.05$), or was not profiled (white box) in each cohort. * indicates CCP score (using all available genes) is prognostic ($P<0.05$).

Acknowledgments

The authors thank Torben Orntoft and Lars Dryskot, Department of Molecular Medicine, Aarhus University Hospital for providing unpublished survival data for GSE5479 and Steve Stone, Myriad Genetics, Salt Lake City, UT, for blinded evaluation of gene expression signatures.

Author Contributions

Conceived and designed the experiments: GMD DT. Performed the experiments: GMD. Analyzed the data: GMD. Contributed reagents/materials/analysis tools: GMD DT. Wrote the paper: GMD DT.

References

1. Beer DG, Kardia SLR, Huang CC, Giordano TJ, Levin AM, et al. (2002) Gene-expression profiles predict survival of patients with lung adenocarcinoma. Nature Medicine 8: 816–824.

2. Rosenwald A, Wright G, Chan WC, Connors JM, Campo E, et al. (2002) The use of molecular profiling to predict survival after chemotherapy for diffuse large-B-cell lymphoma. New England Journal of Medicine 346: 1937–1947.

3. van de Vijver MJ, He YD, van 't Veer LJ, Dai H, Hart AAM, et al. (2002) A gene-expression signature as a predictor of survival in breast cancer. New England Journal of Medicine 347: 1999–2009.

4. Diamandis EP (2010) Cancer Biomarkers: Can We Turn Recent Failures into Success? Journal of the National Cancer Institute 102: 1462–1467.

5. Lauss M, Ringner M, Hoglund M (2010) Prediction of stage, grade, and survival in bladder cancer using genome-wide expression data: a validation study. Clinical cancer research : an official journal of the American Association for Cancer Research 16: 4421–4433.

6. Barrett T, Troup DB, Wilhite SE, Ledoux P, Evangelista C, et al. (2011) NCBI GEO: archive for functional genomics data sets–10 years on. Nucleic acids research 39: D1005–1010.

7. Dyrskjot L, Zieger K, Real FX, Malats N, Carrato A, et al. (2007) Gene expression signatures predict outcome in non-muscle-invasive bladder carcinoma: a multicenter validation study. Clin Cancer Res 13: 3545–3551.

8. Lindgren D, Frigyesi A, Gudjonsson S, Sjodahl G, Hallden C, et al. (2010) Combined gene expression and genomic profiling define two intrinsic molecular subtypes of urothelial carcinoma and gene signatures for molecular grading and outcome. Cancer Res 70: 3463–3472.

9. Lee ES, Son DS, Kim SH, Lee J, Jo J, et al. (2008) Prediction of Recurrence-Free Survival in Postoperative Non-Small Cell Lung Cancer Patients by Using an Integrated Model of Clinical Information and Gene Expression. Clinical Cancer Research 14: 7397–7404.

10. Colo AE, Simoes AC, Carvalho AL, Melo CM, Fahham L, et al. (2011) Functional microarray analysis suggests repressed cell-cell signaling and cell survival-related modules inhibit progression of head and neck squamous cell carcinoma. BMC Med Genomics 4: 33.

11. Mamelle G, Pampurik J, Luboinski B, Lancar R, Lusinchi A, et al. (1994) Lymph-Node Prognostic Factors in Head and Neck Squamous-Cell Carcinomas. American Journal of Surgery 168: 494–498.

12. Miller JA, Cai C, Langfelder P, Geschwind DH, Kurian SM, et al. (2011) Strategies for aggregating gene expression data: the collapseRows R function. BMC Bioinformatics 12: 322.

13. Huang da W, Sherman BT, Lempicki RA (2009) Systematic and integrative analysis of large gene lists using DAVID bioinformatics resources. Nat Protoc 4: 44–57.

14. Ashburner M, Ball CA, Blake JA, Botstein D, Butler H, et al. (2000) Gene ontology: tool for the unification of biology. The Gene Ontology Consortium. Nat Genet 25: 25–29.

15. Kanehisa M, Goto S (2000) KEGG: kyoto encyclopedia of genes and genomes. Nucleic acids research 28: 27–30.

16. Cuzick J, Berney DM, Fisher G, Mesher D, Moller H, et al. (2012) Prognostic value of a cell cycle progression signature for prostate cancer death in a conservatively managed needle biopsy cohort. Br J Cancer 106: 1095–1099.

17. Cuzick J, Swanson GP, Fisher G, Brothman AR, Berney DM, et al. (2011) Prognostic value of an RNA expression signature derived from cell cycle proliferation genes in patients with prostate cancer: a retrospective study. Lancet Oncol 12: 245–255.

18. Lauss M, Ringner M, Hoglund M (2010) Prediction of stage, grade, and survival in bladder cancer using genome-wide expression data: a validation study. Clin Cancer Res 16: 4421–4433.

19. Mosley JD, Keri RA (2008) Cell cycle correlated genes dictate the prognostic power of breast cancer gene lists. BMC Med Genomics 1: 11.

20. Cooperberg MR, Hilton JF, Carroll PR (2011) The CAPRA-S Score A Straightforward Tool for Improved Prediction of Outcomes After Radical Prostatectomy. Cancer 117: 5039–5046.

21. Guo Y, Sheng Q, Li J, Ye F, Samuels DC, et al. (2013) Large scale comparison of gene expression levels by microarrays and RNAseq using TCGA data. PloS one 8: e71462.

22. Hanahan D, Weinberg RA (2011) Hallmarks of cancer: the next generation. Cell 144: 646–674.

23. Segal E, Friedman N, Koller D, Regev A (2004) A module map showing conditional activity of expression modules in cancer. Nature Genetics 36: 1090–1098.

24. Kenfield SA, Stampfer MJ, Chan JM, Giovannucci E (2011) Smoking and prostate cancer survival and recurrence. JAMA 305: 2548–2555.

25. Blaveri E, Simko JP, Korkola JE, Brewer JL, Baehner F, et al. (2005) Bladder cancer outcome and subtype classification by gene expression. Clin Cancer Res 11: 4044–4055.

26. Sanchez-Carbayo M, Socci ND, Lozano J, Saint F, Cordon-Cardo C (2006) Defining molecular profiles of poor outcome in patients with invasive bladder cancer using oligonucleotide microarrays. J Clin Oncol 24: 778–789.

18

Regulation of the Tumor Suppressor FOXO3 by the Thromboxane-A$_2$ Receptors in Urothelial Cancer

Philip M. Sobolesky[1,2], Perry V. Halushka[2,3], Elizabeth Garrett-Mayer[2,4], Michael T. Smith[1], Omar Moussa[1,2]*

1 Department of Pathology and Laboratory Medicine, Medical University of South Carolina, Charleston, South Carolina, United States of America, **2** Hollings Cancer Center, Medical University of South Carolina, Charleston, South Carolina, United States of America, **3** Departments of Pharmacology and Medicine, Medical University of South Carolina, Charleston, South Carolina, United States of America, **4** Department of Public Health Sciences, Medical University of South Carolina, Charleston, South Carolina, United States of America

Abstract

The transcription factor FOXO3 is a well-established tumor suppressor whose activity, stability, and localization are regulated by phosphorylation and acetylation. Previous data by our laboratory demonstrated amplified thromboxane-A$_2$ signaling was associated with poor prognoses in bladder cancer patients and overexpression of the thromboxane-A$_2$ isoform-β receptor (TPβ), but not TPα, induced malignant transformation of immortalized bladder cells *in vivo*. Here, we describe a mechanism of TP mediated modulation of FOXO3 activity and localization by phosphorylation and deacetylation in a bladder cancer cell model. *In vitro* gain and loss of function studies performed in non-transformed cell lines, UROsta and SV-HUC, revealed knockdown of FOXO3 expression by shRNA increased cell migration and invasion, while exogenously overexpressing TPβ raised basal phosphorylated (p)FOXO3-S294 levels. Conversely, overexpression of ERK-resistant, mutant FOXO3 reduced increases in UMUC3 cell migration and invasion, including that mediated by TP agonist (U46619). Additionally, stimulation of UMUC3 cells with U46619 increased pFOXO3-S294 expression, which could be attenuated by treatment with a TP antagonist (PTXA$_2$) or ERK inhibitor (U0126). Initially U46619 caused nuclear accumulation of pFOXO3-S294; however, prolonged stimulation increased FOXO3 cytoplasmic localization. U46619 stimulation decreased overall FOXO3 transcriptional activity, but was associated with increased expression of its pro-survival target, manganese superoxide dismutase. The data also shows that TP stimulation increased the expression of the histone deacetylase, SIRT1, and corresponded with decreased acetylated-FOXO3. Collectively, the data suggest a role for TP signaling in the regulation of FOXO3 activity, mediated in part through phosphorylation and deacetylation.

Editor: Natasha Kyprianou, University of Kentucky College of Medicine, United States of America

Funding: Imaging facilities for this research were supported, in part, by Cancer Center Support Grant P30 CA138313 to the Hollings Cancer Center, MUSC. The research project described was in part supported by grants RO1127905CA, UL1TR000062, and UL1RR029882 from the National Cancer Institute, National Institutes of Health. The funders had no role in study design, data collection and analysis, decision to publish, or preparation of the manuscript.

Competing Interests: The authors have declared that no competing interests exist.

* Email: moussa@musc.edu

Introduction

Bladder cancer is the fifth most prevalent cancer in the United States with superficial transitional cell carcinoma (TCC) being the most commonly diagnosed form [1]. TCC has a high recurrence rate and requires costly lifelong follow-ups, making bladder cancer one of the most expensive cancers to treat over a patient's lifetime [2]. Understanding the mechanisms of oncogenic transformation of urothelial cells is essential to designing effective and novel therapies for the treatment of bladder cancer. We previously identified an inverse association between thromboxane synthase (TXS) expression and survival of bladder cancer patients, suggesting a role for thromboxane prostaglandin (TP) signaling in urothelial tumor progression [3]. TXS is an important enzyme that catalyzes the conversion of prostaglandin H$_2$ to thromboxane A$_2$ (TXA$_2$). The TXA$_2$ ligand, in turn, activates the TP receptor, promoting cell migration, proliferation, and invasion, which are key hallmarks of cellular transformation and the progression of disease [3,4,5,6,7]. Other studies have indicated a role for TXA$_2$

signalling in the tumorigenesis and malignant phenotypes of prostate [8] and breast cancers [9,10].

The human TP receptor gene encodes two isoforms, TPα and TPβ [11]. Both isoforms are seven trans-membrane G protein coupled receptors that differ only at the C-terminal domain [12]. The C-terminal variation allows each isoform to interact with both identical and unique signaling mediators [13]. Expression of the TP receptor isoforms is tissue and cell-type dependent. We previously reported TPβ overexpression in bladder cancer patients was associated with a significant decrease in survival [14]. In addition, the overexpression of TPβ, but not TPα, was sufficient to increase migration, invasion, and proliferation, as well as induce the malignant transformation of an immortalized non-transformed urothelial cell line [14]. The mechanism of transformation induced by TPβ overexpression remains unknown.

The transcription factor forkhead box-O3 (FOXO3) regulates key cell survival processes including oxidative stress resistance, cell cycle arrest, and apoptosis through the regulation of its target genes e.g. manganese superoxide dismutase (MnSOD), p27^{Kip1}, Fas ligand (FasL), and Bim [15,16]. FOXO3 transcriptional activity can be regulated through post-translational modifications (PTM) such as acetylation and phosphorylation. Dysregulation of FOXO3 activity and localization has been associated with cancer initiation and progression, as well as chemotherapeutic resistance [17,18,19]. Acetylation of FOXO3 by the histone acetyl-transferase p300 has been linked to decreased FOXO3 activity, increased cytoplasmic localization, and degradation [20]. Deacetylation by NAD-dependent deacetylase Sirtuin-1 (SIRT1) has been shown to differentially regulate FOXO3 targets by promoting the transcription of p27^{Kip1} and MnSOD, while decreasing transcription of Bim and FasL [21]. Extracellular signal-regulated kinase 1 and 2 (ERK1/2) has been shown to phosphorylate FOXO3 at -S294, -S344, and -S425, and negatively affect its function and stability through murine double minute 2 (MDM2)-mediated FOXO3 degradation [22]. While stimulation of TPβ is known to induce phosphorylation and activation of ERK [23,24,25], to our knowledge no study has examined the effects of TP signaling on FOXO3 modulation.

Here, we identified FOXO3 as a downstream target of the TP receptor pathway and examined the negative effects of TP signaling on FOXO3 localization and function in the bladder-cancer derived cell line UMUC3. Interestingly, overall FOXO3 transcriptional activity was reduced following TP agonist stimulation resulting in reduced expression of an apoptotic target, yet enhanced expression of a stress resistance target. In accordance with previous studies [21], the differential expression of FOXO3 targets following TP agonist stimulation was associated with increased SIRT1 expression and deacetylated FOXO3. Taken together, this study elucidates a mechanism by which TP induced modulation of FOXO3 activity through post-translational modifications contributes to the malignant phenotype of urothelial cells.

Materials and Methods

Cell culture

The UROsta cell line, kindly provided by Dr. Donald Sens (University of North Dakota, Grand Forks, ND) was derived from normal human urothelial cells and immortalized with the SV40 T-antigen [26]. UROsta cells were maintained in a 70:30 mixture of DMEM medium (1 g/L glucose: 4.5 g/L glucose; Mediatech, VA, USA), 10% fetal bovine serum (FBS). The Simian virus 40-immortalized human uroepithelial (SV-HUC), nontransformed urothelial cell line was kindly provided by Dr. Santhanam Swaminathan (University of Wisconsin, Comprehensive Cancer center, Madison, WI) [27,28,29] and cells were cultured in F12K Khaigns modified media supplemented with 10% FBS, insulin, hydrocortisone, and transferrin. The bladder cancer cell line UMUC3 were obtained from American Type Culture Collection and cells cultured in RPMI 1640 medium (Thermo Fisher Scientific, Rockford, IL, USA) containing 10% FBS. Every media contained 1% penicillin/streptomycin. Cell lines were grown at 37°C in 5% CO_2.

Antibodies, reagents, and plasmids

The following antibodies were used according to the manufacturers' recommendations: pFOXO3-S294, p-c-Jun Ser63, c-Jun, pAKT Ser473, pMAPK Thr202/Tyr204, Akt, ERK, p300, Sirt1, Bim, p27^{Kip1} (Cell Signaling Technology, Danvers, MA, USA), FOXO3, GFP (Santa Cruz), Lamin B1 (GeneTex, Irvine, CA, USA) MnSOD (EnzoLife Sciences, Ann Arbor, MI, USA), α-Tubulin (AbD Serotec, Raleigh, NC, USA), GAPDH (Sigma-Aldrich, St. Louis, MO, USA). TP specific agonist, U46619 was purchased from Cayman Chemicals (Ann Arbor, MI, USA). ERK1/2 inhibitor U0126 was purchased from Sigma-Aldrich.

FHRE-luc plasmid was a gift from Michael Greenberg (Addgene plasmid #1789, Cambridge, MA, USA). The GFP-FOXO3^{3A} (Serines-294, -344, and -425 substituted to alanines) and control pEGFP-C_2 plasmid were gifts from Mien-Chie Hung at The University of Texas M.D. Anderson Cancer Center. The GFP-TPβ plasmid was a gift from Jean-Luc Parent from the University of Sherbrooke, Canada.

Western blot analysis

Cells were washed with PBS and harvested in RIPA buffer (Thermo Fisher Scientific) supplemented with Complete Protease Inhibitors Cocktail Tablets and PhosSTOP Phosphatase Inhibitors Cocktail Tablets (Roche Applied Science). Proteins were denatured by boiling in Laemmli buffer (BioRad, Hercules, CA, USA) and resolved by 12% SDS-PAGE. Following protein transfer, the nitrocellulose membrane was blocked with 5% milk in 1× TBST and probed with primary antibody in 5% BSA in 1× TBST overnight at 4°C. Following primary antibody incubation, membranes were washed in 1× TBST and incubated with HRP-linked secondary antibody (Cell Signaling Technology) in 1× TBST. Membranes were washed 5× for 5 min with 1× TBST and detection was visualized using SuperSignal West Pico Chemiluminescent Substrate (Thermo Fisher Scientific). Western blots were quantified using Image Studio Lite Ver. 3.1 following software instructions and graphed on GraphPad Prism 5.

Transfections and generation of stable clones

To generate stable FOXO3 knockdown clones, SV-HUC and UROsta cells were transfected with either pRFP-C-RS control plasmid, pRFP-C-Scrambled or pRFP-c-shRNA to FOXO3 plasmid (HuSH-29; OriGene, Rockville, MD, USA) using FuGENE 6 (Roche Applied Science, Indianapolis, IN, USA). Single clones were selected in media containing 2.5 µg/ml puromycin (Invivogen, San Diego, CA, USA) and knockdown was analyzed by immunoblotting using a FOXO3 specific antibody (H-144; sc-11351; Santa Cruz Biotechnology, Santa Cruz, CA, USA). Transfection of GFP-TPβ into SVHUC cells was performed with TurboFect transfection reagent (Thermo Fisher Scientific) using a ratio of 1.5 µg DNA to 4 µl TurboFect. UROsta cells ($1×10^6$) were electroporated with 3.5 µg GFP-TPβ using the Amaxa Cell Line Nucleofector kit V solution box (cat#: VCA-1003, Lonza, Allendale, NJ, USA) and the Nucleofector 2b device (Lonza) with the pre-programmed protocol T-030. Four hours following electroporation media was aspirated, replaced with complete media, and incubated at 37°C in 5% CO_2. Transfection efficiency was checked 24 hours post-electroporation. To generate stable GFP-FOXO3^{3A} expressing UMUC3 clones, cells in a 6-well plate were transfected using 4 µl X-tremeGENE HP DNA Transfection Reagent (Roche Applied Science) and 1.5 µg plasmid DNA. Single clones were selected in media containing 500 µg/ml of Geneticin Selective Antibiotic (Life Technologies, Grand Island, NY, USA).

Cell migration assay

The BD falcon Cell Culture Insert System containing polyethylene terephthalate (PET) membranes with 8 µm pores (BD Biosciences, Rockville, MD, USA) were used for this assay. The inserts were pre-coated overnight with 5 µg/cm^2 fibronectin at 4°C and equilibrated in water for 2 hours at 37°C prior to usage. Trypsinized cells were collected, counted, and $5×10^4$ cells were resuspended in 250 µl serum-free medium. The upper chamber of the insert was filled with the cell suspension, whereas 750 µl of medium containing 10% FBS were added to the bottom of each well. UROsta cells were allowed to migrate for 16 hours in a humidified environment at 37°C with 5% CO_2. After migration, cells were removed from the upper surface of the membrane by wiping it with a moist cotton swab. The lower surface of the membranes were stained using the Hema-3 Staining kit (Fisher Scientific, Pittsburg, PA, USA). Once the staining was finished the membranes were rinsed in distilled water for excess stain removal and air dried overnight. Percent migration or invasion was calculated by counting and averaging the number of cells invaded in 10 random fields of view at a 40× magnification, divided by the area of the microscope viewing field and then multiplied by the area of the transwell insert. Then divide the previously calculated number by the number of cells seeded and lastly multiply by 100 to get a percent. This experiment was performed independently three times in duplicates.

Cell invasion assay

The BD BioCoat Matrigel Invasion Chamber Cell Culture Insert System containing 8 μm PET membrane (BD Biosciences) with a thin layer of MATRIGEL Basement Membrane Matrix was used for this assay. Trypsinized cells were collected, counted, and resuspended at 5×10^4 cells/ml in serum-free media. The top chamber received 500 μl of the cell suspension, while 750 μl of RPMI with 10% FBS was added to the well. The cells were allowed to invade for 16 hours in a humidified environment at 37°C with 5% CO_2 before cell removal from the upper surface with a moist cotton swab. Membranes were stained using the Hema-3 Staining kit (Thermo Fisher Scientific) and percent invasion was calculated as described in cell migration assay section. This experiment was performed independently three times in duplicates.

Dual luciferase assay

UMUC3 cells were seeded in 6-well plates at 0.3×10^6 cells/well, then transiently transfected within 24 hours using X-tremeGENE HP DNA transfection reagent (Roche Applied Science) with 4 μg of 3× forkhead response element (FHRE) reporter construct (Addgene plasmid #1789) and 0.1 μg pBind Renilla luciferase control vector (Promega, Madison, WI, USA). Transfected cells were incubated for 24 hours in a humidified environment at 37°C with 5% CO_2. Cells were then serum starved overnight and treated with either vehicle control (methyl acetate, Sigma-Aldrich) or 1 μM U46619 (Cayman Chemical) for 30 or 120 minutes. Following treatment cells were washed twice with PBS and harvested in Reporter Lysis Buffer (Promega). Luminescence was measured using a Veritas Microplate Luminometer (Turner BioSystems, Sunnyvale, CA, USA) in 20 μl of each sample for 10 seconds following each injection of 50 μl Luciferase Assay Reagent II then 50 μl Stop and Glow. The average Firefly luciferase expression was adjusted to total protein and control vector Renilla luciferase expression, and then normalized to vehicle control. Results represent the average percent activity of three independent experiments conducted in duplicates, Student t-test (*) $P<0.05$.

Nuclear/cytoplasmic cell fractionation

UMUC3 cells were serum starved overnight, then pretreated with 1 μM Indomethacin (Cayman Chemicals) for 10 minutes to reduce endogenous TXA_2 signaling. Cells were treated with vehicle or 1 μM U46619 for 5, 30, or 120 minutes. Cells were trypsinized, collected, and washed twice with PBS. Fractionation was performed using the Pierce NE-PER Nuclear and Cytoplasmic Extraction Kit (Thermo Fisher Scientific) following the manufacturer's protocol. Extracts were analyzed by Western blot.

Immunoprecipitation

Immunoprecipitation of FOXO3 from UMUC3 cells was performed using the NHS-linked IP/Co-IP kit (Thermo Fisher Scientific) following manufacturers protocol. Briefly, the UMUC3 cells were grown to 80% confluence in 10 cm plates, and then placed in serum free media for 24 hours in a humidified environment at 37°C with 5% CO_2. Cells were then treated with either vehicle control (methyl acetate, Sigma-Aldrich) or 1 μM U46619 (Cayman Chemical) for 30, 60, or 120 minutes. Following treatment cells were washed once with PBS ($-Ca$, $-Mg$) and harvested in ice cold IP lysis/wash buffer supplemented with protease inhibitor EDTA-free cocktail and PhosSTOP inhibitor cocktail (Roche). Collected lysate then centrifuged to remove cell debris and determined protein concentration using BCA protein assay kit (Thermo Fisher Scientific). The NHS-activated magnetic beads were vortexed and 25 μl of slurry was transferred to 1.5 mL tubes per IP reaction. Tubes were placed on the magnet and storage solution was discarded, and then washed with ice-cold 1 mM HCl and gently vortexed for 5 seconds. Beads were collected on magnetic stand and discarded the supernatant.

The antibody solution was prepared by diluting two μg FOXO3 (Santa Cruz Biotechnology) and negative control rabbit immuno-globulin fraction (solid-phase absorbed) (Dako, Carpinteria, CA, USA) to a final concentration of 2 μg antibody in 100 μL of 0.067M borate buffer. Added 100 μl of prepared antibody solution to the activated beads, gently vortexed, and incubated on a rotating platform for 60 minutes at room temperature. Reactions were vortexed every 10 minutes during the incubation to ensure the beads remained in suspension. Beads were collected and supernatant was discarded. Washed beads twice with elution buffer, vortexing tubes each wash to remove non-covalently bound antibody. Quenching buffer was added to the beads and incubated on a rotating platform for 60 minutes at room temperature. Beads were collected on magnetic stand and discarded the supernatant. Prepared and added 0.5 mL of modified borate buffer to each IP and mixed gently by vortex, then beads were collected on magnetic stand and discarded the supernatant. Reactions were washed twice with IP lysis/wash buffer, then incubated each IP reaction with 100 μg lysate in final volume of 500 μL IP lysis/wash buffer supplemented with protease and phosphatase cocktail inhibitors overnight (between 14–18 hours at 4°C on a rotator. The beads were vortexed every 15 minutes the first hour to ensure the beads stayed in suspension. After antigen incubation the beads were collected, washed twice with IP lysis/wash buffer and then transferred to a new 1.5 ml tube. Washed beads with ultrapure water (pH 7.0), then placed on magnetic stand and discarded the supernatant. Proteins were eluted from the beads with low pH elution buffer (pH 2.0) twice and neutralized with Tris-HCl pH 8.5. Eluted proteins were then analyzed by Western blot.

Statistical analysis

Continuous outcomes were compared across conditions using a two-sided two-sample Student's t-test. Experiments containing more than two variables were compared using a one-way ANOVA followed with a Tukey post-hoc test. A P-value <0.05 was considered statistically significant.

Results

Knockdown of FOXO3 Increases Urothelial Migration and Invasion

We previously reported a role for the TPβ receptor in urothelial migration, invasion, and malignant transformation [3,14]. Reduced FOXO3 expression in patients has also been linked with urothelial cancer invasiveness [30]. To determine whether FOXO3 inactivation would be sufficient to induce a malignant phenotype independent of TPβ, low endogenous TPβ expressing UROsta and SVHUC cell lines (previously determined [14]) were stably transfected with FOXO3 specific shRNA (Figure 1A). FOXO3-shRNA transfected cells reduced FOXO3 protein expression over one half compared to scrambled (scr)-shRNA observed by Western blot and validated by examining the downstream target MnSOD (Figure 1A). Compared to scr-shRNA cells knockdown of FOXO3 expression resulted in a 39% and 114% increase in migration, as well as a 63% and 18% increase in invasion of SV-HUC and UROsta cells, respectively, (P<0.05, Figure 1B–C). Since the absence of FOXO3 was sufficient to induce a malignant phenotype in immortalized non-transformed urothelial cells, we examined the effect of TPβ overexpression on FOXO3 inactivation. SV-HUC and UROsta cells transfected with TPβ displayed a 0.5-fold increase in the basal expression of the inactive pFOXO3-S294 protein (Figure 1D–E).

Effects of TP Agonist Stimulation on FOXO3 Phosphorylation, Localization, and Transcriptional Activity

To demonstrate TXA$_2$ signaling is involved in FOXO3 regulation, the phosphorylation status of FOXO3 and its known regulator ERK were examined in UMUC3 cells after TP agonist U46619 stimulation (Figure 2A). The TP agonist mediated phosphorylation of ERK at T202/Y204 was significantly increased (~1-fold) 15 and 30 minutes following stimulation

(Figure 2A and C). Correspondingly, a significant increase in pFOXO3-S294 was observed 15 (5-fold), 30 (7-fold), and 60 (3.5-fold) minutes following TP agonist stimulation (Figure 2A–B). Treatment of UMUC3 cells with the TP antagonist pinane (PTXA$_2$) or ERK inhibitor (U0126) attenuated the U46619 mediated effects of activated ERK and pFOXO3-S294 (Figure 2D–I).

The effects of TP agonist stimulation on FOXO3 transcriptional activity were examined by a dual luciferase assay. UMUC3 cells were transiently transfected with the forkhead response element (FHRE) firefly luciferase reporter construct and Renilla control vector, prior to treatment with vehicle or TP agonist. FOXO3 transcriptional activity was significantly decreased by 36% and 44% at 30 and 120 minutes, respectively, following TP agonist stimulation compared to vehicle control (Figure 3A).

Based on the phosphorylation kinetics of FOXO3, we examined the cellular distribution of FOXO3 in UMUC3 cells treated with vehicle or TP agonist for 5, 30, or 120 minutes. Nuclear and cytoplasmic protein fractions were analyzed by Western blot (Figure 3B) and band densities were quantified using Image Studio Lite Ver 3.1 (Figure 3C). UMUC3 cells stimulated with TP agonist showed an initial increase in nuclear FOXO3 which was also associated with an increase in nuclear pFOXO3-Ser294 (Figure 3C). Prolonged stimulation resulted in a significant increase in total FOXO3 in the cytoplasm (Figure 3C).

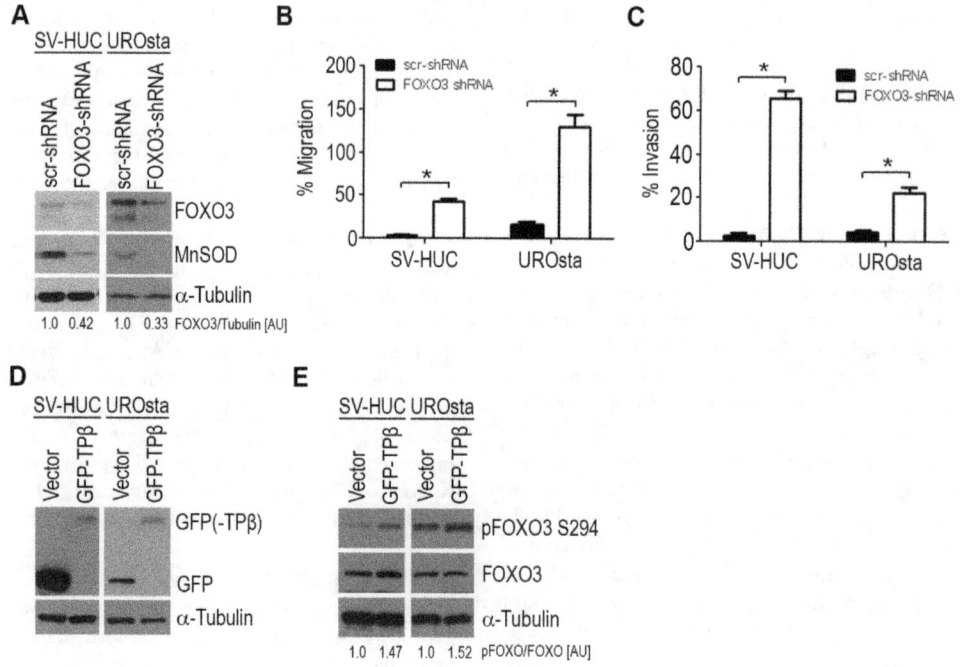

Figure 1. Loss of FOXO3 results in increased cell migration and invasion. (**A**) Western blot of whole cell lysates from SV-HUC and UROsta cells stably transfected with FOXO3-shRNA or control scrambled (scr−) shRNA immunoblotted for total FOXO3 and its known downstream target MnSOD. α-tubulin was applied as loading control. Blots shown are representative of three individual experiments and numbers represent the averaged ratios of FOXO3 to α-tubulin. Ratios quantified using Image Studio Lite Ver.3.1. SV-HUC and UROsta FOXO3 knockdown and control clones were seeded into inserts coated with fibronectin or matrigel and allowed to migrate (**B**) or invade (**C**) for 16 hours. Knockdown of FOXO3 increased SV-HUC and UROsta cell migration (39% and 114%) and invasion (63% and 18%, respectively) compared to scr-shRNA. Data represent three independent assays done in duplicates and expressed as the mean ± SEM. Significance was determined with a two-sided two-sample t-test, (* = P< 0.05, n = 3) compared to scr- control. (**D**) Overexpression of GFP tagged TPβ in UROsta and SVHUC cells increases basal pFOXO3-S294 expression (**E**) compared to vector control (n = 3). Numbers represent the averaged ratios of pFOXO3-S294 to FOXO3. Ratios quantified using Image Studio Lite Ver.3.1. [AU] = arbitrary units.

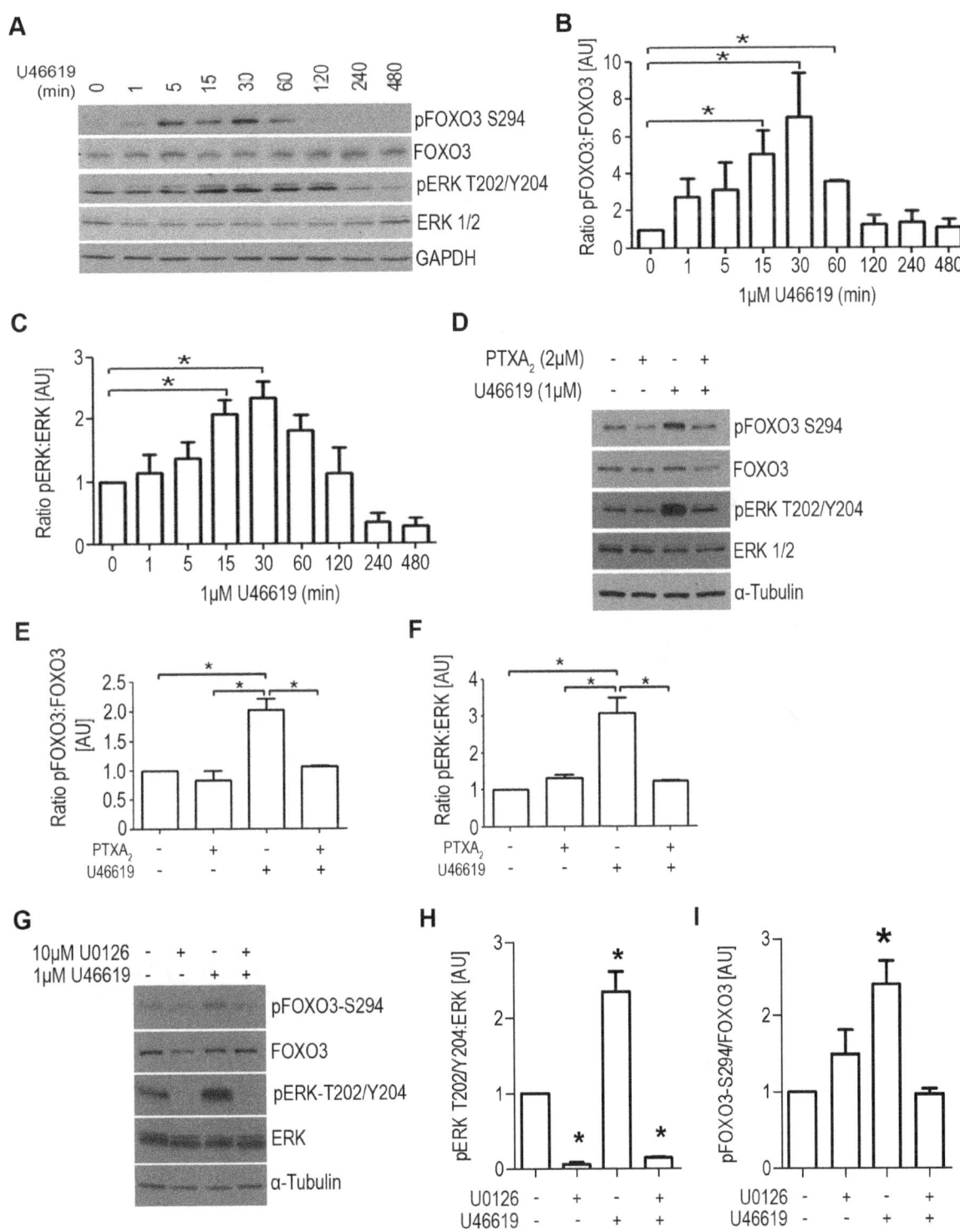

Figure 2. TP agonist activates ERK and increases FOXO3 phosphorylation at –S294. (**A**) UMUC3 cells were treated with 1 μM U46619 for the indicated times. Cell lysates were analyzed by immunoblotting for both total and phosphorylated ERK and FOXO3. GAPDH served as loading control. Blots were quantified and ratios for (**B**) pFOXO3-S294 to FOXO3 and (**C**) pERKT202/Y204 to ERK1/2 were graphed using GraphPad Prism 5. UMUC3 cells pretreated for 15 minutes with (**D**) 2 μM TP antagonist Pinane (PTXA$_2$) or (**G**) 10 μM ERK inhibitor (U0126) attenuated the activation of ERK and phosphorylation of FOXO3 following treatment with 1 μM U46619 for 30 minutes. Cell lysates were immunoblotted for both total and phosphorylated ERK and FOXO3. α-Tubulin served as loading control. Graphs represent quantified ratios for (**E** and **I**) pFOXO3-S294 to FOXO3 and (**F** and **G**) pERKT202/Y204 to ERK1/2 were graphed. Significance was determined for all quantified blots using a repeated measure One-way ANOVA with Tukey post-hoc test. $P<0.05$.

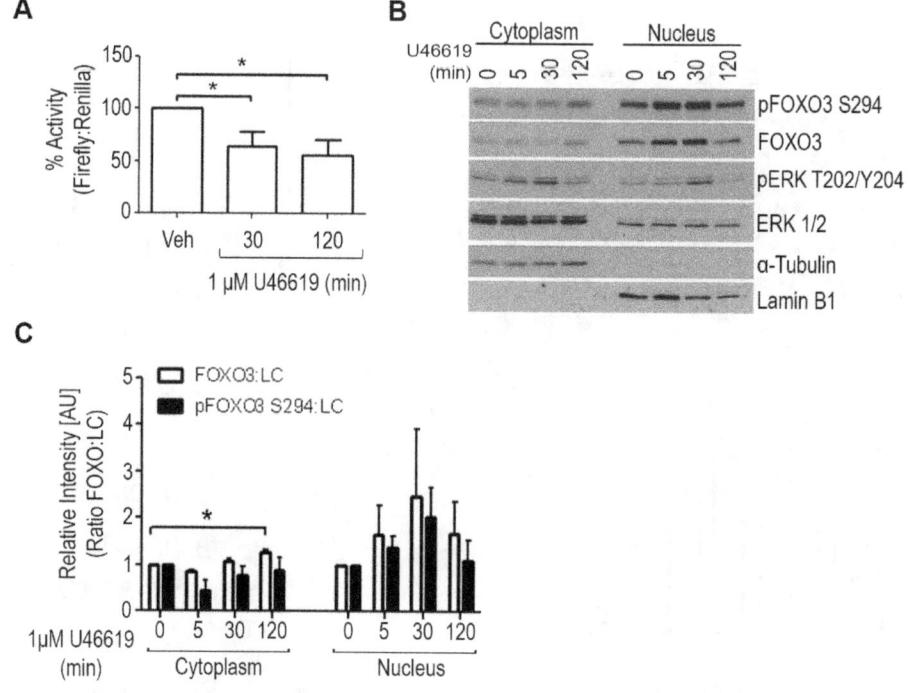

Figure 3. Decreased FOXO3 transcriptional activity and nuclear localization following TP agonist treatment. (**A**) UMUC3 cells transiently transfected with 3× forkhead response element (FHRE) reporter construct and Renilla luciferase control vector were treated with 1 μM U46619 for 30 or 120 minutes and resulted in decreased FOXO3 transcriptional activity. The average Firefly luciferase expression was adjusted to total protein and control vector Renilla luciferase expression before normalization to vehicle control. Results represent the average percent luciferase activity of three independent experiments conducted in duplicates. *P<0.05, One-way ANOVA with Tukey post-hoc test. (**B**) UMUC3 cells were serum starved overnight and pretreated for 15 min. with 1 μM Indomethacin prior to treatment with either vehicle or 1 μM U46619 for 5, 30, or 120 minutes. The cells were subjected to nuclear and cytoplasmic fractionation and proteins were analyzed by Western blot. α-Tubulin and Lamin-B1 served as loading controls for cytoplasmic and nuclear fractions, respectively. (**C**) Densitometry of blots showing prolonged agonist stimulation increased cytoplasmic FOXO3 protein and increased nuclear pFOXO3 proteins compared to vehicle controls. Significance was determined for all quantified blots using a repeated measure One-way ANOVA with Tukey post-hoc test. P<0.05.

TP stimulation increases SIRT1 expression, deacetylation of FOXO3, and affects FOXO3 target expressions

The effect of U46619 stimulation on the expression levels of well characterized FOXO3 targets p27[Kip1], MnSOD, and Bim were examined by Western blot (Figure 4A). UMUC3 cells stimulated with U46619 for 30, 120, and 240 minutes observed decreased p27[Kip1] and Bim proteins, and increased MnSOD protein expression (Figure 4A). Since the expression pattern of FOXO3 targets resembled the pattern observed following overexpression of the histone deacetyltransferase SIRT1 [21], we investigated the effect of U46619 stimulation on SIRT1 expression. UMUC3 cells stimulated with TP agonist displayed increased expression of SIRT1 and decreased expression of p300 compared to vehicle control (Figure 4B–C). To determine if the increased SIRT1 expression in UMUC3 cells stimulated with TP agonist affected FOXO3 acetylation status, FOXO3 was immunoprecipitated from UMUC3 cells treated with either vehicle or U46619, and immunoblotted for acetylated lysine residues. Stimulation of UMUC3 cells with U46619 for 120 and 240 minutes displayed a 48% and 70% reduction in acetylated FOXO3, respectively (Figure 4D–E).

ERK resistant Mutated FOXO3[3A] Reduced TP agonist Mediated Migration and Invasion

UMUC3 cells were stably transfected with a GFP-vector or mutated GFP-FOXO3[3A] construct in which all three ERK phosphorylation residues were substituted for alanine residues to mimic a non-phosphorylated or active state (Figure 5A). To determine if U46619 mediated phosphorylation of FOXO3 by ERK affects cell migration and invasion, the stably transfected cells were allowed to migrate and invade following stimulation with vehicle or U46619. The control GFP-vector cells resulted in a 2-fold increase in cell migration and invasion with U46619 stimulation compared to vehicle control, whereas expression of the GFP-FOXO3[3A] protein reduced U46619 mediated migration and invasion (Figure 5B–C).

To further demonstrate the importance of ERK signalling in TXA_2 mediated cell mobility, we pre-treated with the ERK inhibitor U0126 (10 μM) for 10 minutes before measuring the effect on U46619 mediated migration. UMUC3 cells pre-treated with U0126 did not significantly reduce basal levels of migration (Figure 5D). Pre-treatment with U0126 significantly reduced the U46619 induced cell migration of the UMUC3 cells (Figure 5D).

Discussion

The current study supports the role of TXA_2 signaling in promoting bladder tumorigenesis by modulating the activity of the transcription factor FOXO3 via ERK mediated phosphorylation at −S294 or deacetylation, presumably by SIRT1. We demonstrate the specificity of the effects on FOXO3 are mediated through the TXA_2 pathway by using a pharmacological approach that includes a TP receptor(s) specific agonist and antagonist as well as an ERK inhibitor. We show shRNA mediated knock-down of FOXO3 in immortalized non-transformed bladder cells results

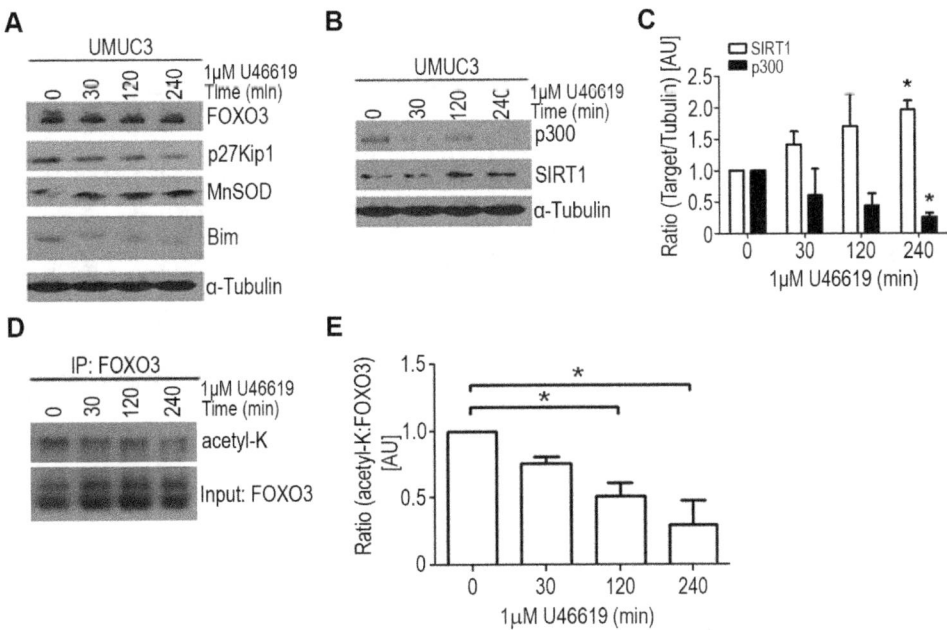

Figure 4. Effect of TP agonist on FOXO3 target proteins expressions and acetylation status. (A) UMUC3 cells treated with vehicle or 1 µM U46619 for 30, 120, and 240 minutes. Cell lysates were collected and analyzed by Western blot for total FOXO3 expression and downstream targets p27^{Kip1}, MnSOD, and Bim. **(B)** Protein expression of p300 and SIRT1 in same cell lysates. α-tubulin served as loading control. **(C)** Quantified values from blots of three independent experiments are graphed. (*) indicates p<0.05, One-way ANOVA, compared to time 0 for each Target ratio. **(D)** Increased SIRT1 expression mediated by U46619 in UMUC3 cells corresponded with decreased acetylated FOXO3. Total FOXO3 was immunoprecipitated from serum starved UMUC3 cells treated with vehicle or 1 µM U46619 for 30, 120, or 240 minutes. Eluted proteins were analyzed by Western blot with antibodies against acetylated lysine residues and FOXO3. Blots are representative of three independent experiments. Blots were quantified and ratios for **(E)** acetylated-lysine (acetyl-K) to FOXO3 were graphed. Significance was determined using repeated measures One-way ANOVA with Tukey post-hoc test. P<0.05.

in malignant phenotypes exhibited thru increases in cell migration and invasion. Thus, elucidating the effects of TXA$_2$ signaling on FOXO3 expression, phosphorylation, and subcellular localization could reveal new chemotherapeutic targets for bladder cancer treatment.

TXA$_2$ non-preferentially signals through the two alternatively spliced TP receptor isoforms, TPα (343 residues) and TPβ (407 residues), for the reason that the first 328 amino acid residues are identical [31]. Due to the short half-life of TXA$_2$ (t½~30 s), we used the TXA$_2$ stable analogue U46619 at a previously established pharmacological concentration [14,32,33,34]. While it is not possible to equate the concentration of U46619 to an *in vivo* concentration, the K$_d$'s for TXA$_2$ and U46619 are in a similar range and when TXA$_2$ is generated it is often synthesized in large amounts so this concentration although pharmacologic could be considered to be in a physiologic range.

Stimulation of TPβ is known to signal through several G-proteins as well as β-arrestin2 to activate multiple pathways resulting in the activation of ERK [14,35,36,37]. Our previous data identified the TPβ receptor isoform as overexpressed in the majority of bladder cancer cases as well as implicated its expression in bladder carcinogenesis and tumor progression [14]. Furthermore, the over-expression of TPβ, but not TPα, in immortalized bladder cells resulted in sustained ERK activation and induced malignant transformation in an in vivo mouse model [38], yet the mechanism for this effect remained unclear. Here, we showed overexpression of TPβ was sufficient to increase the phosphorylation of FOXO3 at Ser-294 implicating the ERK signaling pathway in the TXA$_2$ mediated regulation of FOXO3. As a result, a goal of this research was to focus on the effects of

TXA$_2$ signaling on ERK mediated regulation of FOXO3 in a malignant cell line that expresses TPβ. To select the best cell line for examining the levels of modified FOXO3 protein, we immunoblotted a panel of bladder cancer cell lines for the expression of TPβ and FOXO3 and chose the cell line that expressed the highest levels of both proteins (data not shown). Consequently, the UMUC3 cell line was selected for examining modified FOXO3 protein levels. Moreover, the expression of a mutant FOXO3 protein that is unable to be phosphorylated by ERK, attenuated TP agonist mediated migration and invasion of malignant UMUC3 cells. We also demonstrated that inhibiting ERK pharmacologically is sufficient to attenuate the TP agonist induced migration of bladder cancer cells. Multiple studies have demonstrated the inactivation of FOXO3 by ERK is associated with cell survival and tumorigenesis of multiple cancers [22,39,40], however, this study is the first to experimentally link TXA$_2$ signaling as the source of the effects on FOXO3.

The forkhead transcription factors are emerging as key players in cellular proliferation, migration, apoptosis, adaptation to cellular stress [39], and angiogenesis [41,42,43,44,45]. The subcellular localization of transcription factors can often determine their functionality, potentially making location as important as its overall expression in cancer. For instance, in prostate cancer increased cytoplasmic FOXO3 was associated with increased Gleason grade [19]. In ovarian cancer cells, the overexpression of phosphorylated FOXO3 at Thr-32 correlated with lymph node involvement [46]. In urothelial cancer, decreased FOXO3 expression was associated with increased invasiveness and decreased overall patient survival [30]. While those studies identified the importance of FOXO3 expression in patient

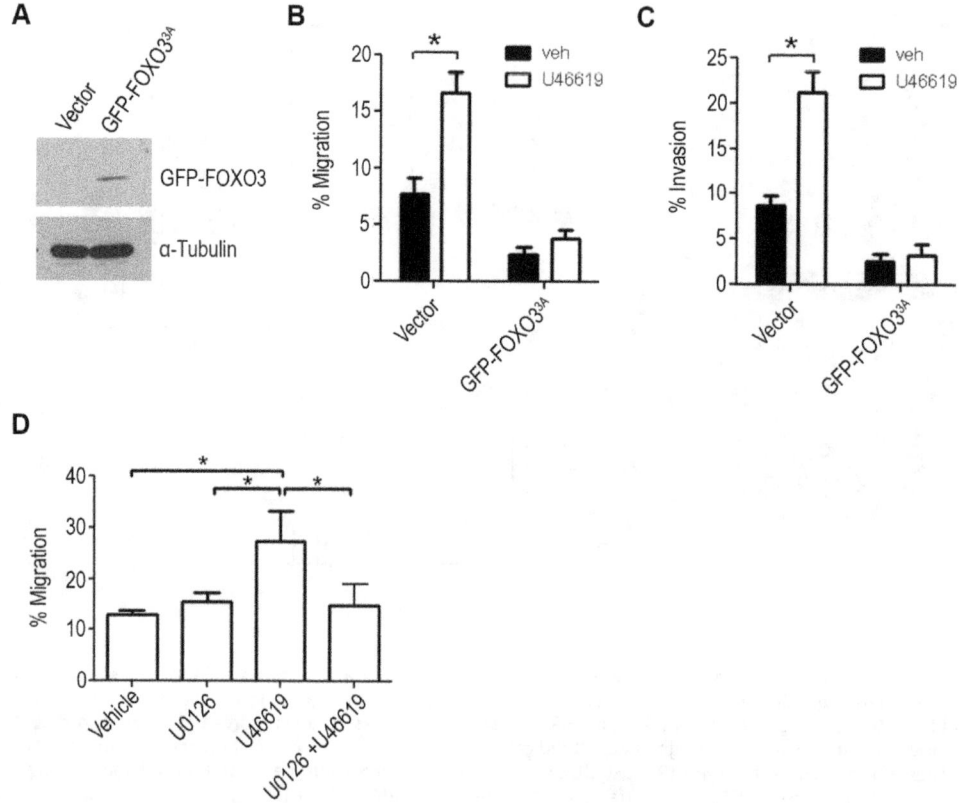

Figure 5. Expression of mutant FOXO3³ᴬ attenuated TP agonist mediated migration of UMUC3 cells. (**A**) GFP-FOXO3³ᴬ or EGFP-C₂ (Vector) was stably transfected into UMUC3 cells and mutant FOXO3 expression was confirmed by immunoblotting for GFP. α-tubulin served as loading control. Cells were seeded into inserts coated with fibronectin for migration or matrigel for invasion in serum free media containing 1 µM U46619 and placed in wells containing complete media with 1 µM U46619. Cells were allowed to migrate (**B**) for 8 hours or invade (**C**) for 16 hours. Significance was determined with a two-sided two-sample t-test, (* = P<0.05, n = 3) compared to GFP-vector control. (**D**) UMUC3 cells were pretreated with 10 µM U0126 for 15 minutes before stimulation with 1 µM U46619 and allowed to migrate for 16 hours. Data represent three independent assays done in duplicates and expressed as the mean ± SEM. Significance was determined with a One-way ANOVA with Tukey post-hoc test. P<0.05.

survival, this study highlights the fact that the localization of FOXO3 and its phosphorylation status may be equally as important in predicting patient outcome.

Since loss or inactivation of FOXO3 activity is associated with tumor progression, drug resistance, and decreased patient survival in multiple cancers [19,46,47,48,49], we investigated the impact of FOXO3 protein loss on cellular migration and invasion of two independent immortalized non-transformed urothelial cell lines, UROsta and SV-HUC. The expression of FOXO3 was silenced with shRNA resulting in increased cell migration and invasion. To implicate the TPβ receptor in affecting FOXO3 function via phosphorylation, we exogenously overexpressed TPβ and observed increased pFOXO3-S294 expression. A key role of ERK phosphorylation in TXA₂ mediated migration was previously demonstrated in human adipose tissue-derived mesenchymal stem cells pretreated with the ERK inhibitor U0126, which abrogated the U46619-induced cell migration, proliferation, and expression of α-smooth muscle actin [32], Similarly, we showed that the pharmacological inhibition of ERK with U0126 or the expression of a mutated FOXO3 that cannot be phosphorylated or inactivated by ERK in UMUC3 cells resulted in decreased TP agonist mediated migration and invasion. Moreover, pre-treatment with the TP antagonist PTXA₂ attenuated U46619 induced activation of ERK. These data indicate that FOXO3 protein is negatively regulating TP mediated cell mobility of bladder cancer

cells in part through phosphorylation by ERK. This suggests that antagonizing the TXA₂ pathway could be an ideal therapeutic target in bladder cancer in part through its ability to prevent FOXO3 modulation.

Agonist stimulation of numerous G-protein coupled receptors (GPCR) has been shown to phosphorylate FOXO3, but result in differential FOXO3-induced cellular effects. For instance, cardio-myocytes treated with hypertrophic GPCR agonists such as angiotensin II, phenylephrine, isoproterenol, and IGF-1 have been shown to phosphorylate FOXO3 and promote its nuclear exclusion, resulting in cellular hypertrophy [50]. Whereas, we demonstrated in a bladder cancer cell model, the TP agonist U46619 induced FOXO3 phosphorylation in a time dependent manner (Figure 2A) and was concurrent with increased activated ERK1/2. The agonist mediated increase in pFOXO3-S294 and pERK1/2 is prevented with TP receptor antagonist PTXA₂ which support the specificity of TP activation on FOXO3 phosphory-lation. To further prove that the effect is specific to ERK1/2 activity, cells were incubated with the ERK inhibitor (U0126). U0126 treatment abolished U46619 mediated increase in both pFOXO3-S294 and pERK1/2 (Figure 2G–I). Although the fold changes in FOXO3 phosphorylation appear modest they were statistically significant and determined to be biologically relevant via its ability to affect U46619 mediated migration and invasion of urothelial cells. Furthermore, this suggests a more complex and potentially cell type dependent mechanism of FOXO3 tumor suppression that may require multiple posttranslational modifications of FOXO3 for the various GPCR mediated effects. Thus, future studies should be aimed at elucidating the signaling mediators upstream of the kinases that phosphorylate FOXO3 which affect its function and localization in response to GPCR stimulation.

Resistance to cisplatin, a common chemotherapeutic drug used to treat bladder cancer, has been associated with decreased FOXO3 expression in urothelial cell lines [18,51]. Interestingly, cisplatin treatment increases renal synthesis of TXA_2, which can lead to impaired renal function [52,53,54]. The use of TP antagonists have been shown to enhance the chemotherapeutic effects of cisplatin [14]. Future studies are needed to examine if the TP antagonist enhanced cisplatin effects are mediated through the regulation of FOXO3.

Dysregulation of oxidative stress resistance genes has been shown to promote carcinogenesis and tumor progression in a variety of cancers [55]. A study in high-grade and advanced stage bladder tumors consistently revealed an inverse relationship in the expression of FOXO3 targets, MnSOD and catalase, [56], which could result in increased cellular hydrogen peroxide levels. Furthermore, deacetylation of FOXO3 by SIRT1 has been reported to have a dual effect on the expression of FOXO3 targets such that SIRT1 expression increases expression of p27^{Kip1} and MnSOD, but inhibits the expression of Bim [21,57]. In this study, a similar FOXO3 target expression pattern was observed following TP agonist stimulation in cells known to endogenously overexpress TPβ [14]. We found TP agonist stimulation increased SIRT1 expression and corresponded with decreased acetylated FOXO3 and increased MnSOD protein. Moreover, TPβ has been shown to be stabilized by hydrogen peroxide [58], the byproduct of MnSOD. This suggests a possible autocrine feedback loop that occurs with elevated TP signaling, such that TP activation results in the specific upregulation of FOXO3 transcriptional target MnSOD which could promote TPβ stability via elevated hydrogen peroxide levels.

Despite numerous studies that have linked decreased TXA_2 synthesis via cyclooxygenase inhibitors with better patient outcomes [59,60,61,62,63,64], there are currently no ongoing clinical trials in the United States that are investigating the effects of TP specific antagonists as adjuvant therapy for the treatment of cancer. In conclusion, we have demonstrated a novel mechanism of FOXO3 regulation through phosphorylation and acetylation mediated by the thromboxane A_2 signaling pathway in bladder cancer. A better understanding of the TXA_2 mediated mechanism of FOXO3 regulation in urothelial cells will promote the identification of new therapeutic strategies such as directly targeting the TP receptors with antagonists. Future studies will be focused on elucidating the differences between the signaling mediators for each TP receptor isoform and determining which mediators facilitate the activation of the kinases responsible for regulating FOXO3 activity.

Acknowledgments

We thank Kayla Hill and Dr. Julia Kuhnert for their valuable comments on the manuscript.

Author Contributions

Conceived and designed the experiments: PMS PVH OM. Performed the experiments: PMS OM. Analyzed the data: PMS EGM MTS. Wrote the paper: PMS.

References

1. Siegel R, Naishadham D, Jemal A (2012) Cancer statistics, 2012. CA: a cancer journal for clinicians 62: 10–29.
2. de Braud F, Maffezzini M, Vitale V, Bruzzi P, Gatta G, et al. (2002) Bladder cancer. Crit Rev Oncol Hematol 41: 89–106.
3. Moussa O, Yordy JS, Abol-Enein H, Sinha D, Bissada NK, et al. (2005) Prognostic and functional significance of thromboxane synthase gene overexpression in invasive bladder cancer. Cancer research 65: 11581–11587.
4. Needleman P, Minkes M, Raz A (1976) Thromboxanes: selective biosynthesis and distinct biological properties. Science 193: 163–165.
5. Sakai H, Suzuki T, Takahashi Y, Ukai M, Tauchi K, et al. (2006) Upregulation of thromboxane synthase in human colorectal carcinoma and the cancer cell proliferation by thromboxane A2. FEBS letters 580: 3368–3374.
6. Moussa O, Riker JM, Klein J, Fraig M, Halushka PV, et al. (2008) Inhibition of thromboxane synthase activity modulates bladder cancer cell responses to chemotherapeutic agents. Oncogene 27: 55–62.
7. Li X, Tai HH (2009) Activation of thromboxane A(2) receptors induces orphan nuclear receptor Nurr1 expression and stimulates cell proliferation in human lung cancer cells. Carcinogenesis 30: 1606–1613.
8. Turner EC, Kavanagh DJ, Mulvaney EP, McLean C, Wikstrom K, et al. (2011) Identification of an interaction between the TPalpha and TPbeta isoforms of the human thromboxane A2 receptor with protein kinase C-related kinase (PRK) 1: implications for prostate cancer. J Biol Chem 286: 15440–15457.
9. Watkins G, Douglas-Jones A, Mansel RE, Jiang WG (2005) Expression of thromboxane synthase, TBXAS1 and the thromboxane A2 receptor, TBXA2R, in human breast cancer. Int Semin Surg Oncol 2: 23.
10. Aitokallio-Tallberg A, Karkkainen J, Pantzar P, Wahlstrom T, Ylikorkala O (1985) Prostacyclin and thromboxane in breast cancer: relationship between steroid receptor status and medroxyprogesterone acetate. Br J Cancer 51: 671–674.
11. Raychowdhury MK, Yukawa M, Collins LJ, McGrail SH, Kent KC, et al. (1994) Alternative splicing produces a divergent cytoplasmic tail in the human endothelial thromboxane A2 receptor. The Journal of biological chemistry 269: 19256–19261.
12. Hirata M, Hayashi Y, Ushikubi F, Yokota Y, Kageyama R, et al. (1991) Cloning and expression of cDNA for a human thromboxane A2 receptor. Nature 349: 617–620.
13. Hirata T, Ushikubi F, Kakizuka A, Okuma M, Narumiya S (1996) Two thromboxane A2 receptor isoforms in human platelets. Opposite coupling to adenylyl cyclase with different sensitivity to Arg60 to Leu mutation. The Journal of clinical investigation 97: 949–956.
14. Moussa O, Ashton AW, Fraig M, Garrett-Mayer E, Ghoneim MA, et al. (2008) Novel role of thromboxane receptors beta isoform in bladder cancer pathogenesis. Cancer research 68: 4097–4104.
15. Weidinger C, Krause K, Klagge A, Karger S, Fuhrer D (2008) Forkhead box-O transcription factor: critical conductors of cancer's fate. Endocr Relat Cancer 15: 917–929.
16. Murphy CT (2006) The search for DAF-16/FOXO transcriptional targets: approaches and discoveries. Experimental gerontology 41: 910–921.
17. Roy SK, Srivastava RK, Shankar S (2010) Inhibition of PI3K/AKT and MAPK/ERK pathways causes activation of FOXO transcription factor, leading to cell cycle arrest and apoptosis in pancreatic cancer. Journal of molecular signaling 5: 10.
18. Shiota M, Yokomizo A, Kashiwagi E, Tada Y, Inokuchi J, et al. (2010) Foxo3a expression and acetylation regulate cancer cell growth and sensitivity to cisplatin. Cancer science 101: 1177–1185.
19. Shukla S, Shukla M, Maclennan GT, Fu P, Gupta S (2009) Deregulation of FOXO3A during prostate cancer progression. International journal of oncology 34: 1613–1620.
20. Bertaggia E, Coletto L, Sandri M (2012) Posttranslational modifications control FoxO3 activity during denervation. American journal of physiology Cell physiology 302: C587–596.
21. Brunet A, Sweeney LB, Sturgill JF, Chua KF, Greer PL, et al. (2004) Stress-dependent regulation of FOXO transcription factors by the SIRT1 deacetylase. Science 303: 2011–2015.
22. Yang JY, Zong CS, Xia W, Yamaguchi H, Ding Q, et al. (2008) ERK promotes tumorigenesis by inhibiting FOXO3a via MDM2-mediated degradation. Nat Cell Biol 10: 138–148.
23. Shankar H, Garcia A, Prabhakar J, Kim S, Kunapuli SP (2006) P2Y12 receptor-mediated potentiation of thrombin-induced thromboxane A2 generation in platelets occurs through regulation of Erk1/2 activation. J Thromb Haemost 4: 638–647.
24. Garcia A, Quinton TM, Dorsam RT, Kunapuli SP (2005) Src family kinase-mediated and Erk-mediated thromboxane A2 generation are essential for VWF/GPIb-induced fibrinogen receptor activation in human platelets. Blood 106: 3410–3414.

25. Zhang W, Zhang Y, Edvinsson L, Xu CB (2009) Transcriptional down-regulation of thromboxane A(2) receptor expression via activation of MAPK ERK1/2, p38/NF-kappaB pathways. J Vasc Res 46: 162–174.

26. Rossi MR, Masters JR, Park S, Todd JH, Garrett SH, et al. (2001) The immortalized UROtsa cell line as a potential cell culture model of human urothelium. Environmental health perspectives 109: 801–808.

27. Christian BJ, Loretz IJ, Oberley TD, Reznikoff CA (1987) Characterization of human uroepithelial cells immortalized in vitro by simian virus 40. Cancer research 47: 6066–6073.

28. Meisner LF, Wu SQ, Christian BJ, Reznikoff CA (1988) Cytogenetic instability with balanced chromosome changes in an SV40 transformed human uroepithelial cell line. Cancer research 48: 3215–3220.

29. Pratt CI, Kao CH, Wu SQ, Gilchrist KW, Oyasu R, et al. (1992) Neoplastic progression by EJ/ras at different steps of transformation in vitro of human uroepithelial cells. Cancer research 52: 688–695.

30. Shiota M, Song Y, Yokomizo A, Kiyoshima K, Tada Y, et al. (2010) Foxo3a suppression of urothelial cancer invasiveness through Twist1, Y-box-binding protein 1, and E-cadherin regulation. Clinical cancer research: an official journal of the American Association for Cancer Research 16: 5654–5663.

31. Miggin SM, Kinsella BT (2002) Regulation of extracellular signal-regulated kinase cascades by alpha- and beta-isoforms of the human thromboxane A(2) receptor. Mol Pharmacol 61: 817–831.

32. Yun DH, Song HY, Lee MJ, Kim MR, Kim MY, et al. (2009) Thromboxane A(2) modulates migration, proliferation, and differentiation of adipose tissue-derived mesenchymal stem cells. Experimental & molecular medicine 41: 17–24.

33. Li L, Jiang J (2011) Regulatory factors of mesenchymal stem cell migration into injured tissues and their signal transduction mechanisms. Frontiers of medicine 5: 33–39.

34. Cartier A, Parent A, Labrecque P, Laroche G, Parent JL (2011) WDR36 acts as a scaffold protein tethering a G-protein-coupled receptor, Galphaq and phospholipase Cbeta in a signalling complex. Journal of cell science 124: 3292–3304.

35. Cho MJ, Pestina TI, Steward SA, Lowell CA, Jackson CW, et al. (2002) Role of the Src family kinase Lyn in TxA2 production, adenosine diphosphate secretion, Akt phosphorylation, and irreversible aggregation in platelets stimulated with gamma-thrombin. Blood 99: 2442–2447.

36. Parent JL, Labrecque P, Orsini MJ, Benovic JL (1999) Internalization of the TXA2 receptor alpha and beta isoforms. Role of the differentially spliced cooh terminus in agonist-promoted receptor internalization. The Journal of biological chemistry 274: 8941–8948.

37. Parent JL, Labrecque P, Driss Rochdi M, Benovic JL (2001) Role of the differentially spliced carboxyl terminus in thromboxane A2 receptor trafficking: identification of a distinct motif for tonic internalization. The Journal of biological chemistry 276: 7079–7085.

38. Moussa O, Ashton AW, Fraig M, Garrett-Mayer E, Ghoneim MA, et al. (2008) Novel role of thromboxane receptors beta isoform in bladder cancer pathogenesis. Cancer Res 68: 4097–4104.

39. Brunet A, Bonni A, Zigmond MJ, Lin MZ, Juo P, et al. (1999) Akt promotes cell survival by phosphorylating and inhibiting a Forkhead transcription factor. Cell 96: 857–868.

40. Plas DR, Thompson CB (2003) Akt activation promotes degradation of tuberin and FOXO3a via the proteasome. The Journal of biological chemistry 278: 12361–12366.

41. Skurk C, Maatz H, Kim HS, Yang J, Abid MR, et al. (2004) The Akt-regulated forkhead transcription factor FOXO3a controls endothelial cell viability through modulation of the caspase-8 inhibitor FLIP. J Biol Chem 279: 1513–1525.

42. Lee HY, Youn SW, Kim JY, Park KW, Hwang CI, et al. (2008) FOXO3a turns the tumor necrosis factor receptor signaling towards apoptosis through reciprocal regulation of c-Jun N-terminal kinase and NF-kappaB. Arterioscler Thromb Vasc Biol 28: 112–120.

43. Lee HY, You HJ, Won JY, Youn SW, Cho HJ, et al. (2007) Forkhead Factor, FOXO3a, Induces Apoptosis of Endothelial Cells Through Activation of Matrix Metalloproteinases. Arterioscler Thromb Vasc Biol 28(2): 302–308.

44. Lee HY, Chung JW, Youn SW, Kim JY, Park KW, et al. (2007) Forkhead transcription factor FOXO3a is a negative regulator of angiogenic immediate early gene CYR61, leading to inhibition of vascular smooth muscle cell proliferation and neointimal hyperplasia. Circ Res 100: 372–380.

45. Kim HS, Skurk C, Maatz H, Shiojima I, Ivashchenko Y, et al. (2005) Akt/FOXO3a signaling modulates the endothelial stress response through regulation of heat shock protein 70 expression. Faseb J 19: 1042–1044.

46. Lu M, Xiang J, Xu F, Wang Y, Yin Y, et al. (2012) The expression and significance of pThr32-FOXO3a in human ovarian cancer. Medical oncology 29: 1258–1264.

47. Hu MC, Lee DF, Xia W, Golfman LS, Ou-Yang F, et al. (2004) IkappaB kinase promotes tumorigenesis through inhibition of forkhead FOXO3a. Cell 117: 225–237.

48. Chen J, Gomes AR, Monteiro IJ, Wong SY, Wu LH, et al. (2010) Constitutively nuclear FOXO3a localization predicts poor survival and promotes Akt phosphorylation in breast cancer. PLoS one 5: e12293.

49. Jin GS, Kondo E, Miyake T, Shibata M, Takashima T, et al. (2004) Expression and intracellular localization of FKHRL1 in mammary gland neoplasms. Acta medica Okayama 58: 197–205.

50. Ni YG, Berenji K, Wang N, Oh M, Sachan N, et al. (2006) Foxo transcription factors blunt cardiac hypertrophy by inhibiting calcineurin signaling. Circulation 114: 1159–1168.

51. Sternberg CN, Calabro F (2000) Chemotherapy and management of bladder tumours. BJU international 85: 599–610.

52. Jariyawat S, Takeda M, Kobayashi M, Endou H (1997) Thromboxane A2 mediates cisplatin-induced apoptosis of renal tubule cells. Biochemistry and molecular biology international 42: 113–121.

53. Blochl-Daum B, Pehamberger H, Kurz C, Kyrle PA, Wagner O, et al. (1995) Effects of cisplatin on urinary thromboxane B2 excretion. Clinical pharmacology and therapeutics 58: 418–424.

54. Remuzzi G, FitzGerald GA, Patrono C (1992) Thromboxane synthesis and action within the kidney. Kidney international 41: 1483–1493.

55. Liou GY, Storz P (2010) Reactive oxygen species in cancer. Free radical research 44: 479–496.

56. Hempel N, Ye H, Abessi B, Mian B, Melendez JA (2009) Altered redox status accompanies progression to metastatic human bladder cancer. Free radical biology & medicine 46: 42–50.

57. Kobayashi Y, Furukawa-Hibi Y, Chen C, Horio Y, Isobe K, et al. (2005) SIRT1 is critical regulator of FOXO-mediated transcription in response to oxidative stress. International journal of molecular medicine 16: 237–243.

58. Valentin F, Field MC, Tippins JR (2004) The mechanism of oxidative stress stabilization of the thromboxane receptor in COS-7 cells. The Journal of biological chemistry 279: 8316–8324.

59. Gustafsson A, Hansson E, Kressner U, Nordgren S, Andersson M, et al. (2007) Prostanoid receptor expression in colorectal cancer related to tumor stage, differentiation and progression. Acta oncologica 46: 1107–1112.

60. Kort WJ, Bijma AM, van Dam JJ, van der Ham AC, Hekking JM, et al. (1992) Eicosanoids in breast cancer patients before and after mastectomy. Prostaglandins, leukotrienes, and essential fatty acids 45: 319–327.

61. Klapan I, Culo F, Culig J, Bukovec Z, Simovic S, et al. (1995) Arachidonic acid metabolites and sinonasal polyposis. I. Possible prognostic value. American journal of otolaryngology 16: 396–402.

62. Han X, Li H, Su L, Zhu W, Xu W, et al. (2014) Effect of celecoxib plus standard chemotherapy on serum levels of vascular endothelial growth factor and cyclooxygenase-2 in patients with gastric cancer. Biomedical reports 2: 183–187.

63. Wang D, Dubois RN (2010) Eicosanoids and cancer. Nature reviews Cancer 10: 181–193.

64. Lanza-Jacoby S, Miller S, Flynn J, Gallatig K, Daskalakis C, et al. (2003) The cyclooxygenase-2 inhibitor, celecoxib, prevents the development of mammary tumors in Her-2/neu mice. Cancer epidemiology, biomarkers & prevention : a publication of the American Association for Cancer Research, cosponsored by the American Society of Preventive Oncology 12: 1486–1491.

19

Prognostic Significance of Lymphovascular Invasion in Radical Cystectomy on Patients with Bladder Cancer

Hwanik Kim, Myong Kim, Cheol Kwak, Hyeon Hoe Kim, Ja Hyeon Ku*

Department of Urology, Seoul National University College of Medicine, Seoul, Korea

Abstract

Purpose: The objective of the present study was to conduct a systematic review and meta-analysis of published literature to appraise the prognostic value of lymphovascular invasion (LVI) in radical cystectomy specimens.

Materials and Methods: Following the PRISMA statement, PubMed, Cochrane Library, and SCOPUS database were searched from the respective dates of inception until June 2013.

Results: A total of 21 articles met the eligibility criteria for this systematic review, which included a total of 12,527 patients ranging from 57 to 4,257 per study. LVI was detected in 34.6% in radical cystectomy specimens. LVI was associated with higher pathological T stage and tumor grade, as well as lymph node metastasis. The pooled hazard ratio (HR) was statistically significant for recurrence-free survival (pooled HR, 1.61; 95% confidence interval [CI], 1.26–2.06), cancer-specific survival (pooled HR, 1.67; 95% CI, 1.38–2.01), and overall survival (pooled HR, 1.67; 95% CI, 1.38–2.01), despite the heterogeneity among included studies. On sensitivity analysis, the pooled HRs and 95% CIs were not significantly altered when any one study was omitted. The funnel plot for overall survival demonstrated a certain degree of asymmetry, which showed slight publication bias.

Conclusions: This meta-analysis indicates that LVI is significantly associated with poor outcome in patients with bladder cancer who underwent radical cystectomy. Adequately designed prospective studies are required to provide the precise prognostic significance of LVI in bladder cancer.

Editor: Ju-Seog Lee, University of Texas MD Anderson Cancer Center, United States of America

Funding: The authors have no support or funding to report.

Competing Interests: The authors have declared that no competing interests exist.

* E-mail: kuuro70@snu.ac.kr

Introduction

Urothelial carcinoma of the bladder is the fifth most common cancer worldwide, with an estimated incidence of 73,510 cases and 14,880 deaths in the United States for 2012 [1]. While the majority of patients present with non-muscle invasive lesions amenable to local resection, radical cystectomy with pelvic lymphadenectomy continues to represent the gold standard for patients with muscle invasive tumors, as well as for patients with high-risk non-muscle invasive disease. Despite recent multidisciplinary advances in its treatment, bladder cancer continues to carry unacceptably high rates of morbidity and mortality. Thus, the identification of patients at high risk of poor outcome is one of the major concerns for clinicians. New strategies, including the administration of innovative and intensive neoadjuvant/adjuvant therapies, may enable improved survival in these patients.

Lymphovascular invasion (LVI) has been documented as a poor prognostic factor in many solid organ tumors [2,3]. In a previous study, we have also demonstrated an association between the presence of LVI and poor prognosis in upper urinary tract urothelial carcinoma [4]. The prognostic value of LVI in bladder cancer has been widely investigated, owing to the fact that this feature exhibited an increasing relevance in clinical practice. Although multiple studies have been conducted on bladder cancer patients, the prognostic significance of LVI in radical cystectomy specimens is still controversial. Therefore, we have conducted an up-to-date meta-analysis to appraise the prognostic value of LVI in bladder cancer.

Materials and Methods

Search Strategy

We conducted and reported this systematic review and meta-analysis following the PRISMA statement [5]. A comprehensive literature search of electronic databases PubMed, SCOPUS, and Cochrane Library were performed using the following keywords: [urinary bladder neoplasms] OR [urinary AND bladder AND neoplasms] OR [bladder AND cancer] OR [bladder cancer] AND [lymphovascular] AND [invasion]. The search concluded in June 2013, and no lower date limit was used. Searches were limited to studies published in English. Conference abstracts were not selected for analysis due to the insufficient data reported.

Study Inclusion/Exclusion Criteria

A study was considered eligible if it met all of the following inclusion criteria: (i) the study included proven diagnosis of urothelial carcinoma; (ii) the study evaluated LVI in radical cystectomy specimens; (iii) the study considered radical cystectomy as a treatment modality; (iv) the study assessed the association between LVI and survival of patients with bladder cancer; and, (v) the study provided a hazard ratio (HR) and 95% confidence interval (CI) directly or presented the data that allows for estimation of the HR and 95% CI. Studies were excluded based on any of the following criteria: (i) review articles, letters to the editor, commentaries, or case reports; (ii) laboratory studies, such as studies on bladder cancer cell lines and animal models; and (iii) duplication of previous publications. All studies were carefully examined to avoid inclusion of duplicate data. When more than one of the same patient populations was included in several publications, only the most recent or most complete study was used to avoid duplication of information. Two reviewers (HK and MK) assessed the eligibility of the screened studies independently. Agreements were reached for discrepant opinions through discussion.

Data Extraction

To rule out subjectivity in the data gathering and entry process, data were extracted independently by two reviewers (HK and MK) for each eligible study. The extracted data were recorded by both investigators independently in separate databases. The two completed databases were compared and discussed between the two investigators to reach a consensus. We did not contact authors of eligible studies for additional data. Pre-specified data parameters to be gathered were as follows: (i) publication data including country, first author's last name, publication year, period of recruitment, study design, inclusion and exclusion criteria, consecutiveness of patient enrollment, definition of LVI, definition of survival, and interpretation of LVI; (ii) demographic data such as sample size, age, gender, treatment, and follow-up period; (iii) tumor data including concomitant carcinoma in situ, variant form, pathological T stage, tumor grade, pathological N stage, and number of lymph nodes retrieved; and (iv) statistical data including the exact data of total and exposed number of subjects in? case and control groups, as well as HRs and their CIs. Multivariate Cox hazard regression analysis data were preferred in our analysis. If this analysis was not available, we extracted univariate Cox hazard regression analysis or Kaplan-Meier survival curves with log-rank p-value of survival outcomes, instead. In studies for which clinical outcomes were estimated using both multivariate and univariate analyses, the results of the multivariate analyses were used to calculate HRs and CIs.

Quality Assessments

Methodological assessment for each of the included studies was performed by three investigators (HK, MK, and JHK), according to three quality scales from the predefined form by De Graeff et al [6], which was adapted from REMARK (Reporting recommendations for tumor MARKer prognostic studies) [7]. The quality scale has seven criteria, and a study with a total score of 8 was considered to have the highest study quality, whereas a score of zero indicated the lowest quality.

Statistical Analysis

We obtained the log-HRs and their 95% CIs from each study and subsequently performed the meta-analysis by a random-effect model. If HRs and the corresponding standard errors were not directly reported, they were estimated according to the available survival data by using the method reported by Palmar et al [8]. An observed HR >1 implied a worse survival for the study group with positive LVI, relative to the reference group. The impact of LVI on outcome was considered statistically significant if the 95% CI did not overlap with 1 and if p<0.05. We also performed subgroup analyses to examine if our pooled estimate of the prognostic value was influenced by publication year, region, number of patients, pathologic N stage, median follow-up, HR estimation, analysis results, and methodological quality scales. To evaluate the robustness of the combined HR and to check the stability of meta-analysis, sensitivity analyses were performed by removing one study at a time. A test of heterogeneity of the combined HRs was carried out using the Chi-square test and Higgins I-squared statistic. P<0.10 was considered to represent substantial heterogeneity between studies. $I^2>50\%$ indicated large heterogeneity among studies, whereas I^2 values between 25% and 50% indicated moderate heterogeneity [9]. Publication bias was evaluated using the funnel plot. The Begg's rank correlation and Egger's linear regression were also applied to assess the potential publication bias. The nomnial level of significance was set at 5%. All 95% CIs were two-sided. The meta-analysis was performed using Review Manager (RevMan) software version 5.0 (RevMan 5; The Nordic Cochrane Center, The Cochrane Collaboration, Copenhagen, Denmark). Publication biases were evaluated by R 2.13.0 (R Development Core Team, Vienna, Austria, http://www.R-project.org).

Results

Study Selection

Of the 389 articles initially identified, 179 articles were excluded as duplicate publications. After screening the titles and abstracts, an additional 88 articles were excluded. The remaining 122 articles were reviewed by full text. After the full text review, 15 were excluded because these studies did not perform survival analysis, eight were excluded because these studies did not provide sufficient data for estimation of HRs, three were excluded because LVI was not assessed for radical cystectomy specimens but for transurethral resection specimens, four were excluded because the assessment was conducted on non-urothelial carcinoma, 11 were excluded because study subjects had been treated with modalities other than radical cystectomy, and 60 were excluded for having overlapping data with another study. At the end of this culling process, 21 articles were selected for the systemic review, which included 12,527 patients, ranging from 57 to 4,257 per study [10–30]. Figure 1 shows a flow diagram of the selection process for relevant studies.

Methodological Quality of the Studies

The median quality score was 3 for the 21 articles reviewed (mean: 3.6, range: 2–5) (Table 1). Ten of the included studies obtained scores of 4 or more in methodolocal assessment, indicating that they were of high quality. There was no significant correlation between study size and quality scores (Spearman's r = −0.002, p = 0.992). There were no statistical differences of quality score according to publication year and median follow-up time. However, there was a significant difference in the quality of studies by study origin (3.2 for Asian countries vs. 4.3 for other countries, p = 0.015).

Study Characteristics

The main features of included studies are listed in Tables 1 and 2. The 21 studies had originated from the United States (9),

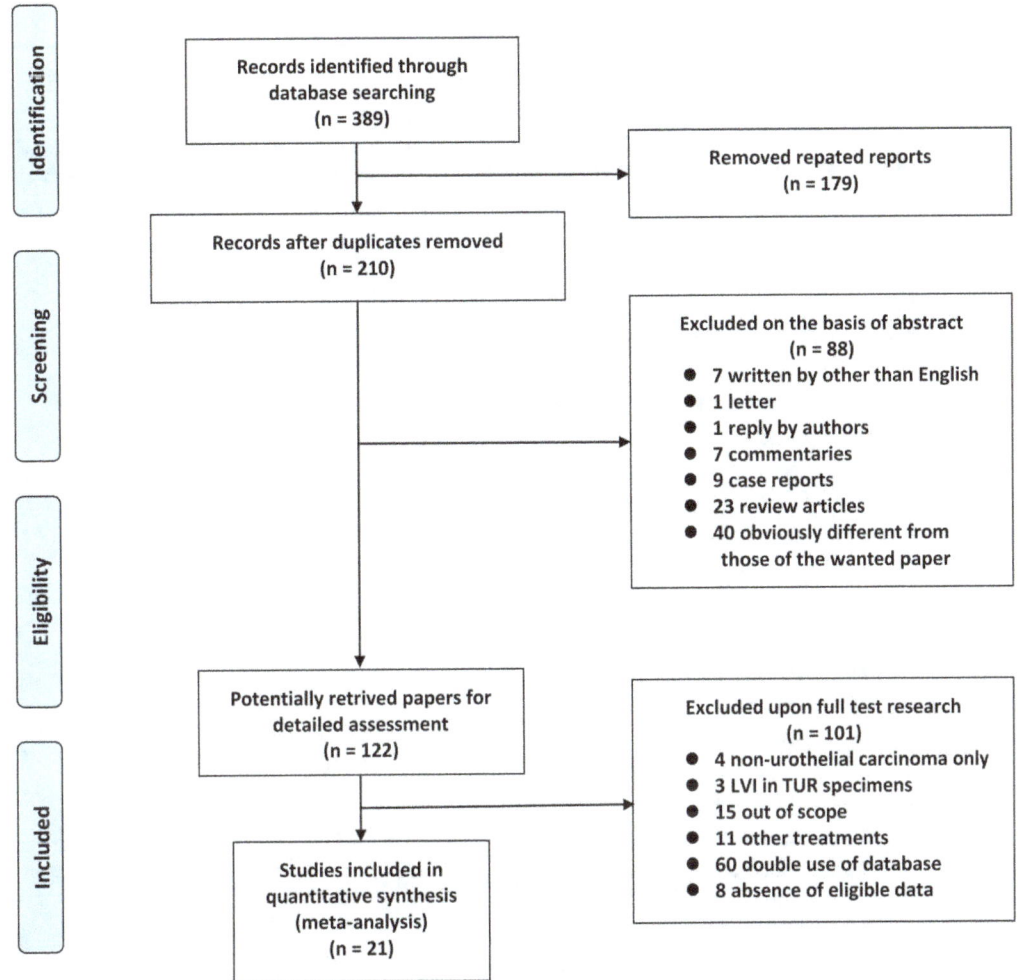

Figure 1. Flow chart of the literature search used in this meta-analysis.

Europe (5), Asia (6), and multiple countries (1). Two studies were based on a prospective cohort design. Four of these studies included <100 patients, and 11 studies had enrolled >200 patients. The median follow-up durations ranged from 18 months to 10.5 years, while three studies did not provide clear follow-up duration. All of the studies were published between 2007 and 2013. Other characteristics such as tumor characteristics and pathologic results are summarized in Table S1. Of the 12,527 patients included in the meta-alaysis, LVI was detected in 34.6% in radical cystectomy specimens. There were higher frequencies of LVI with higher pathological T stages and tumor grades, as well as lymph node metastasis (Table S2). Of the 35 survival analyses, 33 (94.3%) directly reported HRs or p-values with event number for multivariate analysis. In studies using multivariate analysis, the most common cofactors used to assess the risk of mortality was pathologic T stage (Table S3).

Meta-analysis

According to a priori assumptions about the likelihood for heterogeneity between primary studies, the pooled HR estimate of the each study was calculated by the random effect model. Figure 2 demonstrates a forest plot of the individual HRs and results from the meta-analysis. When 10 eligible studies (11 dataset) were pooled into the meta-analysis for recurrence-free survival (RFS),

we found that LVI was significantly associated with worse RFS (pooled HR, 1.61; 95% CI, 1.26–2.06; Z = 3.78). Cochrane Q test (Chi^2 = 68.12; p<0.000001) and test of inconsistency (I^2 = 85%) could not exclude a significant heterogeneity (Fig. 2a). The meta-analysis was performed on 15 studies (16 dataset) assessing the association of LVI and cancer-specific survival (CSS). The pooled HR was 1.67 (95% CI, 1.38–2.01; Z = 5.35) despite the heterogeneity among studies (p<0.00001 for heterogeneity test; I^2 = 87%) (Fig. 2b). Eight studies provided data on overall survival (OS), and meta-analysis of OS suggested that LVI correlated with poor OS (pooled HR, 1.84; 95% CI, 1.27–2.66; Z = 3.25) with a large heterogeneity in the data (p<0.00001 for heterogeneity test; I^2 = 80%) (Fig. 2c).

Subgroup Analysis

Considering the substantial heterogeneity among the studies, we performed subgroup analyses to investigate if there were differences in results by publication year, the country of origin in which the study was conducted, number of patients, pathologic N stage, median follow-up, HR estimation, analysis results, and methodological quality scales (Table S4 to S6). The pooled HR for almost all subgroup analyses again supported LVI as a prognostic marker. However, the association between LVI and worse RFS did not remain statistically significant in studies of Asian subjects

Table 1. Main characteristics of the eligible studies.

Study	Year	Country	Recruitment period	Study design	Inclusion and exclusion criteria	Consecutive patients	Definition of survival	Definition of LVI	Interpretation of LVI	Quality scale
Turkolmez [10]	2007	Turkey	1990–2005	Retrospective	Yes	NA	No	Yes	NA	3
Canter [11]	2008	USA	1988–2006	Retrospective	Yes	NA	No	No	NA	2
Matsumoto [12]	2008	Japan	1990–2004	Retrospective	Yes	Yes	No	Yes	Blind	5
Fairey [13]	2009	USA	1994–2007	Retrospective	Yes	Yes	Yes	No	NA	3
Streeper [14]	2009	USA	1995–2005	Retrospective	Yes	Yes	No	Yes	NA	3
Hugen [15]	2010	USA	1996–2008	Retrospective	Yes	NA	Yes	No	NA	2
Kim [16]	2010	Korea	1986–2005	Retrospective	Yes	NA	No	No	NA	3
Ku [17]	2010	Korea	1991–2000	Retrospective	Yes	Yes	Yes	Yes	NA	4
Manoharan [18]	2010	USA	1992–2008	Retrospective	Yes	NA	No	Yes	NA	2
Palmieri [19]	2010	Italy	1995–2007	Retrospective	Yes	Yes	Yes	Yes	NA	5
Shariat [20]	2010	Multination	1979–2008	Retrospective	No	NA	Yes	Yes	Blind	5
Stephenson [21]	2010	USA	1999–2007	Retrospective	Yes	Yes	No	No	Blind	3
Font [22]	2011	Spain	1991–2007	Retrospective	Yes	NA	No	No	NA	3
Kauffman [23]	2011	USA	2006–2008	Prospective	Yes	Yes	No	No	NA	4
Park(a) [24]	2011	Korea	1999–2009	Retrospective	Yes	NA	Yes	Yes	NA	5
Park(b) [25]	2011	Korea	1991–2008	Retrospective	Yes	Yes	No	No	NA	3
Gondo [26]	2012	Japan	2000–2009	Retrospective	Yes	Yes	No	Yes	NA	4
Otto [27]	2012	Germany	1989–2008	Retrospective	No	NA	Yes	Yes	NA	4
Afonso [28]	2013	Portugal	1996–2005	Retrospective	Yes	NA	Yes	No	NA	4
Eisenberg [29]	2013	USA	1980–2008	Retrospective	Yes	NA	Yes	No	Blind	5
Lotan [30]	2013	USA	2007–2012	Prospective	No	NA	No	No	NA	3

LVI: lymphovascular invasion, NA: not available.

(pooled HR, 1.85; 95% CI, 0.98–3.51; Z = 1.89; p = 0.03 for heterogeneity test; $I^2 = 67$). Notably, many of these subgroup analyses revealed heterogeneities of data.

Sensitivity Analysis

We performed one-way sensitivity analyses by stepwise excluding a single study and calculating again the pooled HR for remaining studies. The pooled HRs and 95% CIs were not significantly altered when any one of the 21 studies was omitted, which indicated that no single study had a significant impact on the combined risk estimates and confirmed the robustness of the result of this meta-analysis. Omitting a certain study did not reduce inter-study heterogeneity significantly in the sensitivity analysis.

Publication Bias

Begg's funnel plot was used to examine publication bias (Fig. 3). No significant publication bias was found in the meta-analysis of survival outcome except for the association between LVI and OS. The funnel plot for OS demonstrated a certain degree of asymmetry, which suggested a slight publication bias. Begg's test indicated no publication bias among these studies regarding HR of OS, CSS and OS with p values of 0.103, 0.6915 and 0.1021, respectively, but Egger's test demonstrated a publication bias (all P<0.05). These results indicated a possibility that publication bias may have played a role in the observed effect.

Discussion

Despite remarkable advances in treatment, the prognosis of bladder cancer remains unsatisfactory at the present time. Identification of the risk of disease recurrence and mortality in bladder cancer is critical to guide surveillance and select adjuvant therapies. Many studies have investigated potential prognostic factors for patients with bladder cancer, in order to guide therapeutic approaches and improve survival outcomes. LVI has been found in association with lymph node invasion, distant metastasis, and poor prognosis in patients with other sold tumors [31,32]. Numerous studies have been performed to assess the prognostic value of LVI, but the results are still controversial and ambiguous in the management of bladder cancer.

To our knowledge, this meta-analysis is the first study to systemically assess the association between LVI and prognosis of bladder cancer. This study aggregated the outcomes of 12,527 bladder cancer patients who underwent radical cystectomy, as they were reported in 21 individual studies. We found that LVI was present in 34.6% of patients treated with radical cystectomy for bladder cancer. The significant associations were found between LVI and pathological parameters such as pathologic T stage, tumor grade, and pathologic N stage. Pooled analysis of the included studies found a significant correlation between LVI and poor survival outcome, suggesting that LVI is a significant predictor for poor survival in these patients. Sensitivity analysis demonstrated that omission of any single study did not have a significant impact on the combined risk estimates, further confirming the prognostic value of LVI in bladder cancer.

Table 2. Patient characteristics of the eligible studies.

Study	No. of patients	Median age, range (yr)	Gender (m/f)	Neoadjuvant chemotherapy	Adjuvant chemotherapy	Median FU, range (mon)
Turkolmez [10]	154	Primary MIBC: 59.8 (mean), NA Secondary MIBC: 60.3 (mean), NA	134/20	NA	NA	Primary MIBC: 77.8 (mean), NA Secondary MIBC: 90.3 (mean), NA
Canter [11]	356	65.5 (mean), NA	285/71	NA	NA	46.4 (mean), NA
Matsumoto [12]	92	63, 40–81	75/17	0	17	25.3, 1.1–196.1
Fairey [13]	468	66 (mean), NA	367/101	0	82	NA, NA
Streeper [14]	126	LVI -: 64.0 (mean), 44–87 LVI+: 64.8 (mean), 35–85	101/25	16	41	LVI -: 1.66 yr, 0.25–10.16 yr LVI+: 1.79 yr, 0.04–10.57 yr
Hugen [15]	260	No recurrence: 64.8 (mean), NA Recurrence: 68.4 (mean), NA	193/67	NA	NA	NA, NA
Kim [16]	406	60.8, 27–79	360/46	0	0	66.3, 3–232
Ku [17]	155	60.2, 32–84	128/27	0	0	34.3, 1.0–162.4
Manoharan [18]	357	NA, NA	285/72	0	NA	NA, NA
Palmieri [19]	265	69, 46–93	218/47	0	0	108, 1–216
Shariat [20]	4257	67, NA	3373/864	0	954	43, 0.1–324.0
Stephenson [21]	134	68, 59–75	102/32	0	90	23, 10–36 (IQR)
Font [22]	57	64, 41–80	54/3	57	NA (RT: 5)	45, 13–190
Kauffman [23]	85	73.5, 41.4–93.8	67/18	17	10*	18 (mean), NA
Park(a) [24]	155	67.8, 38–80	127/28	0	0	36.6 (mean), 12–141
Park(b) [25]	450	pN-: 63, 38–85 pN+: 63, 37–80	408/42	0	86	26.8, 2–204
Gondo [26]	194	70, 38–85	162/32	0	48	26.8, 3.1–131.8
Otto [27]	2483	66.4, 60.1–72.5 (IQR)	1976/507	0	245	42, 21–79 (IQR)
Afonso [28]	81	71, 41–83	66/15	0	0	24, 1–132
Eisenberg [29]	1776	68, 62–75 (IQR)	1464/312	0	131 (RT: 17)	10.5 yr, 7.3–15.3 yr (IQR)
Lotan [30]	216	70, 62–76	171/15	48	29	20, 10–37 (IQR)

*chemotherapy or radiation therapy.
FU: follow-up, MIBC: muscle-invasive bladder cancer, NA: not available, LVI: lymphovascular invasion, IQR: interquartile range, RT: radiation therapy.

Although subgroup analyses also demonstrated similar results, LVI was not significantly correlated with poor RFS for patients living in Asian countries. The characteristics of bladder cancer in different regions might differ because of diverse environmental and genetic factors, As such, the prognostic value of LVI in bladder cancer might differ across study locations. More studies with larger sample sizes in Asian countries are thus needed to further elucidate the prognostic value of LVI.

In addition to lymphatic metastasis, LVI is most likely associated with hematogenous tumor dissemination. Infiltration of the vascular and/or lymphatic structures by tumor cells is an important step in tumor dissemination [33–37]. Malignant cells invade the lymphovascular space, proliferate, and then permeate the local lymphatics or spread more widely [38]. This association is not limited to bladder cancer, and has also been shown in other cancers [39–41]. In addition, LVI is an important prognostic factor in various malignancies such as liver, testis, and penile cancer. In other malignancies [42,43], LVI has been added the TNM staging system, allowing for improved cancer staging and treatment decision-making. Despite the increasing numbers of published studies that have added to the general knowledge about the prognostic role of LVI in bladder cancer, LVI is not a part of the TNM staging system or treatment guidelines for bladder cancer. Upstaging tumors on the basis of LVI might improve the accuracy of prognosis in bladder cancer, and therefore is a worthy consideration.

Several limitations of this meta-analysis should be acknowledged. One weakness of our study was publication bias, which could be seen from the publication bias evaluation of OS outcomes; the reported HR might be an overestimation of the true effect size. Because studies with negative results are less likely to be published than those representing positive data, and even if these results are published, they are more frequently reported in a brief way and not easily available for analysis, meta-analyses of selective reports may often introduce bias. It should be also noted that we could not exclude the bias associated with reviewing articles written in only the English language. Studies with positive results are more frequently published in English language, while studies with negative results tend to be published in the native language of respective authors [44].

The second limitation was heterogeneity. In sensitivity analysis, omission of any individual study did not reduce the heterogeneity. Our meta-analysis relied on publication but not on individual patient data. Studies have differed in baseline characteristics of patients. Though the random effect model takes heterogeneity into account and was used to analyze the studies with heterogeneities, the conclusion drawn in this meta-analysis should be approached with caution.

A.

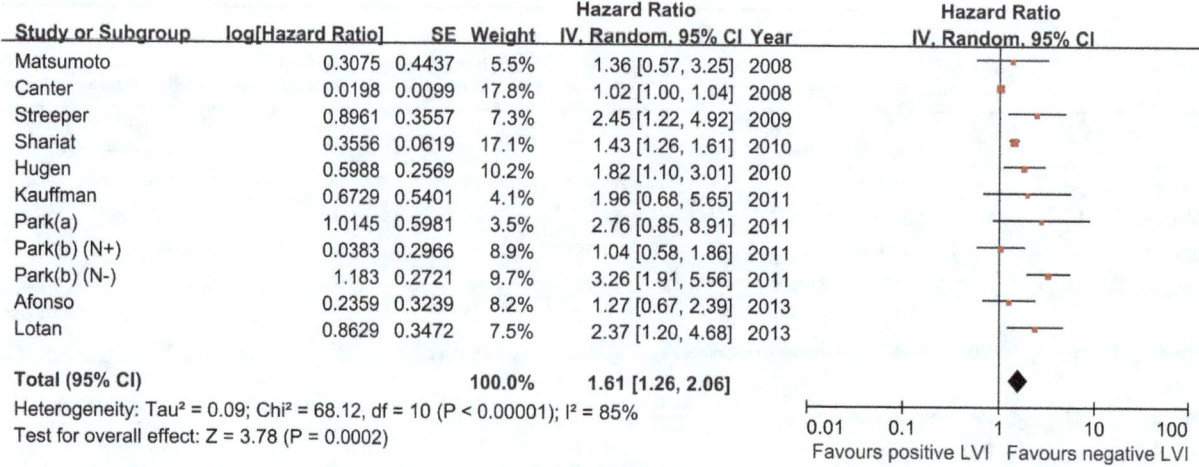

Study or Subgroup	log[Hazard Ratio]	SE	Weight	Hazard Ratio IV, Random, 95% CI	Year
Matsumoto	0.3075	0.4437	5.5%	1.36 [0.57, 3.25]	2008
Canter	0.0198	0.0099	17.8%	1.02 [1.00, 1.04]	2008
Streeper	0.8961	0.3557	7.3%	2.45 [1.22, 4.92]	2009
Shariat	0.3556	0.0619	17.1%	1.43 [1.26, 1.61]	2010
Hugen	0.5988	0.2569	10.2%	1.82 [1.10, 3.01]	2010
Kauffman	0.6729	0.5401	4.1%	1.96 [0.68, 5.65]	2011
Park(a)	1.0145	0.5981	3.5%	2.76 [0.85, 8.91]	2011
Park(b) (N+)	0.0383	0.2966	8.9%	1.04 [0.58, 1.86]	2011
Park(b) (N-)	1.183	0.2721	9.7%	3.26 [1.91, 5.56]	2011
Afonso	0.2359	0.3239	8.2%	1.27 [0.67, 2.39]	2013
Lotan	0.8629	0.3472	7.5%	2.37 [1.20, 4.68]	2013
Total (95% CI)			**100.0%**	**1.61 [1.26, 2.06]**	

Heterogeneity: Tau² = 0.09; Chi² = 68.12, df = 10 (P < 0.00001); I² = 85%
Test for overall effect: Z = 3.78 (P = 0.0002)

B.

Study or Subgroup	log[Hazard Ratio]	SE	Weight	Hazard Ratio IV, Random, 95% CI	Year
Turkolmez	0.8329	0.3319	4.6%	2.30 [1.20, 4.41]	2007
Matsumoto	0.7227	0.47	2.9%	2.06 [0.82, 5.18]	2008
Canter	0.0296	0.01	10.1%	1.03 [1.01, 1.05]	2008
Fairey	0.3507	0.1738	7.6%	1.42 [1.01, 2.00]	2009
Streeper	1.0367	0.3221	4.7%	2.82 [1.50, 5.30]	2009
Manoharan	0.2927	0.2322	6.3%	1.34 [0.85, 2.11]	2010
Palmieri	1.0473	0.2205	6.6%	2.85 [1.85, 4.39]	2010
Kim	0.4253	0.2104	6.8%	1.53 [1.01, 2.31]	2010
Ku	0.9341	0.287	5.3%	2.54 [1.45, 4.47]	2010
Shariat	0.3736	0.0679	9.6%	1.45 [1.27, 1.66]	2010
Park(b) (N-)	0.7227	0.3123	4.9%	2.06 [1.12, 3.80]	2011
Park(b) (N+)	-0.008	0.3295	4.6%	0.99 [0.52, 1.89]	2011
Otto	0.392	0.0821	9.4%	1.48 [1.26, 1.74]	2012
Gondo	0.771	0.3513	4.3%	2.16 [1.09, 4.30]	2012
Eisenberg	0.3365	0.123	8.7%	1.40 [1.10, 1.78]	2013
Lotan	1.0296	0.3954	3.7%	2.80 [1.29, 6.08]	2013
Total (95% CI)			**100.0%**	**1.67 [1.38, 2.01]**	

Heterogeneity: Tau² = 0.09; Chi² = 118.81, df = 15 (P < 0.00001); I² = 87%
Test for overall effect: Z = 5.35 (P < 0.00001)

C.

Study or Subgroup	log[Hazard Ratio]	SE	Weight	Hazard Ratio IV, Random, 95% CI	Year
Canter	0.0488	0.0098	21.4%	1.05 [1.03, 1.07]	2008
Fairey	0.3148	0.1505	18.8%	1.37 [1.02, 1.84]	2009
Stephenson	0.47	0.2936	14.1%	1.60 [0.90, 2.84]	2010
Ku	0.9014	0.281	14.5%	2.46 [1.42, 4.27]	2010
Kauffman	0.7129	0.616	6.5%	2.04 [0.61, 6.82]	2011
Park(a)	1.9012	0.9018	3.6%	6.69 [1.14, 39.20]	2011
Font	1.8116	0.4883	8.8%	6.12 [2.35, 15.94]	2011
Afonso	0.567	0.3442	12.5%	1.76 [0.90, 3.46]	2013
Total (95% CI)			**100.0%**	**1.84 [1.27, 2.66]**	

Heterogeneity: Tau² = 0.17; Chi² = 34.89, df = 7 (P < 0.0001); I² = 80%
Test for overall effect: Z = 3.25 (P = 0.001)

Figure 2. Forest plots of prognosis of lymphovascular invasion. The horizontal lines correspond to the study-specific hazard ration and 95% confidence interval, respectively. The area of the squares reflects the study-specific weight. The diamond represents the pooled results of hazard ratio and 95% confidence interval. (A) Recurrence-free survival. (B) Cancer-specific survival. (C) Overall survival.

A.

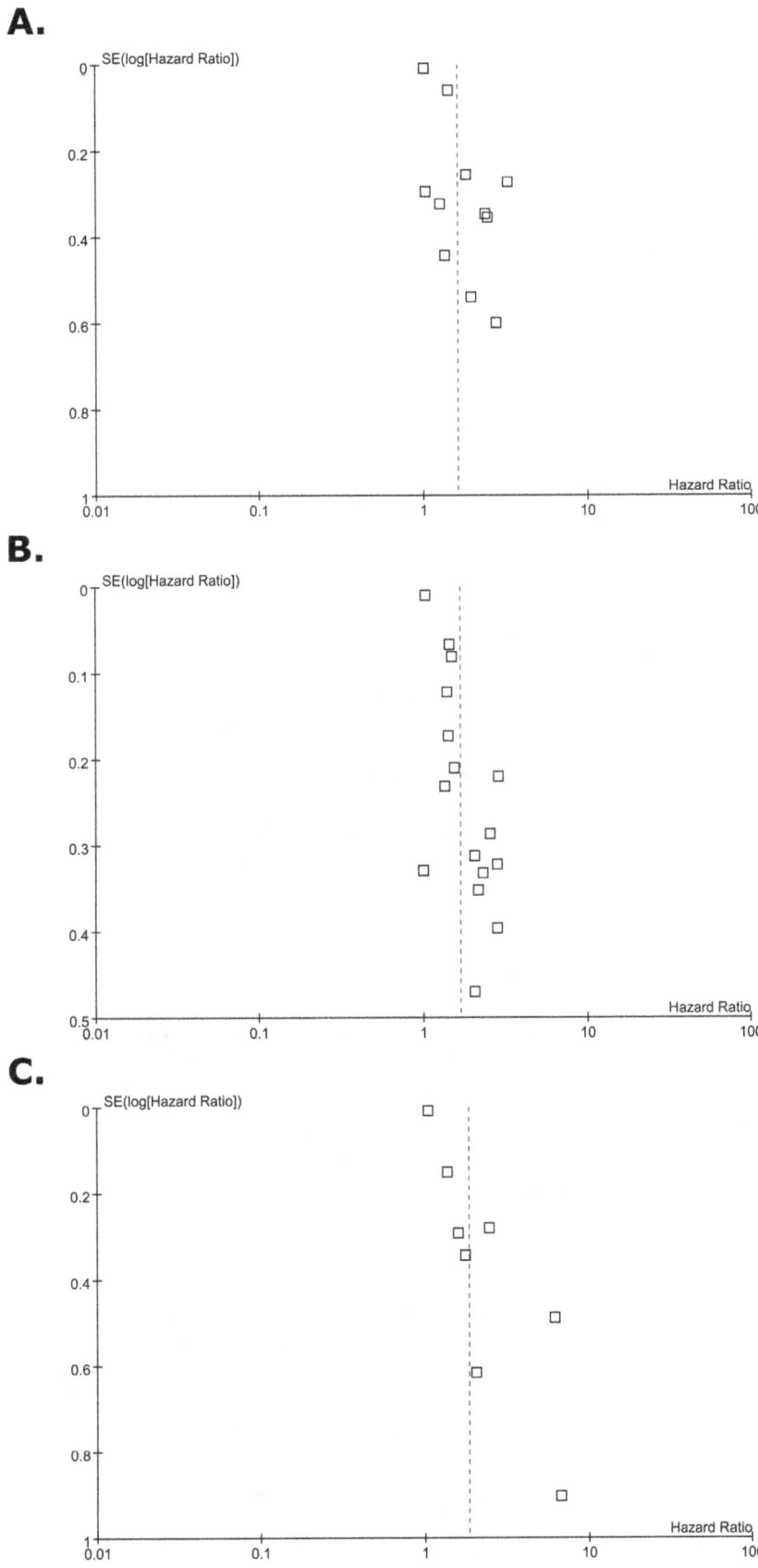

Figure 3. Begg's Funnel plots for publication bias test. Each point represents a separate study for the indicated association. Vertical line represents the mean effects size. (A) Recurrence-free survival. (B) Cancer-specific survival. (C) Overall survival.

Moreover, we admit that meta-analysis of prognostic literature is associated with a number of inherent limitations. One of these key limitations is the general prevalence of retrospective study design in this setting. Only two studies included in the current meta-analysis specified a prospective design, with the remaining studies providing a lower level of evidence. There is a clear need for the initiation of a prospective multicenter trial to provide more definite answers.

In addition to these study limitation, significant differences in the assessment of prognostic factors have been observed among pathologists [45]. Because retraction artifacts in the surrounding stromal tissue can mimic vascular invasion, experts have recommended reporting LVI only in unequivocal cases, using immunohistochemistry if necessary [46]. However, the use of immunohistochemical staining to identify lymphatic vessels remains controversial and is not practical for everyday clinical use [47,48]. It is of utmost importance that strict morphological criteria are established to standardize and render the diagnosis of LVI reproducible, allowing its recommendation in daily clinical settings [33]. In most studies on bladder cancer outcomes, vascular invasion and lymphatic invasion were combined as LVI. One of the reasons for this is that an unequivocal distinction between vascular invasion and lymphatic invasion is often difficult to make without the use of special stains, and that the clinical value of distinguishing vascular invasion from lymphatic invasion to predict bladder cancer outcomes has not been fully investigated. The development of novel markers and further studies are required to examine the significance of the distinction between blood and lymphatic vessels [26].

Conclusions

This meta-analysis indicates that LVI is significantly associated with poorer outcomes in patients with bladder cancer who underwent radical cystectomy. LVI in radical cystectomy speci- mens not only predicts prognosis, but may also be useful in identifying a subgroup of patients who could benefit from adjuvant therapy. Strict criteria to unify the reproducibility of diagnosis as well as adequately designed prospective studies are required to provide a precise prognostic significance of LVI in bladder cancer.

Supporting Information

Table S1   Tumor characteristics of the eligible studies.

Table S2   Lymphovascular invasion according to pathological features.

Table S3   Estimation of hazard ratio.

Table S4   Subgroup analysis for recurrence-free survival.

Table S5   Subgroup analysis for cancer-specific survival.

Table S6   Subgroup analysis for overall survival.

Checklist S1   PRISMA Checklist, page one.

Checklist S2   PRISMA Checklist, page two.

Author Contributions

Conceived and designed the experiments: JHK CK HHK. Analyzed the data: HK MK JHK. Wrote the paper: HK. Critical comments: CK HHK. Quality assessments of articles: MK HK JHK.

References

1. Siegel R, Naishadham D, Jemal A (2012) Cancer statistics, 2012. CA Cancer 62: 10–29.
2. Gasparini G, Weidner N, Bevilacqua P, Maluta S, Dalla Palma P, et al. (1994) Tumor microvessel density, p53 expression, tumor size, and peritumoral lymphatic vessel invasion are relevant prognostic markers in node-negative breast carcinoma. J Clin Oncol 12: 454–466.
3. Herman CM, Wilcox GE, Kattan MW, Scardino PT, Wheeler TM (2000) Lymphovascular invasion as a predictor of disease progression in prostate cancer. Am J Surg Pathol 24: 859–863.
4. Ku JH, Byun SS, Jeong H, Kwak C, Kim HH, et al. (2013) Lymphovascular invasion as a prognostic factor in the upper urinary tract urothelial carcinoma: A systematic review and meta-analysis. Eur J Cancer49: 2665–2680.
5. Moher D, Liberati A, Tetzlaff J, Altman DG; PRISMA Group (2009) Preferred reporting items for systematic reviews and meta-analyses: the PRISMA statement. PLoS Med 6: e1000097.
6. de Graeff P, Crijns AP, de Jong S, Boezen M, Post WJ, et al. (2009) Modest effect of p53, EGFR and HER-2/neu on prognosis in epithelial ovarian cancer: a meta-analysis. Br J Cancer 101: 149–159.
7. McShane LM, Altman DG, Sauerbrei W, Taube SE, Gion M, et al. (2005) Statistics Subcommittee of the NCI-EORTC Working Group on Cancer Diagnostics. REporting recommendations for tumour MARKer prognostic studies (REMARK). Br J Cancer 93: 387–391.
8. Parmar MK, Torri V, Stewart L (1998) Extracting summary statistics to perform meta-analyses of the published literature for survival endpoints. Stat Med 17: 2815–2834.
9. Higgins JP, Thompson SG, Deeks JJ, Altman DG (2003) Measuring inconsistency in meta-analyses. BMJ 327: 557–560.
10. Türkölmez K, Tokgöz H, Reşorlu B, Köse K, Bedük Y (2007) Muscle-invasive bladder cancer: predictive factors and prognostic difference between primary and progressive tumors. Urology 70: 477–81.
11. Canter D, Guzzo T, Resnick M, Magerfleisch L, Sonnad S, et al. (2008) The presence of lymphovascular invasion in radical cystectomy specimens from patients with urothelial carcinoma portends a poor clinical prognosis. BJU Int 102: 952–957.
12. Matsumoto K, Satoh T, Irie A, Ishii J, Kuwao S, et al. (2008) Loss expression of uroplakin III is associated with clinicopathologic features of aggressive bladder cancer. Urology 72: 444–9.
13. Fairey AS, Jacobsen NE, Chetner MP, Mador DR, Metcalfe JB, et al. (2009) Associations between comorbidity, and overall survival and bladder cancer specific survival after radical cystectomy: results from the Alberta Urology Institute Radical Cystectomy database. J Urol 182: 85–92.
14. Streeper NM, Simons CM, Konety BR, Muirhead DM, Williams RD, et al. (2009) The significance of lymphovascular invasion in transurethral resection of bladder tumour and cystectomy specimens on the survival of patients with urothelial bladder cancer. BJU Int 103: 475–479.
15. Hugen CM, Polcari AJ, Fitzgerald MP, Dauw C, Flanigan RC, et al. (2010) Risk factors for recurrence following radical cystectomy for pathologic node negative bladder cancer. J Surg Oncol 102: 334–337.
16. Kim DS, Cho KS, Lee YH, Cho NH, Oh YT, et al. (2010) High-grade hydronephrosis predicts poor outcomes after radical cystectomy in patients with bladder cancer. J Korean Med Sci 25: 369–73.
17. Ku JH, Moon KC, Kwak C, Kim HH (2010) Influence of stage discrepancy on outcome in patients treated with radical cystectomy. Tumori 96: 699–703.
18. Manoharan M, Katkoori D, Kishore TA, Jorda M, Luongo T, et al. (2010) Lymphovascular invasion in radical cystectomy specimen: is it an independent prognostic factor in patients without lymph node metastases? World J Urol 28: 233–237.
19. Palmieri F, Brunocilla E, Bertaccini A, Guidi M, Pernetti R, et al. (2010) Prognostic value of lymphovascular invasion in bladder cancer in patients treated with radical cystectomy. Anticancer Res 30: 2973–2976.
20. Shariat SF, Svatek RS, Tilki D, Skinner E, Karakiewicz PI, et al. (2010) International validation of the prognostic value of lymphovascular invasion in patients treated with radical cystectomy. BJU Int 105: 1402–1412.
21. Stephenson AJ, Gong MC, Campbell SC, Fergany AF, Hansel DE (2010) Aggregate lymph node metastasis diameter and survival after radical cystectomy for invasive bladder cancer. Urology 75: 382–386.
22. Font A, Taron M, Gago JL, Costa C, Sánchez JJ, et al. (2011) BRCA1 mRNA expression and outcome to neoadjuvant cisplatin-based chemotherapy in bladder cancer. Ann Oncol 22: 139–144.

23. Kauffman EC, Ng CK, Lee MM, Otto BJ, Wang GJ, et al. (2011) Early oncological outcomes for bladder urothelial carcinoma patients treated with robotic-assisted radical cystectomy. BJU Int 107: 628–635.

24. Park E, Ha HK, Chung MK (2011) Prediction of prognosis after radical cystectomy for pathologic node-negative bladder cancer. Int Urol Nephrol 43: 1059–1065.

25. Park J, Kim S, Jeong IG, Song C, Hong JH, et al. (2011) Does the greater number of lymph nodes removed during standard lymph node dissection predict better patient survival following radical cystectomy? World J Urol 29: 443–449.

26. Gondo T, Nakashima J, Ozu C, Ohno Y, Horiguchi Y, et al. (2012) Risk stratification of survival by lymphovascular invasion, pathological stage, and surgical margin in patients with bladder cancer treated with radical cystectomy. Int J Clin Oncol 17: 456–461.

27. Otto W, May M, Fritsche HM, Dragun D, Aziz A, et al. (2012) Analysis of sex differences in cancer-specific survival and perioperative mortality following radical cystectomy: results of a large German multicenter study of nearly 2500 patients with urothelial carcinoma of the bladder. Gend Med 9: 481–489.

28. Afonso J, Longatto-Filho A, Martinho O, Lobo F, Amaro T, et al. (2013) Low RKIP expression associates with poor prognosis in bladder cancer patients. Virchows Arch 462: 445–453.

29. Eisenberg MS, Boorjian SA, Cheville JC, Thompson RH, Thapa P, et al. (2013) The SPARC (Survival Prediction After Radical Cystectomy) Score: A Multifactorial Outcome Prediction Model for Patients Undergoing Radical Cystectomy for Bladder Cancer. J Urol 190(6): 2005–10. doi: 10.1016/j.juro.2013.06.022.

30. Lotan Y, Bagrodia A, Passoni N, Rachakonda V, Kapur P, et al. (2013) Prospective Evaluation of a Molecular Marker Panel for Prediction of Recurrence and Cancer-specific Survival After Radical Cystectomy. Eur Urol 64(3): 465–71. doi:10.1016/j.eururo.2013.03.043.

31. Dicken BJ, Saunders LD, Jhangri GS, de Gara C, Cass C, et al. (2004) Gastric cancer: establishing predictors of biologic behavior with use of population-based data. Ann Surg Oncol 11: 629–635.

32. Woo CS, Silberman H, Nakamura SK, Ye W, Sposto R, et al. (2002) Lymph node status combined with lymphovascular invasion creates a more powerful tool for predicting outcome in patients with invasive breast cancer. Am J Surg 184: 337–340.

33. Padera TP, Kadambi A, di Tomaso E, Carreira CM, Brown EB, et al. (2002) Lymphatic metastasis in the absence of functional intratumor lymphatics. Science 296: 1883–1886.

34. Alitalo K, Mohla S, Ruoslahti E (2004) Lymphangiogenesis and cancer: meeting report. Cancer Res 64: 9225–9229.

35. Kikuchi E, Margulis V, Karakiewicz PI, Roscigno M, Mikami S, et al. (2009) Lymphovascular invasion predicts clinical outcomes in patients with node-negative upper tract urothelial carcinoma. J Clin Oncol 27: 612–618.

36. Kikuchi E, Horiguchi Y, Nakashima J, Hatakeyama N, Matsumoto M, et al. (2005) Lymphovascular invasion independently predicts increased disease specific survival in patients with transitional cell carcinoma of the upper urinary tract. J Urol 174: 2120–2123.

37. Akao J, Matsuyama H, Yamamoto Y, Hara I, Kawai Y, et al. (2008) Clinical significance of lymphovascular invasion in upper urinary tract urothelial cancer. BJU Int 102: 572–575.

38. Alexander-Sefre F, Singh N, Ayhan A, Salveson HB, Wilbanks G, et al. (2003) Detection of tumour lymphovascular space invasion using dual cytokeratin and CD31 immunohistochemistry. J Clin Pathol 56: 786–788.

39. Capdet J, Martel P, Charitansky H, Lim YK, Ferron G, et al. (2009) Factors predicting the sentinel node metastases in T1 breast cancer tumor: an analysis of 1416 cases. Eur J Surg Oncol 35: 1245–1249.

40. Lee KB, Ki KD, Lee JM, Lee JK, Kim JW, et al. (2009) The risk of lymph node metastasis based on myometrial invasion and tumor grade in endometrioid uterine cancers: a multicenter, retrospective Korean study. Ann Surg Oncol 16: 2882–2887.

41. Meier I, Merkel S, Papadopoulos T, Sauer R, Hohenberger W, et al. (2008) Adenocarcinoma of the esophagogastric junction: the pattern of metastatic lymph node dissemination as a rationale for elective lymphatic target volume definition. Int J Radiat Oncol Biol Phys 70: 1408–1417.

42. Vauthey JN, Lauwers GY, Esnaola NF, Do KA, Belghiti J, et al. (2002) Simplified staging for hepatocellular carcinoma. J Clin Oncol 20: 1527–1536.

43. Albers P, Siener R, Kliesch S, Weissbach L, Krege S, et al. (2003) German Testicular Cancer Study Group. Risk factors for relapse in clinical stage I nonseminomatous testicular germ cell tumors: results of the German Testicular Cancer Study Group Trial. J Clin Oncol 21: 1505–1512.

44. Egger M, Zellweger-Zähner T, Schneider M, Junker C, Lengeler C, et al. (1997) Language bias in randomised controlled trials published in English and German. Lancet 350: 326–9.

45. Margulis V, Lotan Y, Montorsi F, Shariat SF (2008) Predicting survival after radical cystectomy for bladder cancer. BJU Int 102: 15–22.

46. Chromecki TF, Bensalah K, Remzi M, Verhoest G, Cha EK, et al. (2011) Prognostic factors for upper urinary tract urothelial carcinoma. Nat Rev Urol 8: 440–447.

47. Miyata Y, Kanda S, Ohba K, Nomata K, Eguchi J, et al. (2006) Tumor lymphangiogenesis in transitional cell carcinoma of the upper urinary tract: association with clinicopathological features and prognosis. J Urol 176: 348–353.

48. Straume O, Jackson DG, Akslen LA (2003) Independent prognostic impact of lymphatic vessel density and presence of low-grade lymphangiogenesis in cutaneous melanoma. Clin Cancer Res 9: 250–256.

20

Upregulated UHRF1 Promotes Bladder Cancer Cell Invasion by Epigenetic Silencing of KiSS1

Yu Zhang[1,2*,9], Zhen Huang[2,9], Zhiqiang Zhu[2], Xin Zheng[2], Jianwei Liu[2], Zhiyou Han[3], Xuetao Ma[3], Yuhai Zhang[1*]

1 Department of Urology, Beijing Friendship Hospital, Capital Medical University, Beijing, China, 2 Department of Urology, Beijing You An Hospital, Capital Medical University, Beijing, China, 3 Department of Urology, Dongzhimen Hospital Affiliated to Beijing University of Chinese Medicine, Beijing, China

Abstract

Ubiquitin-like with PHD and RING finger domains 1 (UHRF1), as an epigenetic regulator, plays important roles in the tumorigenesis and cancer progression. KiSS1 functions as a metastasis suppressor in various cancers, and epigenetic silencing of KiSS1 increases the metastatic potential of cancer cells. We therefore investigated whether UHRF1 promotes bladder cancer cell invasion by inhibiting KiSS1. The expression levels of UHRF1 and KiSS1 were examined by quantitative real-time PCR assay in vitro and in vivo. The role of UHRF1 in regulating bladder cancer metastasis was evaluated in bladder cancer cell. We found that UHRF1 levels are upregulated in most clinical specimens of bladder cancer when compared with paired normal tissues, and UHRF1 expression levels are significantly increased in primary tumors that subsequently metastasized compared with non-metastatic tumors. Forced expression of UHRF1 promotes bladder cancer cell invasion, whereas UHRF1 knockdown decreases cell invasion. Overexpression of UHRF1 increases the methylation of CpG nucleotides and reduces the expression of KiSS1. UHRF1 and KiSS1 expression level is negatively correlated in vivo and in vitro. Knockdown of KiSS1 promotes bladder cancer cell invasion. Importantly, forced expression of KiSS1 partly abrogates UHRF1-induced cell invasion. These data demonstrated that upregulated UHRF1 increases bladder cancer cell invasion by epigenetic silencing of KiSS1.

Editor: Hari K. Koul, Louisiana State University Health Sciences center, United States of America

Funding: The authors have no support or funding to report.

Competing Interests: The authors have declared that no competing interests exist.

* Email: zhangyud@hotmail.com (YZ); zhangyuhaizyh@sohu.com (YhZ)

9 These authors contributed equally to this work.

Introduction

Human bladder cancer ranks second in frequency of genitourinary cancer [1], and approximately 50% of patients diagnosed with muscle-invasive bladder cancer (MIBC) develop distant metastases in the lungs and liver, resulting in poor 5-year survival rates [2]. Currently, the advances in suitable therapy for enhancing survival rate are limited because the underlying mechanisms causing cancer metastasis are not well understood. Therefore, it is very important to reveal the molecular mechanism of bladder cancer metastasis for developing effective therapy.

UHRF1, also called ICBP90 in humans and Np95 in mice, is a multidomain protein, which is required for epigenetic regulation of gene expression and chromatin modification [3,4]. UHRF1 increases the G1/S transition as the target of E2F transcription factor [5], and changes in UHRF1 expression level regulates cell cycle progression, cell proliferation and cell migration [6,7]. UHRF1 is upregulated in multiple types of cancers, and overexpression of UHRF1 is involved in tumorigenesis and cancer progression [8,9]. Several reports showed that UHRF1 may be an important biomarker for diagnosis and prognosis of cancers [5]. Unoki et al demonstrated that UHRF1 overexpression is associated with the grade and stage of bladder cancer [10].

Overexpression of UHRF1 in bladder cancer is also correlated with increased risk of cancer progression after transurethral resection [10]. Wang et al showed that UHRF1 is overexpressed in colorectal cancer (CRC) cell lines and clinical specimens [5]. UHRF1 expression levels are correlated with cancer metastasis and poor Dukes staging. UHRF1 knockdown induces cell apoptosis and cell cycle arrest at the G0/G1 phase and suppresses cell proliferation and migration.

UHRF1 is a very important regulator of DNA methylation, and aberrant DNA methylation is a frequent epigenetic event in bladder cancer [6,11]. UHRF1 recognizes hemimethylated DNA generated during DNA replication and recruits DNMT1 (DNA methyltransferase1) to ensure faithful maintenance of DNA-methylation patterns in daughter cells [6]. KiSS1 is identified as suppressing metastases in various cancers, such as bladder cancer, breast cancer cells and melanoma [12]. KiSS1 encodes a 145-amino acid protein that is processed into KiSSpeptins (KP), including KP10, KP13, KP14 and KP54 [12,13,14]. Recent studies showed that KiSS1 is epigenetically silenced by hypermethylation in bladder cancer [15]. Cebrian et al demonstrated that KiSS1 hypermethylation is frequently observed and is correlated with low gene expression, being restored by demethylating azacytidine in bladder cancer cells [12]. Hypermethylation of KiSS1 is also correlated with high tumor grade and stage. Despite these intriguing findings, little is known about whether UHRF1 increases bladder cancer cell invasion by epigenetic silencing of KiSS1.

In the study, we tested whether UHRF1/KiSS1 represents a novel pathway regulating bladder cancer cell invasion. Our results revealed that UHRF1 expression is upregulated in primary tumors that subsequently metastasized, and overexpression of UHRF1 promotes bladder cancer cell invasion by epigenetic silencing of KiSS1.

Materials and Methods

Clinical samples and cell lines

Human bladder tissues were obtained with written informed consent from the Beijing Friendship Hospital affiliated to Capital Medical University. The study was approved by the Ethics Committee of Capital Medical University. 47 specimens (Table 1) of pathologically and normally diagnosed biopsy specimens (≥ 3 cm away from bladder cancer tissues) were collected from patients with bladder cancer, including 22 with non-muscle-invasive [NMI, stage pTa-pT1] and 25 with muscle-invasive [MI, stage ≥T2].Human bladder cancer cells were obtained from the American Type Culture Collection (ATCC, Manassas, VA) and were maintained in RPMI 1640 with 10% FBS (GIBCO, Carlsbad, CA).

Real-time quantitative PCR

Total RNA from bladder cancer cell lines and specimens was extracted using Trizol reagent (Invitrogen, Carlsbad, CA). The RT (reverse-transcription) reaction was performed using an M-MLV Reverse Transcriptase kit (Invitrogen). Real-time quantitative PCR was carried out using a standard SYBR Green PCR Master Mix (Life Technologies) protocol on the StepOne Real-Time PCR System (Applied Biosystems) according to the instructions from the respective manufacturer. β-actin was used as internal control for mRNA. Respective ΔCt values (both UHRF1 and KiSS1) were obtained by normalization to β-actin. Relative expression was calculated with respect to the control. The results were expressed as $2^{-\Delta\Delta Ct}$. $*p<0.05$.

Overexpression and Small interfering RNA

To overexpress UHRF1, plasmid pcDNA-UHRF1 was constructed by introducing a *HindIII-EcoRI* fragment containing the UHRF1 cDNA into the same sites in pcDNA3.1. The UHRF1 gene was amplified by PCR using the forward and reverse primers: cccaagcttgggATGTGGATCCAGGTTCGGACCATGGACGGG and ggaattccTCACCGGCCATTGCCGTAGCCGGGGAAG. pcDNA-UHRF1 was transfected into bladder cancer cell lines by using Lipofectamine 2000 (Invitrogen).

To inhibit endogenous UHRF1 and KiSS1 expression, bladder cancer cells were transfected with 30 nM indicated indicated siRNA or negative control using Lipofectamine 2000. UHRF1-siRNAs (reference sequence, sc-76805) were purchased from Santa Cruz Biotechnology (Santa Cruz Biotechnology, Santa Cruz, CA). The KiSS1-siRNAs (reference sequence, sc-37443) were purchased from Santa Cruz Biotechnology.

Transwell invasion assay

Cell invasion was examined using Transwell invasion assay with inserts of 8-μm pore size (Corning Costar) as described previously [16]. Briefly, bladder cancer cells (RT4 or T24) were suspended in serum free medium, and then seeded onto Matrigel-coated Transwell filters in Biocoat Matrigel invasion chambers. The serum-containing medium was used as a chemo-attractant in the lower chamber. The bladder cancer cells were treated with indicated reagents for 72 h, and then cells that did not invade through the pores were eliminated by using a cotton swab. Cells on the lower surface of the membrane were stained with Crystal violet. The cell numbers were determined by counting of the

Table 1. Associations of UHRF1 level with clinicopathologic characteristics in 47 patients with bladder cancer.

Variable	n	UHRF1 level		P
		low	high	
Age	47			
<60	19	8	11	0.594
≥60	28	12	16	
Gender				
Male	31	14	17	0.365
Female	16	6	10	
Histologic grade				
G1	8	3	5	0.058
G2	29	13	16	
G3	10	4	6	
Depth of invasion				
pTa-pT1	22	10	12	0.042
pT2-pT4	25	10	15	
KiSS1 level				
Low	31	14	17	0.033
High	16	10	6	

Fisher's exact test was used for the statistical analyses.

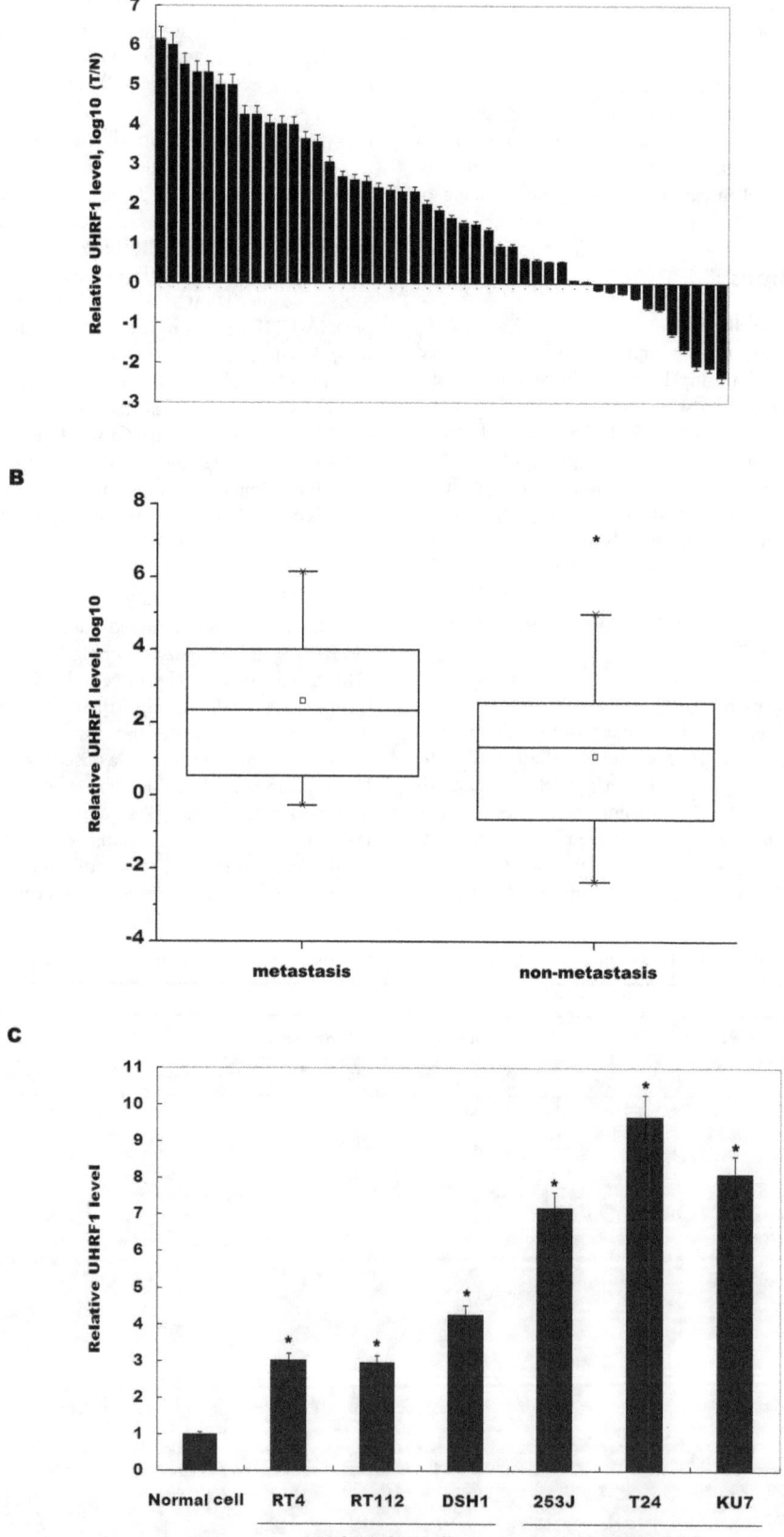

Figure 1. Higher UHRF1 expression is associated with bladder cancer metastasis. (A) The quantitative analysis of UHRF1 expression level was carried out in bladder cancer tissues (n = 47) and adjacent normal tissues. Total RNA was extracted and subjected to real-time PCR to analyze the expression of UHRF1 in each sample. β-actin was used as an internal control. The relative UHRF1 level was calculated by $2^{-\Delta\Delta Ct}$ where $\Delta Ct = Ct$

(UHRF1) – Ct (β-actin) and ΔΔCt = ΔCt (tumor tissue) – ΔCt (adjacent normal tissue). (B) The bladder cancer specimens were divided into two groups based on clinical progression. The UHRF1 levels in the metastasis group (n = 25) were higher than those in the no-metastasis group (n = 22). *$p<0.05$. (C) UHRF1 expression level was assayed by real-time PCR in three noninvasive and three invasive bladder cancer cell lines. Normal urothelial cells were used as control. *$p<0.05$.

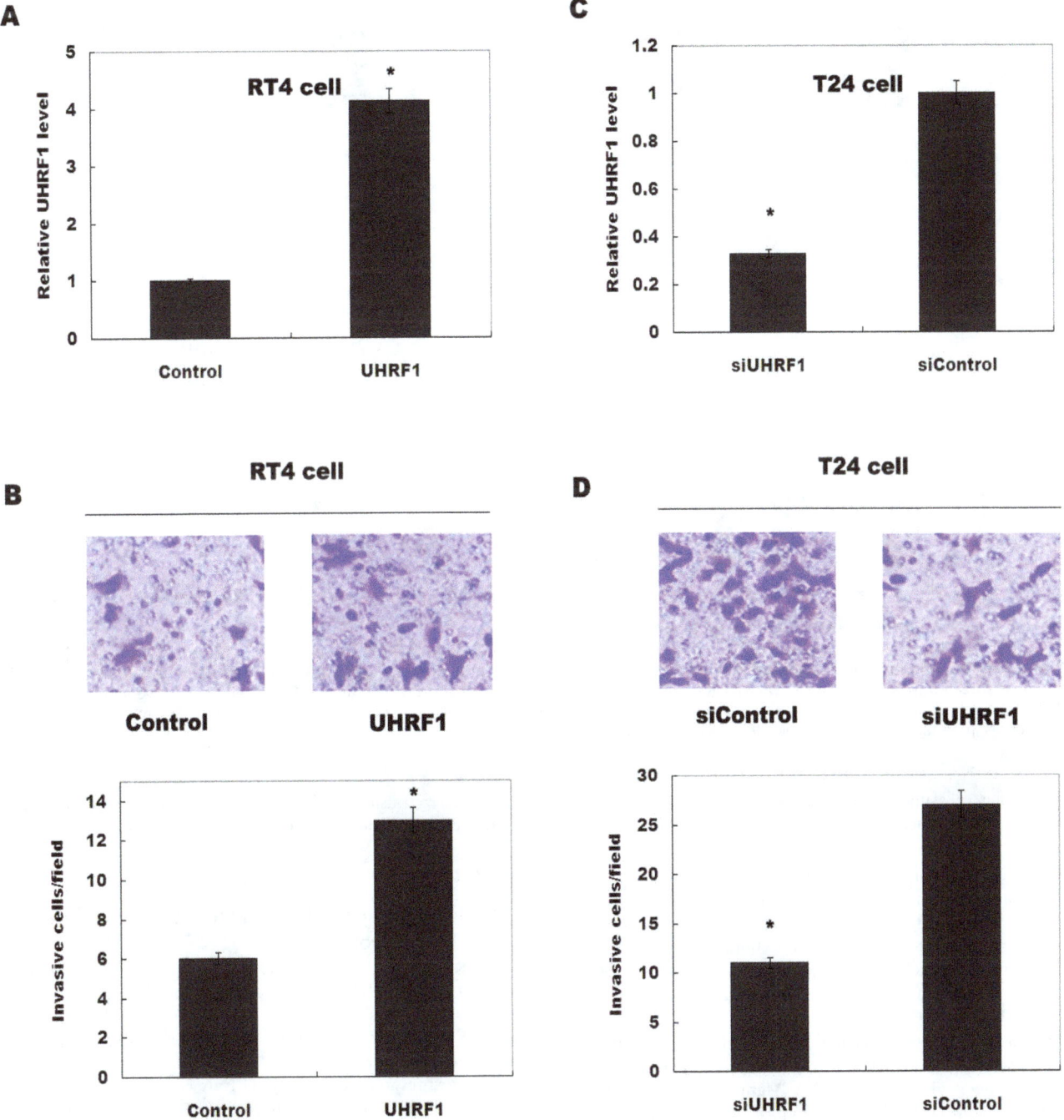

Figure 2. Overexpression of UHRF1 promotes bladder cancer cell invasion. (A) RT4 cells were treated with pcDNA-UHRF1, and the relative level of UHRF1 was assayed by realtime PCR. *$p<0.05$. (B) UHRF1 was overexpressed in RT4 cells, and invasion assay was performed as described in Material and Methods. Representative figures of each experiment are shown. These results show data from five independent experiments, expressed as the mean ±SD. *$p<0.05$. (C) T24 cells were treated with UHRF1-siRNA, and the relative level of UHRF1 was assayed by realtime PCR. *$p<0.05$. (D) Invasion assay was performed after UHRF1 knockdown. Representative figures of each experiment are shown. These results show data from five independent experiments, expressed as the mean ±SD. *$p<0.05$.

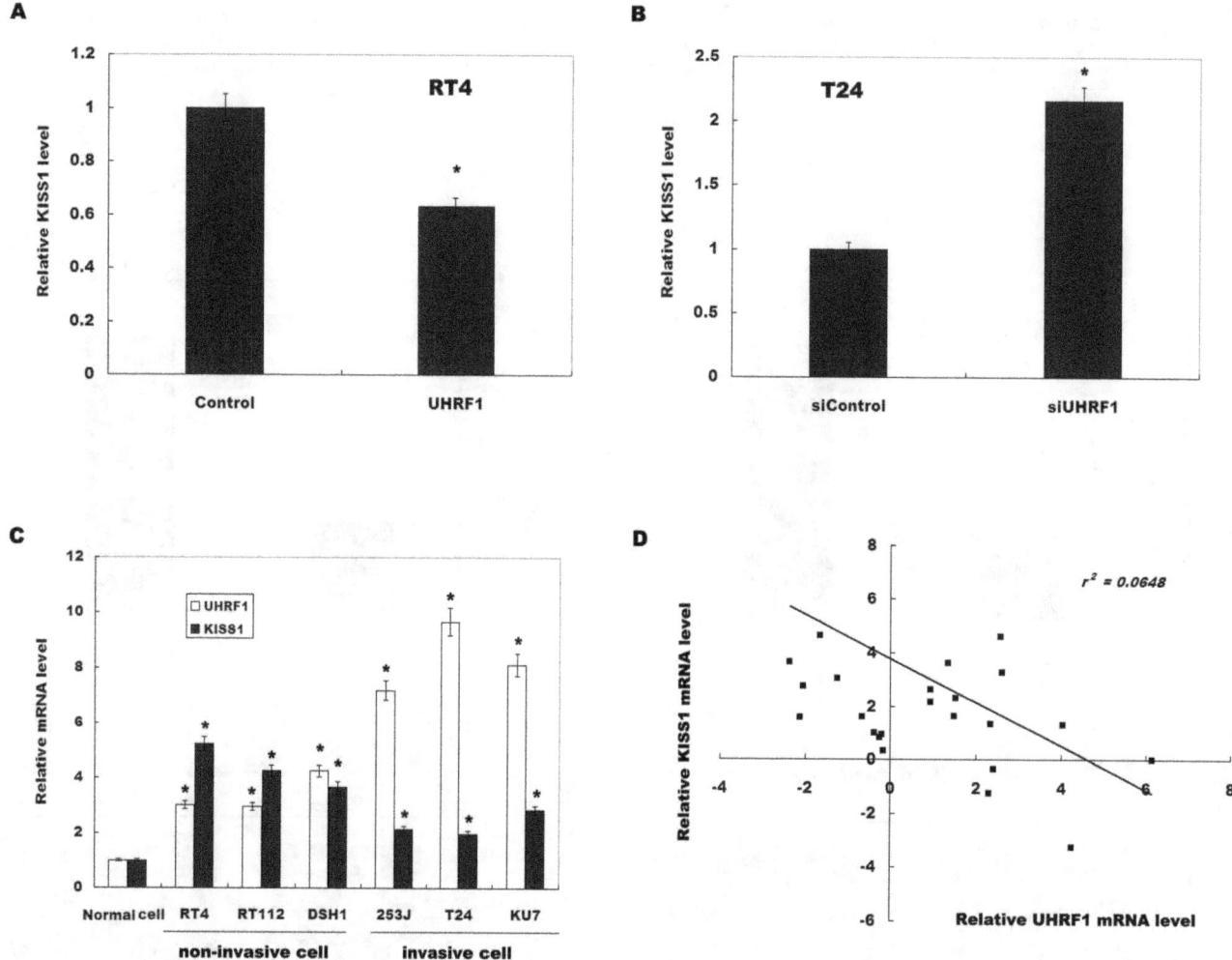

Figure 3. UHRF1 negatively regulates KiSS1 expression. (A and B) KiSS1 expression level was assayed in RT4 cells overexpressed with UHRF1 or T24 cells treated with UHRF1-siRNA. *$p<0.05$. (C) UHRF1 and KiSS1 levels were assayed by real-time PCR in three noninvasive and three invasive bladder cancer cell lines. Normal urothelial cells were used as control. *$p<0.05$. (D) Negative correlation between the UHRF1 mRNA levels and the KiSS1 levels in 24 bladder cancer samples ($r^2 = 0.0648$, $p = 0.0063$).

penetrating cells under a microscope at 200× magnification in random fields in each well.

Methylation Analysis of *KiSS1*

A search for enrichment of CpG in KiSS1 was performed and bisulfite sequencing primers were designed using the CpG Island Searcher online tool (MethPrimer, http://www.urogene.org/methprimer/). The forward primers are GATGGAAGGGGAA-TAGTTTTATTAGA, and the reverse primers are TACAAC-TAAAACTCCTTCCACCTAC [12].

Genomic DNA was prepared from bladder cancer cells using the QiAmp DNA blood Mini kit, and then the genomic DNA was bisulfite modified using EZ DNA Methylation-Gold Kit from Zymo research [17]. The PCR products were cloned into pMD-18T (TaKaRa) according to manufacturer's instructions. 9 positive clones were sequenced. The data were analyzed using the BiQ analyzer software [17].

Statistical Analysis

Data are expressed as mean ±SD (standard deviation) from at least three separate experiments. The differences between groups were analyzed using Student's *t* test. The difference was deemed statistically significant at $p<0.05$.

Results

UHRF1 level is upregulated in metastatic bladder urothelial carcinoma

UHRF1 results in abnormal DNA methylation and cancer metastasis, and UHRF1 expression is correlated with a poor prognosis in several cancers. To assess whether UHRF1 regulates bladder cancer metastasis, we first examined UHRF1 expression in bladder cancer cell lines and cancer tissues. Figure 1A showed that the expression levels of UHRF1 are significantly upregulated in most bladder cancer tissues compared with adjacent normal controls. UHRF1 is remarkably increased expression in 77% (36/47) of bladder cancer tissues (Figure 1A). When the 47 tumor tissues were stratified based on clinical progression, UHRF1 expression is significantly increased in primary tumors that subsequently metastasized compared with non-metastatic tumors (Figure 1B). Then we assayed the expression levels of UHRF1 in both invasive bladder cancer cell lines and noninvasive bladder cancer cell lines. Among the three invasive cell lines (253J, T24

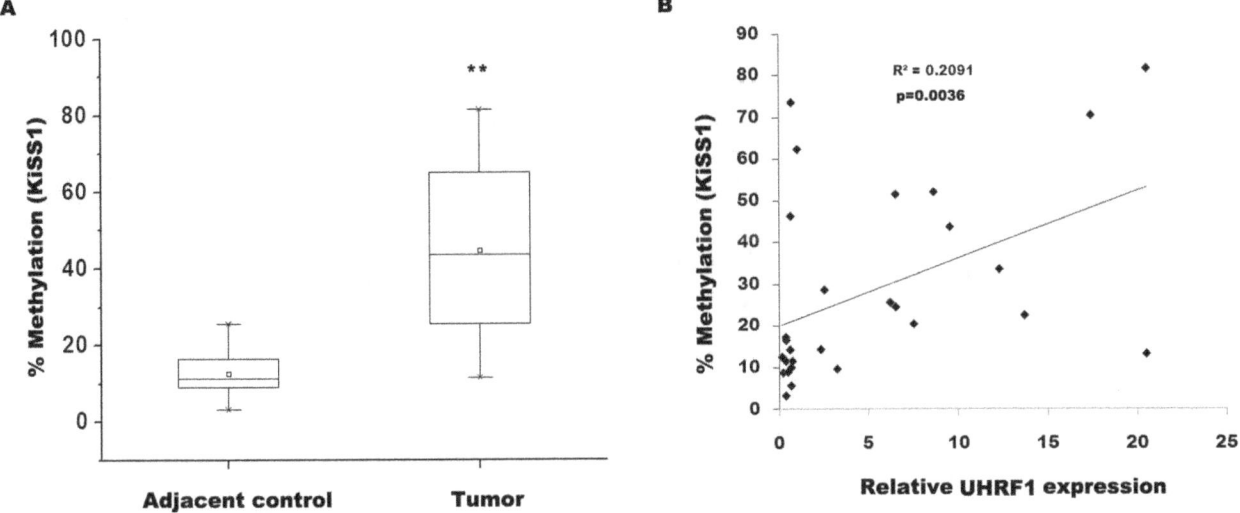

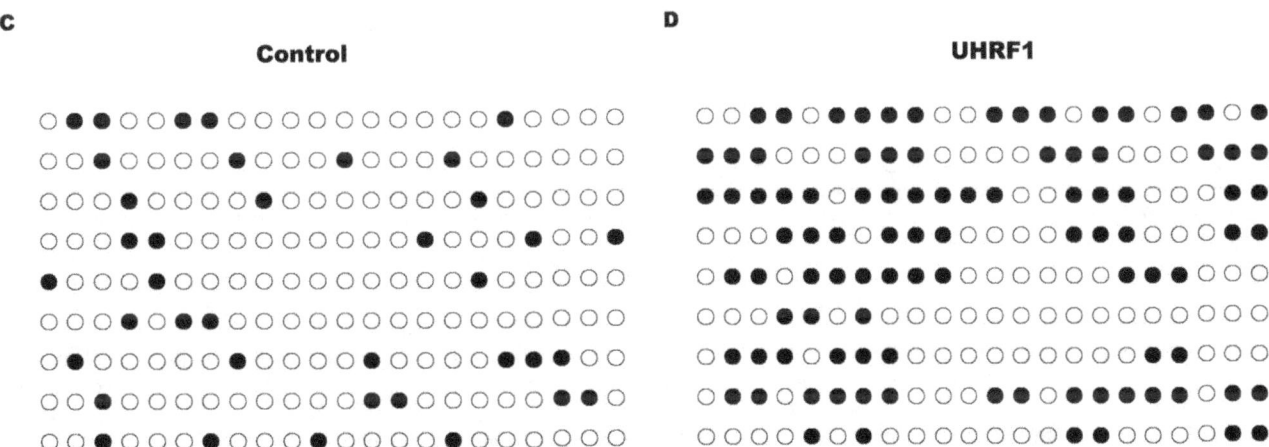

Figure 4. UHRF1 reduces the expression of KiSS1 by increasing the methylation of CpG nucleotides. (A) The methylation analysis of the *KiSS1* gene in 14 bladder cancer tissues and adjacent normal samples. BSQ analysis revealed that *KiSS1* methylation frequency is markedly increased with bladder cancer samples. ** p<0.01. (B) A positive correlation is observed between *KiSS1* methylation and UHRF1 expression ($R^2 = 0.2091$, p = 0.0036). (C and D) CpG island methylation status of KiSS1 was analyzed by bisulfite sequencing in RT4 cells. Nine individual clones were shown per cell line. CpG dinucleotides were represented as dark squares for methylated cytosines and open squares for unmethylated cytosines.

and KU7) the UHRF1 levels are relatively higher than those in the noninvasive ones (Figure 1C). These data suggest that UHRF1 overexpressoin may be related to bladder cancer metastasis.

Upregulated UHRF1 increases bladder cancer cell invasion *in vitro*

To investigate the role of UHRF1 in regulating cell invasion, the bladder cancer cell lines treated with UHRF1-siRNA or pcDNA-UHRF1 were analyzed. We first demonstrated whether RT4 and T24 cells can be used as *in vitro* model to investigate UHRF1 by assaying its expression in RT4 or T24 cells after overexpression or knockdown of UHRF1. Figure 2A and C showed that the pcDNA-UHRF1 treatment significantly increases UHRF1 levels in non-invasive RT4 cells, whereas UHRF1-siRNA treatment decreases UHRF1 expression in invasive T24 cells. Furthermore, upregulation of UHRF1 promotes RT4 cell invasion

(Figure 2B), whereas siRNA-mediated UHRF1 silencing inhibits T24 cell invasion (Figure 2D). These results demonstrated that UHRF1 positively regulates bladder cancer cell invasion.

UHRF1 increases the methylation of CpG nucleotides and reduces the expression of KiSS1

Previous studies showed that KiSS1 is frequently hypermethylated in bladder cancer and is correlated with cancer progression [12]. Here we investigated whether UHRF1 regulates bladder cancer cell invasion by epigenetic silencing of KiSS1. We first assayed whether UHRF1 regulates KiSS1 expression. As shown in Figure 3A and B, forced expression of UHRF1 inhibits KiSS1 expression, whereas knockdown of UHRF1 increases KiSS1 expression. We then assayed the expression level of UHRF1 and KiSS1 in both invasive bladder cancer cell lines and noninvasive bladder cancer cell lines. Figure 3C showed that the UHRF1

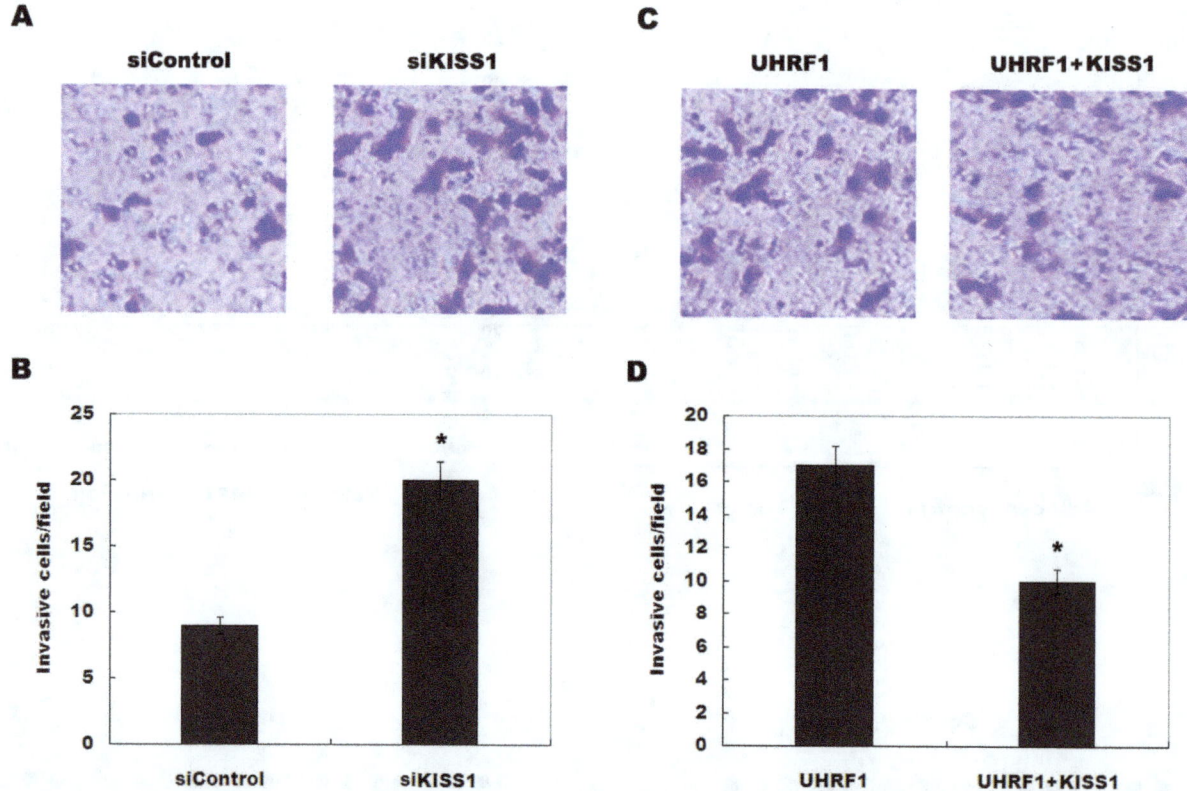

Figure 5. UHRF1 increases bladder cancer cell invasion by inhibiting KiSS1. (A and B) RT4 cells were treated with KiSS1-siRNA and invasion assay was performed after KiSS1 knockdown. Representative figures of each experiment are shown. These results show data from five independent experiments, expressed as the mean $\pm$SD. $*p<0.05$. (C and D) RT4 cells were overexpressed with the UHRF1 or UHRF1 plus KiSS1, and invasion assay was performed. $*p<0.05$.

levels are relatively higher with concurrent low levels of KiSS1 in invasive cell lines. A significant negative correlation is also observed between the UHRF1 mRNA levels and the KiSS1 mRNA levels *in vivo* ($r^2 = 0.0648$, $p = 0.0063$, Figure 3D). We further investigated whether UHRF1 inhibits KiSS1 expression by increasing the methylation of CpG nucleotides of *KiSS1*. We analyzed the methylation status of CpG islands in KiSS1 by bisulfite sequencing, as reported previously [12,15]. The methylation assay results for the *KiSS1* gene in 14 bladder cancer tissues and adjacent normal controls are summarized in Figure 4A. Bisulfite sequencing analysis revealed that *KiSS1* methylation frequency is markedly increased in bladder cancer tissues compared with adjacent controls (Figure 4A). Correlation analysis showed that the *KiSS1* methylation level is positively correlated with UHRF1 expression in both bladder cancer and normal bladder tissues (Figure 4B, $p = 0.0036$, $R^2 = 0.2091$). Bisulfite sequencing analysis further showed that UHRF1 overexpression increases the methylation of CpG nucleotides of *KiSS1* (Figure 4C,D). These results suggest that UHRF1 suppresses KiSS1 expression by epigenetic silencing of KiSS1.

UHRF1 increases bladder cancer cell invasion by inhibiting KiSS1

UHRF1 decreases KiSS1 expression by increasing the methylation of CpG nucleotides of *KiSS*, and downregulation of KiSS1 promotes bladder cancer cell invasion. Therefore we speculated that the role of UHRF1 in regulating cell invasion is partly mediated by KiSS1. We first assayed whether KiSS1 inhibition increases bladder cancer cell invasion. As shown in Figure 5A and

B, knockdown of KiSS1 promotes RT4 cell invasion. More important, KiSS1 overexpression partly inhibits UHRF1-inducing RT4 cell invasion (Figure 5C and D). These results confirm that UHRF1 promotes bladder cancer cell invasion, at least in part, by epigenetic silencing of KiSS1.

Discussion

In mammals, DNA methylation occurs at the C5 position of cytosine in the context of CpG dinucleotides, resulting in 5-methylcytosine (5mC) [18]. The modification of genomic DNA by methylation is an important epigenetic signal, and changes in the pattern of DNA methylation have been a consistent finding in various tumor types [19]. Recent studies showed that epigenetic inheritance of DNA methylation requires UHRF1, which recruits DNMT1 to DNA replication forks through a unique hemimethylated CpG-binding activity [20]. Liu *et al* reported that UHRF1 recruits DNMT1 for DNA maintenance methylation through binding either hemi-methylated CpG or H3K9me2/3, and that the presence of both binding activities ensures high fidelity DNA maintenance methylation [20].

UHRF1 overexpression is associated with the tumor stages and predicts poor prognoses in various cancers [21]. UHRF1 coordinates PPARG (peroxisome proliferator-activated receptor γ) epigenetic silencing and mediates colorectal cancer progression [22]. Knockdown of UHRF1 elicits PPARG re-activation, accompanied by positive histone marks and DNA demethylation, corroborating its role in PPARG silencing. Babbio *et al* showed that UHRF1 contributes to epigenetic gene silencing in prostate cancer progression [23]. In the present study, we found that the expression levels of UHRF1 are significantly increased in most bladder cancer tissues compared with adjacent normal controls. Moreover, UHRF1 expression is significantly increased in primary tumors that subsequently metastasized compared with non-metastatic tumors. We also found that the UHRF1 levels are relatively higher in invasive bladder cancer cell lines than those in the noninvasive ones. Furthermore, upregulated UHRF1 promotes noninvasive RT4 cell invasion, whereas knockdown of UHRF1 inhibits invasive T24 cell invasion. These data demonstrated that upregulation of UHRF1 contributes to bladder cancer cell invasion.

KiSS1 is a tumor metastasis suppressor gene in several cancers. KiSS1 expression is markedly decreased in invasive bladder tumors compared with their respective normal urothelium [24]. Lower KiSS1 level is correlated with overall survival in bladder tumors [24]. KiSS1 is significantly methylated. Inactivation of KiSS1 by promoter methylation is an infrequent event in pancreatic ductal adenocarcinoma (PDAC) [25]. KiSS1 is also epigenetically modified in colorectal cancer, and KiSS1 methylation is associated with tumor grade, predicted recurrence and

overall survival [15]. Here we found that UHRF1 negatively regulates KiSS1 expression. UHRF1 levels are relatively higher with concurrent low levels of KiSS1 in invasive bladder cancer cell lines. A significant negative correlation is also observed between the UHRF1 mRNA levels and the KiSS1 mRNA levels *in vivo*. Bisulfite sequencing analysis showed that UHRF1 inhibits KiSS1 expression by increases the methylation of CpG nucleotides of *KiSS1*. More important, KiSS1 overexpression partly inhibits RT4 cell invasion in UHRF1-overexpressing cells.

Conclusion

Our data showed that upregulated UHRF1 contributes to bladder cancer cell invasion by epigenetic silencing of KiSS1.

Author Contributions

Conceived and designed the experiments: YZ Z. Huang YhZ. Performed the experiments: YZ Z. Huang ZqZ XZ JwL. Analyzed the data: YZ Z. Huang YhZ. Contributed reagents/materials/analysis tools: YZ Z. Huang ZqZ. Wrote the paper: YhZ. Edited the manuscript: Z. Han XtM.

References

1. Hussain SA, James ND (2003) The systemic treatment of advanced and metastatic bladder cancer. Lancet Oncol 4: 489–497.
2. Overdevest JB, Thomas S, Kristiansen G, Hansel DE, Smith SC, et al. (2011) CD24 offers a therapeutic target for control of bladder cancer metastasis based on a requirement for lung colonization. Cancer Res 71: 3802–3811.
3. Chu J, Loughlin EA, Gaur NA, SenBanerjee S, Jacob V, et al. (2012) UHRF1 phosphorylation by cyclin A2/cyclin-dependent kinase 2 is required for zebrafish embryogenesis. Mol Biol Cell 23: 59–70.
4. Unoki M, Bronner C, Mousli M (2008) A concern regarding the current confusion with the human homolog of mouse Np95, ICBP90/UHRF1. Radiat Res 169: 240–244.
5. Wang F, Yang YZ, Shi CZ, Zhang P, Moyer MP, et al. (2012) UHRF1 promotes cell growth and metastasis through repression of p16(ink(4)a) in colorectal cancer. Ann Surg Oncol 19: 2753–2762.
6. Mudbhary R, Hoshida Y, Chernyavskaya Y, Jacob V, Villanueva A, et al. (2014) UHRF1 Overexpression Drives DNA Hypomethylation and Hepatocellular Carcinoma. Cancer Cell 25: 196–209.
7. Jeanblanc M, Mousli M, Hopfner R, Bathami K, Martinet N, et al. (2005) The retinoblastoma gene and its product are targeted by ICBP90: a key mechanism in the G1/S transition during the cell cycle. Oncogene 24: 7337–7345.
8. Jenkins Y, Markovtsov V, Lang W, Sharma P, Pearsall D, et al. (2005) Critical role of the ubiquitin ligase activity of UHRF1, a nuclear RING finger protein, in tumor cell growth. Mol Biol Cell 16: 5621–5629.
9. Bronner C, Achour M, Arima Y, Chataigneau T, Saya H, et al. (2007) The UHRF family: oncogenes that are drugable targets for cancer therapy in the near future? Pharmacol Ther 115: 419–434.
10. Unoki M, Kelly JD, Neal DE, Ponder BA, Nakamura Y, et al. (2009) UHRF1 is a novel molecular marker for diagnosis and the prognosis of bladder cancer. Br J Cancer 101: 98–105.
11. Zhou L, Zhao X, Han Y, Lu Y, Shang Y, et al. (2013) Regulation of UHRF1 by miR-146a/b modulates gastric cancer invasion and metastasis. FASEB J 27: 4929–4939.
12. Cebrian V, Fierro M, Orenes-Pinero E, Grau L, Moya P, et al. (2011) KISS1 methylation and expression as tumor stratification biomarkers and clinical outcome prognosticators for bladder cancer patients. Am J Pathol 179: 540–546.
13. Fernandez-Fernandez R, Martini AC, Navarro VM, Castellano JM, Dieguez C, et al. (2006) Novel signals for the integration of energy balance and reproduction. Mol Cell Endocrinol 254–255: 127–132.
14. Cho SG, Li D, Stafford LJ, Luo J, Rodriguez-Villanueva M, et al. (2009) KiSS1 suppresses TNFalpha-induced breast cancer cell invasion via an inhibition of RhoA-mediated NF-kappaB activation. J Cell Biochem 107: 1139–1149.
15. Moya P, Esteban S, Fernandez-Suarez A, Maestro M, Morente M, et al. (2013) KiSS-1 methylation and protein expression patterns contribute to diagnostic and prognostic assessments in tissue specimens for colorectal cancer. Tumour Biol 34: 471–479.
16. Connor KM, Hempel N, Nelson KK, Dabiri G, Gamarra A, et al. (2007) Manganese superoxide dismutase enhances the invasive and migratory activity of tumor cells. Cancer Res 67: 10260–10267.
17. Karouzakis E, Rengel Y, Jungel A, Kolling C, Gay RE, et al. (2011) DNA methylation regulates the expression of CXCL12 in rheumatoid arthritis synovial fibroblasts. Genes Immun 12: 643–652.
18. Sukackaite R, Grazulis S, Tamulaitis G, Siksnys V (2012) The recognition domain of the methyl-specific endonuclease McrBC flips out 5-methylcytosine. Nucleic Acids Res 40: 7552–7562.
19. Bird A (2002) DNA methylation patterns and epigenetic memory. Genes Dev 16: 6–21.
20. Liu X, Gao Q, Li P, Zhao Q, Zhang J, et al. (2013) UHRF1 targets DNMT1 for DNA methylation through cooperative binding of hemi-methylated DNA and methylated H3K9. Nat Commun 4: 1563.
21. Unoki M, Daigo Y, Koinuma J, Tsuchiya E, Hamamoto R, et al. (2010) UHRF1 is a novel diagnostic marker of lung cancer. Br J Cancer 103: 217–222.
22. Sabatino L, Fucci A, Pancione M, Carafa V, Nebbioso A, et al. (2012) UHRF1 coordinates peroxisome proliferator activated receptor gamma (PPARG) epigenetic silencing and mediates colorectal cancer progression. Oncogene 31: 5061–5072.
23. Babbio F, Pistore C, Curti L, Castiglioni I, Kunderfranco P, et al. (2012) The SRA protein UHRF1 promotes epigenetic crosstalks and is involved in prostate cancer progression. Oncogene 31: 4878–4887.
24. Sanchez-Carbayo M, Capodieci P, Cordon-Cardo C (2003) Tumor suppressor role of KiSS-1 in bladder cancer: loss of KiSS-1 expression is associated with bladder cancer progression and clinical outcome. Am J Pathol 162: 609–617.
25. Mardin WA, Haier J, Mees ST (2013) Epigenetic regulation and role of metastasis suppressor genes in pancreatic ductal adenocarcinoma. BMC Cancer 13: 264.

21

Quantitative Apparent Diffusion Coefficient Measurements Obtained by 3-Tesla MRI are Correlated with Biomarkers of Bladder Cancer Proliferative Activity

Sabina Sevcenco[1], Andrea Haitel[2], Lothar Ponhold[3], Martin Susani[2], Harun Fajkovic[1], Shahrokh F. Shariat[1], Manuela Hiess[1], Claudio Spick[3], Tibor Szarvas[1], Pascal A. T. Baltzer[3]*

1 Department of Urology, Medical University of Vienna, Vienna, Austria, 2 Department of Pathology, Medical University of Vienna, Vienna, Austria, 3 Department of Biomedical Imaging and Image-guided therapy, Medical University of Vienna, Vienna, Austria

Abstract

Purpose: To investigate the association between Apparent Diffusion Coefficient (ADC) values and cell cycle and proliferative biomarkers (p53, p21, Ki67,) in order to establish its potential role as a noninvasive biomarker for prediction of cell cycle, proliferative activity and biological aggressiveness in bladder cancer.

Materials and Methods: Patients with bladder cancer who underwent 3,0 Tesla DW-MRI of the bladder before TUR-B or radical cystectomy were eligible for this prospective IRB-approved study. Histological specimen were immunohistochemically stained for the following markers: p53, p21 and ki67. Two board-certified uropathologists reviewed the specimens blinded to DW-MRI results. Histological grade and T-stage were classified according to the WHO 2004 and the 2009 TNM classification, respectively. Nonparametric univariate and multivariate statistics including correlation, logistic regression and ROC analysis were applied.

Results: Muscle invasive bladder cancer was histologically confirmed in 10 out of 41 patients. All examined tissue biomarkers were significantly correlated with ADC values ($p < 0.05$, respectively). Based on multivariate analysis, p53 and ADC are both independent prognostic factors for muscle invasiveness of bladder cancer ($>/=T2$). ($p = 0.013$ and $p = 0.018$).

Conclusion: ADC values are associated with cell cycle and proliferative biomarkers and do thereby reflect invasive and proliferative potential in bladder cancer. ADC and p53 are both independent prognostic factors for muscle invasiveness in bladder cancer.

Editor: Peter C. Black, University of British Columbia, Canada

Funding: The authors have no support or funding to report.

Competing Interests: The authors have declared that no competing interests exist.

* Email: pascal.baltzer@meduniwien.ac.at

Introduction

Bladder cancer is a malignant disease causing substantial morbidity and mortality. For optimized clinical management of patients with bladder cancer, an accurate prediction of the individual cancers biological behavior is needed. However, standard prognostic factors such as pathological staging and grading are limited in this respect [1].

Therefore, molecular biomarkers taken from tissue specimen have become increasingly investigated in order to overcome these limitations and to accurately predict tumor grade and stage [2]. Previous studies based on cell cycle and tumor proliferation markers (p53, p21, ki67) have shown a prognostic role regarding patient outcome with muscle and non-muscle bladder cancer [1,2]. Computed tomography and magnetic resonance imaging (MRI) are regularly used for local staging of bladder cancer [3].

One of the more recent developments in MRI is the use of Diffusion-Weighted Magnetic Resonance Imaging (DW-MRI). This technique measures water diffusion by insertion of motion probing gradients in a fast T2-weighted Echo Planar Imaging sequence. A water diffusion dependent signal loss caused by spin de-phasing can be quantified by means of the Apparent Diffusion Coefficient (ADC). Recent studies have shown a promising potential of DW-MRI for detection, grading and staging in bladder cancer [4–6]. Microstructural changes in bladder cancers measured by ADC values correlate with the histopathological grade and stage [7,8].

Besides these clinical prognostic factors, a recent study has shown an inverse correlation between ADC value and proliferative activity as measured by Ki67 [9]. Therefore, ADC may be described as a potential biomarker reflecting invasive and proliferative potential in bladder cancer.

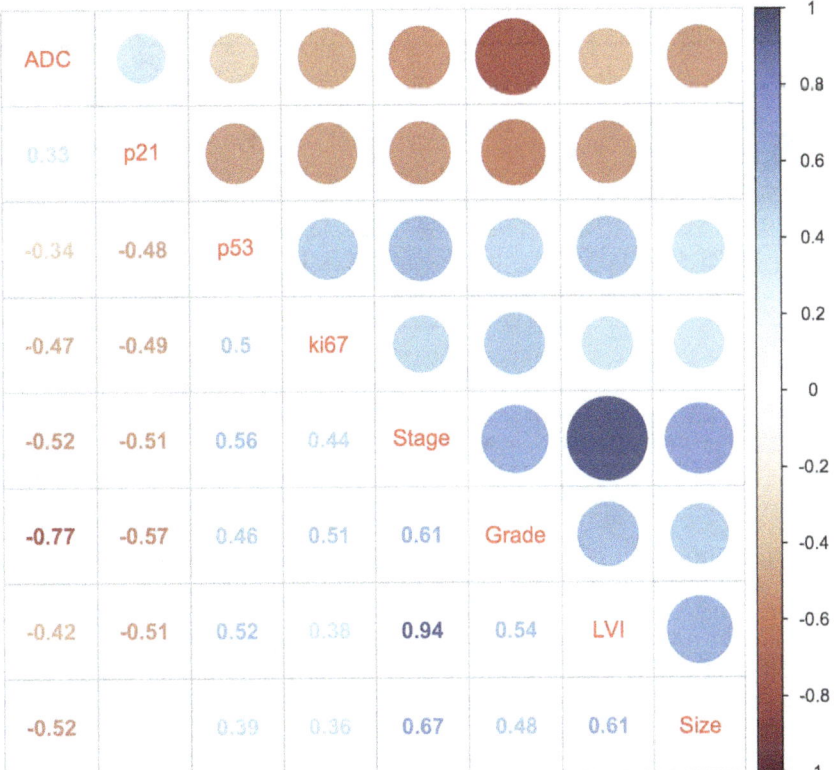

Figure 1. Spearman's correlation coefficient matrix with color-coded correlation coefficients (upper right denotes correlation coefficients as bubble size while lower left provides the actual coefficients as numbers). Blank spaces indicate a nonsignificant correlation defined by a P-value of >0.01.

Consequently, in order to follow this path of research, the aim of this study was to investigate the correlation of ADC values with cell cycle and proliferative biomarkers (p53, p21, Ki67) and to establish its potential role as a noninvasive biomarker for prediction of cell cycle, proliferative activity and biological aggressiveness in bladder cancer.

Materials and Methods

Patients

Patients with suspected bladder cancer that underwent 3.0 Tesla DW-MRI of the bladder before TUR-B and, in case of muscle invasive bladder cancer, subsequent radical cystectomy were eligible for this prospective study which was approved by the ethical review board of the medical university of Vienna

(registration number 1749/2012). Only patients with histopathologically proven bladder cancer were included in our analysis. All patients provided written informed consent for use of anonymised data including medical images for the purpose of this study.

MRI protocol

The examination was conducted using a whole body MRI system at a field strength of 3-Tesla (TIM Trio, Siemens, Erlangen, Germany). Dedicated vendor-supplied phased-array receiver coils were used for image acquisition. The imaging protocol included an Echo-Planar-Imaging based Diffusion Weighted Imaging (DWI) sequence (TR 7500 ms, TE_{eff} 84 ms, 3 b-values: 50, 400, 1000 s/mm^2, parallel imaging using GRAPPA factor 2, receiver bandwidth 1736 Hz, echo spacing 0.92 ms,

Table 1. Mean ADC values stratified by molecular biomarker results.

Prognostic factor	N	ADC (Median)	ADC (IQR)	P-value*
p21≥10%	32	1.101	0.426	0.080
p21<10%	9	0.856	0.324	
p53≥10%	24	0.906	0.489	0.030
p53<10%	17	1.205	0.254	
Ki67>20%	20	0.897	0.415	0.032
Ki67≤20%	21	1.205	0.316	

*derived from two-sided Mann-Whitney-U test.

Table 2. Clinicopathological features stratified by biomarker results.

Prognostic factor	N	Size (median)	Size (IQR)	≥T2+/−(n)	High grade +/−(n)	LVI +/−(n)
p21>10%	32	12	14	4/28	12/20	5/27
p21≤10%	9	24	39	6/3	7/2	6/3
p53>10%	24	14	31	10/14	16/8	11/13
p53≤10%	17	13	13	0/17	3/14	0/17
Ki67>20%	20	19	29	9/11	14/6	9/11
Ki67≤20%	21	10	14	1/20	5/16	2/19

spatial resolution 1.8*1.5*5 mm, acquisition time 6 min.) Pixel-wise monoexponential regression of measured signal intensity values at different b-values was used to calculate Apparent Diffusion Coefficient maps.

Histology and Immunohistochemistry

The histological specimens taken from TUR-B and, in case of muscle invasive bladder cancer, radical cystectomy were immunohistochemically stained for the following markers: p53, p21, and ki67. Two board-certified uropathologists reviewed the stained slices blinded to DW-MRI results. Further, histological grade and T-stage were classified according to the WHO 2004 and the 2009 TNM classification, respectively.

For immunohistochemical stainings on serial sections from paraffin-embedded tumor blocks BenchMark ULTRA IHC/ISH Staining Module (Ventana/Roche) with the following antibodies: p53 (Neomarkers, RM-9105-S, 1:50 for 32 min, pretreatment ULTRA CC1-52 min), p21 (Oncogene, OP64, 1:100 for 32 min, pretreatment ULTRA CC1-36 min), and Ki67 (Novocastra, NCL-Ki67, 1:20 for 1 hour 12 min, pretreatment ULTRA CC1-76 min). 500 nuclei were counted in a hotspot and percentage of positive nuclei per area was evaluated within each specimen. p53 immunoreactivity was considered altered when samples demonstrated at least ≥10% nuclear reactivity [10]. p21 immunoreactivity was considered altered when samples had ≤ 10% staining [11]. Ki67 staining was considered to be altered when samples had >20% reactivity [12] [13][14].

Data analysis

Imaging data was analyzed on a dedicated workstation (Siemens Leonardo MMWP, Munich, Germany) by two independent radiologists experienced in DW-MRI and bladder cancer imaging. Solid parts of the investigated lesions were carefully identified on DWI images and ADC values were measured by placing a small (5–15 pixels) region of interest (ROI) on the ADC map avoiding postsurgical changes, necrosis or cystic tumor parts. In addition, a ROI was placed in the unaffected bladder wall. The mean ADC values were noted for further analysis. Lesion size was measured using electronic calipers on the MRI image.

Statistical analysis

Statistical analysis was performed after testing the normal distribution of data using the Kolmogorov-Smirnoff test. ADC measurement reproducibility was addressed by calculating the coefficient of variation and the intraclass correlation coefficient. Multiple nonparametric spearman correlation analyses of averaged ADC values of both readers with immunohistochemically assessed prognostic factors and clinicopathological features were performed and the results visualized as a color-coded correlation matrix. P-values <0.05 were considered significant in this exploratory correlation analysis. Using clinically usual cut-off values for dichotomization of immunohistochemically measured biomarkers, Mann-Whitney-U tests were performed to prove group differences. For multivariate identification of independent predictors of clinicopathologic prognostic factors, binary logistic regression with forward feature selection based on likelihood ratios

Table 3. Multivariate binary logistic regression models and their according area under the ROC curve (AUC) for prediction of clinicopathological bladder cancer features.

Predicted linicopathological parameter	Selected prognostic factor	Regression coefficient	Standard error	P-value	AUC (95% CI)
					0.926 (0.843–1)
<T2 vs. ≥T2*	ADC	−0.005	0.002	0.013	
	p53	0.007	0.003	0.018	
LVI°	p21	−0.006	0.003	0.039	0.830 (0.687–0.973)
	p53	0.005	0.003	0.070	
Grading+	ADC	−0.014	0.005	0.010	0.981 (0.945–1)
	p21	−0.008	0.004	0.035	
Size <30 mm vs ≥30 mm|	ADC	−0.004	0.002	0.019	0.774 (0.578–0.970)

Method: forward feature selection (likelihood ratios).
Nagelkerke R-squared: *0.574, °:0.445, +: 0.852, |: 0.244.
Hosmer and Lemeshow test: *P = 0.229, °P = 0.901, +P = 0.225, |P = 0.244.

(entry and remove limits of 0.05 and 0.1, respectively) was performed. Nagelkerkes R-squared and the Hosmer and Lemeshow test were calculated in order to demonstrate the validity of the regression models. Predicted probabilities were saved as a variable and the area under the ROC curve (AUC) of each model was calculated using ROC analysis.

All statistical analyses were performed using the software programs R-statistics (version 3.0.3 "Warm Puppy", the R foundation), Medcalc 13 (Medcalc, Mariakerke, Belgium) and SPSS 22 (IBM).

Results

Forty-one patients (mean age 68y, range 41–89 years, 9 female, 31 male) were included. Of these, thirty-seven patients underwent MRI prior to TUR-B. Four patients were examined by MRI one to 27 days after TUR-B prior to cystectomy. All four patients showed bulky residual disease on MRI. There were 20 Ta, 11 T1 and 10 T2 urothelial carcinoma. Eleven patients with stage T1 received BCG therapy for one year and no patient underwent radiation or neoadjuvant chemotherapy. Median lesion size was 13 mm (IQR 19 mm) with a range of 4–80 mm. Median time between TUR-B and MRI was two days, ranging between 28 days prior to 27 days after TUR-B.

The median bladder cancer lesion ADC value was 1.032 (IQR 0.449) $*10^{-3}$ mm^2/s. The coefficient of variation between both readers was 7.7%, the intraclass correlation coefficient was 0.97. The median ADC value of the unaffected bladder wall (1.338, IQR 0.384 $*10^{-3}$ mm^2/s) was significantly higher than the ADC value of bladder cancer (P = 0.000018). We identified significant correlations (P<0.05) between clinicopathological factors, prognostic immunohistochemical markers and ADC values obtained from DW-MRI. Regarding clinicopathological factors, ADC values were inversely correlated with tumor size (P = 0,000277), stage (P = 0,000002), lymphovascular invasion (P = 0.004) and grade (P = $6*10^{-10}$). Regarding molecular biomarkers, a weak positive correlation was observed between ADC and p21 (P = 0.038) and a moderate negative correlation was present between ADC and p53 (0.024) and ki67 (P = 0.007) expression. Details on correlation coefficients are given in a correlation matrix (Figure 1).

Applying clinical cut-off values for immunohistochemically derived prognostic factors, the Mann-Whitney-U test identified significant ADC group differences between p53, and ki67 (Table 1).

Regarding prognostic factors and clinicopathological factors, positive correlations were identified regarding tumor size for p53 (P = 0.013) and ki67 (P = 0.018). Stage, lymphovascular invasion (LVI) and grading were each negatively correlated with p21 (P = 0.001, P = 0.001 and P = 0.0002, respectively) and positively correlated with p53 (P = 0.0005, P = 0.001 and P = 0.0002, respectively) and ki67 (P = 0.001, P = 0.0003 and P = 0.012, respectively; cf Figure 1 and Table 2).

In order to identify independent predictive factors for clinicopathological variables, multivariate logistic regression analysis was performed. ADC and p53 were both independent predictors of muscle invasion (P<0.05, respectively, cf Table 3). Both p21 and p53 were independent predictors for lymphovascular invasion; ADC and p21 were independent predictors of tumor grade. Regarding lesion size, ADC was the only independent variable selected by the regression model (P = 0.019). Detailed regression results are given in Table 3. Representative clinical examples are given in Figure 2, Figure 3 and Figure 4.

Discussion

The present study showed significant correlations between ADC values obtained from DW-MRI and clinicopathological prognostic criteria, specifically histological grade, tumour size and muscle invasiveness. Further, significant correlations between ADC values and the prognostic immunohistochemically derived biomarkers p53, p21 and ki67 were identified. Despite cross-correlations, ADC was one independent predictor for bladder cancer stage and grade as identified by multivariate analysis. Aggressive muscle invasive bladder cancers present with low ADC values and a high fraction of ki67 positive cells. These findings logically fit to each other: an aggressive neoplasm shows a high proliferation rate as reflected by ki67 measurements while the result of this high proliferation rate leads to an increased cellularity, decreasing the proportion of extracellular to intracellular space. ADC measurements reflect water diffusion in the extracellular space and are relatively decreased in highly proliferative tumors [15]. However, the reason why ADC values are decreased in aggressive cancers is not fully understood, as several authors in several organs have demonstrated associations between ADC values and cellularity of the tumor proliferation rate, however, these correlations are weak

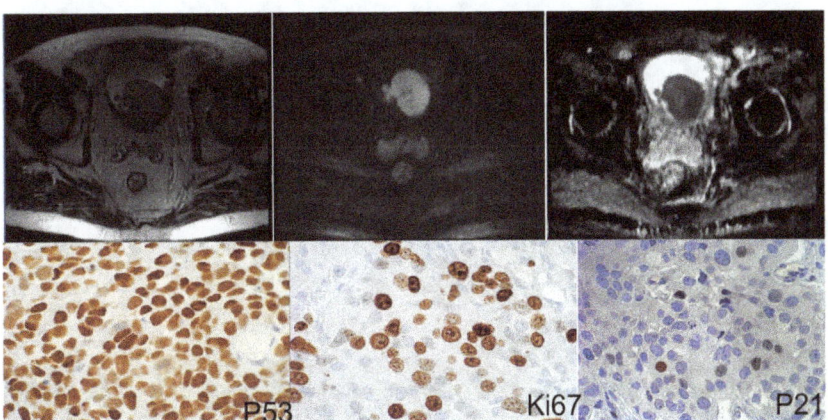

Figure 2. 71 year old male patient. MRI images (upper row, right: T2w, middle: DWI, left: ADC map) show an intravesical mass. ADC value was measured as 0.655 $*10^{-3}$ mm^2/s. Lower row shows immunohistochemical stainings. Percentage of positive cells was 92% (P53), 69% (Ki67) and 1% (P21). Histopathology showed muscle invasive high-grade bladder cancer stage T2a.

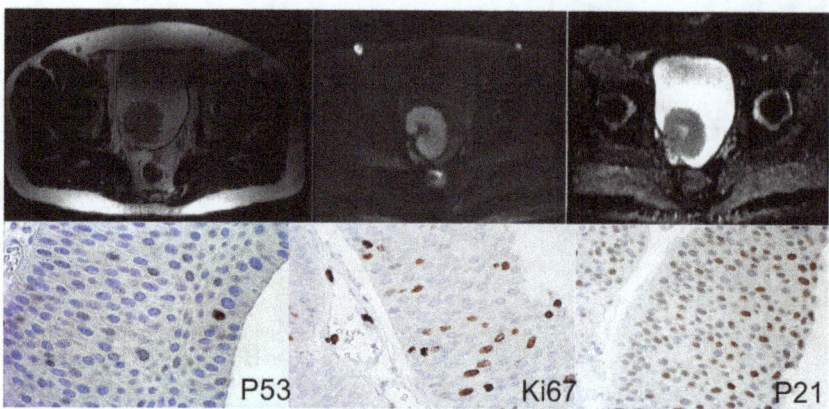

Figure 3. 47 year old male patient. MRI images (right: T2w, middle: DWI, left: ADC map) show an intravesical mass. ADC value was measured as 1.081 *10^{-3} mm^2/s. Lower row shows immunohistochemical stainings. Percentage of positive cells was 6% (P53), 12% (Ki67) and 71% (P21). Histopathology showed non-muscle invasive low-grade bladder cancer stage Ta.

to moderate and thus in good agreement with our own findings [9,16–18]. Further, we investigated p53 and p21: p53 is also associated with tumour stage, pathological tumour grade and lymphovascular invasion. Further studies have reported that p53 over-expression is associated with high grade and higher stage in patients with bladder cancer [19]. It has also been established that p53 is an independent factor for prediction of recurrence progression and mortality in bladder cancer [19]. Recent studies have demonstrated that a combination of cell cycle regulators such as p53, p21, p27 and cyclin e1 provides superior prognostic information as compared to these markers analyzed independently [2]. The association between ADC, ki67, p53 and p21 underlines that ADC values are associated with certain phenotypes of bladder cancer, showing lower values in muscle invasive and high-grade tumors. The reason why we should be interested in another marker of malignancy is obvious: while immunohistochemically derived prognostic markers require invasive tissue sampling and human interaction in selecting representative slides for analysis, ADC values represent the result of a noninvasive, three-dimensional and quantitative test. However, based on our preliminary results, ADC values may also have an incremental prognostic value and are not an replacement for other prognostic

markers. It has been suggested in a recent review, that a combination of prognostic markers in bladder cancer may be needed to provide a complete description of the underlying tumor pathology in this heterogeneous disease [19].

We are not the first to describe associations between ADC values and clinicopathological features in bladder cancer [6,8,9,20,21]. While our results are in good agreement with these previous studies, little is known about the association between ADC values and prognostic biomarkers. To our knowledge, only Kobayashi et al. conducted a study on correlations between ADC, ki67 and clinicopathological features in bladder cancer [9]. Our results go along with this prior study, demonstrating a similar correlation coefficient between ki67 and ADC (−0.47 in our study and −0.57 in the study by Kobayashi et al.). The authors concluded that ADC values are a biomarker for bladder cancer aggressiveness [9]. Our study goes beyond this initial study, as we included further markers of the cell cycle and their associations with both ADC values and clinicopathological factors. Of note, except for lymphovascular invasion, ADC values were independently predictive of all important clinicopathological features such as grade and stage in bladder cancer.

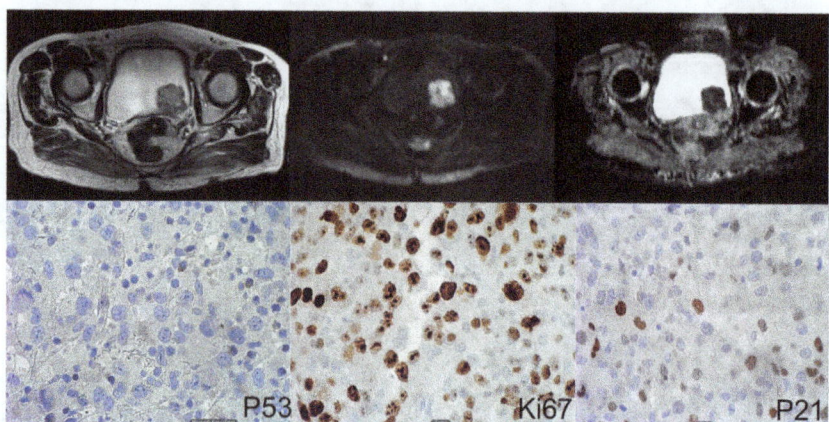

Figure 4. 78 year old female patient. MRI images (right: T2w, middle: DWI, left: ADC map) show an intravesical mass. ADC value was measured as 0.539 *10^{-3} mm^2/s. Lower row shows immunohistochemical stainings. Percentage of positive cells was 0% (P53), 8% (Ki67) and 23% (P21). Histopathology showed non-muscle invasive high-grade bladder cancer stage T1a.

We are obliged to mention limitations of the current study. First, the number of patients included in this study are rather low. This underlines the pilot study character of our research. It has to be stressed that the exploratory multivariate models presented in this text cannot be directly applied in clinical practice as they are not prospectively validated under the same conditions under which the underlying data were collected. However, the positive correlations between the single examined factors and the computed multivariate models have each proven statistical significance and underline the interest in further research on this topic. Further, we did not investigate retest reliability data on the variability of ADC measurements if measured on two different occasions in the same patient. The low variation of ADC measurements in different tumors within this study strongly suggests a low re-test variation. As our study was intended as an exploratory analysis to identify cross-correlations between ADC values and prognostic biomarkers with clinicopathological features. Standardization and reliability analyses are thus beyond the scope of this paper. The coefficient of variation between different readers on the same images was low.

Although we identified correlations with clinicopathological and immunohistochemical prognostic factors, the possible prediction of patient outcomes in terms of disease free and overall survival would be of primary clinical interest. However, the associations identified in our study are very suggestive of a prognostic value of ADC values for patients' outcomes.

In conclusion, ADC values are both correlated with altered proliferative activity in bladder cancer as measured by immunohistochemical biomarkers and, further, correlated with the prognostically relevant clinicopathological presentation of bladder cancer. Multivariate statistics demonstrated ADC values as an independent predictor of BCA grading, size and muscle invasion. Of the investigated immunohistochemical biomarkers, p21 and p53 were predictive of LVI and p53 independently contributed to muscle invasion and tumor grade prediction. Our findings underline the potential role of ADC values as an independent and additive diagnostic biomarker for prediction of bladder cancer biological aggressiveness and provide a basis for further studies validating the utility of these findings for clinical decision-making.

Author Contributions

Conceived and designed the experiments: SS AH LP PATB. Performed the experiments: AH LP MS CS PATB. Analyzed the data: SS AH LP MS HF SFS MH CS TS PATB. Contributed reagents/materials/analysis tools: SS AH LP MS PATB. Contributed to the writing of the manuscript: SS AH LP MS HF SFS MH CS TS PATB. Statistical analysis: PATB.

References

1. Svatek RS, Shariat SF, Novara G, Skinner EC, Fradet Y, et al. (2011) Discrepancy between clinical and pathological stage: external validation of the impact on prognosis in an international radical cystectomy cohort. BJU Int 107: 898–904. doi:10.1111/j.1464-410X.2010.09628.x.

2. Shariat SF, Karakiewicz PI, Ashfaq R, Lerner SP, Palapattu GS, et al. (2008) Multiple biomarkers improve prediction of bladder cancer recurrence and mortality in patients undergoing cystectomy. Cancer 112: 315–325. doi:10.1002/cncr.23162.

3. Witjes JA, Compérat E, Cowan NC, De Santis M, Gakis G, et al. (2014) EAU guidelines on muscle-invasive and metastatic bladder cancer: summary of the 2013 guidelines. Eur Urol 65: 778–792. doi:10.1016/j.eururo.2013.11.046.

4. El-Assmy A, Abou-El-Ghar ME, Refaie HF, Mosbah A, El-Diasty T (2012) Diffusion-weighted magnetic resonance imaging in follow-up of superficial urinary bladder carcinoma after transurethral resection: initial experience. BJU Int. doi:10.1111/j.1464-410X.2012.11345.x.

5. Avcu S, Koseoglu MN, Ceylan K, Bulut MD, Dbulutand M, et al. (2011) The value of diffusion-weighted MRI in the diagnosis of malignant and benign urinary bladder lesions. Br J Radiol 84: 875–882. doi:10.1259/bjr/30591350.

6. Rosenkrantz AB, Mussi TC, Spieler B, Melamed J, Taneja SS, et al. (2012) High-grade bladder cancer: association of the apparent diffusion coefficient with metastatic disease: preliminary results. J Magn Reson Imaging JMRI 35: 1478–1483. doi:10.1002/jmri.23590.

7. Rosenkrantz AB, Haghighi M, Horn J, Naik M, Hardie AD, et al. (2013) Utility of quantitative MRI metrics for assessment of stage and grade of urothelial carcinoma of the bladder: preliminary results. AJR Am J Roentgenol 201: 1254–1259. doi:10.2214/AJR.12.10348.

8. Kobayashi S, Koga F, Yoshida S, Masuda H, Ishii C, et al. (2011) Diagnostic performance of diffusion-weighted magnetic resonance imaging in bladder cancer: potential utility of apparent diffusion coefficient values as a biomarker to predict clinical aggressiveness. Eur Radiol 21: 2178–2186. doi:10.1007/s00330-011-2174-7.

9. Kobayashi S, Koga F, Kajino K, Yoshita S, Ishii C, et al. (2014) Apparent diffusion coefficient value reflects invasive and proliferative potential of bladder cancer. J Magn Reson Imaging JMRI 39: 172–178. doi:10.1002/jmri.24148.

10. Shariat SF, Ashfaq R, Sagalowsky AI, Lotan Y (2007) Predictive value of cell cycle biomarkers in nonmuscle invasive bladder transitional cell carcinoma. J Urol 177: 481–487; discussion 487. doi:10.1016/j.juro.2006.09.038.

11. Stein JP, Ginsberg DA, Grossfeld GD, Chatterjee SJ, Esrig D, et al. (1998) Effect of p21WAF1/CIP1 expression on tumor progression in bladder cancer. J Natl Cancer Inst 90: 1072–1079.

12. Shariat SF, Passoni N, Bagrodia A, Rachakonda V, Xylinas E, et al. (2014) Prospective evaluation of a preoperative biomarker panel for prediction of upstaging at radical cystectomy. BJU Int 113: 70–76. doi:10.1111/bju.12343.

13. Margulis V, Shariat SF, Ashfaq R, Sagalowsky AI, Lotan Y (2006) Ki-67 is an independent predictor of bladder cancer outcome in patients treated with radical cystectomy for organ-confined disease. Clin Cancer Res Off J Am Assoc Cancer Res 12: 7369–7373. doi:10.1158/1078-0432.CCR-06-1472.

14. Margulis V, Lotan Y, Karakiewicz PI, Fradet Y, Ashfaq R, et al. (2009) Multi-institutional validation of the predictive value of Ki-67 labeling index in patients with urinary bladder cancer. J Natl Cancer Inst 101: 114–119. doi:10.1093/jnci/djn451.

15. Padhani AR, Liu G, Koh DM, Chenevert TL, Thoeny HC, et al. (2009) Diffusion-weighted magnetic resonance imaging as a cancer biomarker: consensus and recommendations. Neoplasia N Y N 11: 102–125.

16. Hatakenaka M, Soeda H, Yabuuchi H, Matsuo Y, Kamitani T, et al. (2008) Apparent diffusion coefficients of breast tumors: clinical application. Magn Reson Med Sci MRMS Off J Jpn Soc Magn Reson Med 7: 23–29.

17. Guo AC, Cummings TJ, Dash RC, Provenzale JM (2002) Lymphomas and high-grade astrocytomas: comparison of water diffusibility and histologic characteristics. Radiology 224: 177–183. doi:10.1148/radiol.2241010562.

18. Guo Y, Cai Y-Q, Cai Z-L, Gao Y-G, An N-Y, et al. (2002) Differentiation of clinically benign and malignant breast lesions using diffusion-weighted imaging. J Magn Reson Imaging JMRI 16: 172–178. doi:10.1002/jmri.10140.

19. Kamat AM, Hegarty PK, Gee JR, Clark PE, Svatek RS, et al. (2013) ICUD-EAU International Consultation on Bladder Cancer 2012: Screening, diagnosis, and molecular markers. Eur Urol 63: 4–15. doi:10.1016/j.eururo.2012.09.057.

20. Watanabe H, Kanematsu M, Kondo H, Goshima S, Tsuge Y, et al. (2009) Preoperative T staging of urinary bladder cancer: does diffusion-weighted MRI have supplementary value? AJR Am J Roentgenol 192: 1361–1366. doi:10.2214/AJR.08.1430.

21. Takeuchi M, Sasaki S, Ito M, Okada S, Takahashi S, et al. (2009) Urinary bladder cancer: diffusion-weighted MR imaging—accuracy for diagnosing T stage and estimating histologic grade. Radiology 251: 112–121. doi:10.1148/radiol.2511080873.

22

Fibroblast Growth Factor Receptor 3 Interacts with and Activates TGFβ-Activated Kinase 1 Tyrosine Phosphorylation and NFκB Signaling in Multiple Myeloma and Bladder Cancer

Lisa Salazar[1,◐], Tamara Kashiwada[2,◐], Pavel Krejci[3,4,5], April N. Meyer[6], Malcolm Casale[7], Matthew Hallowell[1], William R. Wilcox[3,5], Daniel J. Donoghue[6,8], Leslie Michels Thompson[1,2,7,9]*

1 Department of Psychiatry and Human Behavior, University of California Irvine, Irvine, California, United States of America, 2 Department of Biological Chemistry, University of California Irvine, Irvine, California, United States of America, 3 Medical Genetics Institute, Cedars-Sinai Medical Center, Los Angeles, California, United States of America, 4 Institute of Experimental Biology, Masaryk University and Department of Cytokinetics, Institute of Biophysics AS CR, v.v.i., Brno, Czech Republic, 5 Department of Pediatrics, UCLA School of Medicine, Los Angeles, California, United States of America, 6 Department of Chemistry and Biochemistry, University of California San Diego, La Jolla, California, United States of America, 7 Department of Neurobiology and Behavior, University of California Irvine, Irvine, California, United States of America, 8 Moores Cancer Center, University of California San Diego, La Jolla, California, United States of America, 9 Chao Family Comprehensive Cancer Center, University of California Irvine, Irvine, California, United States of America

Abstract

Cancer is a major public health problem worldwide. In the United States alone, 1 in 4 deaths is due to cancer and for 2013 a total of 1,660,290 new cancer cases and 580,350 cancer-related deaths are projected. Comprehensive profiling of multiple cancer genomes has revealed a highly complex genetic landscape in which a large number of altered genes, varying from tumor to tumor, impact core biological pathways and processes. This has implications for therapeutic targeting of signaling networks in the development of treatments for specific cancers. The NFκB transcription factor is constitutively active in a number of hematologic and solid tumors, and many signaling pathways implicated in cancer are likely connected to NFκB activation. A critical mediator of NFκB activity is TGFβ-activated kinase 1 (TAK1). Here, we identify TAK1 as a novel interacting protein and target of fibroblast growth factor receptor 3 (FGFR3) tyrosine kinase activity. We further demonstrate that activating mutations in FGFR3 associated with both multiple myeloma and bladder cancer can modulate expression of genes that regulate NFκB signaling, and promote both NFκB transcriptional activity and cell adhesion in a manner dependent on TAK1 expression in both cancer cell types. Our findings suggest TAK1 as a potential therapeutic target for FGFR3-associated cancers, and other malignancies in which TAK1 contributes to constitutive NFκB activation.

Editor: Hari K. Koul, Louisiana State University Health Sciences center, United States of America

Funding: This work was supported by the Multiple Myeloma Research Foundation, Chao Family Comprehensive Cancer Center at UCI, Elsa U. Pardee Foundation, Ministry of Education, Youth and Sports of the Czech Republic (KONTAKT LH12004), Czech Science Foundation (P305/11/0752). The funders had no role in study design, data collection and analysis, decision to publish, or preparation of the manuscript.

Competing Interests: The authors have declared that no competing interests exist.

* E-mail: lmthomps@uci.edu

◐ These authors contributed equally to this work.

Introduction

Cancer is a complex disease arising from the acquisition of somatic mutations that dysregulate signaling pathways central to cell proliferation and survival, angiogenesis, and metastasis. Dysregulation of FGFR3 signaling has been implicated in several cancer types, most notably urothelial cell carcinoma (UC) and multiple myeloma (MM). Urothelial cell carcinomas account for more than 90% of bladder cancers, which have a worldwide incidence of over 350,000 new annual diagnoses and rank as the third most common malignancy in men and the tenth most common in women in the United States [1]. Overexpression or activating mutation of FGFR3 is the most frequent genetic alteration in UC (Reviewed in [2]). Multiple Myeloma, a cancer of terminally differentiated B cells, is the second most common

hematologic cancer with an American Cancer Society estimate of 22,350 new cases for 2013. Among the cases of MM with the poorest prognosis are those 15% with the t(4;14) translocation, which targets both FGFR3 and MMSET (Reviewed in [3–5]). Recent studies indicate that this translocation may be the major clone at diagnosis or, conversely, observed only at the time of relapse [6]. However, the mechanism underlying the aggressiveness of t(4;14) myeloma remains unclear and the relative contribution of FGFR3 and MMSET as putative oncogenes is controversial, as 25% of t(4;14) tumors lack FGFR3 expression. The acquisition of FGFR3-activating mutations (5–10% of t(4;14) cases) with disease progression indicates a role for FGFR3 in MM pathogenesis, and early studies demonstrate the oncogenic potential of activated mutant FGFR3 [4]. It was also more recently demonstrated that wild-type FGFR3, as is expressed in most FGFR3-positive t(4;14) tumors, can contribute to B cell oncogenesis [7]. Furthermore, a wealth of preclinical data demonstrate the effectiveness of receptor tyrosine kinase inhibitors and neutralizing antibody against MM cells expressing FGFR3-activating mutations and wild-type receptor (reviewed in [3–5]). Similarly, inhibition of FGFR3 can induce cell cycle arrest and/or apoptosis in UC [8,9] both *in vitro* and *in vivo*, providing validation that FGFR3 and downstream signaling pathways represent potentially relevant therapeutic targets for the treatment of FGFR3-associated cancers.

FGFR3 is one of four tyrosine kinase receptors that mediate the effects of FGFs on diverse cellular processes, including proliferation, differentiation, and migration. Receptor activation triggers signal transduction pathways implicated in oncogenesis, including the Ras/ERK/MAPK, PLCγ/PKC, PI3K, and STAT pathways [10]. More recent evidence indicates that FGF receptor signaling can also activate NFκB [11,12], the aberrant activation of which is frequently observed in human cancer [13,14] and closely correlates with cancer hallmarks [15]. A key intermediate in NFκB signaling, TGFβ-activated kinase 1 (TAK1), functions downstream of multiple signaling pathways, regulating cell survival, differentiation, and inflammatory responses [16], and stands as a key IKK-kinase of the canonical NFκB pathway [17]. Chemical and genetic inhibition of TAK1 promotes apoptosis in skin tumors [18] and a subset of colon cancers [19], as well as decreasing chemoresistance in breast and colon cancer cells [20] and chemoresistance and NFκB activity in pancreatic cancer cells in culture [21]. Furthermore, suppression of TAK1 signaling reduces NFκB activation in human head and neck squamous cell carcinoma cell lines [22], ovarian carcinoma cells [23], and breast cancer cell lines [24], and blocks breast cancer cell adhesion, invasion, and metastasis in vitro [25]. TAK1 has not been investigated in the context of MM or bladder cancer; however, it's downstream target, NFκB, has emerged as one of the most potent drivers of tumorigenesis in MM, with as many as 82% of MM samples expressing signature activation molecules [26,27]. Consistent with this key oncogenic role, several drugs that are effective against MM, including bortezomib, thalidomide, and lenalidomide, block activation of NFκB (reviewed in [28]). In UC, suppression of NFκB activity potentiates the apoptotic effects of chemotherapeutic agents and cytokines [29,30].

Using a combination of yeast two-hybrid and microarray genetic screening coupled with systems pathway analysis, we identify TAK1 as a novel interactor and target of FGFR3 tyrosine kinase activity. We further demonstrate a role for TAK1 as a positive regulator of NFκB activity downstream of FGFR3 in both multiple myeloma and urothelial cell carcinoma, two cancers with demonstrated FGFR3 involvement [10,31], with modulatory effects on cell adhesion.

Methods

Cell Culture and Transfection

FGFR3-negative (RPMI-8226) and wild-type (LP1) human MM cell lines were obtained from the German Collection of Microorganisms and Cell Cultures [DSMZ; Braunschweig, Germany]; FGFR3 mutant MM cells (KMS-11; Y373C) derived from a MM patient and established at Kawasaki Medical School [32], were generously provided by Dr. P Leif Bergsagel. The mutant FGFR3 bladder cancer cell line, MGHU3 (Y375C), a kind gift from Dr. Margaret Knowles (University of Leeds, Leeds, UK), was derived from a grade 1 tumor [33]. MM and UC cells were maintained in RPMI 1640 (Hyclone; Thermo Scientific, Rockford, IL) and HeLa and HEK293 cells (ATCC) in DMEM

(Hyclone), both media supplemented with 10% fetal bovine serum (Invitrogen). Transient transfection of HeLa and HEK293 cells was achieved using Lipofectamine 2000 (Life Technologies; Grand Island, NY) according to the manufacturer's protocol and MM and UC transfected lines using the Neon system (Life Technologies). Following the manufacturer's procedure, 1×10^6 UC or 2×10^6 MM cells were suspended in 100 µl suspension solution containing 5 µg siRNA (Dharmacon) or plasmid and pulsed under program 3 for UC and program 15 (KMS-11) or 20 (RPMI-8226) for MM cells.

Antibodies and Reagents

FGFR3 antibody (B-9, C-15) and FGFR1/2/4 antibodies were from Santa Cruz Biotechnology, Inc. (Santa Cruz, CA). Antibodies to TAK1, ERK, phospho-ERK, phospho-Tyrosine (4G10), p65 and p84 were from Millipore (Billerica, MA), as was normal rabbit IgG. Recombinant human FGF1 was obtained from R&D Systems (Minneapolis, MN) and PD173074 from Sigma (St. Louis, MO). Non-targeting and TAK1-specific siRNA (both ON-TARGETplus SMART-pool) were purchased from Dharmacon (Thermo Scientific). Human Collagen type IV was from Sigma.

Plasmid Constructs

Untagged or C-terminally FLAG-tagged FGFR3 constructs have been previously described [34], as were constructs for FGFR2, and −4 [35,36]. The vector expressing FGFR1 was generated by cloning full-length human FGFR1 ORF into the pcDNA3.1 vector (Life Technologies), according to the manufacturer's protocol. HA-tagged murine TAK1 was kindly provided by Dr. Hiroaki Sakurai (University of Toyama, Toyama, Japan). NF-κB-Luc was from Agilent Technologies (Santa Clara, CA), and pRL-TK control *Renilla* from Promega (Madison, WI).

Yeast 2-hybrid

A yeast two-hybrid screen was performed as previously described [37]. Briefly, wild-type or constitutively active (K650E) sequences of the human FGFR3 cytoplasmic domain amino acids 399–806) were fused to the LexA DNA-binding domain in the pBTM116 plasmid and used to screen a human chondrocyte library encoding fusion proteins with the Gal4 activation domain (BD Biosciences Clontech, Palo Alto, CA) in the L40 strain of *Saccharomyces cerevisiae*. Transformants were grown 3–4 days on selective media and the resulting colonies subjected to a β-galactosidase filter lift assay. Subsequent domain-mapping was performed similarly, using truncated FGFR3 cytoplasmic domain sequences as bait, paired with full-length or C-terminal TAK1 sequences as prey.

Immunoprecipitation and Immunoblot Analysis

Cells were washed in cold PBS containing 1% sodium orthovanadate and lysed in 1% Nonidet P-40 lysis buffer (20 mMTris-HCl, pH7.5, 137 mM NaCl, 1% Nonidet P-40, 5 mM EDTA, 50 mM NaF, 1 mM sodium orthovanadate, 1 mM phenylmethylsulfonyl fluoride, 10 µg/ml aprotinin). Lysates were pre-cleared with protein A-Sepharose beads (Millipore) and immunoprecipitations performed overnight with 2 µg antibody. Immunoprecipitates were washed 3 times with lysis buffer, boiled 5 min in sample buffer and resolved by 10% SDS-PAGE. Membranes were blocked with Starting Block blocking buffer (Thermo Scientific) and probed as indicated. Antibody binding was detected using SuperSignal West Pico or SuperSignal West Dura chemiluminescent substrate (Thermo Scientific). To reprobe with other antibodies, membranes were stripped of bound antibodies using Restore stripping buffer (Thermo Scientific). Where indicated, densitometry was performed using ImageJ. It should be noted that co-immunoprecipitations from Figure 1E were performed using 30 μl washed Dynabeads (Life Technologies) instead of protein A-sepharose beads and without a preclear step, but were otherwise treated as described above.

Mass Spectrometry Analysis

HEK293 cells were transfected with expression plasmids for TAK1 and constitutively active (K650E) FGFR3. After 24 hours, cell lysates were prepared as described [38,39]. TAK1 immune complexes were precipitated with anti-TAK1 antibody at 4°C overnight, collected with Protein A-sepharose for an additional 2 hours, and then digested with trypsin. Peptides were analyzed by the Proteomics Facility of the Sanford-Burnham Medical Re-

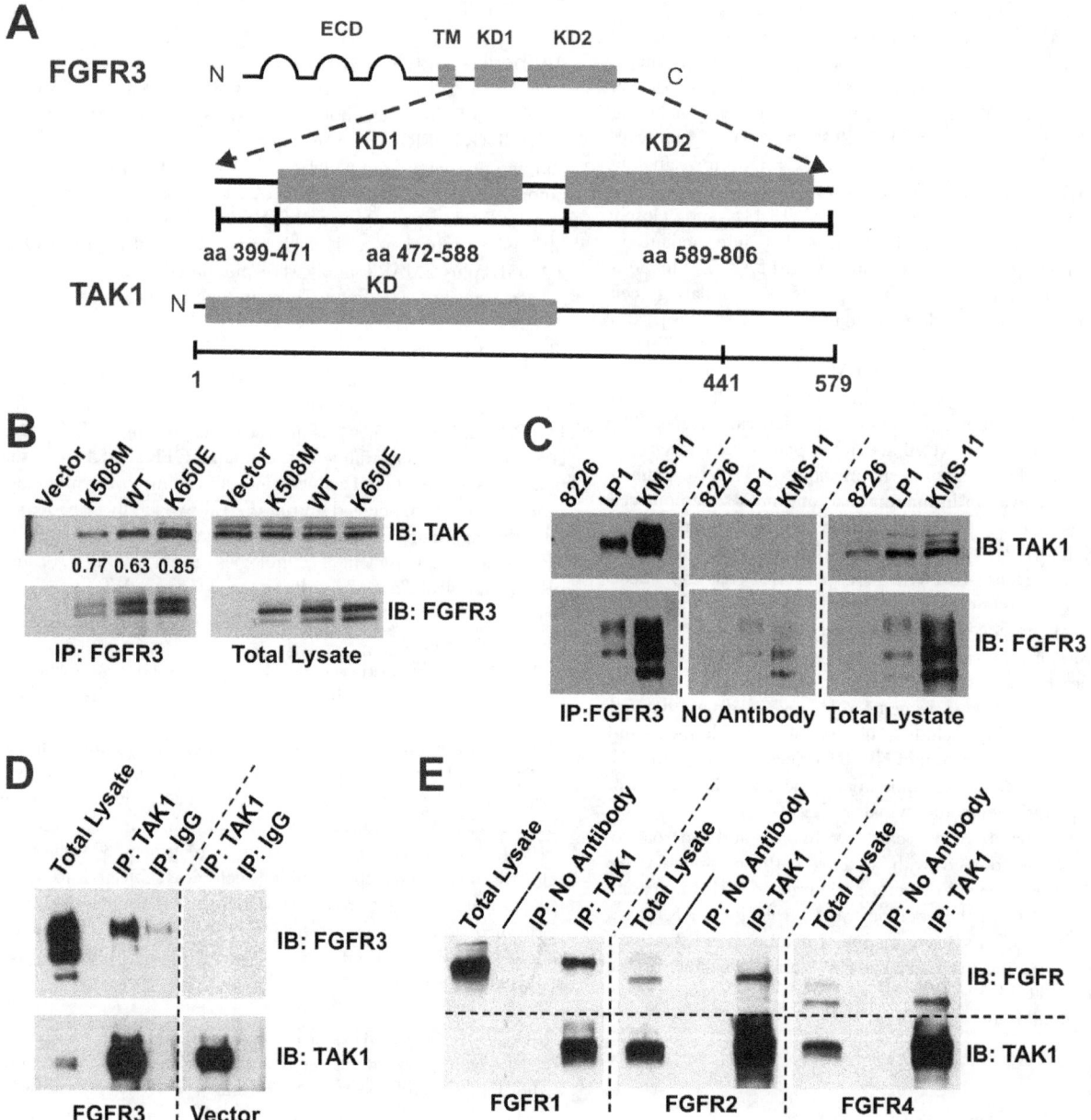

Figure 1. TAK1 interacts with FGFR3. (A) Schematic of FGFR3 and TAK1 domains used for yeast two-hybrid screening and subsequent mapping of the interaction in yeast. **(B)** Endogenous TAK1 interacts with kinase-dead (K508M), wild-type, and constitutively active (K650E) FGFR3 in HeLa cells. Numerical values represent the ratio of TAK1 co-precipitated with FGFR3. **(C)** FGFR3 and TAK1 (both endogenous) interact in LP1 (FGFR3WT) and KMS-11 (FGFR3Y373C) multiple myeloma cell lines. The 8226 line is negative for FGFR3. **(D)** Endogenous TAK1 interacts with FGFR3 in MGHU3 bladder cancer cells transfected with wild-type FGFR3. MGHU3 also express the FGFR3 activating mutation, Y375C. **(E)** TAK1 (endogenous) interacts with overexpressed FGFR1, −2, and −4 in HEK293 cells. TAK1 in the FGFR1-transfected total lysate is detectable upon longer exposure (data not shown). For all blots **(B-E)**, immunoprecipitations were performed from 1mg total lysate using the antibody indicated. Blots were first probed for the interaction partner being tested, then stripped and re-probed for the immunoprecipitated protein. 20 μg total lysate was similarly probed to control for expression and loading. Arrow indicates TAK1. Multiple FGFR3 bands represent various glycosylation intermediates and appear as previously published [45,85]. Four independent experiments were performed for each panel.

search Institute using immobilized metal affinity chromatography/ nano-liquid chromatography/electrospray ionization mass spectrometry (IMAC/nano-LC/ESI-MS) [38,39].

FGFR3 *In-vitro* Kinase Assay

The FGFR3 kinase assays were carried out as previously described [40]. Briefly, kinase reactions were performed in 50 μl of kinase buffer (60 mMHepes-NaOH pH 7.5, 3 mM $MgCl_2$, 3 mM $MnCl_2$, 3 μM Na_3VO_4, 1.2 mM DTT) supplemented with 2.5 μg PEG, 100 μM ATP and recombinant human TAK1 (500 ng; Abnova, Taipei City, Taiwan) as a substrate. The recombinant active FGFR3 intracellular domain (397-End; SignalChem, Richmond, CA) was used at 300 ng per reaction.

Microarray Procedures and Analysis

Cells were transfected with 5 μg non-targeting or TAK1-specific siRNA and allowed to recover overnight. The next day, cells remained untreated or received 100 nM PD173074 for 48 hr before RNA isolation. Each treatment was prepared as triplicate samples. Total RNA was processed as recommended by Affymetrix, Inc. Briefly, RNA was isolated using TRIzol (Life Technologies) and passed through RNeasy spin columns (Qiagen, Valencia, CA) for further clean up. The UCI DNA Microarray Core Facility then quantified total RNA by NanoDrop (Thermo Scientific) and tested for purity using the Agilent Bioanalyzer 2100 (Agilent Technologies). The Ambion WT expression kit (Life Technologies) was used to prepare RNA samples for whole transcriptome microarray analysis. Two ug of the labeled, fragmented single-stranded cDNA was then hybridized to probe sets on a Human AffymetrixGeneChip 1.0ST array. Arrays were scanned using the GeneChip Scanner 3000 7 G and Command Console Software v. 3.2.3. Results are available through the Gene Expression Omnibus (GEO) repository (accession number GSE52452).

Data were imported into Partek Genomics Suite Version 6.6 software with the following operations being done to prepare the data for statistical analysis: 1) RMA Background Correction, 2) Quantile Normalization, 3) Log base 2 transformation, and 4) Summary of Probe sets using mean value. Statistical analysis consisted of one-way ANOVA with a single categorical variable, and gene lists were generated for those genes with fold-change magnitude >2 and p-value with a false discovery rate (FDR) <.05.

Gene lists were then imported into Ingenuity Systems Pathway Analysis (IPA) software, which has functions for generating gene networks, sorting genes into various functional and other categories, and for overlaying genes onto known signaling pathways, coloring by fold change or some other value.

Quantitative RT-PCR

Total RNA was isolated from MGHU3 and KMS-11 cells using TRIzol (Life Technologies) and passed through RNeasy spin columns (Qiagen) for further clean up. Random-primed cDNA synthesis was performed on 1 μg total RNA using the Superscript III RT Kit (Life Technologies). All primer pairs were intron-spanning and a no RT control was included. Primer pairs were as follows: Actin reverse AGGTGTGGTGCCAGATTTTC and forward GGCATGGGTCAGAAGGATT, GAPDH reverse GCCAGTGGACTCCACGAC and forward CAACTACATGGTTTACATG, DFNA5 *reverse* CAGGTTCAGCTTGACCTTCC and *forward* ACCAATTTCCGAGTCCAGTG, GSTA1 reverse CCGTGCATTGAAGTAGTGGA and forward ACGGTGACAGCGTTTAACAA, PSCA reverse GTTCTTCTTGCCCACGTAGT and forward CAGGTGAGCAACGAGGAC, BAMBI reverse GAAGTCAGCTCCTG-

CACCTT and forward TGCACGATGTTCTCTCTCCT, TNFAIP3 reverse CGCTGTTTTCCTGCCATTTC and forward GATAGAAATCCCCGTCCAAGG, SGK1 reverse TGTCAGCAGTCTGGAAAGAGAAGT and forward CGGAATGTTCTGTTGAAGAATGTG.

NFκB Luciferase Assay

Cells were transfected with 5 μg non-targeting or TAK1-specific siRNAs. Twenty-four hours later, cells were transfected with NF-κB-Luc and pRL-TK control *Renilla* at a ratio of 3:1 and were allowed to recover for 24 hours. Where indicated, cells were simultaneously transfected with the indicated FGFR3 plasmids. Cells were then serum starved overnight, followed by an 8 hour treatment with 40 ng/ml FGF1. Luciferase activity was detected using a dual-luciferase reporter assay (Promega: Madison, WI). Differences in NFκB activity following TAK1 silencing under each treatment condition were statistically analyzed using an unpaired two-tailed t-test.

Cell Fractionation

MGHU3 cells were transfected with 5 μg non-targeting or TAK1-specific siRNAs. Forty-eight hours later, cells were serum starved overnight, then treated with 40 ng/ml FGF1 for 0, 5 or 60 minutes. Cells were collected then fractionated, using a protocol adapted from [41].

Cell Adhesion Assay

Cells were transfected with 5 μg non-targeting or TAK1-specific siRNA and allowed to recover overnight. The next day, cells remained untreated or received 50 nM PD173074 for 48 hours before plating of the adhesion assay. Cells treated with FGF1 were serum-starved overnight and treated with ligand 1 hour prior to plating and throughout the duration of the assay. Adhesion assays were performed 72 hours post-transfection. Briefly, ninety-six-well plates were coated overnight at 4°C with 1 μg/ml collagen IV, blocked with 1% BSA for 1 hour at 37°C, and washed twice with PBS and once with serum-free medium. Cells were collected and seeded at 5×10^4 on the pre-coated plates, in the presence of the treatment indicated. Cells were allowed to adhere 3 hours at 37°C, wells were washed 3 times with PBS to remove non-adherent cells, and adherence determined following 4 hour incubation with Calcein-AM (Life Technologies) by measuring fluorescence intensity at Ex/Em 490/520 nm. Statistical analysis of differences in cellular adhesion following TAK1 silencing under each treatment condition was performed using an unpaired two-tailed t-test.

Results

FGFR3 Interacts with TAK1

The identification of protein interactions can provide critical information about specific signaling pathways and identify novel potential therapeutic targets. In MM, the specific role of ectopically expressed FGFR3 in a subset of cases remains controversial, while in bladder cancer, FGFR3 has been recently implicated as an important driver of proliferation [42]. We took a systematic approach to gaining a better understanding of FGFR3 signaling in associated cancers through the identification of new FGFR3 protein interactions using a yeast two hybrid (Y2H) assay. The cytoplasmic domain of human FGFR3 (amino acids 399–806), containing the wild-type sequence or the strongly activating K650E mutation, was used as bait to screen a primary human chondrocyte cDNA library (Fig. 1A) as described [37]. This library was chosen as FGFR3 is highly expressed in chondrocytes, and the strongly activating K650E mutation, present in a subset of both MM and UC [43], is present in the intracellular tyrosine kinase domain. Potential interactions were identified by the filter lift β-galactosidase assay, sequenced, and re-tested for interaction in yeast. Among the interactions identified were signal transduction proteins, including the p85 regulatory subunit of PI3-kinase [37], and TAK1. The yeast prey plasmid consisted of the C-terminal 138 amino acids of TAK1 (amino acids 441–579) indicating that this region of TAK1 is involved in binding FGFR3. We further determined by Y2H using FGFR3 domain constructs (Fig. 1A) that the region encompassing the second half of the tyrosine kinase domain of FGFR3, containing the activation loop of the receptor and C-terminal tail of FGFR3 (amino acids 589–806), is sufficient for the FGFR3-TAK1 interaction. To confirm the FGFR3-TAK1 interaction in mammalian cells and, specifically, FGFR3-associated cancer cell lines, human FGFR3 constructs, including wild-type, kinase-dead and constitutively active (K650E) sequences, were transiently expressed in HeLa cells. TAK1 co-immunoprecipitated with all FGFR3 sequences tested; demonstrating that FGFR3 and TAK1 interact in mammalian cells and that receptor activation is not required (Figure 1B). Endogenous FGFR3 in two t(4;14) MM cell lines, LP-1 (wt) and KMS-11 (Y373C) [44,45], also interacted with TAK1 by co-immunoprecipitation (Figure 1C). As we observed FGFR3 levels were considerably lower in MGHU3 than MM lines, FGFR3^{WT} was overexpressed for adequate detection of a TAK1-FGFR3 interaction in MGHU3 (Figure 1D). Note that the MGHU3 UC cells carry the same FGFR3 mutation as the KMS-11 MM cells. An FGFR3-TAK1 interaction was also evaluated in RT-112 UC cells, which express a truncated wild-type FGFR3 (amino acids 1–758) in fusion with transforming acid coiled coil 3 (TACC3) sequences (residues 433–838) [46]. We were unable to convincingly detect the interaction in this line, further supporting the importance of FGFR3 C-terminal sequences in the interaction with TAK1 (data not shown). Finally, we also utilized mass spectrometry to characterize proteins recovered in TAK1 immunoprecipitates. Following expression of both activated FGFR3-K650E and TAK1 in HEK293 cells, TAK1 immunoprecipitates were analyzed by immobilized metal affinity chromatography/nano-liquid chromatography/electro-spray ionization mass spectrometry (IMAC/nano-LC/ESI-MS) [38,39]. In three independent samples, in addition to significant coverage of TAK1 as expected, FGFR3-derived peptides representing 48% coverage overall were unambiguously identified, as presented in Table 1. Collectively, these results provide evidence of a novel interaction between FGFR3 and TAK1 that does not require activation of the receptor. There is precedence for this with the FRS2 adaptor, which interacts with FGF receptors constitutively, yet only activates downstream signaling (ERK/MAPK) upon receptor activation [47]. We further demonstrate that FGFR1, 2 and 4 transiently expressed in HEK293 cells, also interact with TAK1 (Figure 1E), suggesting that the interaction is broadly relevant to FGF receptor signaling.

FGFR3 can Tyrosine Phosphorylate TAK1 *in vitro*

TAK1 activation requires Ser/Thr phosphorylation at multiple residues in the activation loop (reviewed in [48,49]). Although tyrosine phosphorylation of TAK1 has not been previously reported, FGFR3 functions as a tyrosine kinase; therefore, we evaluated the possibility that FGFR3 might tyrosine phosphorylate TAK1. Indeed, we found that TAK1 was tyrosine phosphorylated in HEK293 cells transiently expressing constitutively active FGFR3 (K650E), but not the kinase-dead receptor (K508M), indicating that activated FGFR3 can either directly or indirectly tyrosine phosphorylate TAK1 (Figure 2A). TAK1 tyrosine

phosphorylation was further observed in a cell-free kinase assay using recombinant TAK1 and the kinase-active intracellular domain of FGFR3, indicating that TAK1 can be a direct target of FGFR3 tyrosine kinase activity (Figure 2B).

Gene Expression Analysis Identifies NFκB as a Signaling Hub for FGFR3 and TAK1 Integration

TAK1 is a key mediator of signaling cascades leading to activation of the NFκB and AP-1 transcription factors, which each modulate expression of genes involved in oncogenesis and apoptosis (Reviewed in [16,50]). To begin to investigate the integration of TAK1 and FGFR3 signaling in cancer cells, we performed a comparative microarray analysis of gene expression in the MGHU3 bladder cancer cell line, which expresses the FGFR3 Y375C activating mutation and exhibits strong responses to the FGF receptor-specific PD173074 inhibitor as assessed by ERK phosphorylation [9]. To identify genes that are dependent on both FGFR3 and TAK1 signals, MGHU3 cells were transfected with non-targeting or TAK1-specific siRNA, and each subset further treated with PD173074, or vehicle control. One way ANOVA with fold change magnitude >2 and p-value with FDR <.05 was used to generate gene lists. TAK1 siRNA versus non-targeting siRNA samples yielded 39 gene changes reflecting TAK1 specific genes in the presence of FGFR3 signaling. TAK1 siRNA plus PD173074 versus non-targeting siRNA plus PD173074 samples yielded 105 gene changes reflecting TAK1 specific genes in the absence of FGFR3 signaling. To discern changes that are dependent on both FGFR3 and TAK1, genes that show statistically significant gene changes arising from TAK1 knockdown only in the presence of FGFR3 signaling but not in its absence were selected. Overlapping genes from the set of 105 TAK1 gene changes in the absence of FGFR3 signaling were removed from the 39 TAK1 gene changes in the presence of FGFR3 activity. The 13 unique genes that remained as significantly altered in these conditions represent genes that reflect both TAK1 and FGFR3 signaling (Table 2).

We chose 6 genes from the list of 13 for validation based on their relevance in cancer, and found that the observed changes were reproducible by qPCR, both in MGHU3 and the KMS-11 MM line treated with TAK1 knockdown and/or FGF receptor inhibition as described above for the microarray analysis (Table 2). The only exception is GSTA1, which has very low levels of expression in MM cells. Finally, input of the list of the 13 genes into Ingenuity Systems Pathway Analysis Tool (IPA) resulted in a single gene network (network score 40) with a major hub around NFκB (Figure 3). These results suggest a critical intersection between FGFR3 and TAK1 signaling that may impact NFκB activation and thus cancer pathogenesis in FGFR3-associated cancers. A second hub focused around PI3K is consistent with our previous results showing an interaction between FGFR3 and the p85 regulatory subunit of PI3K [37].

Activated FGFR3 Positively Regulates NFκB Activity through TAK1

Activation of NFκB contributes to MM pathogenesis, enhancing growth, survival, and metastasis (reviewed in [28]), and also promotes survival of bladder cancer cells [29,30]. Based upon the potential importance of NFκB activity and gene expression profiling results that implicate NFκB signaling as a target for the FGFR3 and TAK1 interaction, we evaluated the combined contribution of FGFR3 and TAK1 to NFκB activity in cancer cells using an NFκB-luciferase reporter assay. As shown in initial assessment of MM lines (Figure 4A), expression of constitutively

Table 1. Mass spec analysis identifies FGFR3 as binding partner of TAK1.

Experiment	Total Independent Spectra	Peptide Sequence	NSP Adjusted Probability	Total Instances	AA Residues
A	360	VAIVAGASSESLGTEQR	0.9998	1	014–030
A	360	IVAGASSESLGTEQR	0.9998	5	016–030
A	360	DGTGLVPSER	0.9999	8	077–086
A	360	VLVGPQR	0.9979	2	087–093
A,C	1460	LQVLNASHEDSGAYSCR	0.9999	69	094–110
A	360	VLCHFSVR	0.9999	10	117–124
A,C	580	VTDAPSSGDDEDGEDEAEDTGVDTGAPYWTRPER	1	26	125–154
A	360	KLLAVPAANTVR	1	4	162–173
A,C	580	LLAVPAANTVR	0.9906	20	163–173
A	360	FRCPAAGNPTPSISWLK	0.9999	2	174–190
A,B,C	677	CPAAGNPTPSISWLK	1	25	176–190
A	360	HQQWSLVMESVVPSDR	1	7	208–223
A	360	GNYTCVVENK	0.9999	1	224–233
A,B,C	677	QTYTLDVLER	1	51	239–248
A	360	HVEVNGSKVGPDGTPYVTVLK	1	2	290–310
A,B,C	897	VGPDGTPYVTVLK	0.9999	56	298–310
B,C	1611	RQVSLESNASMSSNTPLVR	0.9989	21	421–439
A,B,C	2262	QVSLESNASMSSNTPLVR	0.9999	146	422–439
C	220	ASMSSNTPLVR	0.9008	3	429–439
B,C	1611	IARLSSGEGPTLANVSELELPADPK	0.9999	20	440–464
C	440	IARLSSGEGPTLANVSELELPADPKWELSR	0.9999	4	440–469
A,B,C	1628	LSSGEGPTLANVSELELPADPK	0.9994	46	442–464
B,C	220	LSSGEGPTLANVSELELPADPKWELSR	0.9999	7	442–469
B	97	LTLGKPLGEGCFGQVVMAEAIGIDKDR	0.999	1	472–498
A,C	580	AAKPVTVAVK	0.998	3	499–508
A	360	MLKDDATDKDLSDLVSEMEMMK	0.9992	2	509–530
A,C	800	RPPGLDYSFDTCKPPEEQLTFK	0.997	15	571–592
A,B,C	897	DLVSCAYQVAR	0.9999	35	593–603
A,C	360	GMEYLASQK	1	6	604–612
A,B,C	994	NVLVTEDNVMK	0.9999	60	622–632
A	360	IADFGLAR	1	10	633–640
A,C	800	DVHNLDYYK	0.9999	11	641–649
A	360	WMAPEALFDR	1	10	660–669
A	360	MDKPANCTHDLYMIMR	1	2	713–728
A	360	ECWHAAPSQRPTFK	1	12	729–742
A,C	580	QLVEDLDR	0.9982	5	743–750

Mass spectrometry analysis of TAK1 immune complexes prepared from HEK293 cells identifies FGFR3 as a binding partner. The table shows recovered FGFR3 peptides (IPI Protein Index Identifier: IPI00027174,IPI00220253). Amino acid residues refer to the standard FGFR3 protein P22607 (FGFR3_HUMAN) UniProtKB/Swiss-ProtGenBan, 806 aa total length. NSP refers to "number of sibling peptides."

active FGFR3 mutants dramatically increased NFκB transcriptional activity. To determine whether TAK1 is required for NFκB activation by FGFR3, siRNA knockdown of TAK1 was evaluated in MM and UC lines that express endogenous FGFR3. In all lines, whether expressing wild-type or mutant FGFR3, we observed significantly reduced NFκB activation following knockdown of TAK1 (Figures 4 B, C). Addition of ligand enhanced this effect in MGHU3 cells, likely by activating other FGF receptors [42]. As a final test of NFκB activation, nuclear localization of the active p65

subunit of NFκB was evaluated. MGHU3 cells were tested and showed an increase in nuclear p65 upon FGF1 ligand treatment, and levels of nuclear p65 were decreased upon TAK1 knockdown, which is consistent with the NFκB luciferase data (Figure 4D). Notably, TAK1 is not required for the major FGFR3-responsive MAPK signaling pathway, as evidenced by the inability of TAK1 knockdown to alter ERK phosphorylation by FGFR3 (Figure 4E). Taken together, these data suggest a novel signaling pathway in which FGFR3 activates NFκB via TAK1.

A

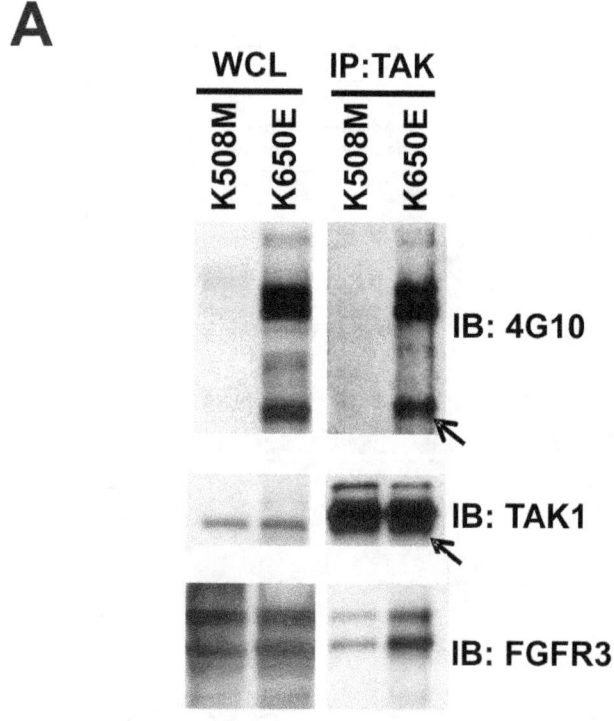

B

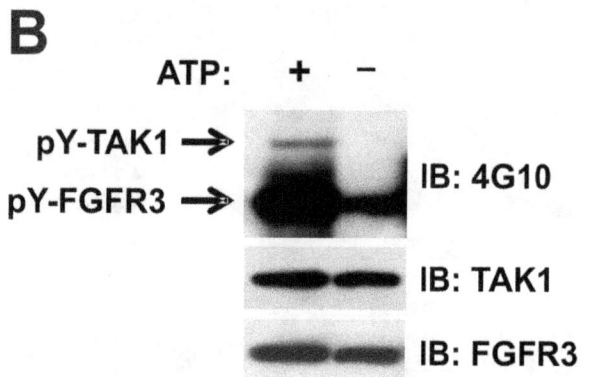

Figure 2. FGFR3 can tyrosine phosphorylate TAK1. (A) HEK293 cells transfected with FGFR3^{K508M} or FGFR3^{K650E}. Twenty-four hours following transfection, cells were lysed and TAK1 immunoprecipitated from 1 mg total lysate. Immunoprecipitates were resolved by SDS-PAGE, blotted, and probed with 4G10 antibody. Arrow indicates TAK1. Representative of six experiments. **(B)** A cell-free kinase assay was performed using recombinant human TAK1 has a substrate for recombinant human FGFR3 (tyrosine kinase domain). Tyrosine phosphorylation was visualized by immunoblotting with 4G10 antibody. Representative of four experiments.

Adhesive Properties of FGFR3 Positive Cancer Cell Lines Change in the Absence of TAK1

Cellular adhesion and migration are critical facets of cancer metastasis, in which altered adhesion to the extracellular matrix allows tumor cells to migrate away from the primary tumor to seed secondary sites [51]. NFκB induces expression of adhesion molecules, including ICAM-1, VCAM-1, and selectins (reviewed in [52]), and NFκB-dependent induction of VCAM-1 was recently reported to promote glioblastoma cell adhesion and invasion [53]. Several reports also define a role for TAK1 [25] and TAK1-NFκB

[54,55] signaling in the promotion of tumor cell adhesion, and FGFR3 mutations have been reported to decrease cellular attachment to extracellular matrix components in benign tumors [56]. As an initial assessment of the functional consequence of TAK1 and FGFR3 signaling, we evaluated cell adhesion in the MGHU3 UC line, based on previous studies using T24 bladder cancer cells [57]. In these cells, FGFR3 inhibition and TAK1 knockdown independently reduce cellular adhesion by approximately 20% (Figure 5). Importantly, simultaneous FGFR inhibition and TAK1 knockdown does not further decrease adhesion, consistent with FGFR3 signaling promoting cellular adhesion through TAK1.

Discussion

This study describes the identification of a novel interaction between FGFR3 and TAK1, a member of the MAPK signaling pathway, both through molecular interaction and at the level of pathway integration. These pathways appear interdependent with selective functional effects on gene expression, NFκB activity and cell adhesion, all involved in oncogenesis. The role of FGFR3 in MM remains controversial, and a recent report implicates FGFR3 as an important driver of UC cell proliferation [42]. This novel interaction and selective effect on NFκB signaling provide new insights into these cancers with therapeutic implications.

The FGFR3-TAK1 interaction was initially identified by yeast two-hybrid screening and subsequently confirmed by Western and mass spectrometric analysis of co-immunoprecipitated proteins from multiple mammalian cell types, including FGFR3-associated malignancies (Figure 1, Table 1). We took a systems approach to examine the signaling integration that might be mediated by this novel FGFR3-TAK1 interaction. Gene expression profiling in UC cells identified 13 unique genes regulated by both TAK1 and FGFR3 (Table 2), which generate a single IPA network (Figure 3) with major hubs implicated in tumorigenesis, including NFκB. Tumor suppressor and other cancer-associated genes were also identified, including TNFAIP3 [58], SGK1 [59], and PSCA [60], which have been implicated in MM or bladder cancer. These findings may provide insight into common underlying mechanisms as well as identify candidates for future study and potential therapeutic development. It is intriguing that higher numbers of TAK1 specific gene changes were identified in the presence of FGFR3 inhibition compared to changes in the presence of active FGFR3. This could suggest that FGFR3 either has a complex impact on TAK1 signaling with both positive and negative effects, or that FGFR3 and TAK1 may also exert independent effects on other downstream pathways. The profiling results suggest that many genes that respond to input from both FGFR3 and TAK1 are associated with NFκB, notably in FGFR3-associated MM and UC. The result is consistent with previous studies indicating NFκB as highly activated and significant to MM pathogenesis [26,61]. Less is known about the role of NFκB in bladder cancer; however, pathway inhibition can induce cell cycle arrest and inhibit proliferation [29], and NFκB nuclear expression is correlated with UC histological grade and T category [62].

We find that TAK1 can activate NFκB nuclear localization (p65) and transcriptional activity downstream of FGFR3 in both MM and bladder cancer cells (Figure 4 A-D). Furthermore, we confirm by qPCR, FGFR3-TAK1-mediated downregulation of TNFAIP3, a known NFκB target gene identified in our microarray analysis (Table 2; [63]). Other TAK1-regulated NFκB target genes identified by our microarray that have also been implicated in FGF signaling include BCL2L11, TNFAIP2, CCND1, CCL20 (MIP-3α), and BCL2L1 (Bcl-xL), the latter two

Table 2. FGFR3 and TAK1 alter gene expression in Bladder Cancer cells.

Gene Symbol	Gene Name	Accession Number	p-value	Direction
ACSL1	acyl-CoA synthetase long-chain family member 1	NM_001995	7.30E-08	Down
VGLL1	vestigial like 1	NM_016267	5.70E-07	Down
ARRB1	arrestin, beta 1	NM_004041	4.82E-07	Down
SCNN1G	sodium channel, non-voltage-gated 1, gamma subunit	NM_001039	1.93E-07	Down
MT2A	metallothionein 2A	NM_005953	1.27E-07	Up
SGK1*	serum/glucocorticoid regulated kinase 1	NM_001143676	5.65E-06	Down
PSCA*	prostate stem cell antigen	NM_005672	2.28E-06	Down
BAMBI*	BMP and activin membrane-bound inhibitor homolog	NM_012342	3.47E-05	Down
TNFAIP3*	tumor necrosis factor, alpha-induced protein 3	NM_006290	1.55E-05	Down
TRIM31	tripartite motif containing 31	NM_007028	1.28E-05	Down
DFNA5*	deafness, autosomal dominant 5	NM_004403	5.18E-04	Up
GSTA1*	glutathione S-transferase alpha 1	NM_145740	1.29E-04	Down
MGAT4A	mannosyl (alpha-1,3-)-glycoprotein beta-1,4-N-acetylglucosaminyltransferase, isozyme A	NM_012214	1.11E-04	Down

A microarray experiment was performed using MGHU3 bladder cancer cells transfected with control or TAK1 siRNA, then treated with or without FGFR inhibitor, PD173074. One way ANOVA with fold change magnitude >2 and a p-value with FDR <0.05 was used to generate gene lists. Lists compared samples transfected with control verses TAK1 siRNA and samples transfected with control versus TAK1 siRNA that were additionally treated with PD173074. Genes common to both comparisons were then removed from the control versus TAK1 siRNA list, and are reflected in the table above. Asterisks indicate further validation done by qPCR in separate experiments using MGHU3 cells or KMS11 MM cells treated as in the original microarray experiment. For TNFAIP3, validation in MM cells was dependent on ligand presence. Expression of GSTA1 in MM cells was not detectable.

shown to be regulated by FGF signaling in an NFκB-dependent manner [64–66]. The ability of FGFR3-TAK1 signaling to activate NFκB is interesting given that we map FGFR3 interaction with TAK1 to the same region (amino acids 441–579 of the C-terminal tail; Figure 1) as the TAB2/3 regulatory proteins (amino acids 479–547) required for TAK1 activation by Ser/Thr phosphorylation [50]. Further, both proteins interact constitutively with TAK1 (Figure 1 and [50]), raising the question of whether FGFR3 and TAB proteins bind TAK1 simultaneously, or whether separate pools of TAK1 with different binding partners exist. Given that TAK1 appears to be a substrate of FGFR3, both in culture and in cell-free kinase assay (Figure 2), it is possible that FGFR3 may activate TAK1 through a mechanism of tyrosine phosphorylation. Phosphotyrosine mapping functional analysis is in progress to address this question. This is the first published evidence of TAK1 tyrosine phosphorylation, although Netphos 2.0 server (http://www.cbs.dtu.dk/services/NetPhos/) has identified three to four tyrosine residues, depending on the TAK1 isoform, with high phosphorylation prediction scores. The importance of these data is further illustrated by the identification of novel FGF receptor-mediated tyrosine phosphorylation of IKKβ, which lies downstream of TAK1 [67,68]. The IKKβ tyrosine phosphorylation, in conjunction with our TAK1 phosphorylation data leads us to propose that NFκB signaling may be a critical component of FGF receptor cellular activity and oncogenic potential.

NFκB activation in MGHU3 bladder cancer cells is further enhanced by addition of ligand (Figure 4C). This is in contrast to the KMS11 and LP1 MM lines (Figure 4B, C) which have FGFR3 overexpression and constitutive activation resulting from the t(4:14) translocation [3–5], as well as elevated NFκB activity due to loss of function mutations in TRAF3, which may account for the dampened ligand responsiveness [26,27]. Ligand responsiveness in MGHU3 cells may result from the stimulation of other FGF receptors, which we have not examined in detail, as FGFR3

is the most relevant FGF receptor for this cancer type. Recent studies demonstrate that FGFR3 and FGFR1 expression in UC cells are restricted to cells which also express epithelial or mesenchymal markers, respectively [42]. FGFR2 and FGFR4 exhibit a similar enrichment in epithelial or mesenchymal cells, respectively, but are expressed at much lower levels. These observations suggest that NFκB responsiveness to FGF1 in MGHU3 cells may be due to stimulation of FGFR2. While such a possibility would be surprising given recent reports that FGFR2 acts as a negative regulator of NFκB activity and suppresses tumor growth in UC cells [68,69], it is consistent with our finding that FGFR2 can also interact with TAK1 (Figure 1E).

Importantly, silencing of TAK1 reduces NFκB activity to similar levels in the presence or absence of added ligand, suggesting that multiple FGF receptors may stimulate NFκB through interaction with TAK1. Indeed, we observe that FGFR1, 2, and 4 can all interact with TAK1 (Figure 1E), and over-activation of all has been associated with various human cancers, including those of the breast, lung, colon, endometrium, and prostate (reviewed in [10,31]). It is therefore possible that TAK1-mediated activation of NFκB may be a common pathway of FGF receptor signaling and potentially relevant to multiple FGF receptor-associated malignancies.

Although FGFR3 can elicit effects on downstream signaling targets of TAK1, we found that TAK1 does not affect downstream FGFR3 signaling, as demonstrated by the inability of TAK1 knockdown to alter the ERK phosphorylation profile (Figure 4E and data not shown). This is in contrast to the effect of knocking down p85 subunits, which does modulate ERK1/2 phosphorylation [37]. These results suggest that the FGFR3/TAK1 effects are novel and distinct from the classically studied ERK/MAPK signaling pathways.

It was recently reported that TGFβ-Smad signaling promotes hepatic fibrosis and carcinogenesis in mice with a hepatocyte-specific deletion of TAK1 [70]. TGFβ is not likely to have the

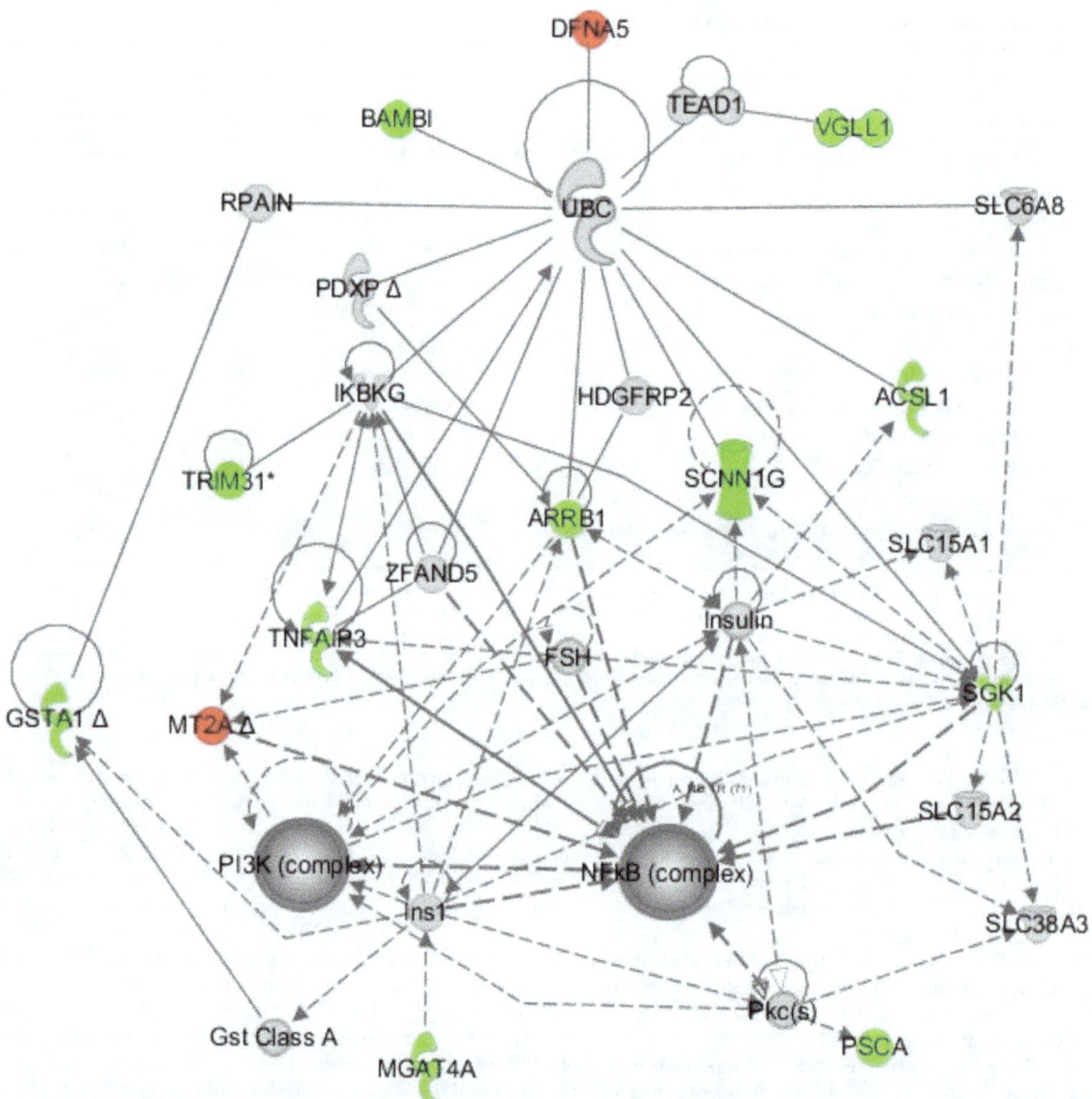

Figure 3. Genes dependent on FGFR3 and TAK1 signaling map to signaling networks with a major hub around NFκB. The 13 unique FGFR3 and TAK1 dependent genes (Table 1) were evaluated by Ingenuity Pathway Analysis (IPA) software, producing a single network (network score of 40) containing major hubs at NFκB and PI3K. IPA molecular shapes include: complex/group (NFκB, PI3K), cytokine/growth factor (IKBKG, SGK1), enzyme (ACSL1, GSTA1, MGAT4A, PDXP, TNFAIP3, UBC), ion channel (SCNNIG), transcriptional regulator (TEAD1, VGLL1), transporter (SLC6A8, SLC15A1, SLC15A2, SLC38A3), and other (ARRB1, BAMBI, DFNA5, FSH, GST Class A, HDGFRP2, Ins1, Insulin, MT2A, PKC(s), PSCA, RPAIN, TRIM31, ZFAND5). IPA Relationships: solid lines indicate direct interaction; dashed lines indicate indirect interaction; filled arrows indicate "acts on"; open arrows indicate "translocates to"; -| indicates "inhibits" and -|► indicates "acts on and inhibits. Green/red indicates genes down/up-regulated in the microarray (Table 1).

same effect here since TGFβ signaling is typically antagonized by FGF signaling through the ERK/MAPK pathway [71–73], and, in the case of MM cells, malignant cells express fewer surface receptors and are resistant to TGFβ signaling [74–77]. FGF signaling through ERK can phosphorylate Smad in some systems [78,79], and TGFβ signaling can increase ERK/MAPK signaling by FGF receptors through downregulation of the negative regulator, Sprouty2 [80]; however, both function to inhibit Smad transcriptional activity, indicating that FGF is not likely to behave similarly to TGFβ in the absence of TAK1. However, this possibility was not evaluated in the current study.

Both FGFR3 mutations [56] and TAK1-NFκB signaling [53–55] have been implicated in the regulation of cell adhesion, alterations of which appear to have a central role in facilitating the metastatic process [51,81]. Our initial evaluation of FGFR3 and TAK1 signals to adhesion of MGHU3 UC indicates that both function to promote cellular adhesion, possibly in a linear manner (Figure 5). These results are consistent both with the roles of FGFR3 and TAK1 in promoting cancer cell adhesion and invasion, and with previous studies which show reduced soft agar colony formation of MGHU3 cells following FGFR3 inhibition by siRNA or drug treatment [82]. However, FGFR1 and FGFR3 are

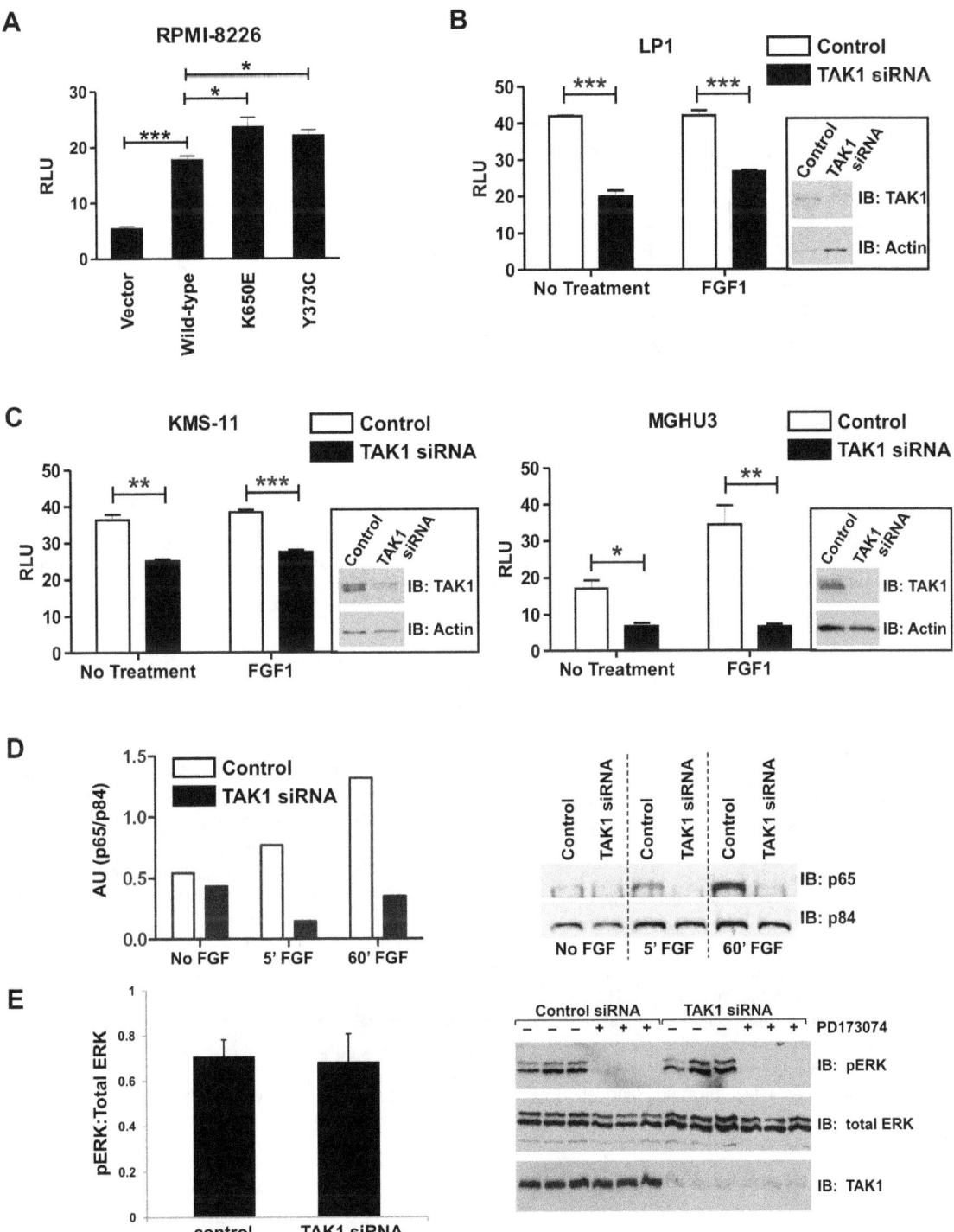

Figure 4. TAK1 knockdown inhibits FGFR3-dependent NFκB activation. (A) 8226 (FGFR3 negative) MM cells were transfected with 5 μg FGFR3 constructs or empty vector, and NF-κB-Luc and pRL-TK control *Renilla* reporter at a ratio of 3:1, respectively for 48 hours. Cells were then lysed and assayed for dual-luciferase activity. **(B, C)** FGFR3-expressing bladder and MM cell lines were transfected with control or TAK1 siRNA, and 24 hours later with κB-Luc and pRL-TK control *Renilla* reporter at a ratio of 3:1. The following day, cells were serum-starved overnight and treated with ligand (FGF1) for 8 hours prior to lysis and dual-luciferase assay. **(D)** MGHU3 cells were transfected with TAK1 or non-targeting siRNA for 48 hours, serum starved overnight then treated with FGF1 ligand for the time indicated. Cells were then fractionated, and 10 μg of nuclear fraction was run on an SDS-page gel and western blotted. Blots were probed with anti-p65 and anti-p84 (nuclear marker) antibodies. Densitometry was performed and p65 measurements were normalized to p84 measurements. **(E)** FGFR3 signaling is not altered by TAK1 knockdown. KMS11 cells were transfected with control or TAK1 siRNA and, 24 hours later, treated with or without FGFR inhibitor, PD173074 for an additional 24 hours. Western blots were probed with p-ERK, total ERK and TAK1 antibodies. Statistical analysis was performed using a t-test; (*) $p < 0.05$; (**) $p < 0.01$; (***) $p < 0.001$. Four independent experiments were performed.

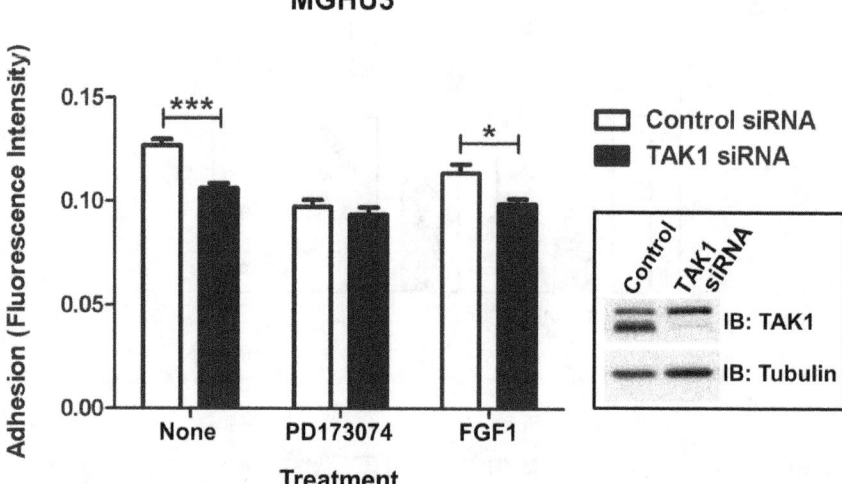

Figure 5. TAK1 knockdown reduces cell adhesion of FGFR3-associated bladder cancer. FGFR3-positive MGHU3 (Y375C) bladder cancer cells were transfected with control or TAK1 siRNA and treated with FGFR3 inhibitor (PD173074) or ligand (FGF1). PD173074 was added 3 hours after transfection and remained present through the duration of the experiment. FGF1-treated cells were serum-starved overnight and FGF1 added 1 hour prior to plating on collagen. Forty-eight hours post-transfection, cells were counted and plated on collagen type IV-coated tissue culture plastic. Cells were allowed to adhere 3 hours and adherence determined by fluorescence intensity following uptake of Calcein-AM. Statistical analysis was performed using a t-test; (*) $p < 0.05$; (***) $p < 0.001$; (****) $p < 0.0001$. Representative of five experiments.

reported to have largely non-overlapping roles in regulating invasion/metastasis or proliferation in UC cells expressing mesenchymal or epithelial markers, respectively [42]. Since we show that TAK1 can interact with FGF receptors 1–4 (Figure 1E), it will be important for future studies to consider the FGF receptor(s) expressed, as well as the cellular context.

Given the nearly identical signaling profiles in terms of ERK, NFκB and gene expression for this newly identified FGFR3-TAK1 pathway, it is likely that similar outcomes will be observed for the two cancers. However, unique outcomes are also possible given the different cell contexts, the tumor type, and the fact that FGFR3 mutations are associated with an early stage and less aggressive form of cancer in the bladder, while in MM, FGFR3 mutations are more associated with cancer progression (Reviewed in [2,4]). Notably, the cellular context in which activating FGFR3 mutations are expressed is implicated in functional outcomes. In chondrocytes, activating FGFR3 mutations induce cell cycle arrest and premature senescence, but drive excessive proliferation in associated tumors, including multiple myeloma and bladder cancer ([83] and reviewed in [84]). These complex roles for FGFR3 in disease suggests that FGFR3 signaling outcomes may

be related to cellular context and highlights the importance of systems wide approaches, such as described here, in understanding mechanisms and identifying therapeutic targets for disease specific treatments.

In this report, we provide evidence of a role for a highly integrated interaction between FGFR3 and TAK1 in bladder cancer and MM cases in which FGFR3 is implicated, laying the ground work for further understanding of these cancers and/or identification of other cancers in which these intersecting pathways are impacted. Finally, the specificity of gene expression modulation and impact on NFκB activation and other relevant oncogenic processes suggest the potential for highly selective therapeutic interventions.

Author Contributions

Conceived and designed the experiments: TK LLS PK ANM DJD LMT. Performed the experiments: TK LLS PK ANM MH DJD. Analyzed the data: TK LLS PK MC ANM DJD WRW LMT. Contributed reagents/materials/analysis tools: WRW DJD LMT. Wrote the paper: TK LLS LMT.

References

1. Siegel R, Naishadham D, Jemal A (2013) Cancer statistics, 2013. CA Cancer J Clin 63: 11–30.

2. Iyer G, Milowsky MI (2012) Fibroblast growth factor receptor-3 in urothelial tumorigenesis. Urol Oncol.

3. Kalff A, Spencer A (2012) The t(4;14) translocation and FGFR3 overexpression in multiple myeloma: prognostic implications and current clinical strategies. Blood Cancer J 2: e89.

4. Chesi M, Bergsagel PL (2011) Many multiple myelomas: making more of the molecular mayhem. Hematology Am Soc Hematol Educ Program 2011: 344–353.

5. Herve AL, Florence M, Philippe M, Michel A, Thierry F, et al. (2011) Molecular heterogeneity of multiple myeloma: pathogenesis, prognosis, and therapeutic implications. J Clin Oncol 29: 1893–1897.

6. Hebraud B, Caillot D, Corre J, Marit G, Hulin C, et al. (2013) The translocation t(4;14) can be present only in minor subclones in multiple myeloma. Clin Cancer Res.

7. Zingone A, Cultraro CM, Shin DM, Bean CM, Morse HC, 3rd, et al. (2010) Ectopic expression of wild-type FGFR3 cooperates with MYC to accelerate development of B-cell lineage neoplasms. Leukemia 24: 1171–1178.

8. Gust KM, McConkey DJ, Awrey S, Hegarty PK, Qing J, et al. (2013) Fibroblast growth factor receptor 3 is a rational therapeutic target in bladder cancer. Mol Cancer Ther 12: 1245–1254.

9. Lamont FR, Tomlinson DC, Cooper PA, Shnyder SD, Chester JD, et al. (2011) Small molecule FGF receptor inhibitors block FGFR-dependent urothelial carcinoma growth in vitro and in vivo. Br J Cancer 104: 75–82.

10. Wesche J, Haglund K, Haugsten EM (2011) Fibroblast growth factors and their receptors in cancer. Biochem J 437: 199–213.

11. Ettelaie C, Fountain D, Collier ME, Elkeeb AM, Xiao YP, et al. (2011) Low molecular weight heparin downregulates tissue factor expression and activity by modulating growth factor receptor-mediated induction of nuclear factor-kappaB. Biochim Biophys Acta 1812: 1591–1600.

12. Lungu G, Covaleda L, Mendes O, Martini-Stoica H, Stoica G (2008) FGF-1-induced matrix metalloproteinase-9 expression in breast cancer cells is mediated

by increased activities of NF-kappaB and activating protein-1. Mol Carcinog 47: 424–435.

13. Chaturvedi MM, Sung B, Yadav VR, Kannappan R, Aggarwal BB (2011) NF-kappaB addiction and its role in cancer: 'one size does not fit all'. Oncogene 30: 1615–1630.

14. Perkins ND (2012) The diverse and complex roles of NF-kappaB subunits in cancer. Nat Rev Cancer 12: 121–132.

15. Hanahan D, Weinberg RA (2000) The hallmarks of cancer. Cell 100: 57–70.

16. Landstrom M (2010) The TAK1-TRAF6 signalling pathway. Int J Biochem Cell Biol 42: 585–589.

17. Hayden MS, Ghosh S (2012) NF-kappaB, the first quarter-century: remarkable progress and outstanding questions. Genes Dev 26: 203–234.

18. Omori E, Matsumoto K, Zhu S, Smart RC, Ninomiya-Tsuji J (2010) Ablation of TAK1 upregulates reactive oxygen species and selectively kills tumor cells. Cancer Res 70: 8417–8425.

19. Singh A, Sweeney MF, Yu M, Burger A, Greninger P, et al. (2012) TAK1 inhibition promotes apoptosis in KRAS-dependent colon cancers. Cell 148: 639–650.

20. Martin SE, Wu ZH, Gehlhaus K, Jones TL, Zhang YW, et al. (2011) RNAi screening identifies TAK1 as a potential target for the enhanced efficacy of topoisomerase inhibitors. Curr Cancer Drug Targets 11: 976–986.

21. Melisi D, Xia Q, Paradiso G, Ling J, Moccia T, et al. (2011) Modulation of pancreatic cancer chemoresistance by inhibition of TAK1. J Natl Cancer Inst 103: 1190–1204.

22. Jackson-Bernitsas DG, Ichikawa H, Takada Y, Myers JN, Lin XL, et al. (2007) Evidence that TNF-TNFR1-TRADD-TRAF2-RIP-TAK1-IKK pathway mediates constitutive NF-kappaB activation and proliferation in human head and neck squamous cell carcinoma. Oncogene 26: 1385–1397.

23. Ataie-Kachoie P, Badar S, Morris DL, Pourgholami MH (2013) Minocycline targets NF-kcyB pathway through suppression of TGF-beta1-TAK1-IkcyB kinase axis in ovarian cancer: in vitro and in vivo studies. Mol Cancer Res.

24. Safina A, Ren MQ, Vandette E, Bakin AV (2008) TAK1 is required for TGF-beta 1-mediated regulation of matrix metalloproteinase-9 and metastasis. Oncogene 27: 1198–1207.

25. Ray DM, Myers PH, Painter JT, Hoenerhoff MJ, Olden K, et al. (2012) Inhibition of transforming growth factor-beta-activated kinase-1 blocks cancer cell adhesion, invasion, and metastasis. Br J Cancer 107: 129–136.

26. Annunziata CM, Davis RE, Demchenko Y, Bellamy W, Gabrea A, et al. (2007) Frequent engagement of the classical and alternative NF-kappaB pathways by diverse genetic abnormalities in multiple myeloma. Cancer Cell 12: 115–130.

27. Keats JJ, Fonseca R, Chesi M, Schop R, Baker A, et al. (2007) Promiscuous mutations activate the noncanonical NF-kappaB pathway in multiple myeloma. Cancer Cell 12: 131–144.

28. Li ZW, Chen H, Campbell RA, Bonavida B, Berenson JR (2008) NF-kappaB in the pathogenesis and treatment of multiple myeloma. Curr Opin Hematol 15: 391–399.

29. Kamat AM, Sethi G, Aggarwal BB (2007) Curcumin potentiates the apoptotic effects of chemotherapeutic agents and cytokines through down-regulation of nuclear factor-kappaB and nuclear factor-kappaB-regulated gene products in IFN-alpha-sensitive and IFN-alpha-resistant human bladder cancer cells. Mol Cancer Ther 6: 1022–1030.

30. Kamat AM, Tharakan ST, Sung B, Aggarwal BB (2009) Curcumin potentiates the antitumor effects of Bacillus Calmette-Guerin against bladder cancer through the downregulation of NF-kappaB and upregulation of TRAIL receptors. Cancer Res 69: 8958–8966.

31. Katoh M, Nakagama H (2013) FGF Receptors: Cancer Biology and Therapeutics. Med Res Rev.

32. Namba M, Ohtsuki T, Mori M, Togawa A, Wada H, et al. (1989) Establishment of five human myeloma cell lines. In Vitro Cell Dev Biol 25: 723–729.

33. Lin CW, Lin JC, Prout GR, Jr. (1985) Establishment and characterization of four human bladder tumor cell lines and sublines with different degrees of malignancy. Cancer Res 45: 5070–5079.

34. Krejci P, Masri B, Salazar L, Farrington-Rock C, Prats H, et al. (2007) Bisindolylmaleimide I suppresses fibroblast growth factor-mediated activation of Erk MAP kinase in chondrocytes by preventing Shp2 association with the Frs2 and Gab1 adaptor proteins. J Biol Chem 282: 2929–2936.

35. Galvin BD, Hart KC, Meyer AN, Webster MK, Donoghue DJ (1996) Constitutive receptor activation by Crouzon syndrome mutations in fibroblast growth factor receptor (FGFR)2 and FGFR2/Neu chimeras. Proc Natl Acad Sci U S A 93: 7894–7899.

36. Hart KC, Robertson SC, Kanemitsu MY, Meyer AN, Tynan JA, et al. (2000) Transformation and Stat activation by derivatives of FGFR1, FGFR3, and FGFR4. Oncogene 19: 3309–3320.

37. Salazar L, Kashiwada T, Krejci P, Muchowski P, Donoghue D, et al. (2009) A novel interaction between fibroblast growth factor receptor 3 and the p85 subunit of phosphoinositide 3-kinase: activation-dependent regulation of ERK by p85 in multiple myeloma cells. Hum Mol Genet 18: 1951–1961.

38. Brill LM, Salomon AR, Ficarro SB, Mukherji M, Stettler-Gill M, et al. (2004) Robust phosphoproteomic profiling of tyrosine phosphorylation sites from human T cells using immobilized metal affinity chromatography and tandem mass spectrometry. Anal Chem 76: 2763–2772.

39. Mukherji M, Brill LM, Ficarro SB, Hampton GM, Schultz PG (2006) A phosphoproteomic analysis of the ErbB2 receptor tyrosine kinase signaling pathways. Biochemistry 45: 15529–15540.

40. Krejci P, Salazar L, Kashiwada TA, Chlebova K, Salasova A, et al. (2008) Analysis of STAT1 activation by six FGFR3 mutants associated with skeletal dysplasia undermines dominant role of STAT1 in FGFR3 signaling in cartilage. PLoS ONE 3: e3961.

41. Hacot S, Coute Y, Belin S, Albaret MA, Mertani HC, et al. (2010) Isolation of nucleoli. Curr Protoc Cell Biol Chapter 3: Unit3 36.

42. Cheng T, Roth B, Choi W, Black PC, Dinney C, et al. (2013) Fibroblast growth factor receptors-1 and -3 play distinct roles in the regulation of bladder cancer growth and metastasis: implications for therapeutic targeting. PLoS One 8: e57284.

43. L'Hote CG, Knowles MA (2005) Cell responses to FGFR3 signalling: growth, differentiation and apoptosis. Exp Cell Res 304: 417–431.

44. Chesi M, Nardini E, Brents LA, Schrock E, Ried T, et al. (1997) Frequent translocation t(4;14)(p16.3;q32.3) in multiple myeloma is associated with increased expression and activating mutations of fibroblast growth factor receptor 3. Nat Genet 16: 260–264.

45. Krejci P, Mekikian PB, Wilcox WR (2006) The fibroblast growth factors in multiple myeloma. Leukemia 20: 1165–1168.

46. Williams SV, Hurst CD, Knowles MA (2013) Oncogenic FGFR3 gene fusions in bladder cancer. Hum Mol Genet 22: 795–803.

47. Ong SH, Guy GR, Hadari YR, Laks S, Gotoh N, et al. (2000) FRS2 proteins recruit intracellular signaling pathways by binding to diverse targets on fibroblast growth factor and nerve growth factor receptors. Mol Cell Biol 20: 979–989.

48. Shinohara H, Kurosaki T (2009) Comprehending the complex connection between PKCbeta, TAK1, and IKK in BCR signaling. Immunol Rev 232: 300–318.

49. Sakurai H (2012) Targeting of TAK1 in inflammatory disorders and cancer. Trends Pharmacol Sci 33: 522–530.

50. Dai L, Aye Thu C, Liu XY, Xi J, Cheung PC (2012) TAK1, more than just innate immunity. IUBMB Life 64: 825–834.

51. Mack GS, Marshall A (2010) Lost in migration. Nat Biotechnol 28: 214–229.

52. Pahl HL (1999) Activators and target genes of Rel/NF-kappaB transcription factors. Oncogene 18: 6853–6866.

53. Zheng Y, Yang W, Aldape K, He J, Lu Z (2013) Epidermal Growth Factor (EGF)-enhanced Vascular Cell Adhesion Molecule-1 (VCAM-1) Expression Promotes Macrophage and Glioblastoma Cell Interaction and Tumor Cell Invasion. J Biol Chem 288: 31488–31495.

54. Harikumar KB, Sung B, Tharakan ST, Pandey MK, Joy B, et al. (2010) Sesamin manifests chemopreventive effects through the suppression of NF-kappa B-regulated cell survival, proliferation, invasion, and angiogenic gene products. Mol Cancer Res 8: 751–761.

55. Xie W, Huang Y, Guo A, Wu W (2010) Bacteria peptidoglycan promoted breast cancer cell invasiveness and adhesiveness by targeting toll-like receptor 2 in the cancer cells. PLoS One 5: e10850.

56. Hafner C, Di Martino E, Pitt E, Stempfl T, Tomlinson D, et al. (2010) FGFR3 mutation affects cell growth, apoptosis and attachment in keratinocytes. Exp Cell Res 316: 2008–2016.

57. ZHANG N, SANDERS AJ, YE L, KYNASTON HG, JIANG WG (2010) Expression of Vascular Endothelial Growth Inhibitor (VEGI) in Human Urothelial Cancer of the Bladder and its Effects on the Adhesion and Migration of Bladder Cancer Cells In Vitro. Anticancer Research 30: 87–95.

58. Zhu YX, Tiedemann R, Shi CX, Yin H, Schmidt JE, et al. (2011) RNAi screen of the druggable genome identifies modulators of proteasome inhibitor sensitivity in myeloma including CDK5. Blood 117: 3847–3857.

59. Fagerli UM, Ullrich K, Stuhmer T, Holien T, Kochert K, et al. (2011) Serum/glucocorticoid-regulated kinase 1 (SGK1) is a prominent target gene of the transcriptional response to cytokines in multiple myeloma and supports the growth of myeloma cells. Oncogene 30: 3198–3206.

60. Elsamman E, Fukumori T, Kasai T, Nakatsuji H, Nishitani MA, et al. (2006) Prostate stem cell antigen predicts tumour recurrence in superficial transitional cell carcinoma of the urinary bladder. BJU Int 97: 1202–1207.

61. Baud V, Karin M (2009) Is NF-kappaB a good target for cancer therapy? Hopes and pitfalls. Nat Rev Drug Discov 8: 33–40.

62. Levidou G, Saetta AA, Korkolopoulou P, Papanastasiou P, Gioti K, et al. (2008) Clinical significance of nuclear factor (NF)-kappaB levels in urothelial carcinoma of the urinary bladder. Virchows Arch 452: 295–304.

63. Krikos A, Laherty CD, Dixit VM (1992) Transcriptional activation of the tumor necrosis factor alpha-inducible zinc finger protein, A20, is mediated by kappa B elements. J Biol Chem 267: 17971–17976.

64. Kim HR, Heo YM, Jeong KI, Kim YM, Jang HL, et al. (2012) FGF-2 inhibits TNF-alpha mediated apoptosis through upregulation of Bcl2-A1 and Bcl-xL in ATDC5 cells. BMB Rep 45: 287–292.

65. Kim YS, Min KS, Jeong DH, Jang JH, Kim HW, et al. (2010) Effects of fibroblast growth factor-2 on the expression and regulation of chemokines in human dental pulp cells. J Endod 36: 1824–1830.

66. Nilsson EM, Brokken LJ, Narvi E, Kallio MJ, Harkonen PL (2012) Identification of fibroblast growth factor-8b target genes associated with early and late cell cycle events in breast cancer cells. Mol Cell Endocrinol 358: 104–115.

67. Drafahl KA, McAndrew CW, Meyer AN, Haas M, Donoghue DJ (2010) The receptor tyrosine kinase FGFR4 negatively regulates NF-kappaB signaling. PLoS One 5: e14412.

68. Wei W, Liu W, Cassol CA, Zheng W, Asa SL, et al. (2012) The breast cancer susceptibility gene product fibroblast growth factor receptor 2 serves as a scaffold for regulation of NF-kappaB signaling. Mol Cell Biol 32: 4662–4673.

69. Ricol D, Cappellen D, El Marjou A, Gil-Diez-de-Medina S, Girault JM, et al. (1999) Tumour suppressive properties of fibroblast growth factor receptor 2-IIIb in human bladder cancer. Oncogene 18: 7234–7243.

70. Yang L, Inokuchi S, Roh YS, Song J, Loomba R, et al. (2013) Transforming growth factor-beta signaling in hepatocytes promotes hepatic fibrosis and carcinogenesis in mice with hepatocyte-specific deletion of TAK1. Gastroenterology 144: 1042–1054 e1044.

71. Cushing MC, Mariner PD, Liao JT, Sims EA, Anseth KS (2008) Fibroblast growth factor represses Smad-mediated myofibroblast activation in aortic valvular interstitial cells. FASEB J 22: 1769–1777.

72. Ramos C, Becerril C, Montano M, Garcia-De-Alba C, Ramirez R, et al. (2010) FGF-1 reverts epithelial-mesenchymal transition induced by TGF-{beta}1 through MAPK/ERK kinase pathway. Am J Physiol Lung Cell Mol Physiol 299: L222–231.

73. van Wijk B, van den Berg G, Abu-Issa R, Barnett P, van der Velden S, et al. (2009) Epicardium and myocardium separate from a common precursor pool by crosstalk between bone morphogenetic protein- and fibroblast growth factor-signaling pathways. Circ Res 105: 431–441.

74. Amoroso SR, Huang N, Roberts AB, Potter M, Letterio JJ (1998) Consistent loss of functional transforming growth factor beta receptor expression in murine plasmacytomas. Proc Natl Acad Sci U S A 95: 189–194.

75. Fernandez T, Amoroso S, Sharpe S, Jones GM, Bliskovski V, et al. (2002) Disruption of transforming growth factor beta signaling by a novel ligand-dependent mechanism. J Exp Med 195: 1247–1255.

76. Isufi I, Seetharam M, Zhou L, Sohal D, Opalinska J, et al. (2007) Transforming growth factor-beta signaling in normal and malignant hematopoiesis. J Interferon Cytokine Res 27: 543–552.

77. Urashima M, Ogata A, Chauhan D, Hatziyanni M, Vidriales MB, et al. (1996) Transforming growth factor-beta1: differential effects on multiple myeloma versus normal B cells. Blood 87: 1928–1938.

78. Sabbieti MG, Agas D, Marchetti L, Coffin JD, Xiao L, et al. (2013) BMP-2 differentially modulates FGF-2 isoform effects in osteoblasts from newborn transgenic mice. Endocrinology 154: 2723–2733.

79. Pera EM, Ikeda A, Eivers E, De Robertis EM (2003) Integration of IGF, FGF, and anti-BMP signals via Smad1 phosphorylation in neural induction. Genes Dev 17: 3023–3028.

80. Ding W, Shi W, Bellusci S, Groffen J, Heisterkamp N, et al. (2007) Sprouty2 downregulation plays a pivotal role in mediating crosstalk between TGF-beta1 signaling and EGF as well as FGF receptor tyrosine kinase-ERK pathways in mesenchymal cells. J Cell Physiol 212: 796–806.

81. Christofori G (2006) New signals from the invasive front. Nature 441: 444–450.

82. Bernard-Pierrot I, Brams A, Dunois-Larde C, Caillault A, Diez de Medina SG, et al. (2006) Oncogenic properties of the mutated forms of fibroblast growth factor receptor 3b. Carcinogenesis 27: 740–747.

83. Krejci P, Prochazkova J, Smutny J, Chlebova K, Lin P, et al. (2010) FGFR3 signaling induces a reversible senescence phenotype in chondrocytes similar to oncogene-induced premature senescence. Bone 47: 102–110.

84. Dailey L, Ambrosetti D, Mansukhani A, Basilico C (2005) Mechanisms underlying differential responses to FGF signaling. Cytokine Growth Factor Rev 16: 233–247.

85. Lievens PM, Liboi E (2003) The thanatophoric dysplasia type II mutation hampers complete maturation of fibroblast growth factor receptor 3 (FGFR3), which activates signal transducer and activator of transcription 1 (STAT1) from the endoplasmic reticulum. J Biol Chem 278: 17344–17349.

23

Targeting of Alpha-V Integrins Reduces Malignancy of Bladder Carcinoma

Geertje van der Horst[1]*, Lieke Bos[1], Maaike van der Mark[1], Henry Cheung[1], Bertrand Heckmann[2], Philippe Clément-Lacroix[2], Giocondo Lorenzon[2], Rob C. M. Pelger[1], Rob F. M. Bevers[1], Gabri van der Pluijm[1]

1 Department of Urology, Leiden University Medical Centre, Leiden, The Netherlands, **2** Galapagos SASU, Romainville, France

Abstract

Low survival rates of metastatic cancers emphasize the need for a drug that can prevent and/or treat metastatic cancer. αv integrins are involved in essential processes for tumor growth and metastasis and targeting of αv integrins has been shown to decrease angiogenesis, tumor growth and metastasis. In this study, the role of αv integrin and its potential as a drug target in bladder cancer was investigated. Treatment with an αv integrin antagonist as well as knockdown of αv integrin in the bladder carcinoma cell lines, resulted in reduced malignancy *in vitro*, as illustrated by decreased proliferative, migratory and clonogenic capacity. The CDH1/CDH2 ratio increased, indicating a shift towards a more epithelial phenotype. This shift appeared to be associated with downregulation of EMT-inducing transcription factors including SNAI2. The expression levels of the self-renewal genes NANOG and BMI1 decreased as well as the number of cells with high Aldehyde Dehydrogenase activity. In addition, self-renewal ability decreased as measured with the urosphere assay. In line with these observations, knockdown or treatment of αv integrins resulted in decreased metastatic growth in preclinical *in vivo* models as assessed by bioluminescence imaging. In conclusion, we show that αv integrins are involved in migration, EMT and maintenance of Aldehyde Dehydrogenase activity in bladder cancer cells. Targeting of αv integrins might be a promising approach for treatment and/or prevention of metastatic bladder cancer.

Editor: Francisco X. Real, Centro Nacional de Investigaciones Oncológicas (CNIO), Spain

Funding: This work is supported by a grant from the Dutch Cancer Society UL 2011-4930. The funders had no role in study design, data collection and analysis, decision to publish, or preparation of the manuscript.

Competing Interests: The authors G. van der Horst, L. Bos, M. van der Mark, H. Cheung, R.F.M Bevers, R.C.M Pelger and G. van der Pluijm declare no conflict of interest. The authors B. Heckmann, P. Cle´ment-Lacroix and G.Lorenzon are employees and stakeholders of Galapagos Sasu.

* Email: G.van_der_Horst@lumc.nl

Introduction

Metastasis is a multistep process including invasion of the surrounding tissue, intravasation, survival in the bloodstream, extravasation and colonization of distant sites [1]. For the first steps in this process, cancer cells frequently switch from a sessile, epithelial phenotype towards a motile, mesenchymal phenotype, a process called epithelial-to-mesenchymal transition (EMT). In cancer, aberrant activation of this latent embryonic program contributes to progression to metastatic disease and therapeutic resistance, enabling cancer cells to become invasive, disseminate, resist apoptosis, stimulate angiogenesis and acquire stem/progenitor cell properties [2–5]. For the later stages of metastasis formation (e.g. colonization of a distant site), however, the reverse process of mesenchymal-epithelial transition (MET) may be required [2–5]. The critical involvement of epithelial plasticity (i.e. EMT and MET) along the metastatic cascade are best illustrated by differences in metastatic potential of phenotypical epithelial or mesenchymal bladder cancer cells in preclinical models *in vivo*. At the orthotopic inoculation site, representative for growth at the primary site and the multistep metastatic process, a mesenchymal phenotype is favorable for metastasis formation. However, after systemic (intracardiac) or intrabone inoculation,

thus circumventing the first steps of metastasis formation, a more epithelial phenotype seems favorable [6].

Accumulating experimental and clinical evidence suggests that EMT can generate cells with stem/progenitor-like properties and enables plasticity between cancer stem cells (CSC) and non-CSC [4,7–9], thus providing a link between EMT and CSCs [10,11].

Tumor progression is driven by a subpopulation of cancer cells, the CSCs or tumor-initiating cells that have the ability to self-renew and to regenerate the phenotypic heterogeneity of the original tumor. Furthermore, CSCs have been shown to be involved in drug resistance, colonization and metastasis of distant organs [12–14]. To date, only a limited number of potential CSC markers have been described [15–21]. Recently, high aldehyde dehydrogenase activity (ALDH[hi]) was added to that list. The ALDH[hi] subpopulation of cancer cells was found to be enriched in CSCs and to be involved in metastasis formation in several solid cancers, including breast [22], ovarian [23] and prostate [24] cancer. In bladder cancer, ALDH[hi] cells showed a 100-fold increased heterogeneous tumor formation after subcutaneous inoculation in immuno-compromised mice as compared to ALDH[low] cells [25].

During the process of carcinogenesis, which is often enabled by EMT, disseminated cancer cells seem to acquire self-renewal capability, similar to that displayed by stem cells [10] [11]. This raises the possibility that the EMT process may also impart a self-renewal capability to disseminated cancer cells. During EMT, epithelial markers - including CDH1 (E-cadherin) - are shed while mesenchymal markers, like VIM (vimentin), CDH2 (N-cadherin) and ITGAV/B5 ($\alpha_v\beta_5$ integrin) are upregulated [3]. ITGAV receptors have been shown to be upregulated in cancer in both carcinoma cells and activated endothelial cells [26].

As shown previously by our group, the EMT process in prostate cancer cells could be reversed by adding an integrin receptor antagonist called GLPG0187 [27]. This non-peptide RGD antagonist blocks 6 integrin receptors; all five known α_v integrin receptors with high affinity and ITGA5/B1 ($\alpha5\beta1$) with lower affinity. Targeting of integrins by GLPG0187 inhibited the *de novo* formation and progression of bone metastases in prostate cancer by antitumor (including inhibition of EMT and the size of the prostate cancer stem cell population), antiresorptive, and antiangiogenic mechanisms [27]. GLPG0187 has also been shown to inhibit formation and progression of metastasis in breast cancer [28]. Integrin receptor antagonists, in the form of RGD-antagonists or antibodies, have been shown to decrease angiogenesis, tumor growth and metastasis in several solid tumor types in which ITGAV is upregulated, including breast cancer, melanoma and prostate cancer. [27,29,30]. Several of these antagonists are currently in phase I and II clinical trials [26,31]. GLPG0187 is currently in phase Ib clinical trial for patients with a variety of solid tumors. The effect of blocking integrin receptors by GLPG0187 were similar to effects of knockdown of ITGAV in prostate cancer cells. These data indicate that ITGAV is functionally involved in the migratory, mesenchymal cellular phenotype of prostate cancer cells. Moreover, ITGAV is important for the acquisition of prostate cancer cells with a metastasis-initiating capacity [32].

Inhibition of α_v integrin might also have therapeutic potential in bladder cancer, since ITGAV is significantly overexpressed in bladder tumors (46%) compared to normal urothelium (13%) and a trend is observed of stage and grade-dependent increase in ITGAV expression [33].

In the present study we determined the effect of functional inactivation of ITGAV (targeting with GLPG0187 or knockdown of ITGAV) on migration, EMT and stemness in bladder cancer using the human bladder carcinoma cell line UM-UC-3 and the human papilloma cell line RT-4.

Functional inactivation of ITGAV in bladder cancer leads to a less malignant phenotype as illustrated by significantly impaired migration, EMT response, clonogenicity and a reduction in the size of the stem/progenitor pool. In line with these *in vitro* observations, knockdown of ITGAV or treatment with GLPG0187 significantly inhibited metastasis and secondary tumor growth (in bone marrow).

These data indicate that ITGAV inhibition represents a novel, promising strategy for the prevention and/or treatment of bladder cancer growth and metastasis.

Materials and Methods

Cell lines and culture conditions

The bladder carcinoma cell line UM-UC-3 and the bladder papilloma cell line RT-4 were obtained from ATCC (catalog no.CRL-1749 and HTB-2). UM-UC-3 cells were routinely cultured in ATCC Eagle's Minimal Essential Medium (ATCC) and RT-4 cells in McCoy's 5A+Glutamax medium (Invitrogen Life Sciences, Bleiswijk, the Netherlands), both supplemented with 10% fetal bovine serum (FBS), 100 units/ml penicillin (Invitrogen) and 50 μg/ml streptomycin (Invitrogen). The UM-UC-3 cell line

was stably transfected with pCAGGS3.1 luciferase 2 (modified pGI4 luciferase 2 vector (Promega, The Netherlands)) as previously described [34], resulting in the UM-UC-3luc2 cell line, which was maintained in medium supplemented with 0.8 mg/ml geneticin (Invitrogen). HEK293T cells were maintained in DMEM containing 10% FBS (Invitrogen). All cell lines were grown in a humidified incubator at 37°C and 5% CO_2 and were regularly tested for mycoplasm.

Suppressing ITGAV expression with a shRNA-lentiviral vector

UM-UC-3luc2 and RT-4 cell lines were transduced with short hairpin RNAi constructs against ITGAV or scrambled non-targeting (NT) shRNA derived from Sigma's MISSION library (table S1). HEK293T cells were transfected with the short hairpin constructs together with the packaging plasmids REV, GAG and VSV in a 1:1:1:1 ratio using Fugene HD (Roche) as transfection reagent. Cells were mixed with 1 ml lentiviruses containing the shRNA-lentiviral vector and 8 μg Polybrene (Sigma) was added. The mixture was incubated for 1–2 hours at RT. Cells stably expressing the shRNA were selected using puromycin (1 μg/ml, Sigma). The effects of ITGAV knockdown described in this manuscript, represent activities of the heterogeneous cell populations transduced with high efficiency by the lentivirus and not single-cell selected clones. The αv kd cell lines will further be referred to as sh clone 1 and 2 and the non-targeting control cell line as UM-UC-3luc2 NT cells and RT-4 NT cells.

Migration assay

6×10^4 pre-starved cells (1% FBS for 16 h) were seeded in the upper chamber of an 8-μm Transwell migration chambers (Costar, Corning incorporated, Corning, NY, USA) [24]. Cells were allowed to attach and then either vehicle or GLPG0187 was added. Cells were allowed to migrate for 6 h towards serum-containing medium in the lower chamber. Subsequently, cells were fixed with 4% paraformaldehyde (Merck, Darmstadt, Germany) and stained with 0.1% crystal violet (2 mg/ml, Sigma-Aldrich, The Netherlands). Four random fields were counted for each well and mean numbers of migrated cells/area of 4 fields were calculated (4 wells/condition, n = 3).

Clonogenic assay

Cells were seeded in a 96-well plate at an average of 1 cell/well. After 14–16 days colonies were clearly visible and the size of the colonies and the mean numbers of colony-containing wells per plate were determined by light microscopy (Zeiss Televal 31, Germany) (3 plates/condition, n = 3).

Urosphere assay

UM-UC-3 cells were seeded 100 cells/cm^2 in an ultra-low attachment plate (Corning) in serum-starved conditions (DMEM F12 supplemented with N2 and B27) [35]. The percentage of cells with sphere forming capacity (P0) was measured after 10 days of culture. P0 spheres were dissociated into single cells and seeded in ultra-low attachment 96 wells. The percentage of cells with sphere forming capacity (subsequently P1–3) was measured 10 days after seeding spheres dissociated into single cells. The area of the spheres was measured with Image J software.

Flow cytometry

Cells surface stainings were performed by labeling cells for 45 min at 4°C in the dark (1:10 in PBS containing 0.1% sodium azide and 1% FBS) (table S2). Intracellular stainings were performed by fixing cells in ice-cold methanol, followed by washing with PBS and incubation with 0.5% saponin. Cells were labelled for 30 min at RT, followed by washing and secondary antibody (goat anti rabbit Alexafluor 488) for 30 min at RT in the dark.

Relative expression levels are measured as % of positive cells * mean fluorescence intensity of each condition compared to either the NT or vehicle treated cells. ALDH activity was measured using the ALDEFLUOR assay kit (Stem cell technologies, Aldagen Inc., Durham, NC, USA) as described before [24] (n = 3).

RNA isolation and real-time qPCR

RNA was extracted using Tripure isolation reagent (Roche Diagnostics GmbH, Manheim, Germany) according to manufacturer's instructions. Real-time qPCR was run and analyzed with a Biorad IQ5 cycler (Biorad, Veenendaal, The Netherlands). For primer sequences see table S3. Gene expression was measured relative to GAPDH expression using the following formula: $\log 2^{-\Delta\Delta Ct}$.

Xenograft experiments

Mouse Strain. Female nude mice (Balb/c nu/nu; Charles River, L'Arbresle, France) were housed in individual ventilated cages under sterile condition according to the Dutch guidelines for the care and use of laboratory animals. The protocol was approved by the Committee on the Ethics of Animal Experiments of the Leiden University, The Netherlands (DEC 11082).

Intracardiac Inoculation. A single cell suspension of 1×10^5 UM-UC-3luc2 cells/100 µl PBS was injected into the left cardiac ventricle of 4-week old nude mice as described previously [34].

Intraosseous inoculation. Two holes, 4 to 5 mm apart, were drilled through the bone cortex of the upper tibia with the aid of a 25-gauge needle (25G $^5/_8$, BD Micro-Fine, Becton Dickinson, Etten-Leur, The Netherlands). Space in the bone marrow was created by flushing out the bone marrow from the proximal end of the shaft using a 30-gauge needle (30G ½, BD Micro-Fine, Becton Dickinson). Subsequently, a single cell suspension of 1×10^5 UM-UC-3luc2 cells/10 µl PBS was injected into the tibia of 4-week old nude mice via a 30-gauge needle (30G ½, BD Micro-Fine). Finally, the cutaneous wound was sutured.

Bioluminescence imaging. Bioluminescence imaging (BLI)-was performed using the IVIS Lumina Imaging System (Caliper LifeSciences, USA) [34]. Images were quantified with Living Image and values expressed as relative light units (RLU). Tumor take was measured as the % of mice with BLI foci.

Statistical analysis

Data are presented as mean ± SEM. Two-way ANOVA's were performed followed by the post-hoc Bonferroni test (SPSS20). A P-value <0.05 was considered significant (*P<0.05, **P<0.01, ***P<0.001).

Results

Characteristics of αv integrin knockdown and GLPG0187 treated bladder cancer cell lines

To determine the effect of α_v integrin on bladder cancer, two cell lines were used; the human carcinoma cell line UM-UC-3, representing invasive bladder tumors, and the human papilloma cell line RT-4, representing non-invasive bladder tumors. UM-UC-3 cells were stably transfected with *firefly* luciferase 2 (luc2), and can be used for sensitive *in vivo* cell tracking [34]. ITGAV (α_v integrin) is expressed both in normal urothelium and carcinoma (respectively Figure S1D and S1E). UM-UC-3luc2 and RT-4 cells

were treated with the non-peptide RGD antagonist GLPG0187 in a concentration range of 0, 0.5, 5, 50 or 500 ng/ml. GLPG0187 treatment resulted in a dose-dependent detachment from the tissue culture plastic within 24 hours in both cell lines (respectively Figure 1A and C). No significant effect on viability was observed (Figure S1G) and the effects of GLPG0187 treatment proved to be largely reversible, as cells regained attachment to the tissue culture plastic when GLPG0187-free medium was provided after 48 h of GLPG0187 treatment (Figure 1B and D).

In parallel, ITGAV expression was blocked with 2 independent lentiviral-mediated shRNA constructs which resulted in 99% knockdown of ITGAV in UM-UC-3luc2 sh clone 1 and in sh clone 2, compared to the cells that were transduced with non-target (NT) shRNA (Figure 1H and Figure S1A and S1B). In RT-4 cell, knockdown was respectively 97% for sh clone 1 and 74% for sh clone 2 (Figure 1L and Figure S1A and S1C). Upon knockdown of ITGAV expression, both cell lines displayed strong morphological changes, closely resembling the effect of the non-peptide RGD antagonist GLPG0187. The cells were no longer adherent to tissue-culture plastic and grew in suspension where they clustered together and formed small clumps of cells (Figure 1 E-G UM-UC-3, I-K RT-4). This offered an additional means of selection, since only the cells with very low levels of ITGAV expression detached from the tissue culture plastic (Figure S1F). This effect was not due to reduced viability, since no significant difference in UM-UC-3luc2 viability was observed using Annexin V/PI apoptosis assays (Figure S1G).

Knockdown of ITGAV did not significantly affect the expression levels of ITGA2 in both UM-UC-3 and RT-4 cells (Figure S6A–C). A small decrease in ITGA6 protein expression was observed in RT-4 cells, whereas no effect on ITGA6 was measured in UM-UC-3 cells (Figure S6D–F).

Effects of αv integrin on proliferation and migratory capacity

Subsequently, the effects of α_v kd and GLPG0187 treatment on characteristics that are required for tumor growth and metastasis formation such as proliferation, migration and clonogenic capacity were evaluated. Proliferative capacity was significantly decreased in the UM-UC-3luc2 sh clones (Figure S1H). A decrease, although not significant was also seen in the proliferative capacity of the RT-4 sh clones compared to NT cells (Figure S1I). GLPG0187 did show a significant decrease in proliferation rates of both cell lines 72 hours after treatment with the highest doses of GLPG0187 (i.e. 50 ng/ml and 500 ng/ml GLPG0187; Figure S1J and S1K).

Furthermore, ITGAV knockdown showed a significant and substantial decrease in migratory capacity in a Transwell Boyden chamber assay in both sh clones of UM-UC-3luc2 and RT-4 cells (Figure 2A). Accordingly, GLPG0187 treatment of UM-UC-3luc2 and RT-4 cells resulted in a dose-dependent and significant decrease in migration, and almost completely inhibited migration with the highest dosage used (Figure 2A).

Effects of αv integrin on epithelial plasticity

Acquisition of an invasive phenotype is a requirement for metastasis where transformed epithelial cells can switch from a sessile, epithelial, to a motile, mesenchymal phenotype by epithelial- mesenchymal transition (EMT). Whether α_v integrin is functionally involved in the EMT-like switch in human bladder cancer has remained largely elusive. Therefore, we examined the effects on EMT of α_v knockdown or inhibition by GLPG0187 on the bladder cancer cells. The CDH1/CDH2 (E-cadherin/N-cadherin) ratio, was measured by flow cytometry. During EMT, epithelial markers, including CDH1, are downregulated and

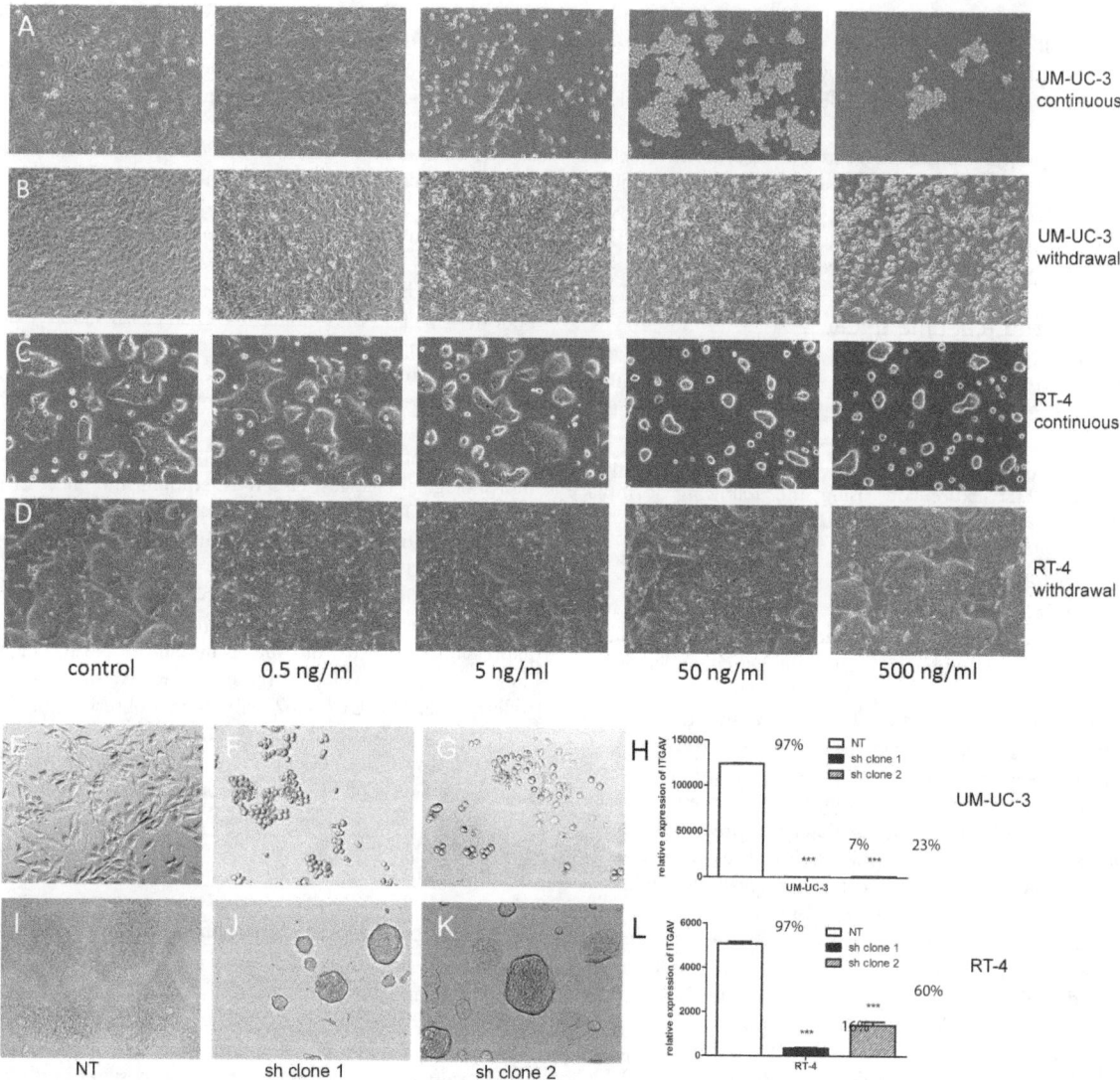

Figure 1. Effects of GLPG0187 and ITGAV knockdown on adherence to tissue culture plastic. Representative images of cells treated for 24 hours with a concentration series of GLPG0187 (dosage between 0–500 ng/ml, indicated underneath the images). Treatment resulted in a dose-dependent loss of adherence to tissue culture plastic in both UM-UC-3luc2 cells (A) and RT-4 cells (C). After 48 hours of GLPG0187 treatment, cells cultured for 4 days in GLPG0187-free medium regained their adherence to the tissue culture plastic in UM-UC-3luc2 cells (B) and RT-4 cells (D). Loss of adherence was also observed in UM-UC-3luc2 and RT4 cells stably transduced with a short hairpin targeted against ITGAV (respectively F–G for UMUC3luc2 sh ITGAV clones 1 and 2 and J–K for RT4 shITGAV clones 1 and 2). As a control, cells stably transduced with a non-targeting short hairpin (NT) were used (UMUC3 (E) and RT4 (I)). Flow cytometric analysis of relative ITGAV expression levels in UM-UC-3luc2 (H) and RT4 (L) cells (% of positive cells * mean fluorescence intensity). Data are presented as mean ± SEM, n = 3, the percentage of ITGAV positive cells is indicated above the bars.

mesenchymal markers, including CDH2, are upregulated, resulting in a decrease of the CDH1/CDH2 ratio. Since EMT is believed to be required for the first steps in metastasis formation, the reverse process of MET, might be the mechanism behind the decreased migratory and clonogenic capacity following α_v kd and GLPG0187 treatment. As expected, CDH1 (E-cadherin) protein levels were relatively high in the epithelial-like RT-4 cells and negligible in the mesenchymal-shaped UM-UC-3 cells. CDH2 (N-cadherin) expression was higher in UM-UC-3 cells compared to RT-4 cells (Figure S2H–I). Hence, base line levels of the CDH1/CDH2 ratio were higher in the RT-4 cell line compared to the UM-UC-3luc2 cell line, corresponding to the more epithelial phenotype of the RT-4 cell line. CDH1/CDH2 ratio was significantly increased as a result of α_v kd in both cell lines (Figure 2B and Figure S2 A–I). CDH1 protein levels increased in

the RT-4 cells and CDH2 protein levels significantly decreased in both cell lines (FACS plots shown in Figure S2A–B and S2H–I). GLPG0187 treatment showed a dose-dependent increase of the CDH1/CDH2 ratio which was significant in the highest dosages used in both UM-UC-3 and RT-4 cells (Figure 2B).

In line with our FACS analysis (Figure S2A), the expression of CDH1 is negligible in the UM-UC3 cells and displays a largely marginal increase in expression (green CDH1, blue DAPI staining of the nucleus, Figure S4A–C). CDH1 protein levels were below the detection limit of our western blot analysis in UM-UC-3 cells (data not shown). Membrane-expression of CDH1 in RT-4 cells increased in the ITGAV knockdown cells ((Figure S4G–H). CDH1 expression was also increased when RT-4 cells were treated with GLPG0187 (Figure S4I).

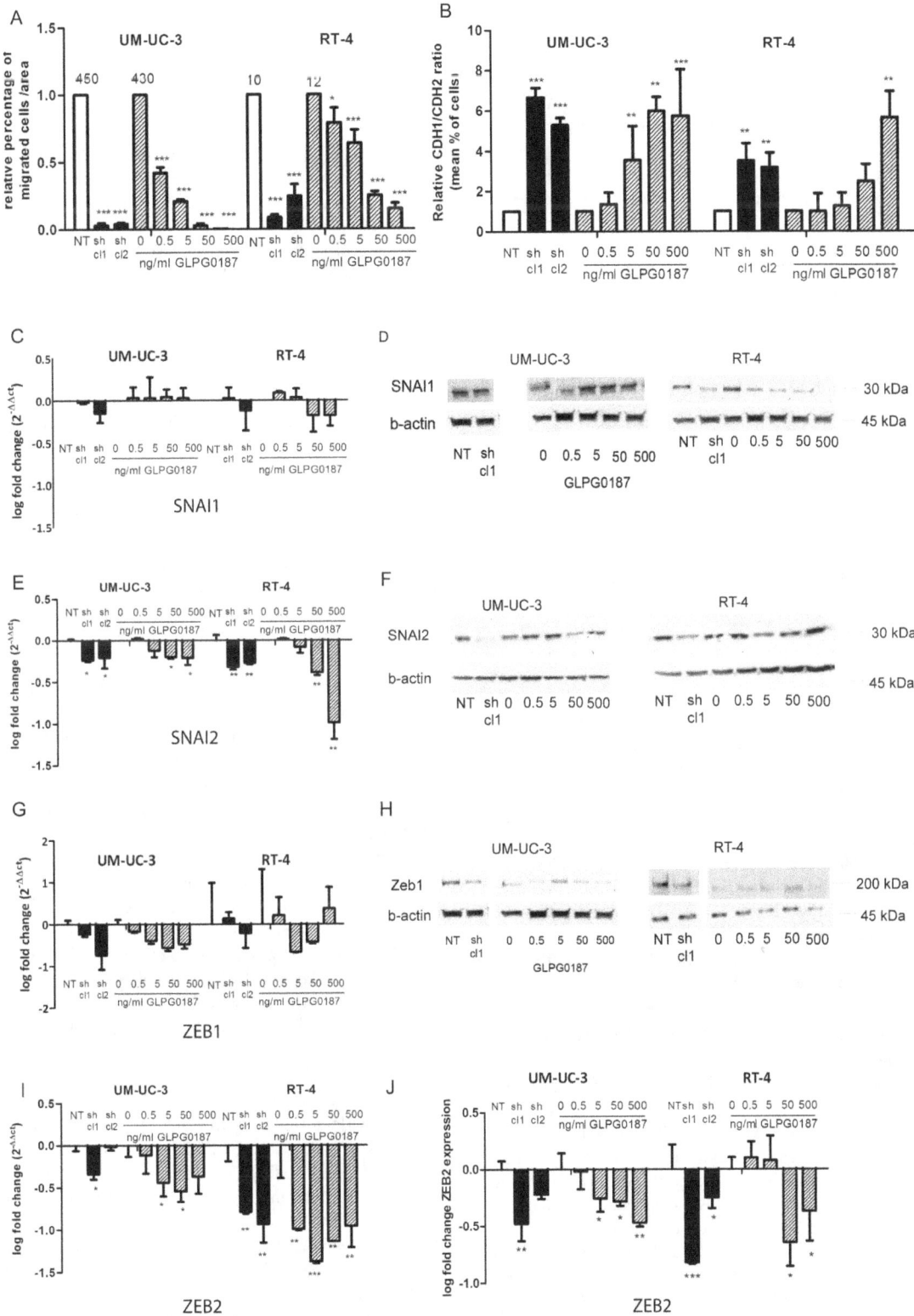

Figure 2. Effects of α_v integrin on migration and EMT. Effects of knockdown of ITGAV and 48 hrs of GLPG0187 treatment on migratory capacity of UM-UC-3luc2 and RT-4 cells as determined by Transwell Boyden chamber migration assays. Mean numbers of migrated cells per area were measured. Mean number of migrated cells of the control NT cells are depicted above the respective bars (A). Effects of ITGAV knockdown and 48 hrs of GLPG0187 treatment on the CDH1/CDH2 ratio (B). Data were normalized to the NT or control conditions (n = 3) and are presented as mean ± SEM. qPCR (C) and protein analysis of SNAI1 (D). qPCR analysis (E) and protein analysis of SNAI2 (F). qPCR analysis (G) and protein analysis of ZEB1 (H). qPCR analysis (I) and protein analysis of ZEB2 (J). Relative expression levels are shown compared to respectively NT or vehicle treated cells. All qPCR values were normalized for GAPDH and presented as mean ± SEM.

Vimentin levels were high in the UM-UC-3 cells, and remained similar in the ITGAV inhibited cells (Figure S4D–F), although the shape of the cells changed considerably. Vimentin levels in the RT-4 cells were markedly lower, and did not display changes upon inactivation of ITGAV. These data are in line with the FACS data using antibodies against CDH1 and Vimentin (respectively Figure S2A–B and S2F–G).

Subsequently, the mRNA and protein expression levels of EMT-inducing transcription factors were determined by real-time qPCR and Western Blot. The expression of SNAI1 was not changed in UM-UC-3 cells following α_v kd or treatment with GLPG0187 and was decreased in RT-4 cells with α_v kd knockdown and upon the GLPG0187 treatment (Figure 2C–D, S3A). SNAI2 mRNA and protein expression levels were significantly downregulated following α_v kd in both cell lines (respectively Figure 2E–F and S3B). Treatment with GLPG0187 showed a slight decrease in both mRNA and protein levels at the highest dosages used in UM-UC-3 cells (respectively Figure 2E–F and S3B). The effect of GLPG0187 on SNAI2 protein expression in RT-4 cells is very mild (Figure 2F).

Zeb1 mRNA was slightly decreased in UM-UC-3 cells upon knockdown and GLPG0187 treatment, and in certain concentrations of GLPG0187 in RT-4 cells (Figure 2G). Western Blot displayed a decrease in ZEB1 protein expression levels in both cell lines in the knockdown conditions (Figure 2H and S3C). GLPG0187 did not alter ZEB1 protein levels. It should be noted that the ZEB1 antibody possesses low specificity and therefore could represent an artefact (Figure S3D).

Zeb2 mRNA levels were significantly downregulated following α_v kd (Figure 2I). Treatment with GLPG0187 showed a slight decrease at the highest dosages used (Figure 2I). ZEB2 protein expression levels were measured with FACS analysis and demonstrated a significant decrease in ZEB2 protein expression in the sh clones in both cell lines (Figure 2J). In addition, the ZEB2 protein expression was dose-dependently decreased upon addition of GLPG0187 in both cell lines (Figure 2J). However, when measuring the protein levels with Western Blot analysis, we repeatedly found a variety of bands unfortunately rendering these experiments non-conclusive (Figure S3D). No significant effect was observed on the expression of TWIST mRNA expression in both cell lines (Figure S3I). In RT-4 cells no expression of TWIST was detected (Ct value>36; Figure S3I).

Effects of αv integrin on clonogenicity, stemness and metastasis markers

Next, we investigated and compared the effect of α_v knockdown on clonogenicity and previously identified bladder cancer stem cell markers. Compared to the UM-UC-3 cell line, RT-4 cell line produced less and smaller colonies in a single cell colony-forming assay, in line with the less malignant phenotype of this cell line. As shown in figure 3A, ITGAV knockdown significantly reduced the clonogenic capacity of both cell lines. Furthermore, the size of the colonies was significantly decreased upon α_v knockdown. Addition of GLPG0187 significantly reduced the clonogenic capacity as well as the size of the colonies in both cell lines (Figure 3A and S5A).

Previously, sphere formation has been described as a characteristic of CSCs that reflects the potential for self-renewal. We have identified a subpopulation of cells with urosphere forming ability within the UM-UC-3 cells. After 10 days of culture in ultra-low attachment plates using serum-starved culture conditions, p0 urospheres were counted (schematic representation in Figure S5B) [35]. The efficiency of urosphere formation (P0) varied and was highest in UM-UC-3 NT cells compared to the cells with ITGAV knockdown ((3.6±0.87% for the UM-UC-3luc2 NT cells versus

2.0±0.72% for the UM-UC-3 ITGAV sh clone1, Figure 3B). In addition, the size of the urospheres was significantly higher in the NT cells compared to the ITGAV knockdown cells (Figure 3D). Furthermore, the self-renewing capacity of these cells was measured by dissociating the obtained primary P0 spheres into single cells and plating one cell per well in anchorage-independent, serum-starved conditions. After 10 days, respectively 15,3% and 10,7% secondary spheres were formed in the (P1) from UM-UC-3 NT cells compared to the cells with ITGAV knockdown. It was also possible to generate further new spheres from single-cell suspension of P1 urospheres (Figure 3C). This clonal self-renewal could be observed for at least 3 passages. These data indicate that UM-UC-3luc2 cells are able to form urospheres, which could be propagated for several passages. ITGAV knockdown decreased the ability of the cells to form urospheres, the size of the formed spheres, and, in addition, decreased the capacity to form secondary spheres.

High ALDH activity (ALDH^{hi}) has recently been proposed to be indicative of cancer stem/progenitor cells in bladder cancer [25]. In line with this, the size of the ALDH^{hi} subpopulation of was significantly smaller in the RT-4 cells compared to the more malignant UM-UC-3luc2 cells (Figure 3E). Both ITGAV knockdown and GLPG0187 treatment significantly decreased the ALDH^{hi} subpopulation in both the UM-UC-3luc2 and RT-4 cells. This effect was most prominent in RT-4 cells (Figure 3E).

Then, the expression of previously identified bladder cancer stem cell markers (POU5F1, BMI1, NANOG, SOX2,) was determined by real-time qPCR in the established control NT and αv kd cell lines as well as in GLPG0187 treated cells. The expression of NANOG and BMI1 was significantly decreased upon ITGAV knockdown and GLPG treatment (Figure 3F–G). The expression of POU5F1 was not affected by ITGAV knockdown or GLPG0187 treatment in either cell line (Figure 3H), whereas the expression of SOX2 only decreased in the RT-4 cells (Figure 3I).

Recently, CD24 has been described as a marker for bladder cancer metastasis formation and was shown to be required for metastasis to the lungs [36]. Interestingly, CD24 protein expression levels were significantly decreased by approximately 80% in α_v kd UM-UC-3 cells, whereas no effect on CD24 expression was observed in α_v kd RT-4 clones (Figure 4A and S6O and S6P). GLPG0187 treatment resulted in a dose-dependent decrease in CD24 expression in UM-UC-3 cells (Figure 4A). Similar to the α_v kd, GLPG0187 treatment did not affect CD24 expression in RT-4 cells (Figure 4A).

No effects were observed on the protein expression of other putative bladder cancer stem cells, e.g. CD133 and CD44v6, by ITGAV knock down or GLPG0187 treatment in either cell line (Figure S6G–K). CD44 protein expression levels slightly decreased, especially in the RT4 cells with ITGAV knockdown (Figure S6L–N).

The expression of CD227 (Mucin-1), a negative marker for basal cells, increased by ITGAV knockdown or treatment with GLPG0187 (dose-dependently) (Figure 4B and S6Q–R). In addition, the expression of KRT20, a keratin which is expressed in differentiated umbrella cells, but not in basal cells or intermediate cells was significantly increased upon ITGAV knockdown or treatment with high doses of GLPG0187 (Figure 4C).

It is important to note that although base line levels of both the migratory and clonogenic capacity of RT-4 cells are much lower than those of UM-UC-3luc2 cells, the percentage of reduction is similar in both cell lines (Figure 2 and 3).

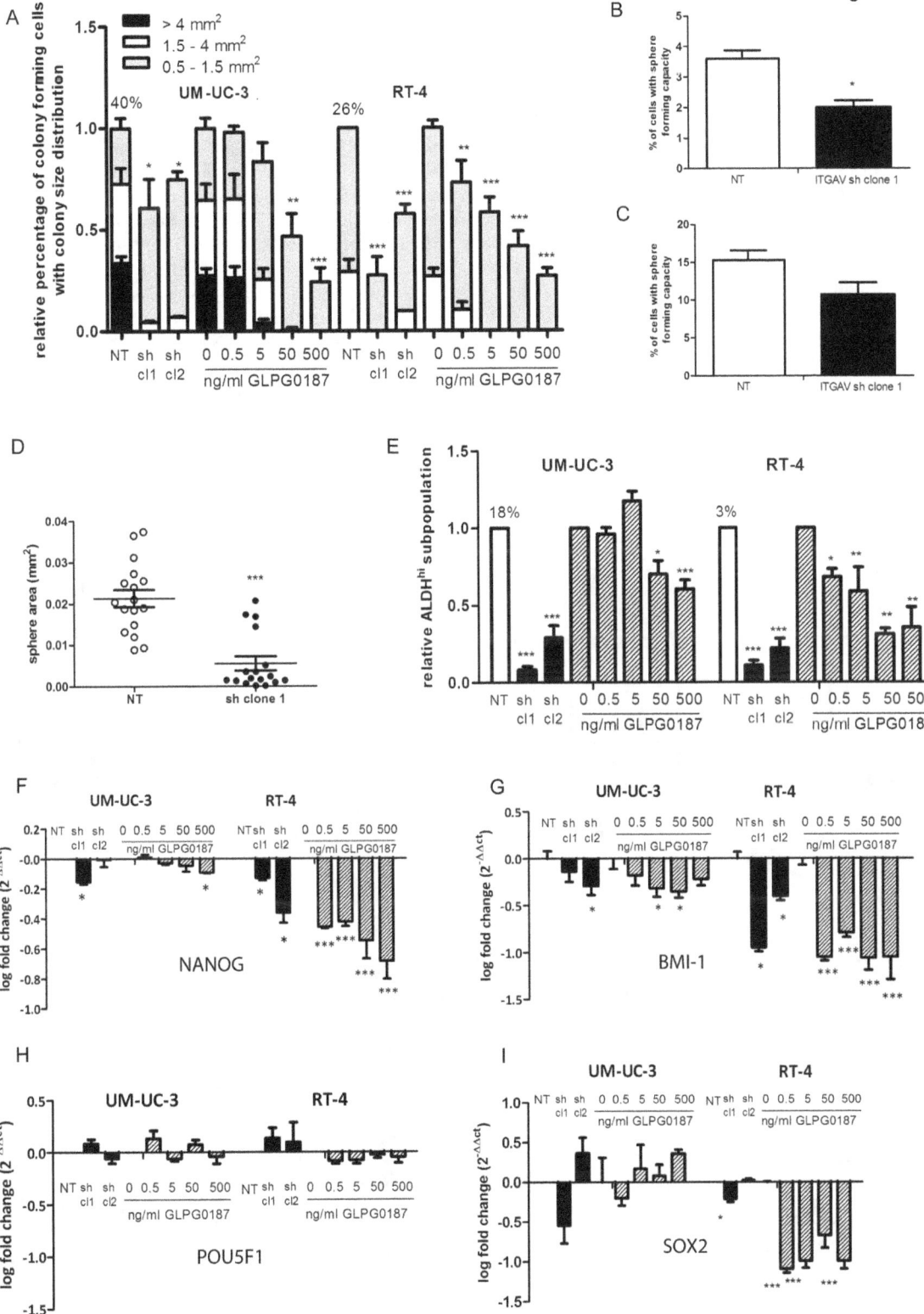

Figure 3. Effects of α_v integrin on clonogenicity and stem cell/metastasis markers. The relative percentage and size distribution of colony-forming cells in a 96-wells plate clonogenic assay of single-cell diluted cultures after 2 weeks in the α_v kd or NT cells and cells treated with a dose range of GLPG0187 for 48 hrs and plated afterwards. The area of the colonies was measured with Image J software and divided according to size. Small colonies are between 0.5 and 1.5 mm^2, medium sized colonies are between 1.5 and 4 mm^2 and large colonies are bigger than 4 mm^2. Data were normalized to the NT or control conditions and are presented as mean ± SEM. Percentage of colony-forming cells in the control NT cells are depicted above the respective bars (A). UM-UC-3 cells were seeded 100 cells/cm^2 in an ultra-low attachment plate in serum-starved conditions. The percentage of cells with sphere forming capacity (P0) was measured after 10 days of culture (B). P0 spheres were dissociated into single cells and seeded in ultra-low attachment 96 wells. The percentage of cells with sphere forming capacity (P1) was measured after 10 days of culture (B). The

area of the spheres was measured with Image J software (D). Percentage of cells with high ALDH activity (ALDH^{hi}) as measured with Aldefluor assay. Data are normalized to the NT or vehicle treated cells. Percentages of ALDH^{hi} cells in the NT and control cells are depicted above the respective bars (F). qPCR analysis of NANOG (F) qPCR analysis of BMI1 (G). Relative expression levels are shown compared to respectively NT or vehicle-treated cells. All values were normalized for GAPDH and presented as mean ± SEM.

In addition to the effects on stemness and epithelial plasticity, functional inactivation of ITGAV by blocking the ITGAV receptor using GLPG0187, dose-dependently induced cellular senescence in UM-UC-3 cells as measured by acidic senescence associated β-galactosidase activity (Figure 4D). ITGAV knockdown resulted in increased senescence in only one of the two short hairpin clones in both cell lines (Figure 4D).

Taken together, both α_v kd and GLPG0187 treatment of UM-UC-3luc2 and RT-4 cell lines, were able to reduce several malignant characteristics *in vitro*.

Effects of αv integrin on tumor growth and metastasis in preclinical *in vivo* models

Subsequently, we analyzed and compared the tumorigenicity and metastatic ability of the αv kd UM-UC-3luc2 cells *in vivo*. We investigated the capacity of the cells to grow in bone marrow, one of the sites of bladder cancer metastasis. The amount of mice displaying metastatic foci, as measured with sensitive bioluminescent imaging of the UMUC3 luciferase 2 cells in real-time after inoculation of the αv kd UM-UC-3luc2 cells in the bone marrow, was strikingly lower compared to the NT cell population (Figure 5A). Moreover, we observed significantly decreased total tumor burden in the mice injected with αv kd cells compared to the mice injected with the NT (Figure 5B–C).

Metastasis formation was significantly decreased in mice inoculated intra-cardiacally with 10,000 αv kd cells vs. NT cells (Figure S7A) [34]. Total tumor burden as well as bone tumor burden was decreased upon ITGAV kd, albeit not significantly (Figure S7B–D).

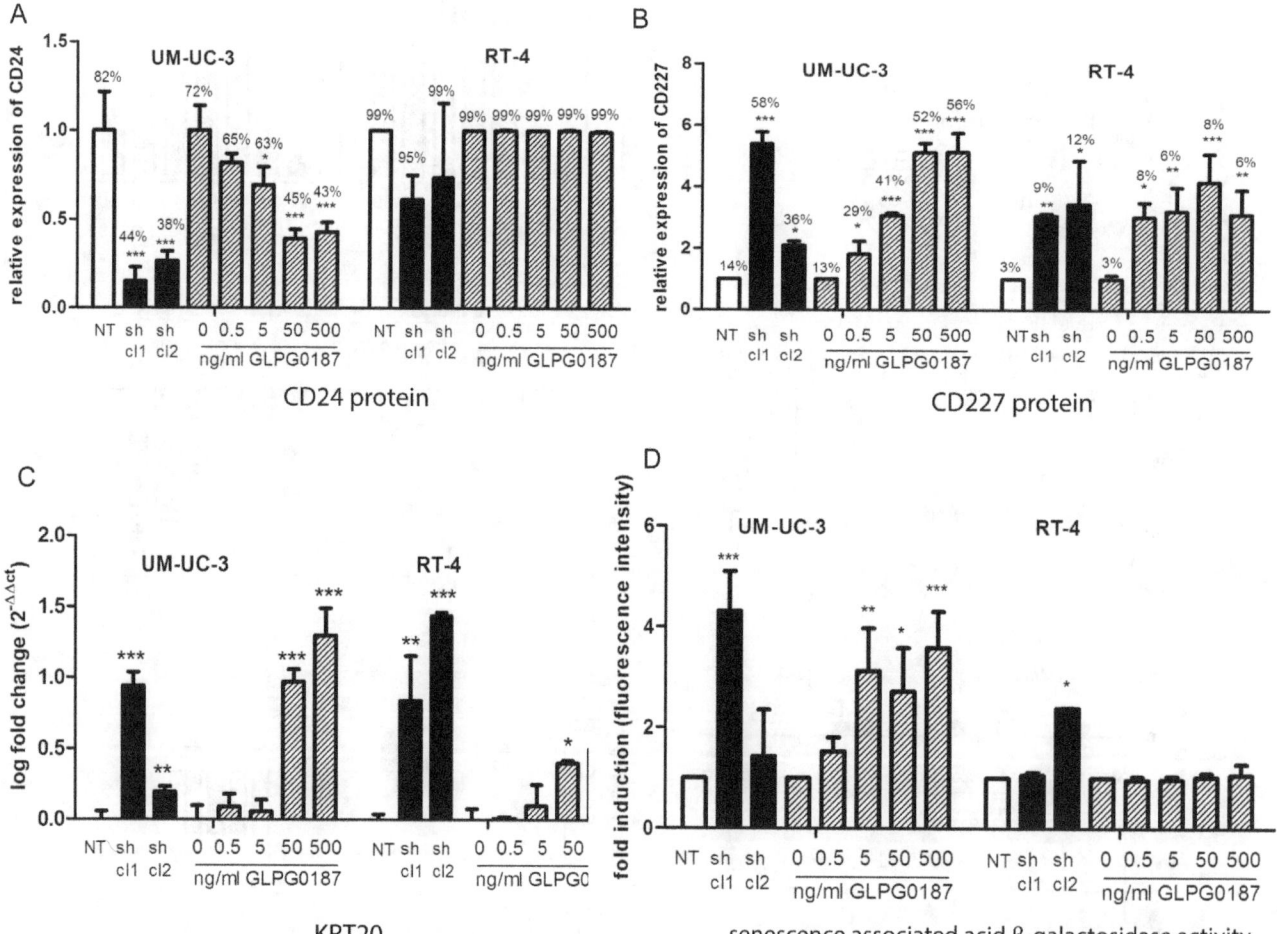

Figure 4. Effect of α_v integrin on expression levels of CD24 and urothelial differentiation markers and on senescence. Relative expression levels of CD24 (A) and CD227 (B). Relative expression levels (% of positive cells * Mean fluorescence intensity) were measured by flow cytometry and normalized to the NT or vehicle treated cells. Data are represented as mean ± SEM. Percentages of positive cells are depicted above the respective bars. qPCR analysis of KRT20. Relative expression levels are shown compared to respectively NT or non-treated cells. All values were normalized for GAPDH and presented as mean ± SEM (C). UM-UC-3 luc2 and RT-4 cells were seeded into a six-well plate and exposed to a concentration series of GLPG0187 (0–500 ng/ml). 48 h after incubation, cells were harvested and senescence associated acid β-galactosidase activity was measured. Data are represented as fold change in fluorescence intensity of the signal (D).

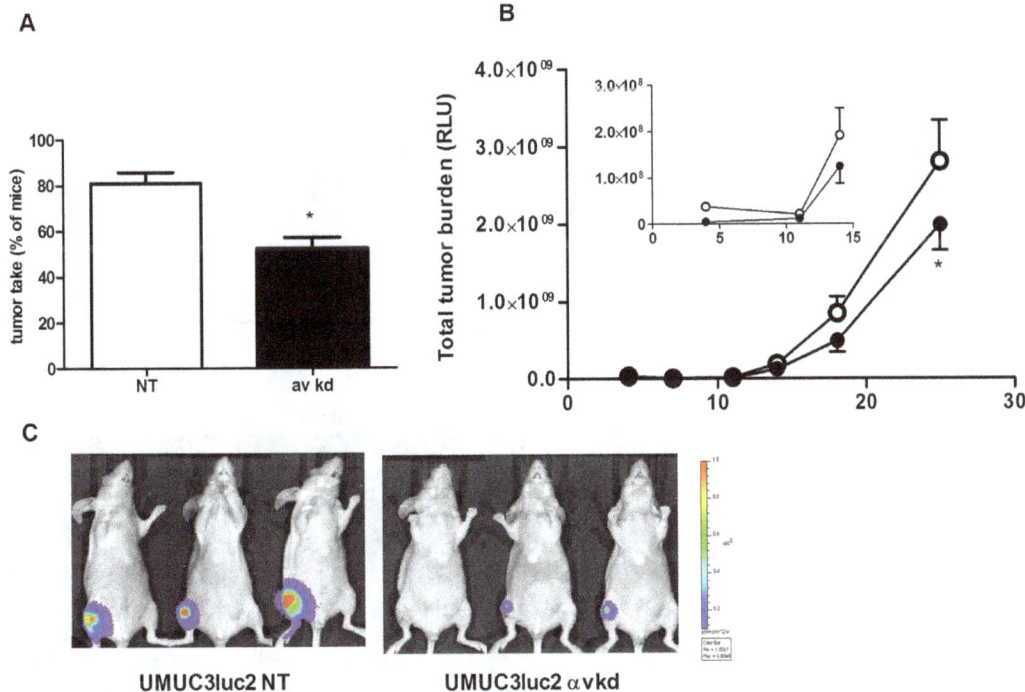

Figure 5. ITGAV knockdown in UM-UC-3luc2 cells affects intra-bone growth in a preclinical model. A) Percentage of mice with tumors after intra-bone inoculation of either α_v-kd-UM-UC-3luc2 or NT-UM-UC-3luc2 cells B) Total tumor burden of the mice injected with α_v-kd-UM-UC-3luc2 (*closed circles*) or NT-UM-UC-3luc2 cells (*open circles*). C) Representative images of mice intra-osseously inoculated with either αv-kd-UM-UC-3luc2 or NT-UM-UC-3luc2 cells 7 days after inoculation ($n = 10$/group *$P < 0.05$).

Next, we investigated whether blocking α_v-integrin can be used to treat experimentally-induced bone metastasis from intracardiacally inoculated UM-UC-3luc2 cells according to a *preventive* protocol (Figure 6A). The number of metastasis (Figure 6B) as well as the total tumor burden (Figure 6C) was significantly decreased in mice daily treated with 100 mg/kg/day GLPG0187 (IP).

In the *curative* protocol, bone metastases were allowed to develop for 21 days (Figure 6E). Subsequently, the mice were treated with a daily dosage of either vehicle or GLPG0187 (100 mg/kg/d IP) to investigate whether blocking α_v-integrin can be used to treat already existing bone metastases. However, no significant effects were found on the amount of metastasis/mouse, total tumor burden or bone tumor burden after 15 days of treatment with 100 mg/kg/d GLPG0187 (Figure 6F–H).

Taken together, knockdown or treatment of α_v integrins resulted in decreased metastatic growth in preclinical *in vivo* models as assessed by BLI.

Discussion

Low survival rates of metastatic bladder cancer emphasize the need for a drug that can prevent and/or treat metastatic cancer. A promising approach that has been explored for these means in breast [29], melanoma [30] and prostate [37] cancer is the targeting of α_v integrins, which has been shown to reduce tumor growth, metastasis and angiogenesis.

In this study, the role of ITGAV, which are highly expressed in bladder carcinomas, and its potential as a drug target in bladder cancer were investigated both by treatment with the ITGAV integrin-inhibitor GLPG0187 and knockdown of ITGAV. RT-4 and UM-UC-3luc2 cells were investigated to determine whether α_v integrin targeted therapies could be beneficial for these different grades of bladder tumors. The rationale for targeting of ITGAV is

their involvement in cell proliferation, migration, invasion, survival and angiogenesis, which are essential processes for primary tumor growth and metastasis formation [26,38,39]. These processes are induced via activation of focal adhesion kinase (PTK2) and src-family kinases (SFKs), that activate the ERK/MAPK, NF-κB and AKT/PKB pathways [40]. Modulating adherence to the extracellular matrix (ECM) by changing the affinity of integrins for their ECM ligands, is important for the motility of cancer cells [41].

Both GLPG0187 treatment and knockdown of ITGAV resulted in loss of adhesion, resembling loss of adherence to the ECM, which might have an inhibitory effect on cell motility and migration. Indeed, a strong decrease in migratory capacity was found after both ITGAV knockdown and GLPG0187 treatment, indicating a less malignant phenotype. However, especially in the knockdown sh clones, we cannot exclude that decreased adhesion and proliferation plays a role in the decreased migratory ability.

Reduced proliferation and clonogenicity upon α_v integrin inactivation provided further evidence for this reduced malignancy. In line with the functional differences, α_v kd and treatment with GLPG0187 resulted in a more epithelial phenotype, as illustrated by an increased CDH1/CDH2 ratio. This indicates that cells have undergone at least partial MET and thus that α_v integrins might be important for the maintenance of a mesenchymal phenotype (EMT). EMT can be regulated by transcription factors including SNAI1, SNAI2, TWIST, ZEB1 and ZEB2, that directly or indirectly repress CDH1 expression, which is considered to be a fundamental event in EMT [42]. In bladder cancer, SNAI1, SNAI2 and TWIST are differentially expressed [43] and TWIST and SNAI2 expression have been shown to play an important role in tumor progression and metastasis formation [44–47]. Since knockdown of ITGAV and to a lesser extent treatment with the GLPG0187 compound in UM-UC-3 and RT-4 cells

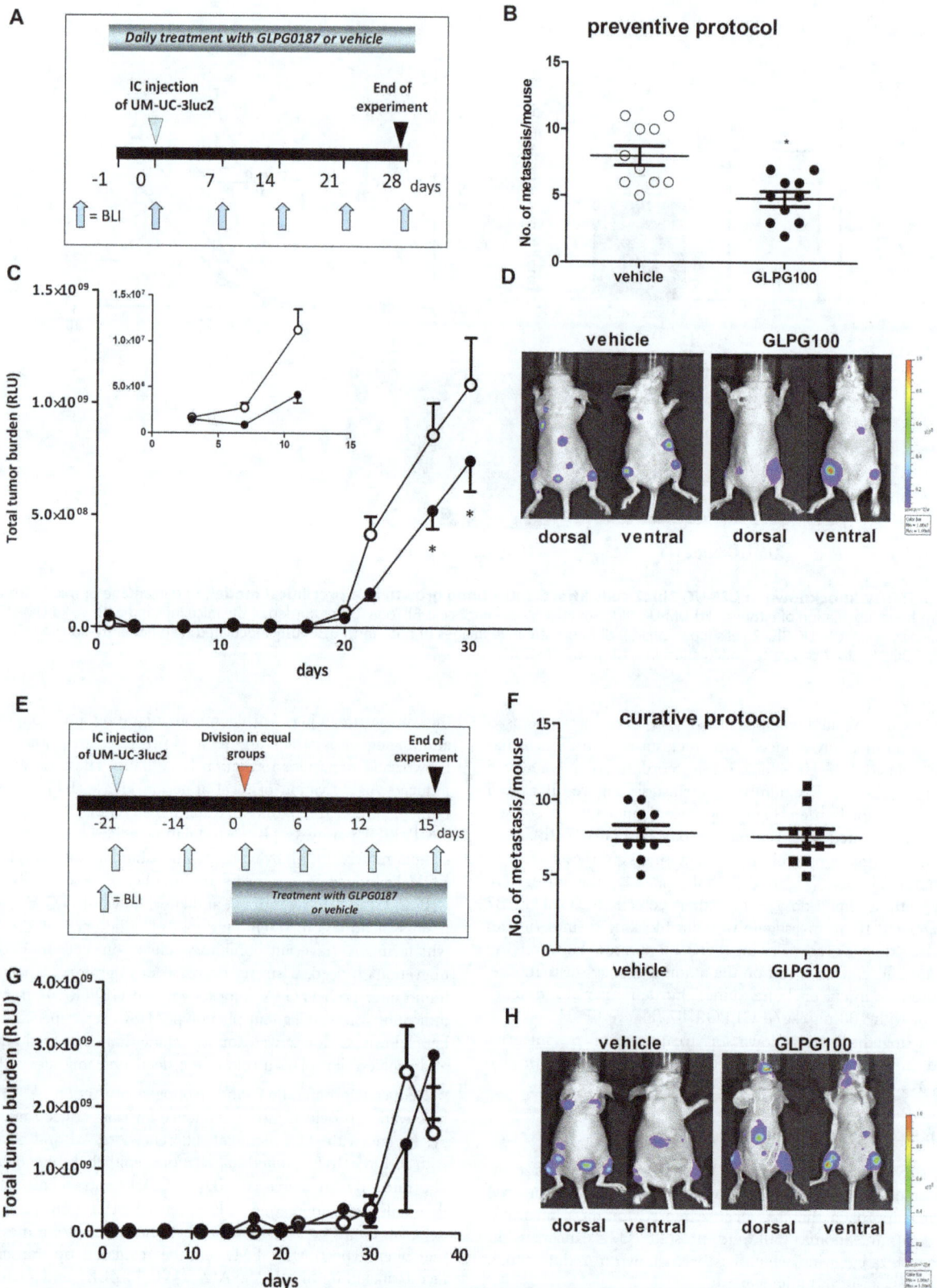

Figure 6. Effect of systemic administration of GLPG0187 on tumor growth and metastasis in a preventive and curative protocol. A) Schematic representation of the *preventive* protocol. Mice were treated daily with either IP administrated vehicle or GLPG0187 (100 mg/kg/day) from day -1 onwards. At day 0, 100,000 UM-UC-3luc2 cells were inoculated into the left heart ventricle and once a week BLI images were taken. B) Number of metastasis per mouse. C) Total tumor burden for the mice treated with 100 mg/kg/day GLPG0187 (closed circles) or vehicle (open circles). In the insert, the first 14 days are shown. D) Representative images of mice treated with vehicle or 100 mg/kg/day GLPG0187 taken at day 28 after inoculation. E) Schematic representation of the *curative* protocol. At day -21, 100,000 UM-UC-3luc2 cells were injected into the left heart ventricle and

once a week BLI images were taken. At day 0, mice were divided into groups with equal total tumor burden. Mice were daily treated with an IP dosage of either vehicle or GLPG0187 (100 mg/kg/day) from day 0 onwards. F) Number of metastasis per mouse. G) Total tumor burden for the mice treated with 100 mg/kg/day GLPG0187 (closed circles) or vehicle (open circles). H) Representative images of mice treated with vehicle or 100 mg/kg/day GLPG0187 taken at day 15 after start of treatment.

resulted in a significant decrease in SNAI2, SNAI2 might play an important role in EMT in bladder cancer. The expression of ZEB1 and 2 also decreased, however, this is not conclusive since the ZEB antibodies possess low specificity.

Recent evidence suggests that EMT generates cells with stem/progenitor-like properties and enables plasticity between CSC and non-CSC [4,7–9]. Therefore, EMT and CSC populations might show a large overlap [48,49]. Furthermore, EMT plays a critical role not only in invasion and metastasis but also in tumor recurrence that is believed to be tightly linked with the biology of cancer stem/progenitor cells. Indeed, the clonogenic capacity significantly decreased upon knockdown of ITGAV or treatment with GLPG0187. In line with these data, ITGAV knockdown and GLPG0187 treatment demonstrated a slight, but significant decrease in the expression of NANOG and BMI1, which have been shown to be regulators of self-renewal in embryonic stem cells [50–52]. Another self-renewal marker, SOX2, was only downregulated in RT-4 cells. In addition, α_v kd and GLPG0187 treatment resulted in a decreased percentage of cells with high ALDH activity. This subpopulation has recently been shown to be involved in stemness and metastasis formation in several solid cancers, including breast [22], ovarian [23], prostate [24] and bladder [25] cancer. A possibility is that α_v integrin functions upstream of ALDH and that the reduction in ALDH activity is responsible for the decreased migratory potential after α_v kd and GLPG0187 treatment.

In this study, α_v kd and GLPG0187 treatment resulted in decreased urosphere area (P0) and decreased self-renewal ability, as assessed with the urosphere assay. However, no effects were found on the mRNA expression levels of POU5F1 (Oct-4), which has been proposed to be a key regulator for pluripotency and self-renewal in embryonic stem cells [53]. POU5F1 has also been shown to have an important role in bladder cancer stem cells, invasion and migration [15,54–56], however, our data suggest that α_v integrin might affect migration through a mechanism independent of POU5F1, for example via NANOG or SOX2. Alternatively, α_v integrin might function downstream of POU5F1.

The decrease in stemness genes coincides with an increase in CD227, a negative marker for basal cells, indicating increased levels of differentiation upon α_v kd and GLPG0187 treatment.

CD24 has recently been proposed as a drug target for anti-metastatic therapy in bladder cancer [36]. The level of expression was shown to be increased in human bladder cancer metastasis compared to primary tumor. In addition, CD24 expression has been correlated with increased metastasis formation of UM-UC-3 cells in a lung metastasis mouse model [36]. In this study, we showed a decrease in CD24 expression in UM-UC-3luc2 cells upon α_v kd and GLPG0187 treatment. Interestingly, acidic senescence associated β-galactosidase activity increased upon functional inactivation of ITGAV, indicating that inhibition of ITGAV increases the amount of senescent cells. Senescent cells do not enter the mitotic cycle even in the presence of growth factors, they are however alive and remain metabolically active. Activating the senescence cell cycle arrest provides a tumor suppressor mechanism that can inhibit cancer growth as shown previously in multiple tumors.

In conclusion, the effects observed with α_v kd and GLPG0187 treatment in both cell lines show that ITGAV inhibition results in

a less malignant phenotype in vitro. α_v integrin appears to be involved in proliferation, migration and clonogenicity through EMT induction, the maintenance of cancer stem/progenitor-like ALDH^{hi} cells and CD24 expression. In line with the in vitro observations, knockdown of ITGAV or treatment with GLPG0187 significantly inhibited metastasis and secondary tumor growth in vivo. One of the models used, the experimental metastasis model, displays the effects of the tumor cells injected into the left cardiac ventricle that subsequently metastasize to the secondary target organs. In this model, the cells have to survive in the bloodstream, extravasate and colonize secondary target organs. The other xenograft transplantation model involves inoculation at the secondary target organ (in this case the bone microenvironment), using this model, the cells have to survive and grow at the secondary site. These data indicate, that in addition to the effects on angiogenesis and osteoclastogenesis [27], GLPG0187 also affects colonization of the metastatic sites and tumor growth.

The effects of GLPG0187 on tumor growth in the curative protocol might be improved by combination therapy with commonly used chemotherapeutics that will target the more differentiated cells in established tumors.

Taken together, we show for the first time that targeting of α_v integrin appears to be a promising approach for treatment and/or prevention of metastatic bladder cancer. Further research should help to elucidate whether GLPG0187 would be beneficial in combination with established therapeutic interventions.

Supporting Information

Figure S1 Expression of ITGAV, effect on viability and proliferation. Real time qPCR analysis of ITGAV (A). Values were normalized for GAPDH and presented as mean ± SEM. Relative expression levels are shown compared to NT cells. Representative images of flow cytometry plots of relative ITGAV expression levels in UM-UC-3luc2 (B) and RT4 (C) transduced with an shRNAi construct targeting ITGAV (sh clone1 and 2) or a non-targeting short hairpin (NT). Tissue sections of normal human bladder urothelium (D) and human bladder carcinoma (E) stained with α_v integrin antibody (data source: www.proteinatlas.org, Novacastra). Relative expression of ITGAV protein expression in NT controls cells (open bars), floating ITGAV knockdown cells (black bars) and in ITGAV knockdown cells that are still attached to the tissue culture plastic (striped bars). At the x-axis, the % of cells with the phenotype is depicted (F). The amount of viable, apoptotic and dead cells in the α_v kd and NT UM-UC-3 and RT-4 cells were measured using the Alexa Fluor 488 annexin V/Dead Cell Apoptosis Kit (Invitrogen). In addition, UM-UC-3 luc2 and RT-4 cells were seeded into a 6-well plate and exposed to a concentration series of GLPG0187 (0–500 ng/ml). 48 h after incubation, cells were harvested and processed for annexin V/PI staining. The percentage of viable (AnnexinV−/PI−), dead (PI+/AnnexinV−), and total apoptotic cells (AnnexinV+) are shown (G). Proliferation rate (mitochondrial activity as assessed with 3-(4,5-dimethylthiazol-2-yl)-2,5-diphenyltetrazolium bromide (optical density at 490 nm)) in the 2 α_v kd clones (respectively closed circles and triangles) and NT (open circles) UM-UC3luc2 (H) and RT-4 (I) cells. The effects of GLPG0187 treatment on proliferation rate of UM-UC-3luc2 (J) and RT-4 cells (K) after 24, 48 and 72 h of treatment was assessed with 3-(4,5-dimethylthiazol-2-yl)-2,5-diphenyltetrazolium bromide (optical density at 490 nm). Data are presented as mean ± SEM (n = 3).

Figure S2   Protein levels of EMT markers. Representative images of flow cytometry plots of relative E-cadherin expression levels in UM-UC-3luc2 (A) and RT-4 (B) cells transduced with an shRNAi construct targeting ITGAV (sh clone1 and 2) or a non-targeting short hairpin (NT). Western Blot analysis of E-cadherin and b-actin in RT-4 cells (C) and densitometry analysis of the relative protein expression levels, measured with western blot analysis, compared to respectively NT or vehicle treated cells and corrected for b-actin expression levels (D). Representative images of flow cytometry plots of relative Vimentin expression levels in UM-UC-3luc2 (F) and RT-4 (G) cells transduced with an shRNAi construct targeting ITGAV (sh clone1 and 2) or a non-targeting short hairpin (NT). Representative images of flow cytometry plots of relative N-cadherin expression levels in UM-UC-3luc2 (H) and RT-4 (I) cells transduced with an shRNAi construct targeting ITGAV (sh clone1 and 2) or a non-targeting short hairpin (NT).

Figure S3   Protein levels of intracellular EMT markers. Densitometry analysis of the relative protein expression levels of SNAI1 (A), SNAI2 (B) and ZEB1 (C), measured with western blot analysis, compared to respectively NT or vehicle treated cells and corrected for b-actin expression levels in UM-UC-3 cells or RT-4 cells (respectively NT, sh clone 1, control and a concentration series of GLPG0187). Whole audiograms of ZEB1 and ZEB2 western blot analysis, displaying multiple additional bands (D). Representative images of cytometry plots of ZEB2 protein expression in UM-UC-3 NT and sh clones 1 and 2 (E) and ZEB2 protein expression in RT-4 NT and sh clones 1 and 2 (F). Representative images of cytometry plots of ZEB2 protein expression in UM-UC-3 cells (G) or RT-4 cells (H) treated with a dose-range of GLPG0187. Real time qPCR analysis of TWIST in UM-UC-3 and RT-4 cells (I). Relative expression levels are shown compared to respectively NT or non-treated cells.

Figure S4   Immunofluorescence of E-cadherin and Vimentin. Representative confocal images of E-cadherin staining in UM-UC-3 NT (A), ITGAV knockdown clone 1 (B) and UM-UC-3 cells treated with 500 ng/ml GLPG0187 for 24 h (C) Representative confocal images of Vimentin staining in UM-UC-3 NT (D), ITGAV knockdown clone 1 (E) and UM-UC-3 cells treated with 500 ng/ml GLPG0187 for 24 h (F). Representative confocal images of E-cadherin staining in RT-4 NT (G), ITGAV knockdown clone 1 (H) and UM-UC-3 cells treated with 500 ng/ml GLPG0187 for 24 h (I) Representative confocal images of Vimentin staining in RT-4 NT (J), ITGAV knockdown clone 1 (K) and RT-4 cells treated with 500 ng/ml GLPG0187 for 24 h (L).

Figure S5   Tumor-initiating cell characteristics. Representative image of a colony in a clonogenic assay of UM-UC-3 cells 14 days after seeding (5x magnification) (A). Schematic representation of the urosphere protocol, adapted from Bisson et al [35]. (B) Representative images of UM-UC-3 NT (C) and ITGAV knockdown (D) P0 urospheres 10 days after seeding. Scale bar represents 50 µm (20x magnification).

Figure S6   Expression levels of markers. Expression levels of ITGAV knockdown clones 1 and 2 were compared to control cells transduced with a non-targeting short hairpin (NT). Cells were treated with GLPG0187 concentration series for 48 h. Data were normalized to the NT or control conditions and are presented as mean ± SEM. Relative expression levels of ITGA2-FITC (percentage of positive cells * mean fluorescence intensity (A) with representative cytometry plot for UM-UC-3 (B) or RT-4 cells (C). Relative expression levels of ITGA6-APC (percentage of positive cells * mean fluorescence intensity (D) with representative cytometry plot for UM-UC-3 (E) or RT-4 cells (F). Relative expression levels of CD133-APC (percentage of positive cells * mean fluorescence intensity (G) with representative cytometry plot for UM-UC-3 (H). Relative expression levels of CD44v6-FITC (percentage of positive cells * mean fluorescence intensity (I) with representative cytometry plot for UM-UC-3 (J) or RT-4 cells (K). Relative expression levels of CD44v6-PE (percentage of positive cells * mean fluorescence intensity (L) with representative cytometry plot for UM-UC-3 (M) or RT-4 cells (N). Representative cytometry plot for CD24 expression in UM-UC-3 (O) or RT-4 cells (P). Representative cytometry plot for CD227 expression in UM-UC-3 (Q) or RT-4 cells (R).

Figure S7   ITGAV knockdown in UM-UC-3luc2 cells affects metastatic growth in a preclinical model. A) Number of metastases/mouse after intra-cardiac inoculation of either α_v-kd-UM-UC-3luc2 or NT-UM-UC-3luc2 cells. B) Total tumor burden and C) tumor burden in long bones after intra-cardiac inoculation of either α_v-kd-UM-UC-3luc2 (closed circles) or NT-UM-UC-3luc2 cells (open circles) D) representative images of mice at day 34 after inoculation.

Table S1   Short hairpin RNAi constructs. UM-UC-3luc2 and RT-4 cell lines were transduced with short hairpin RNAi constructs against ITGAV or scrambled non-targeting (NT) shRNA derived from Sigma's MISSION library.

Table S2   Antibodies with application, supplier and location.

Table S3   Exon-spanning real-time PCR primers. Exon-spanning real-time PCR primers were designed with Primer Express software (Applied Biosystems, Rotkreuz, Switzerland). KRT20 expression was measured with Taqman primer/probe set Hs00300643_m1 from Life Technologies.

Materials and Methods S1 Materials and methods describing Annexin V/Propidium Iodide Apoptosis Assay, proliferation assay and Immunofluorescence staining.

Author Contributions

Conceived and designed the experiments: GP GH LB PCL. Performed the experiments: GH LB MM HC BH PCL GL. Analyzed the data: GH LB MM HC. Contributed reagents/materials/analysis tools: BH PCL GL RP RB. Wrote the paper: GH LB GP.

References

1. Coghlin C, Murray GI (2010) Current and emerging concepts in tumour metastasis. J Pathol 222: 1–15.
2. Kalluri R, Weinberg RA (2009) The basics of epithelial-mesenchymal transition. J Clin Invest 119: 1420–1428.
3. van der Pluijm G (2010) Epithelial plasticity, cancer stem cells and bone metastasis formation. Bone 48(1): 37–43.
4. Polyak K, Weinberg RA (2009) Transitions between epithelial and mesenchymal states: acquisition of malignant and stem cell traits. Nat Rev Cancer 9: 265–273.
5. Bonnomet A, Brysse A, Tachsidis A, Waltham M, Thompson EW, et al. (2010) Epithelial-to-mesenchymal transitions and circulating tumor cells. J Mammary Gland Biol Neoplasia 15: 261–273.
6. Chaffer CL, Brennan JP, Slavin JL, Blick T, Thompson EW, et al. (2006) Mesenchymal-to-epithelial transition facilitates bladder cancer metastasis: role of fibroblast growth factor receptor-2. Cancer Res 66: 11271–11278.
7. Gupta PB, Chaffer CL, Weinberg RA (2009) Cancer stem cells: mirage or reality? Nat Med 15: 1010–1012.
8. Mani SA, Guo W, Liao MJ, Eaton EN, Ayyanan A, et al (2008) The epithelial-mesenchymal transition generates cells with properties of stem cells. Cell 133: 704–715.
9. Morel AP, Lievre M, Thomas C, Hinkal G, Ansieau S, et al. (2008) Generation of breast cancer stem cells through epithelial-mesenchymal transition. PLoS One 3: e2888.
10. Elshamy WM, Duhe RJ (2013) Overview: cellular plasticity, cancer stem cells and metastasis. Cancer Lett 341: 2–8.
11. Chang JT, Mani SA (2013) Sheep, wolf, or werewolf: cancer stem cells and the epithelial-to-mesenchymal transition. Cancer Lett 341: 16–23.
12. Visvader JE, Lindeman GJ (2008) Cancer stem cells in solid tumours: accumulating evidence and unresolved questions. Nat Rev Cancer 8: 755–768.
13. Alison MR, Lim SM, Nicholson LJ (2011) Cancer stem cells: problems for therapy? J Pathol 223: 147–161.
14. Brabletz T, Jung A, Spaderna S, Hlubek F, Kirchner T (2005) Opinion: migrating cancer stem cells - an integrated concept of malignant tumour progression. Nat Rev Cancer 5: 744–749.
15. Bentivegna A, Conconi D, Panzeri E, Sala E, Bovo G, et al. (2010) Biological heterogeneity of putative bladder cancer stem-like cell populations from human bladder transitional cell carcinoma samples. Cancer Sci 101: 416–424.
16. He X, Marchionni L, Hansel DE, Yu W, Sood A, et al (2009) Differentiation of a highly tumorigenic basal cell compartment in urothelial carcinoma. Stem Cells 27: 1487–1495.
17. Chan KS, Espinosa I, Chao M, Wong D, Ailles L, et al. (2009) Identification, molecular characterization, clinical prognosis, and therapeutic targeting of human bladder tumor-initiating cells. Proc Natl Acad Sci U S A 106: 14016–14021.
18. She JJ, Zhang PG, Wang ZM, Gan WM, Che XM (2008) Identification of side population cells from bladder cancer cells by DyeCycle Violet staining. Cancer Biol Ther 7: 1663–1668.
19. Ning ZF, Huang YJ, Lin TX, Zhou YX, Jiang C, et al. (2009) Subpopulations of stem-like cells in side population cells from the human bladder transitional cell cancer cell line T24. J Int Med Res 37: 621–630.
20. Oates JE, Grey BR, Addla SK, Samuel JD, Hart CA, et al. (2009) Hoechst 33342 side population identification is a conserved and unified mechanism in urological cancers. Stem Cells Dev 18: 1515–1522.
21. van der Horst G, Bos L, van der Pluijm G (2012) Epithelial plasticity, cancer stem cells, and the tumor-supportive stroma in bladder carcinoma. Mol Cancer Res 10: 995–1009.
22. Ginestier C, Hur MH, Charafe-Jauffret E, Monville F, Dutcher J, et al (2007) ALDH1 Is a Marker of Normal and Malignant Human Mammary Stem Cells and a Predictor of Poor Clinical Outcome. Cell Stem Cell 1: 555–567.
23. Kryczek I, Liu S, Roh M, Vatan L, Szeliga W, et al. (2012) Expression of aldehyde dehydrogenase and CD133 defines ovarian cancer stem cells. Int J Cancer 130: 29–39.
24. van den Hoogen C, van der Horst G, Cheung H, Buijs JT, Lippitt JM, et al. (2010) High aldehyde dehydrogenase activity identifies tumor-initiating and metastasis-initiating cells in human prostate cancer. Cancer Res 70: 5163–5173.
25. Su Y, Qiu Q, Zhang X, Jiang Z, Leng Q, et al. (2010) Aldehyde dehydrogenase 1 A1-positive cell population is enriched in tumor-initiating cells and associated with progression of bladder cancer. Cancer Epidemiol Biomarkers Prev 19: 327–337.
26. Nemeth JA, Nakada MT, Trikha M, Lang Z, Gordon MS, et al. (2007) Alpha-v integrins as therapeutic targets in oncology. Cancer Invest 25: 632–646.
27. van der Horst G, van den Hoogen C, Buijs JT, Cheung H, Bloys H, et al. (2011) Targeting of alpha(v)-Integrins in Stem/Progenitor Cells and Supportive Microenvironment Impairs Bone Metastasis in Human Prostate Cancer. Neoplasia 13: 516–525.
28. Zhao Y, Bachelier R, Treilleux I, Pujuguet P, Peyruchaud O, et al. (2007) Tumor alphavbeta3 integrin is a therapeutic target for breast cancer bone metastases. Cancer Res 67: 5821–5830.
29. Chen Q, Manning CD, Millar H, McCabe FL, Ferrante C, et al. (2008) CNTO 95, a fully human anti alphav integrin antibody, inhibits cell signaling, migration, invasion, and spontaneous metastasis of human breast cancer cells. Clin Exp Metastasis 25: 139–148.
30. Trikha M, Zhou Z, Nemeth JA, Chen Q, Sharp C, et al. (2004) CNTO 95, a fully human monoclonal antibody that inhibits alphav integrins, has antitumor and antiangiogenic activity in vivo. Int J Cancer 110(3): 326–335.
31. O'Day SJ, Pavlick AC, Albertini MR, Hamid O, Schalch H, et al. (2011) Clinical and pharmacologic evaluation of two dose levels of intetumumab (CNTO 95) in patients with melanoma or angiosarcoma. Invest New Drugs 30(3): 1074–1081.
32. van den Hoogen C, van der Horst G, Cheung H, Buijs JT, Pelger RC, et al. (2011) Integrin alphav expression is required for the acquisition of a metastatic stem/progenitor cell phenotype in human prostate cancer. Am J Pathol 179: 2559–2568.
33. Sachs MD, Rauen KA, Ramamurthy M, Dodson JL, De Marzo AM, et al. (2002) Integrin alpha(v) and coxsackie adenovirus receptor expression in clinical bladder cancer. Urology 60: 531–536.
34. van der Horst G, van Asten JJ, Figdor A, van den Hoogen C, Cheung H, et al. (2011) Real-Time Cancer Cell Tracking by Bioluminescence in a Preclinical Model of Human Bladder Cancer Growth and Metastasis. Eur Urol 60: 337–43.
35. Bisson I, Prowse DM (2009) WNT signaling regulates self-renewal and differentiation of prostate cancer cells with stem cell characteristics. Cell Res 19: 683–697.
36. Overdevest JB, Thomas S, Kristiansen G, Hansel DE, Smith SC, et al. (2011) CD24 offers a therapeutic target for control of bladder cancer metastasis based on a requirement for lung colonization. Cancer Res 71: 3802–3811.
37. Hong H, Yang Y, Zhang Y, Cai W (2010) Non-invasive cell tracking in cancer and cancer therapy. Curr Top Med Chem 10: 1237–1248.
38. Hanahan D, Weinberg RA (2011) Hallmarks of cancer: the next generation. Cell 144: 646–674.
39. Marshall JF, Hart IR (1996) The role of alpha v-integrins in tumour progression and metastasis. Semin Cancer Biol 7: 129–138.
40. Guo W, Giancotti FG (2004) Integrin signalling during tumour progression. Nat Rev Mol Cell Biol 5: 816–826.
41. Hood JD, Cheresh DA (2002) Role of integrins in cell invasion and migration. Nat Rev Cancer 2: 91–100.
42. Thiery JP, Acloque H, Huang RY, Nieto MA (2009) Epithelial-mesenchymal transitions in development and disease. Cell 139: 871–890.
43. Yu Q, Zhang K, Wang X, Liu X, Zhang Z (2010) Expression of transcription factors snail, slug, and twist in human bladder carcinoma. J Exp Clin Cancer Res 29: 119–128.
44. Wallerand H, Robert G, Pasticier G, Ravaud A, Ballanger P, et al. (2010) The epithelial-mesenchymal transition-inducing factor TWIST is an attractive target in advanced and/or metastatic bladder and prostate cancers. Urol Oncol 28: 473–479.
45. Zhang Z, Xie D, Li X, Wong YC, Xin D, et al. (2007) Significance of TWIST expression and its association with E-cadherin in bladder cancer. Hum Pathol 38: 598–606.
46. Fondrevelle ME, Kantelip B, Reiter RE, Chopin DK, Thiery JP, et al. (2009) The expression of Twist has an impact on survival in human bladder cancer and is influenced by the smoking status. Urol Oncol 27: 268–276.
47. Wang X, Zhang K, Sun L, Liu J, Lu H (2010) Short interfering RNA directed against Slug blocks tumor growth, metastasis formation, and vascular leakage in bladder cancer. Med Oncol Suppl 1: S413–422.
48. Floor S, van Staveren WC, Larsimont D, Dumont JE, Maenhaut C (2011) Cancer cells in epithelial-to-mesenchymal transition and tumor-propagating-cancer stem cells: distinct, overlapping or same populations. Oncogene 30: 4609–4621.
49. Kong D, Li Y, Wang Z, Sarkar FH (2011) Cancer Stem Cells and Epithelial-to-Mesenchymal Transition (EMT)-Phenotypic Cells: Are They Cousins or Twins? Cancers (Basel) 3: 716–729.
50. Cavaleri F, Scholer HR (2003) Nanog: a new recruit to the embryonic stem cell orchestra. Cell 113: 551–552.
51. Mitsui K, Tokuzawa Y, Itoh H, Segawa K, Murakami M, et al. (2003) The homeoprotein Nanog is required for maintenance of pluripotency in mouse epiblast and ES cells. Cell 113: 631–642.
52. Chambers I, Colby D, Robertson M, Nichols J, Lee S, et al. (2003) Functional expression cloning of Nanog, a pluripotency sustaining factor in embryonic stem cells. Cell 113: 643–655.
53. Niwa H, Miyazaki J, Smith AG (2000) Quantitative expression of Oct-3/4 defines differentiation, dedifferentiation or self-renewal of ES cells. Nat Genet 24: 372–376.
54. Atlasi Y, Mowla SJ, Ziaee SA, Bahrami AR (2007) OCT-4, an embryonic stem cell marker, is highly expressed in bladder cancer. Int J Cancer 120: 1598–1602.
55. Huang P, Chen J, Wang L, Na Y, Kaku H, et al. (2012) Implications of transcriptional factor, OCT-4, in human bladder malignancy and tumor recurrence. Med Oncol 29(2): 829–834.
56. Chang CC, Shieh GS, Wu P, Lin CC, Shiau AL, et al. (2008) Oct-3/4 expression reflects tumor progression and regulates motility of bladder cancer cells. Cancer Res 68: 6281–6291.

Permissions

All chapters in this book were first published in PLOS ONE, by The Public Library of Science; hereby published with permission under the Creative Commons Attribution License or equivalent. Every chapter published in this book has been scrutinized by our experts. Their significance has been extensively debated. The topics covered herein carry significant findings which will fuel the growth of the discipline. They may even be implemented as practical applications or may be referred to as a beginning point for another development.

The contributors of this book come from diverse backgrounds, making this book a truly international effort. This book will bring forth new frontiers with its revolutionizing research information and detailed analysis of the nascent developments around the world.

We would like to thank all the contributing authors for lending their expertise to make the book truly unique. They have played a crucial role in the development of this book. Without their invaluable contributions this book wouldn't have been possible. They have made vital efforts to compile up to date information on the varied aspects of this subject to make this book a valuable addition to the collection of many professionals and students.

This book was conceptualized with the vision of imparting up-to-date information and advanced data in this field. To ensure the same, a matchless editorial board was set up. Every individual on the board went through rigorous rounds of assessment to prove their worth. After which they invested a large part of their time researching and compiling the most relevant data for our readers.

The editorial board has been involved in producing this book since its inception. They have spent rigorous hours researching and exploring the diverse topics which have resulted in the successful publishing of this book. They have passed on their knowledge of decades through this book. To expedite this challenging task, the publisher supported the team at every step. A small team of assistant editors was also appointed to further simplify the editing procedure and attain best results for the readers.

Apart from the editorial board, the designing team has also invested a significant amount of their time in understanding the subject and creating the most relevant covers. They scrutinized every image to scout for the most suitable representation of the subject and create an appropriate cover for the book.

The publishing team has been an ardent support to the editorial, designing and production team. Their endless efforts to recruit the best for this project, has resulted in the accomplishment of this book. They are a veteran in the field of academics and their pool of knowledge is as vast as their experience in printing. Their expertise and guidance has proved useful at every step. Their uncompromising quality standards have made this book an exceptional effort. Their encouragement from time to time has been an inspiration for everyone.

The publisher and the editorial board hope that this book will prove to be a valuable piece of knowledge for researchers, students, practitioners and scholars across the globe.

List of Contributors

Shuxiong Zeng, Zhensheng Zhang, Ruixiang Song, Rongchao Wei, Junjie Zhao, Linhui Wang, Jianguo Hou, Yinghao Sun and Chuanliang Xu
From the Department of Urology, Changhai Hospital, Second Military Medical University, Shanghai, P. R. China

Xiaowen Yu
From the Department of Geriatrics, Changhai Hospital, Second Military Medical University, Shanghai, P. R. China

Tiewei Cheng and David J. McConkey
Department of Urology, The University of Texas M.D. Anderson Cancer Center, Houston, Texas, United States of America
Department of Cancer Biology, The University of Texas M.D. Anderson Cancer Center, Houston, Texas, United States of America
Experimental Therapeutics Academic Program, The University of Texas-Graduate School of Biomedical Sciences (GSBS) at Houston, Houston, Texas, United States of America

Beat Roth
Department of Urology, The University of Texas M.D. Anderson Cancer Center, Houston, Texas, United States of America

Woonyoung Choi and Colin Dinney
Department of Urology, The University of Texas M.D. Anderson Cancer Center, Houston, Texas, United States of America
Department of Cancer Biology, The University of Texas M.D. Anderson Cancer Center, Houston, Texas, United States of America

Peter C. Black
Department of Urologic Science, The University of British Columbia, Vancouver, British Columbia, Canada

Thomas Reinert, Anders Christiansen, Torben F. Ørntoft and Lars Dyrskjøt
Department of Molecular Medicine, Aarhus University Hospital, Aarhus, Denmark

Michael Borre
Department of Urology, Aarhus University Hospital, Aarhus, Denmark

Gregers G. Hermann
Department of Urology, Frederiksberg Hospital, Copenhagen University, Frederiksberg, Denmark

Anastasia C. Hepburn, Stuart C. Williamson, Huw D. Thomas, Neha Sahay, Craig N. Robson and Alejandra Mantilla
Northern Institute for Cancer Research, Newcastle University, Framlington Place, Newcastle upon Tyne, United Kingdom

Rajan Veeratterapillay
Department of Urology, Freeman Hospital, The Newcastle upon Tyne Hospitals NHS Foundation Trust, Newcastle upon Tyne, United Kingdom

Amira El-Sherif
Department of Pathology, Royal Victoria Infirmary, The Newcastle upon Tyne Hospitals NHS Foundation Trust, Newcastle upon Tyne, United Kingdom

Robert S. Pickard
Department of Urology, Freeman Hospital, The Newcastle upon Tyne Hospitals NHS Foundation Trust, Newcastle upon Tyne, United Kingdom
Institute of Cellular Medicine, Medical School, Newcastle University, Framlington Place, Newcastle upon Tyne, United Kingdom

Rakesh Heer
Northern Institute for Cancer Research, Newcastle University, Framlington Place, Newcastle upon Tyne, United Kingdom
Department of Urology, Freeman Hospital, The Newcastle upon Tyne Hospitals NHS Foundation Trust, Newcastle upon Tyne, United Kingdom

Zhaowei Zhu, Xiaohua Zhang, Zhoujun Shen, Shan Zhong and Xianjin Wang
Department of Urology, Ruijin Hospital, Shanghai Jiaotong University School of Medicine, Shanghai, China

Yingli Lu
Institute and Department of Endocrinology and Metabolism, Shanghai Ninth People's Hospital, Shanghai Jiaotong University School of Medicine, Shanghai, China

Chen Xu
Department of Embryology and Histology, Shanghai Jiaotong University School of Medicine, Shanghai, China
Shanghai Key Laboratory of Reproductive Medicine, Shanghai Jiaotong University School of Medicine, Shanghai, China

Hyung Suk Kim, Myong Kim, Chang Wook Jeong, Cheol Kwak, Hyeon Hoe Kim and Ja Hyeon Ku
Department of Urology, Seoul National University College of Medicine, Seoul, Korea

Yvonne Chekaluk, Yanan Guo and David J. Kwiatkowski
Division of Translational Medicine, Brigham and Women's Hospital, Boston, Massachusetts, United States of America

Chin-Lee Wu, Qishan Dai and Sharron Lin
Department of Pathology, Massachusetts General Hospital, Boston, Massachusetts, United States of America

Jonathan Rosenberg
Division of Genitourinary Oncology, Memorial Sloan-Kettering Cancer Center, New York, New York, United States of America

Markus Riester
Department of Biostatistics and Computational Biology, Dana-Farber Cancer Institute, and Department of Biostatistics, Harvard School of Public Health, Boston, Massachusetts, United States of America

W. Scott McDougal
Department of Urology, Massachusetts General Hospital, Boston, Massachusetts, United States of America

Holger Schwender
Mathematical Institute, Heinrich Heine University Düsseldorf, Düsseldorf, Germany

Silvia Selinski, Meinolf Blaszkewicz, Rosemarie Marchan, Klaus Golka and Jan G. Hengstler
Leibniz Research Centre for Working Environment and Human Factors (IfADo) Dortmund, Germany

Katja Ickstadt
Faculty of Statistics, TU Dortmund University, Dortmund, Germany

Miao-Fen Chen and Wen-Cheng Chen
Department of Radiation Oncology, Chang Gung Memorial Hospital, Chiayi, Taiwan
Chang Gung University, College of Medicine, Taoyuan, Taiwan

Paul-Yang Lin
Chang Gung University, College of Medicine, Taoyuan, Taiwan
Department of Pathology, Chang Gung Memorial Hospital, Chiayi, Taiwan

Ching-Fang Wu
Chang Gung University, College of Medicine, Taoyuan, Taiwan
Department of Urology, Chang Gung Memorial Hospital, Chiayi, Taiwan

Chun-Te Wu
Chang Gung University, College of Medicine, Taoyuan, Taiwan
Department of Urology, Chang Gung Memorial Hospital, Keelung, Taiwan

Shahana Majid, Sharanjot Saini, Varahram Shahryari, Sumit Arora, Mohd Saif Zaman, Inik Chang, Soichiro Yamamura, Takeshi Chiyomaru, Shinichiro Fukuhara, Yuichiro Tanaka, Guoren Deng, Z Laura Tabatabai and Rajvir Dahiya
Department of Urology, VA Medical Center and UCSF, San Francisco, California, United States of America

Altaf A. Dar
Research Institute, California Pacific Medical Center, San Francisco, California, United States of America

Marija G. Matic, Vesna M. Coric, Ana R. Savic-Radojevic, Marija S. Pljesa-Ercegovac, Tatjana I. Djukic and Tatjana P. Simic
Institute of Medical and Clinical Biochemistry, Faculty of Medicine, University of Belgrade, Belgrade, Serbia
Faculty of Medicine, University of Belgrade, Belgrade, Serbia

Petar V. Bulat
Institute of Occupational Health, Belgrade, Serbia
Faculty of Medicine, University of Belgrade, Belgrade, Serbia

Dejan P. Dragicevic
Clinic of Urology, Clinical Center of Serbia, Belgrade, Serbia
Faculty of Medicine, University of Belgrade, Belgrade, Serbia

Tatjana D. Pekmezovic
Institute of Epidemiology, Faculty of Medicine, University of Belgrade, Belgrade, Serbia,
Faculty of Medicine, University of Belgrade, Belgrade, Serbia

Emiel A. M. Janssen
Department of Pathology, Stavanger University Hospital, Stavanger, Norway

Ok Målfrid Mangrud Jan P. A. Baak and Einar Gudlaugsson
Department of Pathology, Stavanger University Hospital, Stavanger, Norway

Clinical Institute-1, University of Bergen, Bergen, Norway

Rune Waalen
Department of Pathology, Innlandet Hospital Trust, Lillehammer, Norway

Ingvild Dalen
Department of Research, Stavanger University Hospital, Stavanger, Norway

Ilker Tasdemir
Department of Urology, Stavanger University Hospital, Stavanger, Norway

Declan J. McKenna, Bernadette A. Doherty, C. Stephen Downes, Stephanie R. McKeown and Valerie J. McKelvey-Martin
Biomedical Sciences Research Institute, University of Ulster, Coleraine, Northern Ireland, United Kingdom

Ding-Zuan Zhang, Eddie S. Y. Chan and Chi-Fai Ng
Division of Urology, Department of Surgery, The Chinese University of Hong Kong, Hong Kong SAR, China

Kin-Mang Lau
Department of Anatomical and Cellular Pathology, The Chinese University of Hong Kong, Hong Kong SAR, China

Gang Wang and Cheuk-Chun Szeto
Division of Nephrology, Department of Medicine and Therapeutic, The Chinese University of Hong Kong, Hong Kong SAR, China

Kenneth Wong and Richard K. W. Choy
Department of Obstetrics & Gynaecology, The Chinese University of Hong Kong, Hong Kong SAR, China

Yan Xu
Department of Obstetrics and Gynecology, Indiana University School of Medicine, Indianapolis, Indiana, United States of America

Hui Cai
Department of Obstetrics and Gynecology, Indiana University School of Medicine, Indianapolis, Indiana, United States of America
Department of Thoracic Oncosurgery, First Affiliated Hospital of Xi'an Jiaotong University, Xi'an, People's Republic of China

Elena G. Chiorean, Michael V. Chiorean, Douglas K. Rex, Bruce W. Robb and Patrick J. Loehrer
Department of Medicine, Indiana University Melvin and Bren Simon Cancer Center, Indiana University School of Medicine, Indianapolis, Indiana, United States of America

Noah M. Hahn
Department of Medicine, Indiana University Melvin and Bren Simon Cancer Center, Indiana University School of Medicine, Indianapolis, Indiana, United States of America
Hoosier Oncology Group, Indianapolis, Indiana, United States of America

Ziyue Liu
Department of Biostatistics, Indiana University School of Medicine, Indianapolis, Indiana, United States of America

Marietta L. Harrison
Medicinal Chemistry and Molecular Pharmacology, Oncological Sciences Center, Purdue University Center for Cancer Research, West Lafayette, Indiana, United States of America

John D. Kelly
Department of Pathology and Cancer Institute, University College London, London, United Kingdom

Tim J. Dudderidge
Department of Pathology and Cancer Institute, University College London, London, United Kingdom
The Royal Marsden National Health Service (NHS) Foundation Trust, London, United Kingdom

Alex Wollenschlaeger
Wolfson Institute for Biomedical Research, University College London, London, United Kingdom

Odu Okoturo
Department of Medicine, Imperial College London, London, United Kingdom

Keith Burling, Fiona Tulloch and Ian Halsall
Department of Clinical Biochemistry, Addenbrooke's Hospital, University of Cambridge, Cambridge, United Kingdom

Teresa Prevost and Joana C. Vasconcelos
Department of Public Health and Primary Care, Centre for Applied Medical Statistics, University of Cambridge, Institute of Public Health, Cambridge, United Kingdom

Andrew Toby Prevost
Department of Primary Care and Public Health Sciences, King's College London, London, United Kingdom

Wendy Robson, Nikhil Vasdev and Robert S. Pickard
Department of Urology, Freeman Hospital, Newcastle upon Tyne, United Kingdom

Hing Y. Leung
Beatson Institute for Cancer Research, University of Glasgow, Bearsden, Glasgow, United Kingdom

Gareth H. Williams and Kai Stoeber
Department of Pathology and Cancer Institute, University College London, London, United Kingdom
Wolfson Institute for Biomedical Research, University College London, London, United Kingdom

Garrett M. Dancik
Mathematics and Computer Science Department, Eastern Connecticut State University, Willimantic, Connecticut, United States of America

Dan Theodorescu
Department of Surgery, University of Colorado, Aurora, Colorado, United States of America Department of Pharmacology, University of Colorado, Aurora, Colorado, United States of America
University of Colorado Comprehensive Cancer Center, Aurora, Colorado, United States of America

Philip M. Sobolesky and Omar Moussa
Department of Pathology and Laboratory Medicine, Medical University of South Carolina, Charleston, South Carolina, United States of America
Hollings Cancer Center, Medical University of South Carolina, Charleston, South Carolina, United States of America

Perry V. Halushka
Hollings Cancer Center, Medical University of South Carolina, Charleston, South Carolina, United States of America
Departments of Pharmacology and Medicine, Medical University of South
Carolina, Charleston, South Carolina, United States of America

Elizabeth Garrett-Mayer
Hollings Cancer Center, Medical University of South Carolina, Charleston, South Carolina, United States of America
Department of Public Health Sciences, Medical University of South Carolina, Charleston, South Carolina, United States of America

Michael T. Smith
Department of Pathology and Laboratory Medicine, Medical University of South Carolina, Charleston, South Carolina, United States of America

Hwanik Kim, Myong Kim, Cheol Kwak, Hyeon Hoe Kim and Ja Hyeon Ku
Department of Urology, Seoul National University College of Medicine, Seoul, Korea

Yuhai Zhang
Department of Urology, Beijing Friendship Hospital, Capital Medical University, Beijing, China

Yu Zhang
Department of Urology, Beijing Friendship Hospital, Capital Medical University, Beijing, China Department of Urology, Beijing You An Hospital, Capital Medical University, Beijing, China

Zhen Huang, Zhiqiang Zhu, Xin Zheng and Jianwei Liu
Department of Urology, Beijing You An Hospital, Capital Medical University, Beijing, China

Zhiyou Han and Xuetao Ma
Department of Urology, Dongzhimen Hospital Affiliated to Beijing University of Chinese Medicine, Beijing, China

Sabina Sevcenco, Harun Fajkovic, Shahrokh F. Shariat, Manuela Hiess and Tibor Szarvas
Department of Urology, Medical University of Vienna, Vienna, Austria

Andrea Haitel and Martin Susani
Department of Pathology, Medical University of Vienna, Vienna, Austria

Lothar Ponhold, Claudio Spick and Pascal A. T. Baltzer
Department of Biomedical Imaging and Image-guided therapy, Medical University of Vienna, Vienna, Austria

Lisa Salazar and Matthew Hallowell
Department of Psychiatry and Human Behavior, University of California Irvine, Irvine, California, United States of America

Tamara Kashiwada
America Department of Biological Chemistry, University of California Irvine, Irvine, California, United States of America

Pavel Krejci
Medical Genetics Institute, Cedars-Sinai Medical Center, Los Angeles, California, United States of America
Institute of Experimental Biology, Masaryk University and Department of Cytokinetics, Institute of Biophysics AS CR, v.v.i., Brno, Czech Republic
Department of Pediatrics, UCLA School of Medicine, Los Angeles, California, United States of America

April N. Meyer
Department of Chemistry and Biochemistry, University of California San Diego, La Jolla, California, United States of America

Malcolm Casale
Department of Neurobiology and Behavior, University of California Irvine, Irvine, California, United States of America

William R. Wilcox
Medical Genetics Institute, Cedars-Sinai Medical Center, Los Angeles, California, United States of America
Department of Pediatrics, UCLA School of Medicine, Los Angeles, California, United States of America

Daniel J. Donoghue
Department of Chemistry and Biochemistry, University of California San Diego, La Jolla, California, United States of America
Moores Cancer Center, University of California San Diego, La Jolla, California, United States of America

Leslie Michels Thompson
Department of Psychiatry and Human Behavior, University of California Irvine, Irvine, California, United States of America

Department of Biological Chemistry, University of California Irvine, Irvine, California, United States of America
Department of Neurobiology and Behavior, University of California Irvine, Irvine, California, United States of America
Chao Family Comprehensive Cancer Center, University of California Irvine, Irvine, California, United States of America

Geertje van der Horst, Lieke Bos, Maaike van der Mark, Henry Cheung, Rob C. M. Pelger, Rob F. M. Bevers and Gabri van der Pluijm
Department of Urology, Leiden University Medical Centre, Leiden, The Netherlands

Bertrand Heckmann, Philippe Clément-Lacroix and Giocondo Lorenzon
Galapagos SASU, Romainville, France

Index

www.ingramcontent.com/pod-product-compliance
Lightning Source LLC
Chambersburg PA
CBHW080412190526
45161CB00003B/208